Handbook of Medical Sociology

HANDBOOK OF MEDICAL SOCIOLOGY

Sixth Edition

CHLOE E. BIRD, PETER CONRAD,
ALLEN M. FREMONT,
AND STEFAN TIMMERMANS
EDITORS

Vanderbilt University Press

Nashville

© 2010 by Vanderbilt University Press
Nashville, Tennessee 37235
All rights reserved
First printing 2010

This book is printed on acid-free paper.
Manufactured in the United States of America

Library of Congress Cataloging-in-Publication Data

Handbook of medical sociology.
— 6th ed. / edited by Chloe E. Bird . . . [et al.].
p.   ; cm.
Includes bibliographical references and index.
ISBN 978-0-8265-1720-3 (cloth : alk. paper)
ISBN 978-0-8265-1721-0 (pbk. : alk. paper)
1. Social medicine—Handbooks, manuals, etc.
I. Bird, Chloe E.
[DNLM: 1. Social Medicine. 2. Sociology, Medical.
WA 31 H236 2010]
RA418.H29 2010
362.1—dc22
2009047976

Contents

Preface to the Sixth Edition

Chloe E. Bird, Peter Conrad,

Allen M. Fremont, and Stefan Timmermans

A revision of *The Handbook of Medical Sociology* has appeared about once a decade since its original publication in 1963. Each edition was comprised of new, specially commissioned chapters reviewing or developing some aspects of medical sociology. As the field of medical sociology grew and diversified, new topics were included and older ones updated, and others continued to be represented by previous editions. When a new editorial team took over the fifth edition (Bird, Conrad, and Fremont 2000), we attempted to maintain the spirit of the earlier editions. We continue here with the sixth edition, reflecting some changes and new vistas in medical sociology, while updating and reconfiguring some perennially important topics.

In 2009 we celebrated the fiftieth year of the Medical Sociology Section of the American Sociological Association. The section has been among the three largest of the ASA's nearly thirty sections. Medical sociology continues to be an expanding and vibrant intellectual field: it is impossible for a single volume to fully represent all the changes and new directions, as well as include the discipline's core topics. For this edition, we asked authors to go beyond reviews of the literature and focus on a number of key questions and issues.

This edition reflects important changes in the study of health and illness. In addition to updated and reconceived chapters on the social impacts of gender, race, and socioeconomic inequalities on health, new chapters examine the influence of social networks, neighborhoods, and social capital. This configuration reflects new directions for medical sociology, and increased interest in how

social connections affect health and illness. While we included two chapters on social perspectives on illness experience in the previous edition, we here offer a section that more deeply examines illness experience and trajectories and emphasizes social constructionist approaches. In addition to focusing on macro issues like medicalization and illness contestation, the chapters in the section look at the subjective experience of illness, both as this research tradition has developed in sociology and in light of the profound impact of the Internet. We also offer chapters on sociological perspectives on disability and a sociological rendering of dying and the right to die, an increasingly salient issue.

The final two sections address new topics that have increased in significance or that merit an update since the last edition, as well as some classic sociological matters. Chapters in the third section recount shifts in the organization of health-care delivery and in the balance of power among institutional actors seeking to control it. These chapters pay particular attention to developments in the decade since the last edition of the handbook, including new efforts to reform the system, with special emphasis on emerging actors that warrant sociological attention, such as pharmaceutical companies. Additional chapters in the third section highlight the growing pervasiveness and impact of evolving models of care and policy that are driven by a conviction that greater use of evidence-based medicine and far more emphasis on care quality and safety are crucial to improving care and health outcomes. Chapters in the final section of the book focus on recent and expanding medical sociological interests, as well as on new and future directions for medical sociological work. Health social movements and genetics, while very different, are not only affecting our understandings of illness and disease but also becoming significant sociological research concerns. The issues surrounding religion and spirituality as they relate to health, while not nearly as well developed in our discipline, seem to be returning to the scene. Medical sociologists, along with sociologists of science, continue to shed light on the effects of biotechnology in medicine—its genetic-environment interactions, the impact of biotechnological interventions, or, since 9/11, the threats of bioterrorism. Topics like these may be a harbinger of the future, when medical sociologists may increasingly examine not just how social and cultural organization affect health and illness, but how interactions among culture, organization, and technology contribute to our understanding of and interventions for health and illness. It is likely that sociological research will continue to be eclectic and diverse in its approaches, yet as our own research technologies improve, we may be increasingly able to link sociological factors with changing biomarkers as we attempt to better understand the development of illness and disease.

As rich and wide-ranging as we believe the topics in this edition to be, as in earlier editions we do not, for example, delve deeply into issues of mental health. We do not include a chapter on national health policy, since the proposals and changes would likely be out of date by the book's publication. For benchmarks in areas not included in this sixth edition, we recommend examining the 2000 edition, consulting, for example, chapters on the impact of the environment on health, doctor-patient relations, complementary and alternative medicine (CAM), and medical education, as well as the several chapters on the interdisciplinary potentials of medical sociology and its related health-focused social science disciplines.

Part I

The eight chapters of Part I, "Social Contexts and Health Disparities," address a long-standing focus of medical sociology, the role of social factors in health and illness, here focusing on many of the ways in which social inequality and social contexts shape health and create and recreate health disparities. Taken together, these chapters provide a nuanced perspective on the persistent social patterning of health and longevity.

In Chapter 1, Bruce Link and Jo Phelan address an issue central to medical sociology: how and why social and economic inequality is a fundamental cause of health disparities. This sociological perspective on health disparities was initially developed in response to the risk-factor approach, which directs attention to proximal causes of ill health—modifiable risk factors. Link and Phelan argue that the unequal distribution of socioeconomic resources inevitably leads to health inequalities as those with more resources use them to obtain and act on new and better information—for example, by consuming healthier diets and avoiding known hazards—in order to protect and improve their health. Consequently, interventions aimed at the proximal causes of health disparities will never be sufficient to close the gaps.

In Chapter 2, Ichiro Kawachi brings the social world into the discussion by shifting the focus from the individual to the community as he articulates the impact of social capital on health. He presents the application of resources as a group-level construct, where to a certain extent individuals perceive the world and act collectively. As advantages thus accrue and flow across networks, one's network becomes another resource that provides, among other things, information, perceived efficacy, and norms for behavior, all of which can directly and indirectly impact health. This focus introduces some of the many ways in which opportunities are structured, building from Granovetter's concept of "the strength of weak ties" (Granovetter 1973) and Coleman's work on "informal social control" (Coleman 1990).

In Chapter 3, Catherine Ross and John Mirowsky make the case that education, operating as both human capital and a commodity, is the key to socioeconomic differentials in health. Although one might argue that education contributes to both in that it shapes our social networks. Ross and Mirowsky note that most U.S. policy makers do not view education as a means to improve population health, despite evidence that it is effective in this arena. The authors also consider evidence that health care cannot and does not improve population health.

Patricia Rieker, Chloe Bird, and Martha Lang in Chapter 4 examine the patterns and trends in gender differences in health and consider how social and biologic factors interact to produce paradoxical differences in men's and women's health. They present constrained choice as a conceptual framework for understanding how the social structure and associated contexts in which we live shape our opportunities to pursue a healthy life, exploring the ways structural constraints narrow the opportunities and choices available to individuals. The authors also offer constrained choice as an alternative framework that goes beyond socioeconomic disparities and discrimination to explain health disparities, including those at the intersection of race, class, and gender.

Gina Lovasi, jimi adams, and Peter Bearman provide a refreshing and strikingly different take in Chapter 5 on the ways in which social networks shape health. Whereas Kawachi focused on social capital as a network or community resource, Lovasi, adams, and Bearman examine more broadly how and why our social ties with individuals and organizations affect our health. They illustrate the role of social networks by focusing on social support, sexual behavior, and food consumption as each relates to health. Moreover, they consider the complexity of both assessing network effects and using networks to promote health. This chapter also brings us back to a consideration of how contexts affect the impact of networks on health.

David Takeuchi, Emily Walton, and Man-Chui Leung explore in Chapter 6 the role of segregation as a social process that contributes to differential exposure to particular environments and contexts, weaving together many of the themes touched upon in preceding chapters and introducing the concept of place. In particular, they consider how opportunity structures and community structures influence health in part by shaping social processes—again raising the issue of how contexts and networks interact.

In Chapter 7, Tamara Dubowitz, Lisa Bates, and Dolores Acevedo-Garcia shed light on the long-standing "Latino health paradox," the recognition that Hispanics/Latinos have higher life expectancy than would be expected given their disproportionate representation among the poor. Dubowitz and colleagues consider how the sociopolitical context and patterns of migration contribute to health and discuss the role of immigration and Latino ethnicity in shaping Latino health and go on to suggest ways that studies can better tease apart these factors by examining immigrants and their acculturation.

Finally, in Chapter 8, Stephanie Robert, Kathleen Cagney, and Margaret Weden present a new way to think sociologically about neighborhoods and place effects as they bring together the concepts of life course and neighborhood, articulating new questions and approaches for understanding the ways neighborhood effects on health may vary over the life course both of individual residents and of neighborhoods themselves. The authors incorporate an appreciation of how neighborhoods change and age over time not only in what may be predictable ways but also, more importantly, in ways that would be expected to impact the health and well-being of their residents.

Taken together, these chapters cover a broad and diverse literature on how individual lives are socially patterned in ways that differentially allocate opportunities and resources, which in turn patterns health and health disparities. Moreover, the authors consider from multiple perspectives how individual resources such as education, as well as network or community resources such as social capital, shape even the ability or skills to call upon and apply particular resources.

Part II

While the chapters in Part I focus on social factors related to the development of diseases in populations and individuals, Part II, "Health Trajectories and Experiences," deals with the social construction and meaning of illness. The five chapters address the trajectory of illness, from its definition to its experience to particular trajectory outcomes. The first three chapters take generally social constructionist/interactionist perspectives about the meaning and experience of illness; the last two focus more on issues around particular aspects of potential trajectories, disability, and dying.

In Chapter 9, Kristin Barker reviews the development and usefulness for understanding illness of the constructionist perspective, which looks beyond biology to human activities for the meanings of disease and illness. This approach leads to new understandings of the creation and uses of biomedical knowledge and the development of illness categories. Barker explores as exemplars constructionism in the important conceptions of medicalization and contested illness. Medicalization focuses on how conditions become defined as illnesses (e.g., ADHD, obesity, menopause), while contested illnesses typically occur when a constituency of sufferers' claim that their ailments are illnesses is not accepted by the medical profession (e.g., fibromyalgia, multiple chemical sensitivity disorder, chronic fatigue syndrome). Studies highlight cultural and contentious aspects of illness definitions, and increase our understandings of how social activities may create illnesses.

Sociologists have investigated the subjective experience of illness for four decades, focusing on how people go on with their everyday lives with and in spite of illness. Using Talcott Parsons's classic work on the sick role as a touchstone and a foil, in Chapter 10 David Rier examines the development and constitution of the experience of illness perspective. This perspective takes seriously individuals' subjective perspectives and expands the notions of being sick or well. The illness trajectory today reaches from healthy, to risk for disease—what Charles Rosenberg (2007) calls "proto illness"—to being ill, to recovering (or not), to what Arthur Frank (1995) dubs "the remission society." Rier sees specific challenges for sociologists in understanding the experiences of Alzheimer's, mental illness, and critical illnesses; our current knowledge of the lived experience of these disorders is sparse.

Peter Conrad and Cheryl Stults in Chapter 11 note two consistent findings from experience of illness studies until the last decade: with few exceptions, no illness subcultures existed, and illness was a profoundly privatizing experience. Except in hospital settings, the ill did not interact with one another; even people with chronic illnesses typically had no contact with others who had the same illness or disorder. The Internet has changed this. It is now common for individuals with both common and rare disorders to have visited Internet sites (e.g., bulletin boards, chat rooms, network groups) where they can contact others with the same illness either actively (by posting) or passively (by lurking). Conrad and Stults agree with Reir that the Internet has revolutionized the experience of illness for many individuals. Thousands of illness subcultures (e.g., Internet support groups) exist, new sources of lay knowledge have emerged, and illness has been transformed from a private to a public experience. Sociologists are just beginning to understand the ramifications of this phenomenon.

Gary Albrecht, in Chapter 12, traces the transformation in the experience of disability in the past two decades (marked by the American with Disabilities Act in 1990), as well as the way sociological researchers have analyzed it. In the past three decades, disability has come to the fore as an important social policy issue, as the disability movement has sought a shift from viewing disability as a medical problem to approaching it as a social access issue. Albrecht shows that current sociological issues around disability—including social networks, sociology of the body, social inequalities, human rights, and changing social and physical environments—reflect how the conceptions of disability have made this shift, affecting a range of social frameworks.

Clive Seale, in Chapter 13, explores the individual and family experience of dying in our society, with an emphasis on the subjective aspects of the process and a focus on palliative care, such as hospice, and on the right to die, both of which are responses to the medicalization of dying (i.e., the ideology of doing all that can be done to keep someone alive and using life extending technology in an institution like a hospital). Seale connects these experiential dilemmas to policy issues like the legalization of assisted dying and even euthanasia. With modern technological medicine, end-of-life decision-making becomes an increasingly significant area for sociological investigation.

Part III

The chapters in Part III, "Health-Care Organization, Delivery, and Impact," indicate the extent of the change in these arenas since the last edition of the handbook. Some provide an essential update and fresh perspectives on topics familiar to sociology, such as professions and markets; others, such as the assessment of evidenced-based medicine, introduce or elaborate on emerging actors and dynamics that are having dramatic effects on health care and warrant increased attention by medical sociologists.

Renee Anspach's discussion in Chapter 14 of the role of gender in health care and delivery links to issues raised in Parts I and II and views from a gendered perspective topics elaborated on by other authors in this section. Her primary focus is the ways gender shapes the medical division of labor, medical treatment decisions, and the social construction of illness.

Peter Mendel and Richard Scott portray changes in the organization of U.S. health care from an institutional theory perspective in Chapter 15. Their review of changes in the system over the last fifty years establishes a foundation for understanding the recent health-care turmoil, and they go on to make a persuasive case that what may appear to be institutional disarray may instead reflect a flurry of innovation in models of organization and strategies to reconcile competing actors, logics, and structures held over from earlier eras.

In Chapter 16, Donald Light also combines a historical view with analyses of contemporary events in his chapter on health-care professions, markets, and countervailing powers, emphasizing the broader ecological context in which shifts in power and influence occur over time. He traces the emergence of several sources of lost trust in the profession of medicine, and observes how this loss of trust has also triggered changes in the profession that, ironically, may strengthen physicians' position, particularly as a bulwark against market forces. An alarming account of a growing threat to professionalism, the pharmaceutical industry, concludes Light's review.

John Abraham in Chapter 17 elaborates on the pharmaceutical industry's increasing power and influence, extending the discussion to include the increasing influence of consumers and the broader society on health and medical decisions by physicians. He argues that the growing use of pharmaceuticals reflects less the advances in biomedicine than the increasing medicalization process driven by the medical profession. However, he notes that other sociological factors—such as the political economy of the pharmaceutical industry, consumerism, and deregulatory state ideology—are uniquely salient to the process he calls "pharmaceuticalization."

Chapters 18 and 19 deal with two forces more beneficial than pharmaceuticalization of which medical sociologists should be aware: the evidenced-based medicine (EBM) and quality/patient safety movements, which are reshaping health care in ways that are generally underappreciated. In Chapter 18, which addresses evidence-based medicine, Stefan Timmerman observes that "it is difficult to exaggerate the resonance of EBM in contemporary health care." The formalization, rapid ascendance, and proliferation of EBM throughout nearly every aspect of health-care delivery and related policy has forced fundamental shifts in routine practice. Precisely what EBM is and the sociological implications of the changes it is creating are the focus of Timmerman's engaging discussion.

In Chapter 19, Teun Zuiderent-Jerak and Marc Berg examine the rapid growth and institutionalization of quality of care and patient safety movements. The focus on patient safety and its link to quality of care, a recent development, has exposed persistent gaps and shortcomings in care delivery. The increased concern about quality and safety, together with emerging information technologies that may allow us to monitor all aspects of care and outcomes, have prompted efforts to fundamentally alter both formal structural features and informal cultural aspects of care delivery. Though Zuiderent-Jerak and Berg raise doubts about the extent to which the rhetoric of the quality and safety movements is matched by intended changes in care and outcomes, they acknowledge that the challenges facing improvement experts and health-care providers are extremely complex. The authors conclude that given the complexity and sociological forces at work, medical sociologists can and should play an active role in applied research and efforts to improve quality, safety, and outcomes of care.

Part IV

As the organization of this handbook reflects, sociologists tend to regard the medical arena as divided into illness experiences, health-care organizations and health services, and the broad social context of health. The chapters in Part IV, "Crosscutting Issues," cut across such divisions as they examine the expansion of health into new domains, charting intriguing, rapidly developing, and occasionally contested sites of social action that are redefining what health is about, where it should be located, and who should take jurisdiction over it.

In Chapter 20, Wendy Cadge and Brian Fair map the sociological intersections of religion, spirituality, health, and medicine, detailing two main research areas: the health benefits of religion, and chaplaincy, an overlooked area in health care. A number of cross-sectional, observational studies report health benefits related to religious beliefs and some medical subareas—e.g., oncology, palliative care, and addiction treatment—have incorporated religious or spiritual beliefs as health promoting. Yet, this literature has trouble dealing with selection bias and reverse causality. A fundamental issue within this research stream is that advocating religion as part of health care seems to require a justification of its efficacy. In terms of religion as serving a cultural rather than a medical function—in the sense that it provides meaning in times of suffering and death—Cadge and Fair explore the work of chaplains, to date little studied, who have been institutionalized by hospital certification agencies in health-care settings and who claim professional status, including "evidence-based chaplaincy" (O'Connor 2002).

In Chapter 21, Stephen Collier and Andrew Lakoff review an emerging field of expertise that deals with biosecurity threats, particularly those addressed since September 11, 2001, by public health, local and federal governmental agencies, and the media—that is, nations' preparedness to combat infectious diseases, food-born diseases, and bioterrorism. This is very much an area in flux. International and national health and defense organizations offer blueprints for responses, biosecurity experts propose draconian health surveillance measures to mount a full-scale defense

against an as yet unknown threat, and decisions often stall under the weight of political debate over civil liberties and funding priorities.

In Chapter 22, Phil Brown, Crystal Adams, Rachel Morello-Frosch, Laura Senier, and Ruth Simpson examine the role of health social movements, embracing a community-based participatory research approach—that is, an approach in which one advocates on behalf of a constituency for health-related issues, often in collaboration with other scientists. Health social movements reflect the social spillover effect of the most intricate epistemological aspects of health, affecting the creation and dissemination of biomedical knowledge from diagnosis to treatment. Activists may work for recognition of contested illnesses or specific disabilities, document health effects of environmental pollution, and advocate for greater access to health services. One of the challenges of this approach to sociology of health and illness is that health advocacy requires a more eclectic approach to rigorous research, including studying health effects with accepted biological measures.

In Chapter 23, Regina Shih, Meenakshi Fernandes, and Chloe Bird address the exciting possibilities of including biomarkers in sociological research to map physiological pathways over the life course. To examine how populations differentially acquire the risk of disease or death, biomarkers might complement or replace self-reported data about health either as a baseline for research or as an indicator of health outcomes over time. As the authors report, to date most of the sociological research using biomarkers is limited to stress research, yet biomarkers set the stage for a physiological evaluation of well-established sociological processes and for closely mapping the effects of physiological events on social outcomes. The nearly endless possibilities for sociological inquiry, from conversation analysis to population health, open up new avenues of communication with health researchers and policy makers.

Besides their use in stress research, biomarkers have taken hold in the study of gene-environment interaction, as Sara Shostak and Jeremy Freese detail in Chapter 24. Biomedical and increasingly social researchers gather genetic markers of diseases such as the APOE gene associated with Alzheimer's diseases to further elucidate causal pathways. Experience with genetic markers demonstrates the complexity of the interaction between the biological and the social—"the pervasive interpenetration of genes and environments in disease etiology"—popularly illustrated by phenylketonuria (PKU), which the authors describe as "a genetically determined condition whose consequences medical science has transformed to being largely environmentally determined." Meanwhile, skeptics point to the limited track record of genetics, even for purely genetic conditions, in disease diagnosis and treatment and the multiple factors that mediate genetic expression.

Finally, as Bryan Turner notes in his sociological critique on issues of biotechnology and the prolongation of life, Chapter 25, the aspiration for immortality "tells us a lot about the society in which we live, especially its subjective individualism, its obsession with technological solutions and its overwhelming confidence in scientific advance." As Turner shows, even undeveloped immortality technologies affect our conceptions of mind and body, and some developed technologies

in this area have become routine medical practice. The author further points to the economic, political, and normative consequences of the growing disparity in average life span within and among countries, which highlight the gaps between resources and needs and the social shifts required to address them.

References

Bird, Chloe E., Peter Conrad, and Allen M. Fremont. 2000. *Handbook of Medical Sociology.* Upper Saddle River, N.J.: Prentice Hall.

Coleman, James S. 1990. *Foundations of Social Theory.* Cambridge, Mass.: Harvard University Press.

Frank, Arthur W. 1995. "The Remission Society." In *The Wounded Storyteller: Body, Illness, and Ethics,* ed. A. Frank, 8–13. Chicago: University of Chicago Press.

Granovetter, Mark S. 1973. "The Strength of Weak Ties." *American Journal of Sociology* 78(6): 1360–80.

O'Connor, Thomas S. 2002. "The Search for Truth: The Case for Evidence Based Chaplaincy." *The Journal of Health Care Chaplaincy* 13(1): 185–94.

Rosenberg, Charles E. 2007. *Our Present Complaint: American Medicine, Then and Now.* Baltimore: Johns Hopkins University Press.

PART I

Social Contexts and Health Disparities

1

Social Conditions as Fundamental Causes of Health Inequalities

Bruce Link, Columbia University and New York State Psychiatric Institute

Jo Phelan, Columbia University

We review in this chapter developments over the past fifteen years in the theory of fundamental social causes of health disparities, specify some issues that arise when the theory is applied to specific as opposed to general health outcomes (i.e., incidence or mortality due to a particular disease versus self-rated health and all-cause mortality), identify evidence that evaluates the theory, and indicate that we view the theory as a sociological "theory of the middle range" (Merton 1968).

Explicating the Theory

Can the Risk-Factor Model Account for Health Inequalities?

The theory of fundamental social causes of health inequalities emerged in the 1990s in response to the powerful and very successful risk-factor approach that dominated medicine and epidemiology at the time (House 2002). The risk-factor model's explanation for health inequalities proceeds according to a seemingly persuasive logic: social conditions are related to health because of their influence on a host of risk factors that lie between social conditions and disease in a chain of causality. Today we might think of intervening risk factors associated with diet, smoking, exercise,

pollution, and preventive health behaviors. To improve health and eliminate health inequalities, the risk-factor model tells us to focus on "modifiable" intervening risk factors like these. If we do, two important accomplishments will be ours. First, if we identify all the intervening risk factors, we will understand why social conditions are related to health. We will be able to tell our colleagues, inform our families, and help our students understand why some social groups are healthier than others. Second, our work will offer the medical and public-health communities actionable evidence about which risk factors are the major culprits in producing health inequalities. Then, our model tells us, if we can eliminate these intervening risks, health inequalities will disappear.

The risk-factor approach and public-health initiatives based on it have been enormously successful in at least one way—interventions based on more proximal, behavioral, and biomedical factors have had a very positive effect on population health. Although we cannot be sure which aspects of new knowledge or which specific interventions are accountable, human health has improved dramatically over the past century or so. Huge declines in the infectious disease killers of the nineteenth century were followed by equally impressive declines in major chronic disease killers such as heart disease, stroke, and, since the

1990s, cancers (NCHS 2006). But with respect to health inequalities, the risk-factor model comes up short in at least two important ways.

First, social conditions powerfully shape the capacity to modify or eliminate identified risk factors, rendering less than fully effective an approach that addresses only risk-factor mechanisms. Instead we need to also address what Rose (1992) called the "causes of causes" and what Link and Phelan (1995) deemed factors that put people "at risk of risk." Put simply, the reason a risk-factor model fails to address health inequalities is that it is difficult to decouple the identification of risk and protective factors and the deployment of knowledge and technology based on those factors from social conditions.

Second, in an ironic twist, rather than addressing health disparities, the identification of risk factors can actually increases such disparities (Link and Phelan 1995; Phelan et al. 2004). As we develop the ability to control disease and death, the benefits of this newfound capacity are not distributed equally throughout the population, but are instead harnessed more securely by individuals and groups who are less likely to be exposed to discrimination and who have greater access to knowledge, money, power, prestige, and beneficial social connections. Accordingly, whatever health differences between advantaged and disadvantaged groups might have existed before a health-enhancing discovery, the uneven distribution of new knowledge and technology results in a powerful social shaping of health disparities. From this vantage point, major health disparities by race, ethnicity, and socioeconomic status are social products, brutal facts that we create (Link 2008; Link and Phelan, in press).

Why Are Social Conditions Fundamental Causes of Health Inequalities?

The short answer to this question is that connections between social conditions and health are reliably reproduced under circumstances that involve vastly different risk and protective factors and completely different diseases. Their persistence under changing circumstances tells us that the observed connections are not reduc-ible to the risk-factor mechanisms that happened to link them in any particular circumstance. It is this feature that led us to deem social conditions fundamental causes of health inequalities. This reasoning is supported by evidence from the history of epidemiology.

To begin, consider the well-established and robust association between mortality and educational attainment, occupational standing, and income (Antonovsky 1967; Sorlie, Backlund, and Keller 1995; Kunst et al. 1998). Biological mechanisms are clearly involved in the SES-disease association. Just as clearly, other mechanisms involving behaviors and environmental exposures must also be present: disease does not flow directly from income, education, or occupational status into the body. Nevertheless, we cannot understand the effect of SES on mortality by focusing solely on the mechanisms that happen to link the two at any particular time.

To show why, we turn to one of the most striking features of the connection between socioeconomic status and mortality: its persistence across time and place. The association was demonstrated in Mulhouse, France, in the early nineteenth century, in Rhode Island in 1865, and in Chicago in the 1930s, and occurs in Europe and the United States today (Antonovsky 1967; Sorlie, Backlund, and Keller 1995; Lantz et al. 1998; Kunst et al. 1998; Chapin 1924; Coombs 1941). Given the vast differences in life expectancy, risk factors, diseases, and health-care systems characterizing these different places and times, the persistence of the SES-mortality association is remarkable.

It is remarkable in the following sense. Imagine a causal model with SES as the distal factor linked to death by more proximal risk factors. If the proximal risk factors are eliminated, we would expect the SES-mortality association to disappear. However, in several important instances, SES disparities in mortality persisted even though major proximal risk factors were eliminated. In the nineteenth century, for example, overcrowding, poor sanitation, and widespread infectious diseases such as diphtheria, measles, typhoid fever, tuberculosis, and syphilis appeared to explain higher mortality rates among less advantaged persons. But the virtual elimination of those conditions and diseases in developed countries did not diminish SES inequalities in mortality (Rosen 1979). In the twentieth century, countries created national health programs providing free medical care to all with the express purpose of radically altering another important link between SES and health—differential access to care. While such programs addressed important mechanisms and may have kept disparities from growing even larger, SES disparities in mortality nevertheless remained undiminished decades later (Black et al. 1982). The reproduction of the connection between SES and mortality in vastly different circumstances speaks to its irreducibility and is the justification for calling social conditions "fundamental" causes of health inequalities.

How Does the Fundamental-Cause Process Work? The Role of Flexible Resources

The reason that the connection between socioeconomic status and mortality reemerges in different places and at different times is that another set of mediating risk and protective factors replaces the preceding one. At first blush this explanation seems to invoke a diabolical magic that reliably works to the detriment of disadvantaged people. So why would new and different intervening mechanisms emerge in disparate places and times?

Fundamental-cause theory claims that new mechanisms arise because persons of higher socioeconomic status are able to deploy a wide range of resources—including knowledge, money, power, prestige, and beneficial social connections—that can be used individually and collectively in different places and at different times to avoid disease and death. Because they can be applied in very different circumstances, we call them flexible resources. Thus when new knowledge about risk and protective strategies emerges, people use the resources available to them to harness the benefits of that new knowledge. People with more resources are able to benefit more, thereby creating a new mechanism linking social conditions to morbidity and mortality.

Consider two examples. Screening for several deadly cancers has become possible over the past few decades, making it feasible to detect cancer or its precursors earlier, thereby helping prevent mortality from these cancers. Since the screening procedures represent relatively recent technological advances, one can imagine a time when resources had no bearing on access to cancer screening because the procedures did not exist. There was no mechanism linking SES → Access to Screening → Health. But after the screening procedures were developed, people with more resources could use those resources both individually and collectively to gain access to the life-saving screens. Link et al. (1998) presented evidence from the Behavioral Risk Factor Survey to show that screens for cervical and breast cancer were indeed associated with education and income. A new mechanism—access to life-saving screens—had emerged to link social conditions to health outcomes.

Another example is that of smoking knowledge and behavior. Scientific evidence strongly linking smoking to lung cancer emerged in the early 1950s with initial reports from case control studies in 1950 and more definitive prospective studies in 1954. To assess changes that may have occurred in the decades following the production of this new knowledge, Link analyzed multiple public opinion polls assessing smoking beliefs and behaviors. Evidence from the first surveys conducted just as the scientific evidence was emerging in 1954 showed that while most people had heard about the findings, only a minority believed that smoking was a cause of lung cancer and no educational gradient in this belief was evident. Nor was smoking behavior strongly linked to educational attainment in 1954. Over the next forty-five years, as people began to believe that smoking is a cause of lung cancer, sharp educational gradients opened up in both this belief and the behavior of being a current smoker (Link 2008). A new and very powerful mechanism linking indicators of SES to an important health behavior had emerged.

The idea, then, is that this process extends beyond these two examples to many others. Examples include gaining access to the best doctors; knowing about and asking for beneficial health procedures; having friends and family who support healthy lifestyles; quitting smoking; getting flu shots; wearing seat belts; and eating fruits and vegetables. Other examples include exercising regularly; living in neighborhoods where garbage is picked up often, interiors are lead-free, and streets are safe; having children who bring home useful health information from good schools; working in safe occupational circumstances; and taking restful vacations.

Do Fundamental-Cause Processes Operate at the Individual Level, the Contextual Level, or Multiple Levels?

At the individual level the flexible resources implicated by the theory of fundamental causes can be conceptualized as the "causes of causes" or "risks of risk" that shape individual health behaviors by influencing whether people know about, have access to, can afford, and receive support for their efforts to engage in health-enhancing or health-protective behaviors. Second, resources shape access to broad contexts that vary dramatically in associated risk profiles and protective factors. For example, a person with many resources can afford to live in a high-status neighborhood where neighbors are also of high status and where, collectively, enormous clout is exerted to ensure that crime, noise, violence, pollution, traffic, and vermin have been kept at a minimum and that the best health-care facilities, parks, playgrounds, and food stores are conveniently located nearby. Once a person has used SES-related resources to locate in an advantaged neighborhood, a host of health-enhancing circumstances comes along as a package deal. Similarly, a person who uses educational attainment and credentials to procure a high-status occupation inherits a package deal that is more likely to include robust and enduring health benefits and less likely to involve dangerous situations and toxic exposures. In both these circumstances people benefit in numerous ways that do not depend on their own initiative or ability to personally construct a healthy situation—it is an add-on benefit operative at the contextual level. And, of course, the same sort of add-on benefit applies in other important contexts such as in social networks, families, and marriages. Thus the processes implied by the fundamental-cause perspective operate at both individual and contextual levels.

Does Fundamental-Cause Theory Predict Unchanging Associations between Fundamental Causes and Health Outcomes?

The theory of fundamental social causes is sometimes read to predict that associations between fundamental causes and general indicators of health do not change but rather can be expected to express themselves the same way in very different circumstances (Krieger et al. 2008; Olafsdottir 2007). While the theory seeks to explain why associations between fundamental causes and health emerge under vastly different circumstances, it does not suggest that the association will always be of the same magnitude. Nor does it suggest that we must be nihilistic about the possibilities of reducing the association between SES and health should we muster the will to do so. The fundamental-cause theory suggests three major ways in which health inequalities might be expected to vary.

First, and most importantly, if inequalities in the flexible resources of knowledge, money, power, prestige, and beneficial social connections change, fundamental-cause theory predicts that health inequalities will also change. Consider, for example, the United States as it moved from the horrendous conditions of racial segregation and resource inequality in the first half of the twentieth century to some positive changes in these factors as a consequence of the civil rights movement and the War on Poverty. To the extent that race differences in flexible resources narrowed somewhat over this period, we would expect race differences in general health indicators to narrow as well—a prediction that appears to concur with empirical facts from one study, at least (Krieger et al. 2008).

Second, some interventions do not require the deployment of the key flexible resources of knowledge, money, power, prestige, and beneficial social connections to procure their benefits. Interventions like these, which benefit everyone regardless of the resources they possess or the health behaviors they manifest, will not contribute to the production of health disparities and will improve overall population health. Consider, for example, air bags rather than seatbelts to reduce road fatalities (even though using both is arguably best). Seat-belt use requires people to secure their own belts, and ample evidence shows that people with higher educational attainment are more likely to do so. To the extent that seat belts are effective, highly educated people benefit more than less educated people, thereby contributing to a gradient in a health-related outcome. If they are in all cars, air bags will help everyone and will not lead to a gradient by educational level. From the same vantage point, in the following list of intervention/policy options, the first option in each case is more likely to create a health inequality than the second: (a) warning parents to keep their children away from paint chips, versus (b) requiring by law that lead paint be removed from the environment; (a) providing vaccinations and health screening through private physicians, versus (b) providing these interventions to everyone in schools, workplaces, and other community settings; (a) advising parents to monitor their children's play around windows, versus (b) requiring window guards in all high-rise apartments; (a) instituting educational initiatives concerning the harms of trans fat, versus (b) banning the use of trans fat in the production of food products; (a) advising consumers to wash cutting boards and cook meat thoroughly, versus (b) inspecting meat thoroughly before consumers buy it; and (a) exhorting people to brush often with fluoridated toothpaste, versus (b) fluoridating water supplies. If we create more interventions/policies that are like the second options, we can improve population health without creating the conditions for health disparities to emerge.

Third, in keeping with the exhortation in fundamental-cause theory that we must be attentive to what puts people at risk of risk, SES gradients can be diminished to the extent that attention is directed to the chain of circumstances that leads to the presence of risks or the absence of protective factors. If we intervene not just by providing information about risks or news about the availability of protective factors, but seek to understand and act upon the factors that influence the uptake of new knowledge and technology—especially as it applies to people with fewer resources—we will diminish associations between fundamental causes and health outcomes.

In each of these instances the key ingredient in fundamental-cause theory, the deployment of flexible resources, changes. In the first instance the resources themselves are made more equal. In the second, resources are irrelevant (or less relevant) to the procurement of a health benefit if policy (b) is enacted. In the third, we seek to make flexible resources less consequential by intervening in ways that mitigate the effects of these resources. Fundamental-cause theory does not predict a uniform or unchanging association between fundamental causes and health outcomes but instead predicts that the association will vary depending on how key flexible resources are addressed in particular contexts.

What Are the Critical Components of Fundamental-Cause Theory?

The foregoing reasoning identifies four important features of a fundamental cause. First, a fundamental cause is related to multiple disease outcomes. For example, SES was related to cholera, tuberculosis, and diphtheria in the nineteenth century and is now related to heart disease, stroke, and many types of cancer. Second, such causes operate through multiple risk-factor mechanisms, including but not limited to items like those mentioned as examples in the preceding paragraphs. Third, new intervening mechanisms reproduce the association between fundamental causes and health over time. Finally, the "essential feature of fundamental social causes is that they involve access to resources that can be used to avoid risks or to minimize the consequences of disease once it occurs" (Link and Phelan 1995, 87).

Fundamental-Cause Theory Applied to Specific Outcomes

Whereas the theory of fundamental causes concerns the amalgamation of effects across many specific processes and many specific conditions, it implies a consistent social shaping that should be observable in individual instances. Lutfey and Freese (2005) make this explicit by indicating that fundamental relationships can generally be expected to be "ho-lographic," that is, the general relationship should be found in most subdomains. The word "most" is critical here. Fundamental-cause theory does indeed require the SES → modifiable risk factor and the SES → disease associations to be present in most instances. But equally important, as we indicate later, these associations need not always be present. In some circumstances the theory actually predicts instances in which SES should be unrelated to disease. In other relatively rare instances, high SES individuals can have faulty knowledge or priorities that place the achievement of goals other than health above the goal of a healthy lifestyle. We give examples of each of these possibilities later in the chapter.

When Will Associations between SES (or Other Social Conditions) and Health-Related Outcomes Differ from the General Inverse Association?

In the fundamental-cause theory, people use flexible resources, both individually and collectively, to garner a health advantage. This proposition suggests three instances in which the theory predicts that resources will be either relatively useless or actually harmful. The first is when extant knowledge and technology is so sparse that the deployment of resources can have little benefit—there is no health advantage to procure. Some diseases like brain cancer and pancreatic cancer approach this state of affairs, in that knowledge of how to prevent or cure these diseases is scant.

The second is when extant information or common practice is incorrect, so that what current knowledge says is good for people is in fact harmful. A recent example is hormone-replacement therapy, which moved from what was thought to be a beneficial treatment with add-on benefits for heart disease to what is now thought to be a dangerous risk factor for cancer. Fundamental-cause theory would predict that during the era when hormone replacement therapy was considered beneficial, higher-SES women would use it more commonly than lower-SES women, as they deployed their knowledge, money, power, prestige and beneficial social connections to

obtain this presumed benefit. But to the extent that HRT is actually harmful, high-SES women would fare worse than low-SES women with respect to cancer risk due to HRT (Carpiano and Kelly 2007).

The third instance occurs when knowledge about a modifiable risk factor exists but acting on the knowledge would be detrimental in other ways. Thus for example, having children relatively early in life is known to be a protective factor for the development of breast cancer in women. But for high-SES women who desire high-status occupations requiring extensive training, having children early might be disruptive to career plans.

These examples describe situations in which we would not expect the commonly observed inverse association between SES and health-related outcomes (risk factors, protective factors, and diseases). Three important points follow from these examples. First, each instance indicates a circumstance in which the basic drivers in fundamental cause theory—flexible resources—are blocked in their capacity to deliver health benefits. This occurs either because there are no extant risk and protective factors for the flexible resources to act upon, because presumed risk and protective factors are based on incorrect information, or because acting on health-relevant knowledge strongly jeopardizes other outcomes people desire. Second, as exceptions to the general rule, they present important empirical reference points for testing the theory of fundamental causes. Indeed, as we will see, a very useful approach to testing the theory is to accurately predict, using the theory, circumstances in which an SES association with a health outcome is expected to be either much less pronounced, nonexistent, or in the opposite direction. Third, exceptions to the general relationship bring the key feature of fundamental-cause theory into clearer focus—people use resources to act on health-relevant information to improve health, thereby generating health disparities. By analogy, factors that cause outcomes discrepant with this general shaping influence are like fall leaves blown upward against the more fundamental force of gravity. The upward trajectories of the leaves are empirical facts, but they do not discount the more general process at work.

Health-enhancing knowledge and technology emerge in the context of preexisting conditions. The prototype that most clearly exemplifies how fundamental-cause processes operate is a situation in which we know nothing about how to prevent or cure a disease, and so there is no association between SES and morbidity and mortality due to that disease. Then, upon discovery of modifiable risk and protective factors, an association between SES and the disease in question emerges, because people with more resources are more able to gain access to and act upon the new health-enhancing knowledge and technology. But preexisting situations that differ from this prototype are not only possible but to be expected. One reason is that in the absence of knowledge of risk and protective factors, a disease may be influenced by factors as yet unplumbed by humans that are nevertheless associated with SES—either directly or inversely. Second, new knowledge and technology often arrive subsequent to discoveries that have already shaped the SES association with a health outcome.

To make informed inferences about the processes implied by fundamental-cause theory, we need to consider the preexisting association between SES and health-related outcomes. The reason is that the new knowledge or technology will help those who have the disease or the risk factor (or could have the risk factor). As a consequence, the distribution of the risk factor or disease by SES prior to the availability of the new knowledge or technology will influence the SES association after the new knowledge or technology arrives. An example will clarify what we mean. Consider the SES and smoking example we referred to earlier, but imagine different scenarios concerning its realization, as portrayed in Figure 1.1. On the left is the situation in the early 1950s before the new knowledge about the harmful effects of smoking was available. Here we consider different initial associations between SES and smoking—null, positive, and negative. At a second time point, after the new knowledge is available, we consider

a variable we call "quitting effort," and then at a third time point, we consider subsequent smoking behavior. We portray the association between SES and quitting effort as positive, with the idea that people of higher SES are more likely (for many reasons, i.e., because of many causes of causes) to engage in quitting efforts. We also portray a positive association between smoking at time 1 and subsequent quitting effort because the new knowledge is about a risk factor that smokers have and that is therefore especially applicable to them. Then quitting efforts at time 2 reduce subsequent smoking behavior, and there is a positive association between smoking at time 1 and subsequent smoking.

If the initial association between SES and smoking is null, a case much like the actual situation we described earlier, an inverse association between SES and smoking emerges over time through the SES → Quitting Effort → Smoking pathway.

If the initial association between SES and smoking is positive, such that people of higher SES are more likely to smoke, then two pathways—(1) SES → Quitting Effort → Smoking, and (2) SES → Smoking T1 → Quitting Effort → Smoking T3—will contribute to an inverse association between SES and smoking at T3. At the same time a third path, SES → Smoking T1 → Smoking T3, will contribute to the maintenance of a positive association between SES and smoking because people who initially smoked, more of whom were of high SES, are more likely to continue to do so. If this latter path is strong, a positive association between SES and smoking would remain at T3 but would be weaker than the SES smoking association at T1.

Finally, if the initial association between SES and smoking is negative, such that people of lower SES are more likely to smoke, something unexpected can occur. Two pathways lead to expectable results—(1) SES → Quitting Effort → Smoking, and (2) SES → Smoking T1 → Smoking T3; that is, either will contribute to an inverse association between SES and smoking T3. However, the pathway SES → Smoking T1 → Quitting Effort → Smoking T3 ($- * + * - = +$) will contribute to a positive association between SES

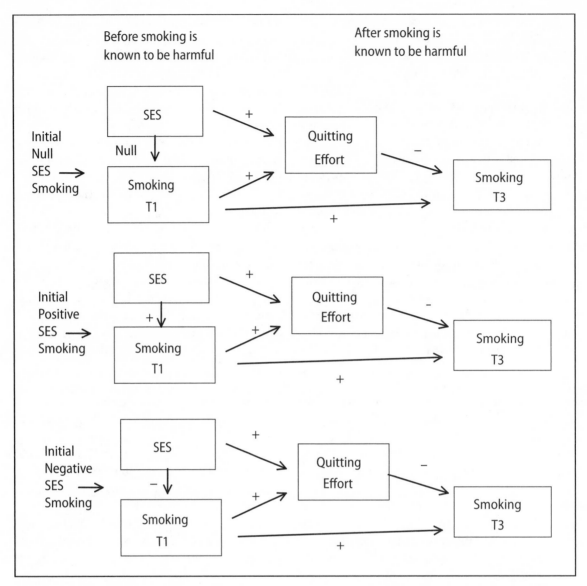

Figure 1.1. The importance of SES disparities prior to the introduction of health-enhancing knowledge or technology

and smoking at T3. The reason this occurs is that the new health-enhancing information that leads to quitting efforts benefits more people of low SES because more of them smoke at T1. If this pathway is strong, it could overwhelm the pathways driving an inverse association and lead us to conclude that the new knowledge (and resultant quitting behavior response) reduces disparities.

We call this a "give-back" effect, because the initial negative SES → disease association provides a starting point that allows the new knowl-edge about the disease to give back some equality, even though it may also exemplify a fundamental-cause process in which the knowledge is not dis-tributed equally across socioeconomic groups. Importantly, from a fundamental-cause perspec-tive, if the knowledge had appeared earlier, before a SES → disease association emerged, and if the knowledge had been maldistributed by SES at that time, the knowledge would have contributed to an inverse association between SES and the disease.

The foregoing considerations highlight several important points for pursuing fundamental-cause theory. Specifically, in examining the impact of any new knowledge or technology on the association between SES and any particular disease, it is critical to take into account the nature of the SES association before the knowledge and technology were implemented. Only this way is it possible to know whether a process consistent with fundamental cause has been operative in the context of a positive association between SES and some risk factor or disease. It is also necessary for the identification of potential give-back effects that occur when even a maldistributed form of knowledge or technology reduces disparities because the preexisting disparities were so pronounced.

Testing Fundamental-Cause Theory

In constructing a rationale for the theory of fundamental social causes, we employ facts that appear congenial with that theory. We find that the SES association with morbidity and mortality has been reproduced under vastly different historical circumstances in terms of risk factors, protective factors, and the diseases afflicting human beings. Further, we observe changes in the SES association with major risk factors like smoking (Link 2008) and with protective factors like access to cancer screens (Link et al. 1998) that are consistent with the theory. Facts like these are critical because it would not have made sense to construct such a theory if they had not been present. At the same time, there are theories that differ from ours in both how they explain health inequalities and what they suggest as means of reducing those inequalities. We have already addressed one of these—the risk-factor approach—in which the implicit theory is that disparities are eliminated by identifying the intervening risk factors and modifying those risk factors. But other theories exist as well. Marmot (2004) and Wilkinson (2005) see the source of the SES-health association in the stress of lower placement in a social hierarchy. Gottfredson (2004) proposes intelligence as the key flexible resource driving both SES attainment and the wise governance of individual health. More recently, Heckman

(2006, 2008) has proposed that noncognitive traits such as conscientiousness, perseverance, and time horizon strongly determine both SES attainment and health. These theories point to different processes and to different flexible resources than those emphasized in the fundamental-cause theory. Because alternative explanations have been proposed, it is important to find "risky tests" (Link 2003) that will either increase or decrease confidence in particular explanations. The following are some ways in which fundamental-cause theory has been tested.

Are SES Associations Stronger for High-Preventability versus Low-Preventability Causes of Death?

As mentioned earlier, flexible resources are relatively useless in the case of potentially fatal diseases that we do not know how to prevent or treat. If access to resources is critical in prolonging life, then when resources associated with higher status are relatively useless, high SES should confer less advantage and the usually robust SES-mortality association should weaken. This leads to the prediction that the SES association will be stronger for diseases which we have a substantial capacity to prevent or cure than for ones where our knowledge is less robust. This prediction makes a risky test of the theory possible. If SES associations are equally strong for diseases in which death is low in preventability and in diseases in which death is highly preventable, the theory would be strenuously challenged.

Phelan and colleagues (2004) implemented this test using the National Longitudinal Mortality Study and ratings they developed of the preventability of death from specific causes. The National Longitudinal Mortality Study (Sorlie, Backlund, and Keller 1995) is a large prospective study that uses combined samples of selected Current Population Surveys (CPS) that are then linked to the National Death Index to determine occurrences and causes of death in a follow-up period of approximately nine years. Reliable ratings (intraclass correlation .85) of the preventability of death were made by two physician-epidemiologists. Causes were categorized into high-preventability and low-preventability groups with common high-preventability causes being cerebrovascular diseases, chronic obstructive pulmonary disease, ischemic heart disease, malignant neoplasm of the trachea, bronchus, and lung, and pneumonia and influenza, and common low-preventability causes being arrhythmias and malignant neoplasms of the pancreas, female breast, and prostate. Gradients according to SES indicators of education and income were then examined separately for high- and low-preventability causes. Consistent with predictions derived from the fundamental-cause theory, Phelan and colleagues found the SES-mortality association substantially stronger for highly preventable causes of death than for less preventable causes (Phelan et al. 2004).

Before and after this study was conducted, a series of other studies focused on what has been called avoidable versus unavoidable mortality or amendable versus nonamenable causes of death (Dahl, Hofoss, and Elstad 2007; Korda et al. 2007; Mackenbach, Stronks, and Kunst 1989; Marshall et al. 1993; Piers et al. 2007; Song and Byeon 2000; Westerling, Gullberg, and Rosen 1996; Wood et al. 1999). None of these studies was developed to test the fundamental-cause theory but rather to evaluate how well treatment systems were functioning in reducing amendable or avoidable causes of death and for which groups. As a result, the studies present only some pieces of evidence that are relevant to fundamental-cause theory. Moreover, the studies differ from Phelan and colleagues' in generally using a somewhat narrower definition of preventable deaths. Nevertheless, the studies provide three sets of facts that have some bearing on fundamental-cause theory.

The first two sets of facts are not strong tests of the theory but are useful in evaluating it because they provide evidence that could potentially be inconsistent with it. Three studies examine whether preventable death rates decline more rapidly than less preventable ones. Fundamental-cause theory rests on the premise that people use new knowledge and technology to prevent disease and death. If preventable and nonpreventable death rates declined at equal rates, this aspect of fundamental-cause theory would be strenuously challenged. Of the three studies that reported

evidence on this issue (Korda et al. 2007; Mackenbach, Stronks, and Kunst 1989; Piers et al. 2007), all three found that preventable causes of death declined more rapidly than less preventable ones. The second and most commonly reported set of facts presented in these studies provides evidence of whether there is an SES gradient in preventable causes of death. For fundamental-cause theory the absence of an association in preventable causes would challenge the theory's assertion that SES gradients are evident when humans develop the capacity to address disease and death to some extent. Of the seven studies we found that provided this evidence, all showed an inverse association between SES and preventable causes of death (Dahl, Hofoss, and Elstad 2007; Korda et al. 2007; Marshall et al. 1993; Piers et al. 2007; Song and Byeon 2000; Westerling, Gullberg, and Rosen 1996; Wood et al. 1999). Finally, the third set of facts provides evidence concerning whether the SES association is stronger for preventable as compared to nonpreventable causes of death. As mentioned, fundamental-cause theory predicts that the SES-mortality association will be weaker in circumstances in which humans are less able to deploy flexible resources to gain a health advantage. Consistent with fundamental-cause theory, all three studies that reported evidence on this issue found that the SES-mortality association was stronger for preventable as opposed to less-preventable causes of death (Dahl, Hofoss, and Elstad 2007; Marshall et al. 1993; Song and Byeon 2000).

What Happens to Health Inequalities as Health-Relevant Knowledge and Technology Produce the Capacity to Avoid Disease and Death?

Another way to test fundamental-cause theory is to examine the association between SES and specific diseases over long periods of time. Whatever the association between SES and a particular disease is before some new life-saving knowledge or technology emerges, that association should move toward a stronger inverse association when the new knowledge and technology begin to influence patterns of morbidity and mortality. Phelan and Link (2005) provide a preliminary examination of this approach to testing fundamental-cause theory by examining selected causes of death in which great strides have been made and comparing race and SES gradients in those causes to gradients for causes of death where little progress was made over the same period of time. Health inequalities emerge over time in heart disease, lung cancer, and colon cancer where great progress has been made, but not in diseases like brain cancer, ovarian cancer, and pancreatic cancer, where much less progress has been made.

A more comprehensive test along these lines is provided by Glied and Lleras-Muney (2008), who operationalize the development of life-saving knowledge and technology, which they refer to as innovation, in two ways. In the first, they use the rate of change in mortality over time to indicate progress in addressing mortality due to particular diseases—the assumption being that the greater the decline in mortality, the greater the progress that has been made. In the second, Glied and Lleras-Muney use the number of active drugs approved to treat particular diseases with the assumption that more progress has been made where more new drugs have been developed to treat disease. Using both national mortality statistics and data from the Surveillance Epidemiology and End Result (SEER) cancer registry, they find, consistent with the theory of fundamental social causes, that education gradients become larger for diseases where greater innovation has occurred.

Can Intelligence or Other Personal Characteristics Replace Knowledge, Money, Power, Prestige, and Beneficial Social Connections as the Key Flexible Resources That Produce Health Inequalities?

Once we have the idea that broadly serviceable resources are required to understand the emergence and reemergence of health inequalities across places and times, we see that a resource other than the social resources identified in the fundamental-cause approach is possible. Intelligence or cognitive ability can also be conceptualized as a broadly serviceable resource that enhances people's abilities to deal with life situations, including situations that have health implications. Theory to support the prominence of intelligence

begins with the observation that the management of health, like so many other aspects of modern life, has become exceptionally complex. Massive amounts of new health-relevant information have become available, and gaining access to that information, absorbing its content, assessing its salience, and constructing a plan to act on the information received is a daunting task. Simply put, a strain is placed on the capacity to fully grasp and effectively deploy health-relevant information, whether it is to address a health crisis or to prevent one from occurring. It follows that individuals who are more intellectually adept are better able to grasp any health situation they confront, ferret out the relevant information required to address the circumstance they experience, and creatively construct a plan to maximize their chances for a healthy outcome. As Gottfredson (2004, 189) puts it: "Health self-management is inherently complex and thus puts a premium on the ability to learn, reason and solve problems." Based on this reasoning, she proposes intelligence may be the "elusive 'fundamental cause' of social class inequalities in health."

The research issue concerning the role of cognitive ability is relatively straightforward. In fundamental-cause theory, social and economic resources of knowledge, money, power, prestige, and beneficial social connections are critical, whereas for Gottfredson the psychological resource of intelligence is the source both of the socioeconomic-related resources and of health. Critical facts that separate these two interpretations hinge on the importance of cognitive ability for health with SES controlled, and the role of SES for health with cognitive ability controlled. To investigate these relationships, Link and colleagues (2008) located two large public-access data sets—the Wisconsin Longitudinal Study and the Health and Retirement Survey—that provided the requisite measures of SES and IQ to assess these differing views. The analysis found little evidence of a direct effect of intelligence on health once adult education and income are held constant. In contrast, the significant effects of education and income on health change very little when intelligence is controlled. Although further research is needed before definitive conclusions can be drawn, this evidence is inconsistent with the claim that intelligence is the fundamental cause of health disparities and instead supports the idea that the flexible resources people actively use to gain a health advantage are SES-related resources like knowledge, money, power, prestige, and beneficial social connections.

Whatever one concludes about the role of intelligence in health disparities based on this and other research, a new potential challenge to fundamental-cause theory is emerging. For example, in a series of articles Heckman (2006, 2008) has emphasized the critical role of what he calls noncognitive traits or socioemotional factors in both socioeconomic attainment and health determination. Examples of the noncognitive traits he identifies are perseverance, motivation, time preference, risk aversion, self-esteem, self-control, and preference for leisure. According to Heckman, these and other personality traits are related to both socioeconomic attainment and health in such a way as to suggest that key aspects of socioeconomic status are simple "proxies" for such personality traits. As Heckman (2008, 13252) puts it: "The evidence that personality traits affect educational attainment helps to explain how education, as a proxy, helps reduce disease gradients by socioeconomic class." While the evidence concerning the role of noncognitive traits in socioeconomic attainment is arguably strong, the evidence linking them to health, particularly with adequate consideration of socioeconomic status, is both thin and weak. Since these noncognitive traits have been put forward to pose a potential challenge to fundamental-cause theory, in much the same way that Gottfredson (2004) raised intelligence as such a challenge, rigorous evaluations of the impact of these noncognitive traits are necessary in evaluating fundamental-cause theory.

One reason that such evaluations are needed is that imagining that cognitive and noncognitive personal attributes lie at the root of health inequalities could support the rationale to expend enormous resources to address "deficits" in these factors in disadvantaged groups. But if the imagined importance of these factors for health inequalities is incorrect, health inequalities will not dissipate with such additional support, and resources that could have been used to address such inequalities will be diverted from approaches that might have been effective.

Considerations on the Scope of Fundamental-Cause Theory

Is Fundamental-Cause Theory a Grand Theory or a Theory of the Middle Range?

Despite the ambitious name that Link and Phelan affixed to the theory (for reasons indicated earlier in this chapter), fundamental-cause theory is decidedly a theory of the middle range. In explicating his concept of middle-range theory, Merton (1968, 5) proposed the need for theories "intermediate to the minor working hypotheses evolved in abundance during the day-by-day routine of research, and the all inclusive speculations comprising a master conceptual scheme." For Merton, the day-to-day hypotheses fell short in their ability to produce robust synthetic explanations, whereas what he termed "grand theories" were too speculative and too far removed from the possibility of empirical testing to be useful. Fundamental-cause theory is a middle-range theory in that it resides above day-to-day hypotheses such as, Is SES causally related to disease x, to disease y, or to disease z? or Is SES linked to disease x through risk factor a, b, or c? Instead, fundamental-cause theory provides an explanation for why SES might be related to many diseases and why such an association might be reproduced in multiple contexts and at different times. At the same time, fundamental-cause theory resides below grand theory in that it identifies a relatively specific phenomenon it seeks to explain—connections between health and social factors like SES and discrimination. Further unlike the prototype of grand theory that Merton describes, fundamental-cause theory generates empirical predictions that can yield evidence bearing on the theory's utility. Some empirical tests have been described here, others are in process, and still others await imaginative formulation of new strategies for evaluating the theory.

Implicit in the idea that fundamental-cause theory is a theory of the middle range is that it must join with other theories to account for the social distribution of health and illness. Within medical sociology, other middle-range theories that need to be engaged are of course social-stress theory, theory concerning health lifestyles, and an emerging sociological theory of health selection, among others. Moreover, in some instances empirical facts make this apparent, as is true with the social patterning of morbidity and mortality by gender and immigration status. Men and people born in the United States are generally thought to have the advantage of high status when compared to women and immigrant populations. With respect to gender, while it is true that women report worse health in a manner consistent with fundamental social cause theory, they also enjoy a robust longevity advantage over men in a way that fundamental-cause theory, at least as elaborated so far, does not explain. Similarly, some immigrant groups enjoy better health than do native-born Americans—at least in the early years of their tenure in the United States. Again this is a fact that fundamental-cause theory as it has been formulated so far does not explain. At the same time, within these categorical divisions (gender and immigration status) SES gradients in health outcomes are usually evident, suggesting the possibility that fundamental social cause processes are at work but need to join with other theories to achieve a more complete accounting of the full pattern of health outcomes.

There also exists substantial evidence that other middle-range theories in medical sociology need to embrace fundamental-cause theory to account for some empirical findings that they have not adequately explained. Much of the evidence for fundamental-cause theory appears here, but two sets of facts speak to the necessity of the perspective, because these facts are consistent with fundamental-cause theory but have not been explained by other middle-range theories in medical sociology. One such fact is the emergence of health inequalities by race and SES over the fifty years or so in major killers such as heart disease, lung cancer, and colon cancer, where significant progress has been made in knowledge and technology relevant to the prevention or cure of these conditions. Whereas at one time death rates from

these diseases tended to be higher in advantaged groups, they are now higher in disadvantaged groups. The second such fact is a relatively stable set of differences between advantaged and disadvantaged groups in age-adjusted mortality rates for diseases like brain, ovarian, and pancreatic cancer, where little knowledge or technology relevant to prevention or cure has developed. This set of facts is consistent with fundamental-cause theory but is difficult to explain from the vantage point of stress theory or a theory of health selection, as neither predicts these changes in patterns of mortality over time.

Conclusion

Over the past fifteen years, the fundamental-cause theory of health inequalities has been elaborated and some tests have been developed and implemented. We now see the theory as a theory of the middle range that helps us understand the social patterning of disease and death from a distinctly sociological vantage point.

References

Antonovsky, Aaron. 1967. "Social Class, Life Expectancy, and Overall Mortality." *Milbank Memorial Quarterly* 45:31–73.

Black, Douglas, J. N. Morris, Cyril Smith, and Peter Townsend. 1982. *Inequalities in Health: The Black Report*. Middlesex, England: Penguin.

Carpiano, Richard M., and Brian C. Kelly. 2007. "Scientific Knowledge as Resource and Risk: What Does Hormone Replacement Tell Us about Health Disparities." Paper presented at the American Sociological Association Meetings, New York City, August.

Chapin, C. V. 1924. "Deaths among Taxpayers and Non-taxpayers Income Tax, Providence, 1865." *American Journal of Public Health* 4:647–51.

Coombs, L. C. 1941. "Economic Differentials in Causes of Death." *Medical Care* 1:246–55.

Dahl, Espen, Dag Hofoss, and Jon I. Elstad. 2007. "Educational Inequalities in Avoidable Deaths in Norway: A Population Based Study." *Health Sociology Review* 16:146–59.

Glied, Sherry, and Adriana Lleras-Muney. 2008. "Technological Innovation and Inequality in Health." *Demography* 45:741–61.

Gottfredson, Linda. 2004. "Intelligence: Is It the Epidemiologists' Elusive 'Fundamental Cause' of Social Class Inequalities in Health?" *Journal of Social and Personality Psychology* 86:174–99.

Heckman, James. 2006. "Skill Formation and the Economics of Investing in Disadvantaged Children." *Science* 312:1900–1902.

———. 2008. "The Economics, Technology, and Neuroscience of Human Capability Formation." *Proceedings of the National Academy of Sciences of the United States of America* 104:13250–55.

House, James S. 2002. "Understanding Social Factors and Inequalities in Health: 20th-Century Progress and 21st-Century Prospects." *Journal of Health and Social Behavior* 43:125–42.

Korda, Rosemary, James R. G. Butler, Mark S. Clements, and Stephen Kunitz. 2007. "Differential Impacts of Health Care in Australia: Trend Analysis and Socioeconomic Inequalities in Avoidable Mortality." *International Journal of Epidemiology* 36:157–65.

Krieger, Nancy, David H. Rehkopf, Jarvis T. Chen, Pamela D. Waterman, Enrico Marcelli, and Malinda Kennedy. 2008. "The Fall and Rise of U.S. Inequities in Premature Mortality, 1960–2002." *PLoS Medicine/Public Library of Science* 5(2): e46.

Kunst, Anton E., Groenhof Feikje, and Johan P. Mackenbach, EU Working Group on Social Inequalities and Health. 1998. "Occupational Class and Cause-Specific Mortality in Middle-Aged Men in 11 European Countries: Comparison of Population-Based Studies." *British Medical Journal* 316:1636–42.

Lantz, Paula M., James S. House, James M. Lepkowski, David R. Williams, Richard P. Mero, and Jieming Chen. 1998. "Socioeconomic Factors, Health Behaviors, and Mortality: Results from a Nationally Representative Prospective Study of U.S. Adults." *Journal of the American Medical Association* 279:1703–8.

Link, Bruce G. 2003. "The Production of Understanding." *Journal of Health and Social Behavior* 44:457–69.

———. 2008. "Epidemiological Sociology and the Social Shaping of Population Health." *Journal of Health and Social Behavior* 49(4): 367–84.

Link, Bruce G., and Jo C. Phelan. 1995. "Social Conditions as Fundamental Causes of Disease. *Journal of Health and Social Behavior* (extra issue): 80–94.

———. In press. "The Social Shaping of Smoking and Health." *Drug and Alcohol Dependence.*

Link, Bruce G., Mary E. Northridge, Jo C. Phelan, and Michael L. Ganz. 1998. "Social Epidemiology and the Fundamental Cause Concept: On the Structuring of Effective Cancer Screens by Socioeconomic Status." *Milbank Memorial Quarterly* 76:375–402.

Link, Bruce G., Jo C. Phelan, Richard Miech, and Emily Leckman. 2008. "The Resources That Matter: Fundamental Social Causes of Health Disparities and the Challenge of Intelligence." *Journal of Health and Social Behavior* 49:72–91.

Lutfey, Karen, and Jeremy Freese. 2005. "Toward Some Fundamentals of Fundamental Causality: Socioeconomic Status and Health in the Routine Clinic Visit for Diabetes." *American Journal of Sociology* 110:1326–72.

Mackenbach, Johan P., Karien Stronks, and Anton E. Kunst. 1989. "The Contribution of Medical Care to Inequalities in Health: Differences between Socioeconomic Groups in Decline of Mortality from Conditions Amenable to Medical Intervention." *Social Science and Medicine* 29:369–76.

Marmot, Michael. 2004. *The Status Syndrome: How Social Standing Affects Our Health and Longevity.* New York: Henry Holt.

Marshall, Stephen W., Ichiro Kawachi, Neil Pearce, and Barry Borman. 1993. "Social Class Differences in Mortality from Diseases Amenable to Medical Intervention in New Zealand." *International Journal of Epidemiology* 22:255–61.

Merton, Robert K. 1968. *Social Theory and Social Structure.* New York: Free Press.

NCHS [National Center for Health Statistics]. 2006. *Health United States 2006: With Chartbook on Trends in the Health of Americans.* Hyattsville, Md.: NCHS.

Olafsdottir, Sigrun. 2007. "Fundamental Causes of Health Disparities: Stratification, the Welfare State, and Health in the United States and Iceland." *Journal of Health and Social Behavior* 48:239–53.

Phelan, Jo C., and Bruce G. Link. 2005. "Controlling Disease and Creating Disparities: A Fundamental Cause Perspective." *Journals of Gerontology* 60B (special issue II): 27–33.

Phelan, Jo C., Bruce Link, Ana Diez-Roux, Ichiro Kawachi, and Bruce Levin. 2004. "Fundamental Causes of Social Inequalities in Mortality: A Test of the Theory." *Journal of Health and Social Behavior* 45:265–85.

Piers, Leonard S., Norman J. Carlson, Kaye Brown, and Zahid Ansari. 2007. "Avoidable Mortality in Victoria between 1979 and 2000." *Australian and New Zealand Journal of Public Health* 31:1–12.

Rose, Geoffrey. 1979. "The Evolution of Social Medicine." In *The Handbook of Medical Sociology,* 3rd ed., ed. Howard E. Freeman, Sol Levine, and Leo G. Reeder. Englewood Cliffs, N.J.: Prentice Hall.

———. 1992. *The strategy of preventive medicine.* Oxford: Oxford University Press.

Song, Yun-Mi, and Jai Jun Byeon. 2000. "Excess Mortality from Avoidable and Non-Avoidable Causes in Men of Low Socioeconomic Status: A Prospective Study in Korea." *Journal of Epidemiology and Community Health* 54:166–72.

Sorlie, Paul D., Eric Backlund, and Jacob B. Keller. 1995. "U.S. Mortality by Economic, Demographic, and Social Characteristics: The National Longitudinal Mortality Study." *American Journal of Public Health* 85:949–56.

Westerling, Ragnar, Anders Gullberg, and Mans Rosen. 1996. "Socioeconomic Differences in Avoidable Mortality in Sweden, 1986–1990." *International Journal of Epidemiology* 25:560–67.

Wilkinson, Richard G. 2005. *The Impact of Inequality: How to Make Sick Societies Healthier.* New York: New Press.

Wood, Evan, Anthony M. Sallar, Martin T. Schechter, and Robert S. Hogg. 1999. "Social Inequalities in Male Mortality Amenable to Medical Intervention in British Columbia." *Social Science and Medicine* 48:1751–58.

2

Social Capital and Health

Ichiro Kawachi, Harvard School of Public Health

Social capital has been hailed as one of the most popular exports from sociology into the field of population health. At the same time, the application of the concept to explain variations in population health has been greeted with spirited debate and controversy (Kawachi et al. 2004). The debates have ranged from the very definition of social capital—whether it ought to be understood as an individual-level attribute or as a property of the collective—to skepticism about the utility of applying the concept to the health field as a health promotion strategy (Pearce and Davey Smith 2003; Navarro 2004). As Szreter and Woolcock (2004) noted, social capital has become one of the "essentially contested concepts" in the social sciences, like class, race, and gender.

Definitions of Social Capital

In modern sociology, the origins of social capital are most closely identified with the writings of Pierre Bourdieu and James Coleman. Bourdieu defined social capital as "the aggregate of actual or potential resources linked to possession of a durable network" (1986, 248). Coleman defined the concept via a more functionalist approach, as in: "Social capital is defined by its function. It is not a single entity, but a variety of different entities having two characteristics in common: They all consist of some aspect of social structure, and they facilitate certain actions of individuals who are within the structure" (1990, 302). As examples of the forms that social capital could

take, Coleman cited the trustworthiness of social environment, which makes possible reciprocity exchanges; information channels; norms and effective sanctions; and "appropriable" social organizations, that is, associations established for a specific purpose (for example, a neighborhood block group established to fight crime) that can later be appropriated for broader uses (304–12).

Following these contrasting definitions set forth by Bourdieu and Coleman, the empirical literature on social capital has been split according to those who treat the concept from a network perspective (à la Bourdieu) and those who define the concept from a social cohesion perspective (i.e., emphasizing the forms of social capital highlighted by Coleman such as trust, reciprocity exchanges, norms, and sanctions). Within the field of population health, the social cohesion school has been so far dominant—and has been criticized for paying insufficient attention to network-based definitions of social capital (Moore et al. 2005; Carpiano 2008).[1] According to Carpiano (2008), Bourdieu's network approach to social capital offers a couple of nuances that are not highlighted in the social cohesion-based approaches. First, by conceptualizing social capital as "the resources available through social networks," the approach explicitly recognizes that inequalities can arise in between-individual and between-group access to social capital, since networks are not all the same—some networks are more powerful than others by virtue of the stocks of material and symbolic resources available to their members. Second, the network perspective opens the way to begin considering the negative effects (the "dark side") of social capital, which critics point out have tended to be neglected in the social cohesion literature.

A further critical distinction in the literature lies between those who consider social capital a characteristic of individuals and those who treat social capital as a characteristic of the collective (such as residential neighborhoods or workplaces). Methodological individualists tend to view individual actors within a social structure as either possessing or lacking the ability to secure benefits by virtue of their membership in networks. For example, Nan Lin's (2001) Position Generator is an example of a measurement approach to social capital that inquires about the individual's ability to access resources through personal connections to others with valued occupational positions, such as lawyers, physicians, or bank managers. By contrast, the practice of treating social capital as a collective characteristic treats it as an extraindividual, contextual influence on health outcomes. This practice is in turn reflected by measurement approaches that emphasize the degree to which social cohesion exists within a group (or alternatively, if one hews to the network-based definition of social capital, by attempts to describe group characteristics through whole network analysis). As Coleman noted, the "social" aspect of social capital is aptly chosen because "as an attribute of the social structure in which a person is embedded, social capital is not the private property of any of the persons who benefit from it" (1990, 315).

The main reason population health researchers tend to treat social capital as a group characteristic is that a rich empirical tradition already exists within the field of investigating individual-level access to social support as an influence on health outcomes (Berkman and Glass 2000). In other words, it seems redundant to replace an existing term ("an individual's access to instrumental and emotional social support") with another, albeit fancier term ("social capital").

Mechanisms through Which Social Capital Influences Health Outcomes

Social capital, considered as a group-level construct, is hypothesized to influence population health outcomes through at least four distinct mechanisms (Kawachi and Berkman 2000). First, more cohesive groups are better equipped to undertake collective action. Examples relevant to population health include the ability of a community to organize to protest the closure of a local hospital, the passage of local ordinances to restrict smoking in public places, or the use of zoning restrictions to prevent the incursion of fast-food outlets. The residents' perceived ability to mobilize to undertake collectively desired actions is referred to as "collective efficacy," and validated survey instruments have been developed to tap this form of social capital, for example, in the Project on Human Development in Chicago Neighborhoods (Sampson, Raudenbush, and Earls 1997).

A second pathway through which social capital influences health consists of the ability of the group to enforce and maintain social norms. For example, when adults within a community feel empowered to step in to intervene when they observe instances of deviant behavior by adolescents (such as underage smoking and drinking), it is referred to as "informal social control." The power of informal social control consists in the ability of the community to enforce desired norms without resort to the police or schoolteachers. It is a collective characteristic in the sense that the parents of the offending minors need not be involved; instead their neighbors can be relied upon to step in to admonish the offenders on their behalf. Groups with a strong sense of informal social control are often characterized by high degrees of "network closure"—another form of social capital cited by Coleman (1990). Network closure occurs when not only children A and B are connected via friendship, but also their parents are in close contact. An instance of such network closure used to be found in Japan, where parents (primarily mothers) were connected to each other through volunteering in local PTAs. Adolescent smoking in Japanese society remained fairly uncommon (by Western standards) until the 1980s despite the ubiquitous presence of cigarette-vending machines on virtually every street corner. One reason Japanese schoolchildren observed the legal prohibition of smoking under the age of twenty was because if any child surreptitiously bought and smoked a cigarette on the way home from school, his mother was likely to learn about it from a neighbor before he reached home.[2] As network closure has declined with the retreat of PTA membership in urban Japanese communities, the rate of adolescent smoking has climbed in tandem.

A third mechanism through which social capital influences health is via reciprocity exchanges between members of a network. As Coleman (1990) pointed out, norms of reciprocity are established when actor A does a favor for actor B and trusts that the recipient will return the favor at a later point in time. A's expectation that B will repay the debt creates an obligation on the part of B to keep the trust. As these "credit slips" begin to multiply and to extend to other members of the network, the result is a community where people are constantly helping each other out. An instance of such a system of reciprocity exchanges is described in Hideo Okuda's 2005 novel *Southbound* about an island community in Okinawa, where the locals use the term *yuima¯ru* to describe the norms of mutual aid. When a new family arrives on the island, a steady procession of neighbors gathers on their doorstep to help the newcomers refurbish their dwelling, lend them farming equipment, and donate food.[3] The maintenance of reciprocity exchanges in turn depends upon two key elements: the trustworthiness of the social environment, and the ability of the group to enforce sanctions against free riders.

Finally, social capital is linked to health through the diffusion of innovations via information channels that exist within network structures. As Granovetter (1973) pointed out in his influential paper on "the strength of weak ties," the diffusion of information need not occur through close social contacts. Indeed, the potential to glean new information from intimate relationships is often low, because by definition such people are likely to share the same information. In Granovetter's study of job seekers, individuals were more likely to find out about jobs from friends of friends. In other words, the diffusion of information and other resources from the outside into the network depends upon the presence of network bridges, individuals who serve as channels that connect disparate, unconnected groups of actors (Lakon, Godette, and Hipp 2008). The diffusion of innovations via "connectors," "mavens," and "salesmen" was popularized by Malcolm Gladwell's *The Tipping Point* (2000). For a more formal treatment of sociometric approaches to investigate the spread of health-related innovations, see Valente, Gallaher, and Mouttapa 2004.

Although the discussion of the mechanisms linking social capital to health so far has focused on the positive (i.e., benign and beneficial) aspects of social capital, each mechanism described is equally applicable to the so-called downsides of social capital. Thus, a community with high levels of collective efficacy could just as easily use those resources to oppress and discriminate against outsiders (the South Boston riots during the busing and forced desegregation of schools during the 1960s come to mind). The flip side of informal social control is a community that is often controlling and intolerant of diversity, with restrictions on individual freedom that nonconformists might chafe at. A dense system of reciprocity exchanges is often associated with excessive obligations on the part of group members who are called upon to provide aid to others, sometimes at high personal cost. And not all information that diffuses through a dense social network is good or beneficial. The spread of malicious rumors via social networking sites (cyber-bullying) is a case in point.

Finally, social capital researchers—particularly those who hew to the social cohesion school—have been accused of yearning for a romanticized vision of "community" as it existed in a bygone era, or perhaps only in the imagination (Muntaner, Lynch, and Davey Smith 2001). This is a straw-man argument—the aim of social capital studies is not to turn the clock back or to advocate the transformation of American suburbia into Okinawan society, but to attempt to identify resources within social relations that can be practically mobilized in contemporary settings to promote health; as well as to understand and manage the situations in which social cohesion can lead to deleterious consequences (such as the spread of misinformation and rumors).

The Measurement of Social Capital

The measurement of social capital hinges on the way in which the investigator defines the concept—as an individual attribute or a collective attribute, or from a network-based perspective or a cohesion-based perspective. Four broad approaches to measurement have been applied: surveys of individuals or groups, sociometric methods, experimental elicitation of trust and cooperation, and qualitative approaches.

Surveys

Survey-based approaches are the commonest method encountered in the field of population health for assessing social capital either at the individual or the collective level. At the individual level, Lin's Position Generator (2001) is an instrument that inquires about whether the respondent has access to people with high-prestige occupations (e.g., doctor, lawyer). The assumption is that knowing people with high-prestige occupations correlates with the ability of the individual to access a variety of resources, such as instrumental support, information and advice, or symbolic status. Responses to the instrument can be then used to generate measures of social capital such as the highest level of accessed prestige ("upper reachability") or the range in accessed prestige (the difference in prestige between the highest and lowest occupations accessed). Upper reachability is akin to the concept of linking social capital, which refers to resources accessed across socioeconomic gradients—as contrasted with bonding social capital, which describes resources accessed within groups that are similar with respect to class, race, and ethnicity (Szreter and Woolcock 2004).

As is evident from its emphasis on occupational prestige, the Position Generator has been used to examine the instrumental uses of social capital—how individuals can use their social connections to get ahead in society. When it comes to studying the potential influence of social capital on health outcomes, the Position Generator has some limitations. For example, accessing occupational prestige is not relevant for all types of resources—receiving emotional support from a surgeon is not necessarily better than receiving it from a priest. Likewise, some positions are not assigned official job prestige, such as homemakers, yet they provide valued resources from a health perspective (van der Gaag and Webber 2008).

An alternative approach to measuring individual social capital is exemplified by van der Gaag and Snijders's Resource Generator (2005). This validated instrument provides a checklist of different kinds of social resources that respondents can potentially access through their networks. Items are phrased in the form: "Do you know anyone who ___," with examples of resources such as "can repair a car," "owns a car," "has knowledge about financial matters," "can baby sit for your children." As is evident from the foregoing description, the Resource Generator closely parallels the survey instruments already used in the public health literature to tap into individual access to social support. The Resource Generator has been reported to correlate well with health outcomes (e.g., Webber and Huxley 2007), which might be expected given the resemblance of the instrument to measures of social support, and the well-established associations of social support with health outcomes.

From a social cohesion perspective, researchers have sought to measure social capital through surveys inquiring about what people feel (their values and perceptions), as well as what people do (participation in formal and informal contacts) (Harpham 2008). The responses to such surveys can be then analyzed at the individual level (as in residents' perceptions of the cohesiveness of their neighborhood) or aggregated up to the group level and analyzed as a contextual influence on individual health outcomes. Table 2.1 illustrates these distinctions.

Community surveys have been the mainstay in health research to assess neighborhood

Table 2.1. Typology of measurement approaches to social capital

Definition of social capital	Level of analysis	
	Individual	Group
Network based	Position generator, resource generator	Whole social network analysis
Cohesion based	Individual perceptions (e.g., trustworthiness of neighbors) and behaviors (e.g., participation in civic associations)	Survey responses aggregated to the group level

characteristics such as social cohesion, collective efficacy, and informal social control. For example, instruments that measure social cohesion typically consist of multi-item scales that inquire about the trustworthiness of neighbors, norms of reciprocity and mutual aid, and the extent to which residents share the same values. A number of psychometrically validated instruments have been developed for use in field studies (see Harpham 2008).

A frequent criticism leveled at survey instruments is that they often include elements that are not properly part of social capital, but rather are antecedents or consequences of it (Harpham 2008; De Silva 2006). Examples include residents' satisfaction with their neighborhood or perceptions of safety from crime. On occasion, when survey data are lacking, researchers have resorted to the use of proxies such as crime rates obtained from Justice Department statistics or voting participation. The problems with these approaches are that they lay the practice open to charges of "conceptual stretching," where social capital begins to lose meaning, and that they conflate the consequences of social capital with its measurement, which risks tautology ("a community with low crime rates must have high social capital because it has low crime rates") (Portes 1998).

Social Network Analysis

An altogether different approach to measuring social capital is via whole network (sociometric) analysis. Within the public health literature it is quite common to see social networks assessed from the individual (egocentric) perspective (e.g., "How many friends do you have, and how often do you see them?") (Berkman and Glass 2000). In contrast to the ego-centered network assessment approach, the sociometric approach seeks to characterize the whole network by interviewing all the alters nominated by the ego and, in turn, all of their alters, until saturation is reached. As the description makes clear, the limiting step for initiating such studies is establishing the boundary of the network. While boundaries are readily identifiable in settings like schools or companies or within subcultures such as injection drug users, they are less straightforward in contexts like

neighborhoods, which may explain why few studies so far have applied sociometric network analysis to the investigation of social capital and health. However, as Lakon, Godette, and Hipp (2008) illustrate, several measures derived from sociometric analysis have direct relevance for the concept of social capital, including network-based analogs of cohesion, bonding, and bridging social capital (more about this later).

Experimental Approaches

Experimental approaches to measure constructs related to social capital (such as trust and cooperation) have been advocated by economists who inherently distrust survey responses to questions inquiring about perceptions, opinions, and attitudes. For example, Glaeser and colleagues (2000) have suggested that instead of relying on survey-based measures of trust, researchers should attempt to directly elicit observable behavioral measures of trust such as the envelope drop. In this approach, subjects are told that the experimenter will intentionally drop a money-filled envelope addressed to the sender, say, in the middle of Harvard Square. If the subject places a high value on the dropped envelope, the economist infers that the subject is more likely to trust the anonymous stranger who will find the envelope and mail it.

Another experimental approach to studying trust and cooperation is the trust game, in which subject A is given a sum of money and offered the opportunity to pass some, all, or none of it to partner B. The experimenter then increases the transferred amount by some multiple before passing it on to B. Finally, B has the opportunity to return some, none, or all of the money to A. In this experiment, the amount initially transferred by A is interpreted as a measure of trusting behavior. Anderson and Mellor (2008) describe other versions of the trust experiment, including the public-goods game, a version of the prisoner's dilemma. Some of these experiments have found that individuals who self-report greater trust of others or higher participation in voluntary groups (two survey-based indicators of social capital) are also more likely to exhibit trusting and cooperative behaviors in experimental situations (Anderson, Mellor, and Milyo, 2004), thereby suggesting convergent validity between survey-based and experimental measures of social capital.

Qualitative Approaches

Finally, qualitative approaches to investigating social capital have yielded important insights into the complexity and nuances of the links between social capital and health that quantitative studies do not reveal. In a systematic review of qualitative studies, Whitley (2008) concluded that they had been instrumental in drawing attention to the downsides of social capital, as well as in reminding us of the existence of broader historical and structural forces that shape the health of community residents.

Empirical Evidence Linking Social Capital to Health

The relationship between social capital and health has been investigated through a variety of study designs, including ecological, individual-level, multilevel, and qualitative approaches. As mentioned earlier, the majority of studies in the population health realm have focused on the health effects of social cohesion. From the perspective of social capital as a contextual influence on health, the most convincing design is the multilevel study in which relationships of social capital to individual health can be examined after controlling for potential confounding by individual-level compositional variables. In other words, the merit of the multilevel study is being able to test the counterfactual question, "If two individuals with exchangeable characteristics (i.e., the same sociodemographic characteristics, occupying the same socioeconomic position, with the same level of social ties and trust of others) were observed in a high social capital community and in a low social capital community, would their health outcomes differ, all other things equal?" The limitation of ecological studies is that any difference observed in average health status across communities with different levels of social capital could

be confounded by the characteristics of residents who belong to each place. Controlling for the aggregated characteristics of residents will not solve the problem, since in an ecological study, by definition, we do not know the distribution of confounders (the common prior causes of social capital and health) among individual residents.

When we turn to individual-level studies of social capital and health, they tend to be limited by common method bias: individuals' perceptions of the trustworthiness of their neighbors are potentially contaminated by unobserved characteristics such as personality and negative affectivity that simultaneously influence health status. This problem is particularly salient in studies that have used self-reported health outcome measures as the endpoint of interest. Similarly, an association between individual-level participation in associational activity and health outcomes is likely to suffer from endogeneity bias. The direction of the bias can theoretically cut in both directions—either healthier people are more likely to volunteer in groups (positive selection) or sick people are more likely to join some groups (adverse selection). This bias may partly account for the contradictory findings in the literature when social participation is used as an indicator of social cohesion (Ellaway and Macintyre 2007).

With these caveats in mind, we find that systematic reviews of social capital and health have identified fairly consistent evidence of associations between markers of social cohesion and health outcomes, including physical health (e.g., mortality and self-rated health; Kim, Subramanian, and Kawachi 2008), mental health (e.g., depressive symptoms; Almedom and Glandon 2008), and health-related behaviors (smoking, drinking, high-risk sexual behavior; Lindstrom 2008b).

The preponderance of evidence suggests that there is something there, although strong causal claims are premature due to the number of gaps in the existing literature, as noted by the systematic reviews. These include: (a) the cross-sectional design of most studies so that temporal ordering cannot be established; (b) the reliance of many studies on secondary analyses of survey data that were not specifically designed to measure social capital (De Silva 2006); (c) the reliance of many studies on single indicators of social capital (often a single item on social trust, at that); (d) residual confounding by omitted variables such as personality and negative affectivity in studies that examined correlations between individual-level perceptions of trust and reciprocity and self-reported health outcomes; and (e) the preponderance of evidence from Western countries (North America and Europe) and the sparseness of studies conducted in other cultural contexts.

A major source of heterogeneity across studies arises in the choice of scale for examining the effects of social capital on health, which ranges from cross-national comparisons (e.g., Lynch et al. 2001) to U.S. state-level analyses (Kawachi et al. 1997) to municipalities (Islam et al. 2006a) and neighborhoods (e.g., within Chicago, see Lochner et al. 2003). Critics have complained that this breadth of application illustrates another instance of "conceptual stretching" (Portes 1998), although from a social cohesion perspective, plausible arguments could be raised in defense of theorizing that whole societies as well as neighborhoods can be characterized as cohesive (or not). Nonetheless, as a general principle, the further the researcher moves away from proximal processes linking exposures to health outcomes, the greater the number of plausible confounders, and the higher the likelihood that we lose our grasp of the causal steps linking the "exposure" variables to the outcomes of interest (Zimmerman 2008).

A further pattern remarked in the literature is that the associations between social cohesion and health outcomes seem stronger and more consistently observed in less egalitarian societies (e.g., with high levels of economic inequality) compared to more egalitarian societies marked by the presence of strong welfare states and safety-net provisions (Islam et al. 2006b). Thus, for example, the intraclass correlation (ICC, corresponding to the percent of variation in outcomes explained at the area level) was considerably higher in a U.S. study of neighborhood influences on violent crime and homicide (7.5 percent) than the corresponding ICCs observed in studies from Sweden and Canada (0–2 percent) (Islam et al. 2006b). This pattern seems to argue against the strand of political theory that posits that strong welfare states tend to crowd out associational activities and norms of mutual assistance. If anything, social cohesion

would appear to be even more salient in explaining the health variations among citizens belonging to societies with weak safety-net provisions, for example, in health care, public education, and unemployment protections (Rostila 2007)

With regard to the potential diversity of settings in which social cohesion could be observed and assessed, the systematic reviews reveal that the bulk of studies to date—whether quantitative or qualitative—have focused on residential neighborhoods. This is understandable given the burgeoning interest in neighborhood influences in population health (Kawachi and Berkman 2003). However, social capital can be transported to other settings such as schools or workplaces. A recent example is a prospective study of more than thirty-three thousand Finnish public-sector employees that sought to examine the relationships between workplace social cohesion and the risk of incident depression (Kouvonen et al. 2008). Workplace social capital was measured by a scale developed by the authors that inquired about cohesion (trust and cooperation) between employees, as well as relations between employees and supervisors. The eight-item scale had good internal consistency reliability (Cronbach alpha = 0.87) (Kouvonen et al. 2006). While lower individual-level perceptions of workplace social capital was associated with a 20–50 percent higher risk of depression during follow-up, the study found no association in multilevel analyses between aggregate workplace social cohesion and depression. Thus the study did not find a significant contextual influence of workplace social capital on the risk of depression, and even the individual-level findings could have been artifacts of reverse causation (i.e., negative emotions leading to lower perceptions of workplace social cohesion). Nevertheless, the study points to a novel direction for empirical studies of social capital and health, especially since workplaces (as compared to neighborhoods) are where people in midlife spend an increasing part of their time engaged in social interactions. In a thoughtful commentary accompanying the Finnish study, Lindstrom (2008a) suggested additional directions in which research on workplace social capital could be advanced, including: (a) drawing the distinction between so-called horizontal social capital (cohesion between employees occupying similar levels of employment grade) and vertical social capital (cohesion between workers and their supervisors); and (b) examining the interactions between social capital in the workplace and social capital outside the workplace. In other words, as workers seek to maintain work/family balance, their health is likely to be shaped by the simultaneous and interactive influences of workplace, family, and neighborhood social environments. Extensions of the multilevel approach—so-called cross-classified models—are well equipped to handle such analytical complexity (Subramanian, Jones, and Duncan 2003).

Lastly, a relatively underexplored dimension of social cohesion and health is the potential for cross-level interactions between aggregate-level cohesion and individual characteristics. Multilevel analysis permits the explicit testing of such cross-level interactions. For example, Subramanian, Kim, and Kawachi (2002) found in an analysis of the U.S. Social Capital Benchmark Survey that community levels of social cohesion (as proxied by aggregate levels of trust) were not statistically significantly associated with residents' self-rated health after controlling for individual-level compositional characteristics, including individual reports of trust in others. However, in the same study the authors found evidence of a significant cross-level interaction whereby individuals reporting high levels of trust report better health when their neighbors were also trusting. On the other hand, individuals reporting low levels of trust tended to fare worse when they were surrounded by more-trusting neighbors. This result echoes the observations made in qualitative studies that social capital does not uniformly affect the health of all individuals within the same community (Whitley 2008). While social capital can be beneficial for some individuals, it may harm others.

Future Directions in Social Capital Research

While the use of multilevel analysis has become fairly standard in investigations of the health effects of social capital, this is in one sense only the starting point of methodological sophistication required for strengthening causal inference. Aside from the need for more prospective data, as well as the application of network-based approaches to studying social capital already alluded to, future research needs to engage more seriously with thornier issues such as unobserved heterogeneity and endogeneity. Multilevel analysis is quite good at dealing with compositional confounding and partitioning the variance in health outcomes at different levels of influence (individual versus the community). However, additional approaches are called for to deal with issues such as the selective sorting of different individuals into different contexts, as well as the reciprocal and dynamic relationships among social cohesion, individual social interactions, and health.

The problem of nonrandom sorting of residents into different types of residential areas is already familiar to researchers who study neighborhood effects on health (Oakes 2004; Subramanian, Glymour, and Kawachi 2007). Suppose we demonstrate in a multilevel analysis that more cohesive neighborhoods are associated with better health outcomes for individual residents even after controlling for individual-level characteristics (such as SES); this still does not prove causation. If trusting and sociable individuals selectively move into areas where they are surrounded by neighbors who share the same preferences, an association between social cohesion and health merely proves that cohesive neighborhoods have more sociable residents who are healthier by virtue of their proclivities. It does not necessarily follow that if we relocate a socially isolated individual from a less cohesive to a more cohesive neighborhood, her health status will improve. This type of confounding could be controlled by adjusting for those individual characteristics (e.g., sociability, trust). However, such data may not be available, and life is too short (as well as resources finite) to keep going back to the study sample to measure and control for every unobserved characteristic. In this type of situation, it has been suggested that techniques such as instrumental variable (IV) estimation could improve causal inference (Glymour 2006).

The idea of instruments is to find variables that cause exogenous variation in the treatment (or exposure) of interest—in this instance, neighborhood social cohesion—without directly affecting the values of the outcome variable (individual health status). In other words, instruments are natural experiments that randomly assign individuals into different social contexts, for instance, neighborhoods with high or low social cohesion. High population density, high immigrant concentration, and income polarization are each plausible instruments for social cohesion within a community (e.g., Alesina et al. 2003). Provided that these variables are not independently associated with differences in individual health status, they may serve as instruments to identify the causal effect of social cohesion on health.[4] For example, an individual residing in an area with high immigrant concentration will be more likely to find himself in a low-cohesion environment (this can be checked empirically within the data). Provided that immigrant concentration does not predict health status—other than through its influence on levels of social cohesion—the causal effect of social capital can be obtained by comparing the difference in health status of individuals who reside within high- versus low-cohesion neighborhoods induced by the fact that they "happen" to be living in areas with high or low immigrant concentration.[5] Although clearly not a panacea for solving the thorny issues of causal inference, instruments represent a hitherto underutilized approach (at least within the field of social capital and health) for squeezing more out of observational data without going to the extent of launching a randomized controlled trial.

A more direct approach to utilize natural experiments would be to observe real-life scenarios such as the evacuation and resettlement of residents into different neighborhoods following a natural disaster—such as Hurricane Katrina—or to examine changes in the health status of residents who happen to live near a newly opened community center where people can congregate. Taking advantage of such scenarios relies upon serendipity, foresight (i.e., the measurement of the health of residents both at baseline as well as following the natural experiment), or both. In the example of Hurricane Katrina, the opportunity to study the natural experiment (residents from the same neighborhoods in New Orleans being relocated to neighborhoods with different levels of social capital) was unfortunately lost because the Federal Emergency Management Agency failed to keep records of the addresses to which people

were evacuated. In the example of the opening of a new community center, the natural experiment would not work if the decision to locate the center in a particular neighborhood was influenced by lobbying by the residents, or if residents deliberately moved into the neighborhood to be closer to the new facility. These caveats notwithstanding, it seems likely that such natural experiments are being repeated on a regular basis throughout the social world, and causal inference would be strengthened by taking advantage of them.

The gold standard of causal inference is to directly manipulate the treatment—either through cluster-randomized community trials (e.g., opening senior centers in one set of randomly selected communities, and rolling out the same intervention at a later time in a control set of communities), or by randomizing residents to move into different communities, such as happened in HUD's Moving to Opportunity (MTO) Demonstration Project (Lieberman, Katz, and Kling 2004).

A separate set of challenges to causal inference is posed by studies in which individual-level measures of social capital (such as perceptions about the trustworthiness of neighbors, or the perceived availability of resources within one's network) are linked to self-reported health outcomes, such as mental health. Two kinds of biases are possible: (a) common method bias, where unmeasured individual characteristics such as negative affectivity may influence individuals' ratings of social capital as well as their reported health status; and (b) confounding by omitted variables such as early life circumstances or genetic factors, which may predispose an individual to being hostile, mistrusting, and unhealthy. That is, variations in individual characteristics such as attachment styles, sociable personality, and trusting attitudes are likely to be shaped by early family experiences. In the absence of data that permit the investigator to control for these characteristics, studies among twins can help to mitigate these concerns. Not only do twins share genetic and perinatal factors, but also often their family environment during childhood. In the twin fixed-effects design, the investigator is able to examine health differences between twin pairs who are discordant with respect to their reported perceptions of social capital, thereby canceling the potential confounding influences of the unmeasured genetic and personality traits, as well as shared early life circumstances.

In an analysis of 944 adult twin pairs (37 percent monozygotic and 63 percent dizygotic) enrolled in the National Survey of Midlife Development in the U.S., Fujiwara and Kawachi (2008) examined the associations between individual-level perceptions of social capital (trust of neighbors and neighborhood cohesion) and self-reported behavioral indicators of community participation and voluntarism, in relation to a set of health outcomes that included perceived physical and mental health, depressive symptoms, and physician-diagnosed major depression. When the analyses were carried out ignoring the discordant twin design, each indicator of social capital was significantly associated with health outcomes in the expected direction (e.g., more community participation = lower risk of major depression). However, when the analyses were repeated using the twin fixed-effects design, most of the associations became statistically nonsignificant. Only the association between trust of neighbors remained strongly associated with perceived physical health among both monozygotic and dizygotic twins. Notably, no associations remained between any of the measures of social capital and the diagnosis of major depression.

In summary, much work remains to be carried out in shoring up the empirical evidence base linking social capital to health outcomes. There is a need to improve the measurement of social capital by applying reliable and valid survey instruments, or by attempting whole network–based approaches. Panel data, objective assessment of health status, and multilevel analysis are good starting points for methodological rigor, but in addition, research needs to strengthen causal inference by incorporating more rigorous study designs and analytical methods, such as propensity score matching, instrumental variable approaches, and the use of natural experiments (Subramanian, Glymour, and Kawachi 2007).

Policy Implications of Social Capital for Health Promotion

Critics of social capital have voiced skepticism about the utility of applying the concept as a health promotion strategy (Pearce and Davey Smith 2003). They point out that: (a) social capital is an unwarranted distraction from more pressing policy agendas such as the elimination of poverty;[6] (b) attributing the poor health status of disadvantaged communities to the lack of social capital only serves to blame the victims for their unfortunate predicament (Muntaner, Lynch, and Davey Smith 2001); and (c) even if interventions could be mounted to successfully build social capital, the results might be counterproductive to health because of the unintended side effects of social cohesion, which tend to be ignored or downplayed by overenthusiastic advocates.

These are all cogent arguments that dictate caution in how social capital should be exported and adapted to the population health realm. As Szreter and Woolcock (2004) point out, the discourse on social capital in the policy realm needs to be more productively directed toward how to optimize community cohesion and network-based resources under specific circumstances to improve health, rather than focusing on mindless calls to citizens to behave more nicely toward each other. These considerations tend to rule out mass media campaigns based on generic slogans that exhort citizens to "practice random acts of kindness," as well as spraying oxytocin from overhead helicopters to promote trust among strangers.

For social capital to contribute usefully to population health improvement, two questions need to be answered: (1) Can interventions effectively build social capital? and (2) If we strengthen social capital, will health improve? Regarding the first question, suggestions abound but demonstrations remain sparse. The political scientist Robert Putnam (2000), who has been more effective than any other academic in popularizing the concept of social capital, suggests several directions for such efforts, including expanding funding for community service programs, providing incentives to private sector employers to introduce flexible work arrangements that facilitate employees to invest in the social capital of their families and communities, and incorporating Social Capital Impact Assessments (modeled after Health Impact Assessments) to forecast the consequences of social policies for levels of social capital within society. While each of these prescriptions has the merit of plausibility, they remain somewhat generic and several steps removed from influencing the health outcomes of individuals.

A more concrete demonstration of building social capital is provided by the Experience Corps, originally piloted as a randomized trial in Baltimore, Maryland, but subsequently scaled up across communities in the United States (Glass et al. 2004; Fried et al. 2004). The program places older volunteers in public elementary schools in roles designed to meet the schools' needs and to increase the social, physical, and cognitive activity of the volunteers. In other words, the program builds intergenerational social capital, and it has been described as providing a win/win outcome for the seniors whose functional abilities are improved through social engagement, physical activity, and cognitive stimulation, as well as for the pupils (who are primarily in resource-scarce public school settings) for whom academic performance is improved.

Additional grassroots-based ideas for boosting community social capital have been suggested by advocacy groups such as the Saguaro Seminar of the Kennedy School of Government at Harvard University (Sander and Lowney 2005). The Saguaro Seminar advocates making a series of so-called smart bets based upon established principles of community organizing, such as encouraging the formation of neighborhood associations. However, it remains to be proven through rigorous evaluation whether organizing neighborhood associations, book clubs, or carpooling (all examples cited in the Seminar's "Toolkit") can boost social capital in a sustainable manner. More importantly, before rushing off to organize a block party, it is critical to reflect that it is not only the overall level of social capital that matters, but also the *type* of social capital that matters for different purposes. For example, widely scattered weak ties are more effective at disseminating information, whereas strong and dense connections are more effective for collective action (Chwe 1999). As Sobel (2002, 151) cautions: "People apply the notion of social capital to both types of situation. Knowing what types of networks are best for generating social capital requires that one be specific about what the social capital is going to be used to do." For example, it would not be

sufficient (and possibly counterproductive) to encourage reciprocity between residents of a highly disadvantaged community. Residents of disadvantaged communities are often already maxed out on assisting each other as a survival strategy, and launching a campaign to encourage stronger bonding ties within such a setting might only add to that strain. The type of social capital called for in such a situation would be of the bridging kind, which connects disadvantaged residents with credit counselors, employment agencies, or loan officers.

As the foregoing example illustrates, there is a critical distinction to be drawn between so-called bonding social capital and bridging social capital (Gittell and Vidal 1998; Szreter and Woolcock 2004; Kawachi 2006). Bonding capital refers to resources that are accessed within social groups whose members are alike (homophilous) in terms of their social identity, such as class or race. By contrast, bridging capital refers to the resources accessed by individuals and groups through connections that cross class, race/ethnicity, and other boundaries of social identity. Although few empirical studies to date have gone to the trouble of distinguishing between these two types of capital, growing evidence suggests that a deeper understanding of the consequences of each form of capital may prove to be helpful in avoiding some of the downsides of social cohesion. Hence, bonding capital represents part of the day-to-day survival strategy for residents of disadvantaged communities. As documented in Carol Stack's (1974) ethnographic study of a poor African American community, the mutual exchange of resources through kinship networks is the primary mechanism for getting by in such communities. At the same time, bonding capital extracts a cost from the network members in the mental and financial strain associated with providing support for others in need. Consistent with this notion, Mitchell and LaGory (2002) found that in a small study of a disadvantaged minority community in Birmingham, Alabama, high levels of bonding social capital (measured by the strength of trust and associational ties with others of a similar racial and educational background as the respondent) were paradoxically associated with higher levels of mental distress. By contrast, individuals in the same study who reported access to high levels of bridging social capital (ties to others who were unlike them with respect to race and class) were less likely to experience mental distress.

Yet another instance of the importance of distinguishing between bonding and bridging social capital is illustrated by Ashutosh Varshney's (2002) study of sectarian violence across cities of India. According to Varshney, cities in India are characterized by marked variations in the outbreak of violence between Hindus and Muslims, even though they superficially resemble each other in terms of ethnic makeup. The difference between peaceful and violence-wracked localities, according to Varshney, can be attributed to the presence of bridging social capital in the former. In cities that are able to maintain the peace, bridging capital takes the form of integrated civic organizations—business groups, trade unions, and even reading circles based in local libraries—that include both Muslims and Hindus among their members. Such organizations, Varshney maintains, have proved extremely effective both at preventing the outbreak of violence by maintaining channels of communication across ethnic groups, and at quelling rumors that troublemakers often initiate within a community to incite riots.

Distinguishing between bonding and bridging forms of social capital may thus assist in answering the second question posed at the beginning of this section: If you build social capital, will it improve health? Social capital, like any form of capital (e.g., financial capital), can be deployed for both good ends and bad ends, and bonding capital may be particularly susceptible to both uses. For example, in India, belonging to the local branch of the Bharatiya Janata Party promotes a member's sense of Hindu nationalism, while belonging to the Muslim League promotes the sense of Muslim nationalism. Both are forms of bonding capital. A generic, one-size-fits-all prescription to boost social capital by encouraging membership in local organizations may not end up promoting the greater good if it simply drives people to join these highly bonding but divisive manifestations of social cohesion.

Social capital has been an active topic of research throughout the social sciences for some time, including in mainstream sociology, economics, and political science. Population health is a relative newcomer to the field, with the first study linking social capital to health outcomes appearing circa 1997 (Kawachi et al. 1997). Social capital serves to remind us that population health is determined by more than access to health care, genetics, lifestyles, money, and schooling. The social world also matters a great deal, and our ties to family, friends, coworkers, and neighbors constitute a credit bank—a form of capital—that we can rely upon to promote health. And even though much work remains to be carried out in filling in both the theories and empirical evidence linking social capital to population health outcomes, few would deny the intuitive appeal of the concept in bringing together diverse fields of inquiry in medical sociology, including studies of social relationships and networks, social stratification, and health disparities, as well as neighborhood and other contextual influences on health.

Notes

1. According to Moore et al. (2005), the public health literature on social capital has tended to exhibit an uncritical acceptance of the definition offered by the political scientist Robert Putnam (1993, 2000), who defined social capital as "the features of social organization, such as trust, norms, and networks, that can improve the efficiency of society by facilitating coordinated actions" (Putnam 1993, 167). Interestingly, Putnam himself cites his source as Coleman, not Bourdieu.

2. By contrast, smoking prevalence among Japanese males jumps to over 30 percent as soon as they reach the legal age. Indeed, twenty years ago, it was not uncommon for free cigarettes to be distributed at local town halls across the nation on Adults' Day, where fresh batches of twenty-year-olds were formally inducted into adulthood by local functionaries.

3. Okinawa was—at least until comparatively recently—renowned as the prefecture with the highest average life expectancy in Japan, a nation with notably high longevity. According to the researchers of the Okinawa Centenarian Study, a major key to the islanders' longevity is their diet, followed by their close family ties (Wilcox, Wilcox, and Suzuki 2001). A social epidemiologist would switch the order of the emphasis on these factors. A similar literary example of community mutual

aid can be found in Flora Thompson's *Lark Rise to Candleford* (1939, 2000), about a rural Oxfordshire village in early twentieth-century England.

4. On the other hand, if the proposed instruments are, in fact, associated with the outcomes of interest, they will fail. For instance, income polarization has been proposed as an independent determinant of health, although the hypothesis is controversial (Subramanian and Kawachi, 2004). However, in empirical studies, income inequality is more consistently associated with health outcomes at larger levels of spatial aggregation such as states, and much less at lower levels of aggregation such as neighborhoods. If this is true, income polarization may still serve as an instrument for studies of social cohesion at the neighborhood level. One of the downsides of the IV approach is that the validity of the instrument is often untestable and must rest on prior knowledge and theory.

5. In regression, this is accomplished by a two-stage least squares procedure.

6. The apparent cooption of social capital by third-way politicians as a cheap way to solve the problems of poverty is often cited as an instance of distracting the gullible public (Fine 2001; Muntaner, Lynch, and Davey Smith 2001; Navarro 2002).

References

Alesina, A., A. Devleeschauwer, W. Easterly, S. Kurlat, and R. Wacziarg. 2003. "Fractionalization." *Journal of Economic Growth* 8:155–94.

Almedom, Astier M., and Douglas Glandon. 2008. "Social Capital and Mental Health: An Updated Interdisciplinary Review of Primary Evidence." In *Social Capital and Health*, ed. Ichiro Kawachi, S. V. Subramanian, and Daniel Kim, 191–244. New York: Springer.

Anderson, Lisa R., Jennifer M. Mellor, and Jeffrey Milyo. 2004. "Social Capital and Contributions in a Public Goods Experiment." *American Economic Review Papers and Proceedings* 94(2): 373–76.

Anderson, Lisa R., and Jennifer M. Mellor. 2008. "The Economic Approach to Cooperation and Trust: Lessons for the Study of Social Capital and Health." In *Social Capital and Health*, ed. Ichiro Kawachi, S. V. Subraminian, and Daniel Kim, 117–36. New York: Springer.

Berkman, Lisa F., and Thomas Glass. 2000. "Social Integration, Social Networks, Social Support, and Health." In *Social Epidemiology*, ed. Lisa F. Berkman and Ichiro Kawachi, 137–73. New York: Oxford University Press.

Bourdieu, Pierre. 1986. "The Forms of Capital." In *The Handbook of Theory: Research for the Sociology of Education*, ed. J. G. Richardson, 241–58. New York: Greenwood Press.

Carpiano, Richard M. 2008. "Actual or Potential Neighborhood Resources for Health: What Can Bourdieu Offer for Understanding Mechanisms Linking Social Capital to Health?" In *Social Capital and Health*, ed. Ichiro Kawachi, S. V. Subramanian, and Daniel Kim, 83–93. New York: Springer.

Chwe, M. S. 1999. "Structure and Strategy in Collective Action." *American Journal of Sociology* 105:128–56.

Coleman, James S. 1990. *Foundations of Social Theory.* Cambridge, Mass.: Harvard University Press.

De Silva, Mary. 2006. "A Systematic Review of the Methods Used in Studies of Social Capital and Mental Health." In *Social Capital and Mental Health*, ed. Kwame McKenzie and Trudy Harpham, 39–67. London: Jessica Kingsley.

Ellaway, Anne, and Sally Macintyre. 2007. "Is Social Participation Associated with Cardiovascular Disease Risk Factors?" *Social Science and Medicine* 64(7): 1384–91.

Fine, Ben. 2001. *Social Capital versus Social Theory: Political Economy and Social Science at the Turn of the Millennium.* London: Routledge.

Fried, L. P., M. C. Carlson, M. Freedman, K. D. Frick, T. A. Glass, J. Hill, S. McGill, G. W. Rebok, T. S. Seeman, J. Tielsch, B. A. Wasik, and S. Zeger. 2004. "A Social Model for Health Promotion for an Aging Population: Initial Evidence on the Experience Corps Model." *Journal of Urban Health* 81(1): 64–78.

Fujiwara, Takeo, and Ichiro Kawachi. 2008. "Social Capital and Health: A Study of Adult Twins in the U.S." *American Journal of Preventive Medicine* 35(2): 139–44.

Gittell, Ross J., and Avis Vidal. 1998. *Community Organizing: Building Social Capital as a Development Strategy.* Thousand Oaks, Calif.: Sage.

Gladwell, Malcolm. 2000. *The Tipping Point.* Boston: Little, Brown.

Glaeser, E. L., D. I. Laibson, J. A. Scheinkman, and C. L. Soutter. 2000. "Measuring Trust." *Quarterly Journal of Economics* 115(3): 811–46.

Glass, T. A., M. Carlson, M. Freedman, et al. 2004. "Experience Corps: Design of an Intergenerational Health Promotion Program to Boost Social Capital." *Journal of Urban Health* 81(1): 79–93.

Glymour, Maria M. 2006. "Natural Experiments and Instrumental Variable Analyses in Social Epidemiology." In *Methods in Social Epidemiology*, ed. J. Michael Oakes and Jay S. Kaufman, 429–60. San Francisco: Jossey-Bass.

Granovetter, Mark S. 1973. "The Strength of Weak Ties." *American Journal of Sociology* 78(6): 1360–80.

Harpham, Trudy. 2008. "The Measurement of Community Social Capital through Surveys." In

Social Capital and Health, ed. Ichiro Kawachi, S. V. Subramanian, and Daniel Kim, 51–62. New York: Springer.

Islam, M. K., J. Merlo, I. Kawachi, M. Lindstrom, K. Burstrom, and U-G. Gerdtham. 2006a. "Does it Really Matter Where You Live? A Panel Data Multilevel Analysis of Swedish Municipality-Level Social Capital on Individual Health-Related Quality of Life." Health Economics, Policy and Law 1 (Pt 3): 209–35.

Islam, M. K., J. Merlo, I. Kawachi, M. Lindstrom, and U-G. Gerdtham. 2006b. "Social Capital and Health: Does Egalitarianism Matter? A Literature Review." International Journal of Equity in Health 5(1): 3.

Kawachi, I. 2006. "Commentary: Social Capital and Health—Making the Connections One Step at a Time." International Journal of Epidemiology 35(4): 989–93.

Kawachi, I., and L. F. Berkman. 2000. "Social Cohesion, Social Capital, and Health." In Social Epidemiology, ed. Lisa F. Berkman and Ichiro Kawachi, 174–90. New York: Oxford University Press.

———, eds. 2003. Neighborhoods and Health. New York: Oxford University Press.

Kawachi, I., B. P. Kennedy, K. Lochner, and D. Prothrow-Stith. 1997. "Social Capital, Income Inequality, and Mortality." American Journal of Public Health 87:1491–98.

Kawachi, I., D. J. Kim, A. Coutts, and S. V. Subramanian. 2004. "Reconciling the Three Accounts of Social Capital." International Journal of Epidemiology 33(4): 682–90.

Kawachi, I., S. V. Subramanian, and D. Kim, eds. 2008. Social Capital and Health. New York: Springer.

Kim, Daniel, S. V. Subramanian, and Ichiro Kawachi. 2008. "Social Capital and Physical Health: A Systematic Review of the Literature." In Social Capital and Health, ed. Ichiro Kawachi, S. V. Subramanian, and Daniel Kim, 139–90. New York: Springer.

Kouvonen, A., M. Kivimäki, J. Vahtera, et al. 2006. "Psychometric Evaluation of a Short Measure of Social Capital at Work." BMC Public Health 6:251.

Kouvonen, A., T. Oksanen, J. Vahtera, M. Stafford, R. Wilkinson, J. Schneider, A. Väänänen, M. Virtanen, S. J. Cox, J. Pentti, M. Elovainio, and M. Kivimäki. 2008. "Low Workplace Social Capital as a Predictor of Depression: The Finnish Public Sector Study." American Journal of Epidemiology 167(10): 1143–51.

Lakon, Cynthia M., Dionne C. Godette, and John R. Hipp. 2008. "Network-Based Approaches for Measuring Social Capital." In Social Capital and Health, ed. Ichiro Kawachi. S. V. Subramanian, and Daniel Kim, 63–81. New York: Springer.

Lieberman, Jeffrey B., Lawrence F. Katz, and Jeffrey R.

Kling. 2004. Beyond Treatment Effects: Estimating the Relationship between Neighborhood Poverty and Individual Outcomes in the MTO Experiment. Princeton, N.J.: Princeton Industrial Relations Section.

Lin, Nan. 2001. Social Capital: Theory and Research. New York: Aldine de Gruyter.

Lindstrom, Martin. 2008a. "Invited Commentary: Social Capital, Social Contexts, and Depression." American Journal of Epidemiology 167(10): 1152–54.

———. 2008b. "Social Capital and Health-Related Behaviors." In Social Capital and Health, ed. Ichiro Kawachi, S. V. Subramanian, and Daniel Kim, 215–38. New York: Springer.

Lochner, K., I. Kawachi, R. T. Brennan, and S. L. Buka. 2003. "Social Capital and Neighborhood Mortality Rates in Chicago." Social Science and Medicine 56(8): 1797–1805.

Lynch, J. W., G. Davey Smith, M. M. Hillemeier, M. Shaw, T. Raghunathan, and G. A. Kaplan. 2001. "Income Inequality, the Psychosocial Environment, and Health: Comparisons of Wealthy Nations." Lancet 358:194–200.

Mitchell, C. U., and M. LaGory. 2002. "Social Capital and Mental Distress in an Impoverished Community." City and Community 1:195–215.

Moore, S., A. Shiell, P. Hawe, and V. A. Haines. 2005. "The Privileging of Communitarian Ideas: Citation Practices and the Translation of Social Capital into Public Health Research." American Journal of Public Health 95:1330–37.

Muntaner, C., J. Lynch, and G. Davey Smith. 2001. "Social Capital, Disorganized Communities, and the Third Way: Understanding the Retreat from Structural Inequalities in Epidemiology and Public Health." International Journal of Health Services 31(2): 213–37.

Navarro, V. 2002. "A Critique of Social Capital." International Journal of Health Services 32(3): 423–43.

———. 2004. "Commentary: Is Capital the Solution or the Problem?" International Journal of Epidemiology 33:672–74.

Oakes, J. M. 2004. "The (Mis)estimation of Neighborhood Effects: Causal Inference for a Practicable Social Epidemiology." Social Science and Medicine 58:1929–52.

Okuda, Hideo. 2005. Southbound (in Japanese). Tokyo: Kadokawa.

Pearce, N., and G. Davey Smith. 2003. "Is Social Capital the Key to Inequalities in Health?" American Journal of Public Health 93(1): 122–29.

Portes, Alejandro. 1998. "Social Capital: Its Origins and Application in Modern Sociology." Annual Reviews of Sociology 24:1–24.

Putnam, Robert D. 1993. *Making Democracy Work: Civic Traditions in Modern Italy.* Princeton, N.J.: Princeton University Press.

———. 2000. *Bowling Alone: The Collapse and Revival of American Community.* New York: Simon and Schuster.

Rostila, Mikael. 2007. "Social Capital and Health in the Swedish Welfare State." In *Health Inequalities and Welfare Resources: Continuity and Change in Sweden,* ed. Johan Fritzell and Olle Lundberg, 157–77. Bristol: Policy Press.

Sampson, R. J., S. W. Raudenbush, and F. Earls. 1997. "Neighborhoods and Violent Crime: A Multilevel Study of Collective Efficacy." *Science* 277:918–24.

Sander, Thomas H., and Kathleen Lowney. 2005. "Social Capital Building Toolkit, Version 1.1." Cambridge, Mass.: Harvard University John F. Kennedy School of Government. ksg.harvard.edu/saguaro/pdfs/skbuildingtoolkitversion1.1.pdf.

Sobel, J. 2002. "Can We Trust Social Capital?" *Journal of Economic Literature* 40:139–54.

Stack, Carol B. 1974. *All Our Kin: Strategies for Survival in a Black Community.* New York: Harper and Row.

Subramanian, S. V., Maria M. Glymour, and Ichiro Kawachi. 2007. "Identifying Causal Ecological Effects on Health: A Methodological Assessment." In *Macrosocial Determinants of Population Health,* ed. Sandro Galea, 301–31. New York: Springer.

Subramanian, S. V., Kelvyn Jones, and Craig Duncan. 2003. "Multilevel Methods for Public Health Research." In *Neighborhoods and Health,* ed. Ichiro Kawachi and Lisa F. Berkman, 65–111. New York: Oxford University Press.

Subramanian, S. V., and I. Kawachi. 2004. "Income Inequality and Health: What Have We Learned So Far." *Epidemiologic Reviews* 26:78–91.

Subramanian, S. V., D. J. Kim, and I. Kawachi. 2002. "Social Trust and Self-Rated Health in U.S. Communities: Multilevel Analysis." *Journal of Urban Health* 79(4), Suppl. 1: S21–34.

Szreter, S., and M. Woolcock. 2004. "Health by Association? Social Capital, Social Theory, and the Political Economy of Public Health." *International Journal of Epidemiology* 33(4): 650–67.

Thompson, Flora. 1939 (2000). *Lark Rise to Candleford.* London: Penguin Modern Classics.

Valente, T. W., P. Gallaher, and P. Mouttapa. 2004. "Using Social Networks to Understand and Prevent Substance Use: A Transdisciplinary Perspective." *Substance Use and Misuse* 39:1685–1712.

Van der Gaag, M., and T. A. B. Snijders. 2005. "The Resource Generator: Measurement of Individual Social Capital with Concrete Items." *Social Networks* 27:1–29.

Van der Gaag, M., and M. Webber. 2008. "Measurement of Individual Social Capital. Questions, Instruments, and Measures." In *Social Capital and Health,* ed. Ichiro Kawachi, S. V. Subramanian, and Daniel Kim, 29–49. New York: Springer.

Varshney, Ashutosh. 2002. *Ethnic Conflict and Civic Life: Hindus and Muslims in India.* New Haven, Conn.: Yale University Press.

Webber, M. P., and P. J. Huxley. 2007. "Measuring Access to Social Capital: The Validity and Reliability of the Resource Generator-UK and Its Association with Common Mental Disorder." *Social Science and Medicine.* 65(3): 481–92.

Whitley, Rob. 2008. "Social Capital and Health: Qualitative and Ethnographic Approaches." In *Social Capital and Health,* ed. Ichiro Kawachi, S. V. Subramanian, and Daniel Kim, 95–115. New York: Springer.

Wilcox, Bradley J., Craig D. Wilcox, and Makoto Suzuki. 2001. *The Okinawa Program: How the World's Longest-Lived People Achieve Everlasting Health—and How You Can Too.* New York: Clarkson Potter.

Zimmerman, F. J. 2008. "A Commentary on 'Neo-materialist Theory and the Temporal Relationship between Income Inequality and Longevity Change.'" *Social Science and Medicine* 66:1882–94.

3

Why Education Is the Key to Socioeconomic Differentials in Health

Catherine E. Ross, University of Texas

John Mirowsky, University of Texas

People with higher socioeconomic status have better health than lower-status individuals, and inequalities in health grow with age. Education creates most of the association between higher socioeconomic status and better health because education is a root cause of good health. A great deal of evidence suggests that educational attainment leads to better health. Education increases physical functioning and subjective health among adults of all ages and decreases the age-specific rates of morbidity, disability, and mortality.[1] The question is, Why?

The mediators include: (1) work and economic conditions, such as employment status, creative and autonomous work, and income and economic hardship; (2) social psychological resources, including the sense of personal control and social support; and (3) health lifestyle, including patterns of smoking, exercising, walking, drinking, weight, and use of medical services. We contrast two theories that attempt to explain why education improves health: education as human capital and learned effectiveness, and education as a commodity. These theories are not mutually exclusive but emphasize different primary links between education and health. Theories of learned effectiveness posit that education improves health apart from the economic resources it brings; they focus on creative work, sense of personal control, and health lifestyle as mediators. Commodity

theories focus on household income and access to medical care and health insurance as primary mediators. The debate about mediators contrasts learned effectiveness theories, which focus on human capital, with commodity theories, which focus on income and the things it can buy (Lynch 2006; Pampel and Rogers 2004; Reynolds and Ross 1998; Schnittker 2004).

Pathways Linking Education to Health

How does education foster health? The concept of human capital implies that education improves health because it increases effective agency on the part of individuals, that is, education develops habits, skills, resources, and abilities that enable people to achieve a better life (Mirowsky and Ross 1998, 2003; Sen 1997, 1999). To the extent that people want health, education develops the means toward creating that end through a lifestyle that promotes health. Thus health is not just a lucky but unintended consequence of the prosperity that is contingent on education. Human capital theory posits an effect of education on health over and above the good jobs that pay well and provide health insurance and the other economic benefits that stem from education. It describes a causal model which posits that education enables people to coalesce health-producing behaviors into a coherent lifestyle, and that a sense of control over outcomes in one's own life encourages a healthy lifestyle and conveys much of education's effect in part because education boosts the sense of personal control directly and in part indirectly by providing access to creative and autonomous work.

Commodity theories focus on material assets. Education is a credential that employers use in allocating good jobs (Ross and Mirowsky 1999). Degrees, especially college degrees, are markers that employers use to hire. Without a college degree, it is difficult to get a job that pays well. Commodity theories focus on earnings, income, wealth, and health insurance. Education helps a person buy the things that maintain health. Commodity theories and human capital theories are not mutually exclusive, but their primary pathways between education and health differ. Like the human capital theory, the commodity theory of education and health is causal—in contrast to selection or spurious models of education and health, which posit that education does not have a causal effect on health but is simply a marker for socioeconomically advantaged family background.

Most research suggests that the positive association between educational attainment and health is largely due to the effects of education on health, not vice versa (Doornbos and Kromhout 1990; Wilkinson 1986), despite the suggestion of some economists that the association is spurious. Although genetic traits like IQ lead to higher levels of education and to better health, stringent tests of unmeasured spuriousness still find effects of education on health and mortality (Lleras-Muney 2005).

More realistic life-course analyses posit paths in both directions: early childhood conditions, social and genetic, predispose people to better health and higher levels of education, and better childhood health leads to more education (Haas and Fosse 2008). In turn, higher levels of education improve adult health, independent of childhood traits, and also link some of the effect of childhood conditions to adult health (Best, Hayward, and Hidajat 2005; Elo and Preston 1992; Hayward and Gorman 2004; Mirowsky and Ross 1998).

Conditions Moderating Education's Effect on Health

Current debate concerning moderators focuses on issues relating to cumulative advantage and disadvantage over the life course and to other disadvantaged social statuses such as female gender and low income.

Learned Effectiveness as a Mediator

Formal education represents an investment in human capital—the productive capacity developed, embodied, and stocked in human beings themselves. According to theory, formal education develops skills and abilities of general value rather than firm-specific ones of value to a particular employer (Becker 1964; Schultz 1962). On the most general level, education teaches people to learn. It develops the ability to write, communicate, solve problems, analyze data, develop ideas, and implement plans. It develops broadly useful analytic skills such as mathematics, logic, and, on a more basic level, observing, experimenting, summarizing, synthesizing, interpreting, classifying, and so on. In school one encounters and solves problems that are progressively more difficult, complex, and subtle. The more years of schooling, the greater the cognitive development, characterized by flexible, rational, complex strategies of thinking. Higher education teaches people to think logically and rationally, see many sides of an issue, and analyze problems and solve them. Education also develops broadly effective habits and attitudes such as dependability, judgment, motivation, effort, trust, and confidence, as well as skills and abilities. In particular the process of learning creates confidence in the ability to solve problems. Education instills the habit of meeting problems with attention, thought, action, and perseverance. Thus education increases effort, which like ability is a fundamental component of problem solving. Apart from the value of the skills and abilities learned in school, the process of learning builds the confidence, motivation, and self-assurance needed to *attempt* to solve problems. Because education develops competence on many levels, it gives people the ability and motivation to shape and control their lives (Hyman and Wright 1979; Kingston et al. 2003; Pascarella and Terenzini 1991; Mirowsky and Ross 1989, 2003; Wheaton 1980).

Sociologists studying social differences in health (Mirowsky and Ross 1998, 2003, 2005; Ross and Mirowsky 1999) and economists studying international development (Sen 1997, 1999) emphasize the importance of education to health and well-being within nations and among them. Both groups argue for a second and broader revival of the concept of human capital. Sen calls the broader view of human capital "human capability," while Mirowsky and Ross call it "learned effectiveness." This theory suggests that education shapes a sense of personal control that encourages a healthy lifestyle and conveys much of education's effect.

HEALTHY LIFESTYLE

The human capital theory of learned effectiveness suggests that educated, instrumental people merge otherwise unrelated habits and ways into a healthy lifestyle that consequently behaves as a coherent trait. In theory, education makes individuals more effective users of information. Education encourages individuals to acquire information with intent to use it. Thus the more educated may assemble a set of habits and ways that are not necessarily related except as effective means toward health.

Purposeful individuals may coalesce a healthy lifestyle from otherwise incoherent or diametric practices allocated by subcultural forces. Individuals tend to do whatever others like them do, particularly if it distinguishes the people they identify with from the ones they do not. Some of those things make health better and some make it worse. For example, men exercise more frequently than women; women restrict body weight more closely than men; young adults smoke more than older adults but also exercise more (Hayes and Ross 1986; Ross and Bird 1994; Ross and Wu 1995). Individuals putting together a healthy lifestyle must adopt the healthy habits of men and women, young and old. In doing so they create positive correlations among traits that otherwise might be uncorrelated or even negatively correlated.

Evidence supports the ideas that education encourages healthy behaviors and pulls together the healthy elements from the lifestyles of various subpopulations. Compared to those with little schooling, the well educated are more likely to exercise, more likely to walk, more likely to drink moderately rather than abstain or drink heavily, and less likely to smoke or be overweight (Mirowsky and Ross 1998, 2003, 2005; Ross and Bird 1994; Ross and Wu 1995). Interestingly, the healthy behaviors associated with higher education show little consistent relationship to other sociodemographic traits. Only education correlates positively and consistently with healthy behaviors. In turn, each aspect of lifestyle has significant independent effects on health, adjusting for the other indicators and all other sociodemographic variables. Smoking and being overweight significantly worsen health; moderate drinking, walking, and exercising significantly improve health (Mirowsky and Ross 1998; Ross and Wu 1995).

SENSE OF PERSONAL CONTROL

The better educated may enjoy better health in part because education increases the agency and personal control that motivates people to design a healthy lifestyle. The theory of learned effectiveness converges with the theory of personal control in many ways. Through formal education people learn to solve problems and to be active and effective agents in their lives (Mirowsky and Ross 1989, 2007b; Wheaton 1980). People who feel in control of their lives seek information by which to guide their lives and improve their outcomes. Logically, then, people who feel in control of their lives tend to adopt a lifestyle that produces health. By developing personal control and effectiveness, education develops individuals who seek and discover a healthy lifestyle.

The sense of personal control therefore may form an important link between education and health. Belief in personal control is a learned expectation that outcomes depend on one's choices and actions (Mirowsky and Ross 1991, 1998, 2003). The individual believes that he or she can master, control, or effectively alter the environment. On the other end of the continuum, a perceived lack of control is the learned expectation that one's actions do not affect outcomes. Concepts related to perceived control appear in the scientific literature in a number of related forms under various names, including mastery (Pearlin et al. 1981), instrumentalism (Wheaton 1980), personal efficacy or self-efficacy (Gecas 1989), personal autonomy (Seeman and Seeman 1983), internal locus of control (Rotter 1966); and, related to perceived lack of control, fatalism (Wheaton 1980), powerlessness (Seeman 1983), perceived helplessness (Elder and Liker 1982; Rodin 1986), and external locus of control (Rotter 1966).

Beliefs about personal control generally represent realistic perceptions of objective conditions (Mirowsky and Ross 2003). High levels of education increase the sense of personal control (Pearlin et al. 1981; Ross and Mirowsky 1992; Wheaton 1980). In contrast, the poorly educated may not posses the resources necessary to achieve their goals, which produces a sense of powerlessness, fatalism, and helplessness (Wheaton 1980). Education increases learned effectiveness; its absence produces learned helplessness.

A sense of personal control improves health in part by way of health-enhancing behaviors. Compared to people who feel powerless to control their lives, people with a sense of personal control know more about health, they are more likely to initiate preventive behaviors like quitting smoking, exercising, or moderating alcohol consumption and body weight, and they have better self-rated health, fewer illnesses, and lower rates of mortality (Mirowsky and Ross 1998, 2003, 2007b; Seeman and Lewis 1995; Seeman and Seeman 1983; Seeman, Seeman, and Budros 1988; Grembowski et al. 1993). These pathways are summarized in Figure 3.1.

PRODUCTIVE AND CREATIVE WORK

Work—productive activity, paid or not—also links education to health. Mirowsky and Ross (2007a) compare the health consequences of control over one's work (autonomy and creativity), control over the work of others (managerial authority), safety, and occupational attributes like prestige. Education is positively associated with autonomy, creativity, authority, prestige, and safety. Creativity, in turn, has the largest positive impact on health, followed by autonomy. Managerial authority and occupational attributes such as prestige, complexity, direction, control, and planning influence autonomy and creativity but otherwise have little or no impact on health. Although the well educated are much less likely to work at physically strenuous and dangerous jobs than those with less education, this is not a major pathway to health. Postindustrial work risks associated with monotonous and sedentary jobs probably now outweigh the work risks associated with dangerous industrial jobs (Mirowsky and Ross 2007a).

Creativity and autonomy both improve health. Creativity's impact is larger, more statistically significant, and found in follow-up models as well as cross-sectional ones. The difference in health between persons in the sixtieth and fortieth percentiles of creative work is equivalent to the former being 6.7 years younger. Creative and autonomous work boost the sense of personal control, which improves health (Bird and Ross 1993; Kohn and Schooler 1982; Ross and Wright 1998; Ross and Mirowsky 1992, 1996); creative work (as compared with tedious and repetitious work) could affect health by way of energy, fitness, and recovery; it may represent manageable challenges that ultimately improve health by way of anabolic hormones that increase muscle growth, relaxation, and energy, promote healing, and lead to quicker cortisol habituation (Epel, McEwen, and Ickovics 1998); and creative work may stimulate the prefrontal cortex (Mirowsky and Ross 2007a).

Studies of employed persons often combine measures of autonomy and creativity into a single measure of job control, which typically improves health (Cheng et al. 2000; Karasek and Theorell 1990; MacDonald et al. 2001; Wickrama et al. 1997). That can be a convenient simplification when all the respondents are employed, although it blurs the distinction between the two. When the focus broadens to include persons without paid jobs, these indexes are misleading, since paid employees have lower autonomy but higher creativity, as discussed next.

Education increases the likelihood of paid employment (Ross and Wu 1995; Ross and Van Willigen 1997). Interestingly, education benefits health in part by minimizing the trade-off between paid work and autonomous, creative

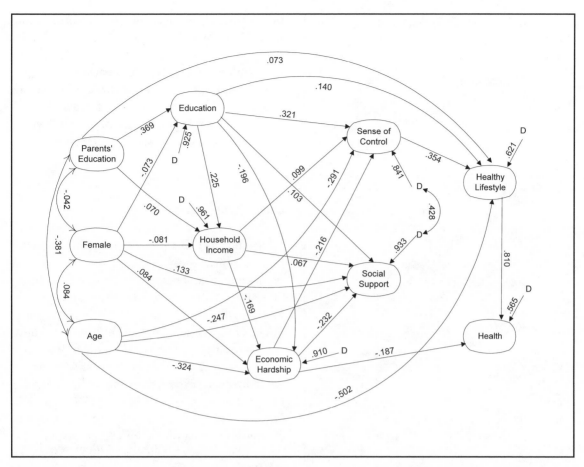

Figure 3.1. Education and health: structural model with standardized coefficients (Mirowsky and Ross 1998)

self-expression. In working for others, employees almost always trade freedom for money. Education reduces the trade-off, providing access to autonomous and creative paid work, which benefits health. Education reduces the amount of autonomy lost in employment and thus reduces any health trade-off (see Figure 3.2). The well educated are much more likely to be employed for pay than are the poorly educated, and paid work benefits health directly and indirectly through two paths. First, although paid employees report less autonomy than do people who are not employed, at high levels of education the gap in autonomy is small. Second, compared to the nonemployed, paid employees report that their work is more creative.

Creative work is a link between education and health. To explain why we consider creative work a component of learned effectiveness requires

distinguishing creative work from its theoretical source, autonomous work. Autonomy is the condition or state of being self-directed, self-governing, and not controlled by others (Mirowsky and Ross 2003). Autonomous work is free from close supervision and provides decision-making independence. Some degree of autonomy is necessary for creativity. Creative work is complex, challenging, and fulfilling (Mirowsky and Ross 2003, 2007a; Ross and Wright 1998). In creative work, people solve problems, figure things out, learn new things, use their skills in the design and production of something of value; they do lots of different things in different ways; the work is interesting, challenging, complex, nonroutine, and enjoyable. Autonomy provides the opportunity for creative work but doesn't guarantee it.

On the other end of the continuum, opportunities for creative work are limited by a lack of

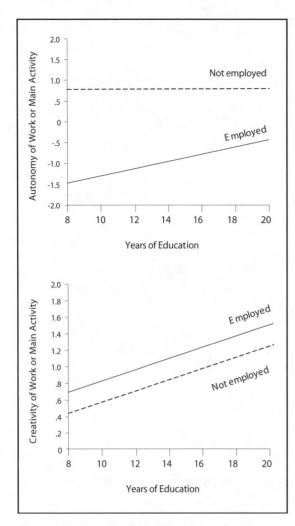

Figure 3.2. Autonomy and creativity of work or daily activity by education and employment (Mirowsky and Ross 2007)

product, being engaged in one's work, learning something new, or solving a problem is something the worker must do. Someone else can teach, give information, encourage, and provide the opportunity to learn, but the individual either learns or does not. Creative work inheres both in the person and in the opportunities made available by the circumstances and situation (Mirowsky and Ross 2007a).

Commodities as Mediators

Education may also provide economic resources that help buy health. A commodity is a material resource that can be bought and sold. The theory of learned effectiveness suggests that education improves health by enhancing effective agency. However, education might simply allocate individuals to social positions with more or less access to society's wealth. A higher education increases an individual's expected income, thus reducing the likelihood of severe economic deprivation. Poverty clearly undermines health and increases the rates of impairment, disability, disease, and death (Angell 1993; Schnittker 2004; Mirowsky and Hu 1996; Pappas et al. 1993; Rogers 1992; Rogers, Hummer, and Nam 2000: Sorlie, Backlund, and Keller 1995; Williams 1990). Indeed, poverty may be defined as lack of the means to provide for material needs (Mirowsky and Hu 1996). Effects of education on health mediated by economic well-being are consistent with a learned effectiveness theory, because high income is one consequence of the human capital acquired in school, but support for learned effectiveness theories must show independent effects of personal control and health lifestyle, while support for commodity theories must show independent effects of income and access to medical care. Thus, adjudicating among primary mediators requires distinguishing the effects of education, personal control, and health lifestyle from those of work, economic well-being, and insurance.

Some research on SES and health uses education and income as interchangeable indicators of socioeconomic status (Williams 1990). In contrast, we argue that education and income indicate different underlying concepts. School-

autonomy. If a supervisor tells workers exactly what to do and how to do it; if they must follow impersonal procedures, rules, and standards; or if their activities are governed by an assembly line, there is little room for innovation and creativity. Some degree of freedom is necessary for creativity. Oppressive work is not likely to be creative.

By our definition, creative work cannot be given to a worker in the same sense that one can award a position of authority, a safe workplace, or freedom from close supervision. What organizations, supervisors, or situations provide is the opportunity or lack of opportunity to engage in creative work; producing a useful or innovative

ing means something apart from socioeconomic status. According to the perspective of learned effectiveness, education indicates the accumulated knowledge, skills, and resources acquired in school. Income indicates economic resources available to people. Both likely affect health, but for different reasons. Further, education and income are not on the same causal level. Combining variables from different causal levels obscures processes. Part of education's effect may be mediated by economic status, but if education's sole value to health is due to economic resources then the learned effectiveness theory is not supported. To understand the processes by which socioeconomic status affects health, the effects of education and income must be distinguished from one another.

INCOME, ECONOMIC HARDSHIP, STRESS, AND HEALTH

Compared with the poorly educated, the well educated have high household incomes because they are more likely to be employed, they earn more, and they are more likely to be married. Household income, in turn, has a diminishing positive association with health, that is, the size of the improvement in health with each additional step up in level of income gets smaller and smaller (Schnittker 2004). The biggest improvements in health are on the low end, moving up from the bottom of the economic ladder to the middle. Beyond forty thousand dollars, the differences in average health with increased level of income get small, and beyond sixty thousand dollars they nearly vanish. Below the twentieth percentile, health problems decline sharply with rising levels of income, but above the twentieth percentile, additional income has little effect (Mirowsky and Hu 1996). Figure 3.3 shows the pattern for physical impairment, which is very similar to that of self-rated health and chronic conditions (Mirowsky and Ross 2003).

The shape of the relationship between income and health is an important clue about why income influences health. First, in terms of policy it suggests that a nation's overall level of health might improve more by raising income at the bottom end than by raising it across the board. Indeed, when nations are compared to others

with similar per capita gross national product, the countries with greater equality of income tend to have higher life expectancy and lower infant mortality (Evans 1994; Hertzman, Frank, and Evans 1994). Theorists suspect this happens because a smaller fraction of the population is down at the low end of income, where even modest increases would improve health substantially. Likewise, a smaller fraction is up at the high end, where even large increases in income would have little or no impact on health.

Second, in terms of theoretical explanations for income's effect on health, the shape of the relationship between income and health suggests that economic hardship drives the association. This is supported empirically, since adjustment for economic hardship renders household income's effect insignificant (Mirowsky and Ross 1998, 2003). Why does economic hardship undermine health? Material privation may be part of the answer. Privation is lack of the basic necessities of life. In wealthy countries such as the United States, few families go without the basic minimum of food, clothing, and shelter needed to stay alive and functioning (Evans, Hodge, and Pless 1994; Mayer 1997). Mostly low income limits housing options to dilapidated buildings, frequently in squalid and threatening neighborhoods, dwellings plagued by a host of problems that increase exposure to infection, injury, toxins, carcinogens, and physical stress from excessive heat or cold. The problems include infestation with insects and rodents that can carry infectious diseases, plumbing that fails to work or leaks, leaky roofs, damp basements or other interior areas growing mold and mildew, heating systems that break down or can't keep up or release allergens and dusts and hazardous gasses such as carbon monoxide, hot water that does not get hot enough to clean and disinfect well, uninviting bathtubs or showers, poor ventilation, little or no natural light, no air conditioning, no washer and dryer, no electric dishwasher, electrical wiring that is frayed or overburdened, stairs and banisters in bad repair, lights in halls and stairways that are burned out or don't work, poorly maintained or filthy stoves and ovens, disgusting refrigerators that can't keep food sufficiently cold, broken windows or doors, torn or nonexistent

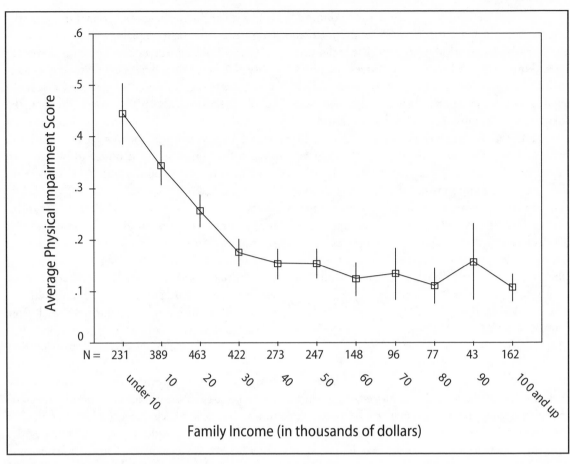

Figure 3.3. Physical impairment scores: mean and 95 percent confidence interval, by level of household income in 1994 (Mirowsky and Ross 2003)

screens, poor insulation to keep heat in and noise out, and decaying surfaces shedding paint and other chemicals. Further, dilapidated apartments and homes often are located in neighborhoods that add biophysical exposures such as heavy traffic, abandoned vehicles and buildings, sanitary sewers that leak or back up into storm sewers that back up into streets, garbage and trash left on the streets or dumped in abandoned lots, excrement, stray dogs and cats, the nests and guano of pigeons or other birds that harbor parasites, rats, or abandoned industrial facilities with old spills and dumps of hazardous chemicals or materials (Mirowsky and Ross 2003).

The litany of risky exposures that are more common in low-cost housing and poor neighborhoods paints a grim picture. The material privations and risky exposures resulting from low

income and economic hardship can get as extreme as the full list implies. Usually, though, individual households face some of the privations and risks but not most. The material wealth of the United States is so great that even households at the bottom of the economic ladder often have amenities once considered luxuries of the well to do. In her study of childhood poverty, Mayer reports the percentage of children living in homes with various design or maintenance problems and various amenities or durable goods. In households at the bottom 10 percent in terms of income, only 31.3 percent had any of the eight problems on her list: incomplete bathroom, no central heat, no electrical outlets in one or more rooms, exposed wires, holes in the floor, open cracks in the wall or ceiling, leaky roof, and signs of rats or mice. Only 14.1 percent had at least two of the problems, and only 5.8 percent had at least four of them. On the other hand, in those same households at the bottom 10 percent of income, 13.9 percent had at least two bathrooms, 16.5 percent had a dishwasher, 17.3 percent had two or more motor vehicles, 37.5 percent had a clothes dryer, 52.3 percent had air conditioning, 57.3 percent had a motor vehicle, 57.8 percent had a clothes washer, and 68.7 percent had a telephone (Mayer 1997, tables 6.2, 6.3).

Clearly, some households suffer from material privations that a wealthy society need not accept. Nevertheless, material privation probably does not account for most of the impact on health of low income and economic hardship in the United States. There are good reasons to suspect that relegation to substandard housing or a bad neighborhood may degrade health for reasons that go beyond material privation. Perhaps more to the point, economic hardship typically means something other than a leaky roof and rats in the walls. Even for the great majority of adults in their comfortable homes and decent neighborhoods, economic hardship signals inadequacy and failure, laced with a threat that one may lose what one has.

Biomedical research shows that threatening situations produce physiological responses that may impair health in several ways: by creating symptoms experienced as illness, by increasing susceptibility to pathogens and pathological conditions, and by accelerating the degradation of critical physiological systems (Fremont and Bird 2000). Perceived threats trigger a primitive, biological, fight-or-flight response. To some extent, low income and economic hardship degrade health by limiting housing options to squalid and threatening neighborhoods. Those conditions probably do arouse the fight-or-flight response frequently and intensely, as well as exposing individuals to pathogens. Nevertheless, statistical analyses suggest that they account for only about 5 to 10 percent of the effects of low income and economic hardship on health (Mirowsky and Ross 2003). Being in an economically strained household has a far greater negative correlation with health than does living in a neighborhood rife with signs of disorder and decay (the standardized coefficient for economic hardship is about 2.6 times greater than that for neighborhood social and physical disorder).

Economic hardship poses a direct threat to one's well-being and that of one's family. As a result, people exposed to economic hardship probably experience frequent, intense, and prolonged activation of the physiological stress response, with consequences for their health (Fremont and Bird 2000; Hill, Ross, and Angel 2005; Marmot and Mustard 1994). An endless and sometimes losing struggle to pay the bills and feed and clothe the family is stressful: it exacts both alarm and exhaustion. Anxious arousal alternates with depressed collapse. Gnawing worries make sleep restless and drain the joy from life. Tense, restless dread partners with listless, prostrate hopelessness. Susceptibility to disease increases when life becomes a relentless, unending struggle to get by.

INCOME, ACCESS TO FORMAL CARE, AND HEALTH

Money goes a long way toward buying relief from economic hardship, which is stressful and impairs health. What else does money buy that could improve health? Most people think that it buys access to needed medical care. Commodity theories propose that something that can be bought and sold—a commodity—must form the bridge between household income and health. However, a number of findings cast doubt on the effectiveness of medical access as a health-producing commodity that might explain the effects of income and economic hardship on health. In this section we review those findings. Money can indeed buy access to medical care, but it is questionable whether buying more access improves health (Evans 1994; Marmor, Barer, and Evans 1994). In particular, the differences in health across levels of income apparently do not result from differences in access to medical care (Ross and Mirowsky 2000).

Access to medical care and population health. Many people think that the health and longevity of modern populations are the result of increasingly sophisticated medical treatments. Given that belief, it seems to make sense that wealthier individuals are healthier than others because they obtain more treatments, particularly the newest, best, and most expensive ones. This idea builds on the premise that advances in medical treatments created the health and longevity enjoyed by modern, industrialized societies, but historical epidemiology finds that the rise of modern life expectancy cannot be attributed to the medical and surgical treatment of disease, because most of the declines in mortality rates preceded the advent of effective medical treatments for the declining causes of death (Cutler and Miller 2005; Evans 1994; McKinlay and McKinlay 1977). In the United States, most of the mortality decline may be attributed to clean water (Cutler and Miller 2005). Surprisingly few studies directly test the general proposition that consumption of medical services accounts for the better health of wealthier populations. However, the existing studies show consistent results: on the aggregate level, medical expenditures and medical resources like doctors and hospitals do not account for differences in mortality across counties or states (Kim and Moody 1992; Lee and Paxman 1997).

National health care systems and socioeconomic differences in health. Based on the belief that medical treatments create healthy populations, many countries such as Great Britain instituted national health care systems that provide universal access to treatment. Doing so reversed the social gradient in the use of services. Before the National Health Service existed, Great Britain's lower socioeconomic strata used far fewer medical services than did those in higher socioeconomic classes, but since its institution they use more. Even so, the National Health Service did not reduce the socioeconomic gradient in health and survival (Angell 1993; Evans 1994; Hollingsworth 1981; MacIntyre 1997; Marmot, Kogevinas, and Elston 1987; Morris 1990; Wagstaff, Paci, and van Doorslaer 1991). Indeed, socioeconomic status mortality differentials are stable or growing in countries with national health care systems, just as in the United States (Blaxter 1987; Diderichsen 1990; Evans 1994; Hertzman, Frank and Evans 1994; Kunst, Looman, and Mackenbach 1990; Kunst and Mackenbach 1994; Lagasse et al. 1990; Lahelma and Valkonen 1990; LaVecchia et al. 1987; Pamuk 1985, 1988; Pappas et. al. 1993; Pearce, Davis, Smith, and Foster 1985; Siskind, Copeman, and Najman 1987;

Townsend, Davidson, and Whitehead 1992). Evidence that social inequalities in health have been stable or increasing since the advent of universal access to medical care implies that the causes of socioeconomic differentials in health lie outside the medical system (Kawachi and Kennedy 1997; Wilkinson 1986, 1997).

Socioeconomic status and use of medical services. Despite the absence of universal medical coverage in the United States, the use of medical services increases as social status decreases, in large part because lower-status persons have more health problems. "Associations of good health with access to insurance and medical care lead some to believe that better health in people of high socioeconomic status is a result of more frequent interactions with the health care system and that improved access to care is the primary approach to improving the health of persons of low socioeconomic status. However, persons of low socioeconomic status currently use medical services more often than persons of high socioeconomic status" (Pincus 1998, 407)

On the surface of it, the use of preventive services seems as if it might account for some of the status differences in health. Higher socioeconomic status increases the likelihood of getting check-ups, or secondary prevention—catching and treating disease early (Ross and Wu 1995). Yet the benefits to overall health of screening, check-ups, or secondary prevention are uncertain. Yearly check-ups have little effect on health; screening often entails some risk, such as exposure to small amounts of radiation; and the risks and side effects of treatment often outweigh the benefits for low-level disease, which may get better if left untreated (Bailar 1976; Cairns 1985; Canadian Task Force on the Periodic Health Examination 1988; Kaiser Foundation Health Plan 1976; U.S. Preventive Services Task Force 1989; Deyo 1998; Deyo, Cherkin, Conrad, and Volinn 1991; Epstein 1996; Johansson et al. 1997; Roos and Roos 1994; Ross and Wu 1995; Verrilli and Welch 1996; Wennberg et al. 1996).

Clearly, differential access to medical care cannot explain the differences in health and survival across levels of socioeconomic status. Williams notes that variable quality of care might yet account for some of those differences (1990). Some evidence exists that, compared to insured patients, uninsured patients suffer higher rates of medical injuries in the hospital, are more frequently hospitalized for conditions that could have been treated on an outpatient basis, are more seriously ill upon hospitalization, and are more likely to die while hospitalized (Billings and Teicholz 1990; Burstin, Lipsitz, and Brennan 1992; Hadley, Steinberg, and Feder 1991; U.S. Congress 1992). Others find insurance unrelated to early prenatal care or outcomes following myocardial infarction (Kreindel et al. 1997; Parchment, Weiss, and Passannante 1996). The poor and poorly educated may gain least from the services they receive and suffer the most iatrogenic (doctor-caused) disease.

Private and public medical insurance and health. Thus far, indirect evidence indicates that health is not something that can be bought. People cannot buy medical services that make them and their families healthy. Some of the clearest evidence of this likelihood comes from research that examines the effect of medical insurance on health.

The substantial association between income and medical insurance coverage gives the impression that lack of coverage accounts for much of the poor health in low-income households, and that government programs soften some of that deleterious effect. Our analyses show that this cannot be true, for two reasons: private medical insurance does not improve adult health, and public insurance seems to make it worse (Ross and Mirowsky 2000). This statement may seem surprising. Most people probably assume that the beneficial effect of medical insurance on health is so great that scientists stumble across it all the time. On the contrary, surprisingly few published studies have attempted to measure the effect of medical insurance on health. Studies that compare individuals in three broad categories—those with private medical insurance provided as a benefit of current or past employment (including the spouse's) or purchased directly (including supplements to Medicare); those with public insurance from Medicaid (which goes primarily to the poor or medically indigent) or Medicare (available to seniors) with no private supplement; and no

medical insurance—all find essentially the same thing. People with private medical insurance have the best health, those with only public medical insurance have the worst, and those with no medical insurance are in-between but close to the privately insured (Hahn and Flood 1995; Rogers, Hummer, and Nam 2000; Short and Lair 1994; Sorlie et al. 1994). This pattern holds for the full range of health measures, from subjective health to mortality rates. What does it mean?

The belief that people need access to medicine is very strong. Sometimes research reports try to explain away their own findings by arguing that the benefits of public medical insurance may be obscured by traits of those who must rely on it. Notably, only the poor or very unhealthy qualify for Medicaid and typically only the poorest retirees with Medicare rely on it alone. Thus it is important to adjust for health status, sex, race, age, education, income, and so on. Possibly other selection processes bias the estimated effects of medical insurance on health. For instance, a person's health may influence whether they get medical insurance. Probably young people who feel healthy and have no impairments or chronic conditions have less motivation to buy private medical insurance or to find a job that provides it. Adjusting for factors that select people into different categories of insurance is crucial: those adjustments reduce the apparent negative effect of public insurance, *but they also reduce the apparent positive effect of private insurance.* In the end the reports typically say that perhaps more complete adjustments for background, socioeconomic status, and health-care needs would reveal a clear beneficial effect of public medical insurance on health (Rogers, Hummer, and Nam 2000).

Ross and Mirowsky's (2000) analysis of medical insurance on health provides the most thorough set of adjustments yet and eliminates selection biases in several ways. First, it relates insurance status to subsequent changes in health, which cannot influence whether a person had medical insurance at the outset, or whether the insurance was private or public. Second, it adjusts for baseline health. In essence, the model compares the effect of insurance on the subsequent changes in health of individuals with similar initial levels of subjective health, physical impairment, and chronic conditions. Thus it tests the idea that medical insurance keeps healthy people from getting unhealthy and keeps unhealthy people from getting worse. Third, it adjusts for initial demographic and economic statuses that might influence medical insurance status and might also influence the rate of deterioration in health over time for reasons unrelated to medical insurance. These include age, sex, race, education, employment, marital status, income, and economic hardship at the beginning of the period. Finally, it adjusts for changes in the household that might be influenced by initial insurance status and might produce changes in health for reasons that have little or nothing to do with the medical services provided. For example, among persons with health problems the ones with medical insurance might better avoid increases in economic hardship over time, thereby recovering faster for reasons that have nothing to do with the medical services used. The models adjust for changes in employment, marital status, household income, and economic hardship.

Our results find no differences between those with private medical insurance and those with no medical insurance in their changes in subjective health, physical impairment, and diagnosed chronic conditions over a three-year period. In other words, private medical insurance shows no sign of preserving or improving health. The better health seen among individuals with private medical insurance results entirely from their high levels of education, employment, marriage, and economic well-being that preserve and improve health directly and also increase the likelihood of having private medical insurance. Our results find a more complicated pattern for public insurance compared to no insurance. Public insurance has no effect on subsequent changes in physical impairment, but it increases the accumulation of diagnosed chronic conditions and decreases subjective health over time. The results just summarized clearly imply that lower rates of medical insurance cannot explain the high levels of health problems found among persons with low socioeconomic standing. The health outcomes of the privately insured do not differ significantly from those of the uninsured, and over time, those on public insurance have more diagnosed chronic conditions and feel less healthy compared to the uninsured. Medical insurance cannot account for any appreciable part of the socioeconomic differences in health. The one benefit of medical insurance that we found is that it helps protect the household from economic hardship, which is stressful and erodes health.

What does money buy? Income in itself has no value, but money allows us to buys things. There is little evidence that the access to medical care that comes with high income has a positive effect on health or that it constitutes a link between SES and health, but we need more research examining this question directly. Most research assumes, but does not test, the idea that access to medical care improves health. Money buys relief from the stress of economic hardship, and money buys relief from the health-eroding sense of helplessness and powerlessness that comes with not being able pay the bills and the rent. When most people think of money, though, they think of material things. What material things could money buy that might improve health? It seems that the things money buys are just as likely to be health risks as health benefits. Healthy fruits and vegetables may be expensive, but so are processed food and restaurant food, which are high in fat. Money can buy a safe car, but it can also buy a fast car. Money can buy alcohol, cigarettes, beef, doughnuts, drugs, flat-screen TVs, and other unhealthy pleasures of life in addition to the healthy pleasures. One underresearched hypothesis is that money allows people to buy a home rather than rent, which could be health promoting by mechanisms yet to be identified.

The Economic Link: Stress, Not Commodity

Economic well-being forms a link between education and health, but mostly not in support of the commodity perspective. Individuals and societies cannot get healthier buying more or better medical interventions. However, poverty and economic hardship are stressful in themselves and they bring a sense of powerlessness, helplessness, and failure. Low income and difficulty paying bills or buying necessities make individuals feel they are victims of merciless forces. The sense of helplessness undermines the motivation to find and adopt healthy lifestyles, while the sense of dread spawns cycles of agitation and depletion that feel like illness, compromise immune response, cultivate pathologies such as high blood pressure or atherosclerosis, and instigate crises such as heart attacks (see Figure 3.1). Education increases household income (largely by way of personal and spouse's employment and earnings), and income in turn decreases economic hardship. Economic hardship directly undermines health. Household income also boosts the sense of personal control, which is associated with a healthy lifestyle, and in turn with good health. Thus, education increases the sense of personal control directly and indirectly by way of household income.

Conclusion

Higher educational attainment is associated with better health, measured as better self-reported health, better physical functioning, fewer chronic conditions, and fewer psychophysiological symptoms. A large part of the reason the well educated experience good health is that they engage in a lifestyle that includes walking, exercising, and drinking moderately and avoiding being overweight and smoking. High levels of personal control among the well-educated account for much of the reason they engage in a healthy lifestyle. Well-educated parents further supply their children with resources of all kinds, including healthy habits (Mirowsky and Ross 1998; Hayward and Gorman 2004). Education also decreases economic hardship. It increases household income, and at the same income level, the better educated have less trouble paying the bills and paying for household food, shelter, and clothing than do the poorly educated (Mirowsky and Ross 2003). Under conditions of general prosperity, lifestyle may have the dominant effect on health, but that does not minimize the stressful and health-damaging effects of economic hardship for those who suffer it.

"Structured disadvantage" and "individual responsibility" are often considered rival explanations of health. Researchers who see health as a function of a social structure that allocates resources unequally sometimes criticize the view

that health is determined by lifestyle characteristics such as exercise and smoking (Knowles 1977). In the theory of learned effectiveness, a low sense of personal control, smoking, being overweight, and a sedentary lifestyle are not explanatory alternatives to structural disadvantage. A low sense of personal control and an unhealthy lifestyle form the mechanism of structural disadvantage connecting low education to poor health (Mirowsky and Ross 1998, 2003; Ross and Wu 1995).

We end with two questions: First, does the influence of education on health increase as people age? The cumulative advantage hypothesis predicts that the gap between the well educated and poorly educated increases with age, but the age-as-leveler hypothesis predicts that the gap eventually levels off and then closes sometime in older age (Herd and House 2004; House et al. 1994; Lauderdale 2001; Lynch 2003; Mirowsky and Ross 2005, 2008; Ross and Wu 1996). Second, is the influence of education on health larger or smaller among people who are otherwise disadvantaged compared to the more advantaged? The resource substitution hypothesis predicts that education has the biggest benefit among the otherwise disadvantaged compared to the advantaged—women, the poor, or people whose parents were poorly educated—while the resource multiplication hypothesis predicts a larger impact among the advantaged (Ross and Mirowsky 2006).

Some may think (or hope) that in old age, after years of increasing growth in the health gap between the well educated and the poorly educated, things get more equal (House et al. 1994), but the evidence indicates that this is probably not the case. More research is needed, although most (Lynch 2006; Pampel and Rogers 2004; Mirowsky and Ross 2008) but not all (Herd and House 2004) shows that the health disadvantages of the poorly educated grow with age. These disadvantages occur on many levels, from bioaccumulators like high blood pressure, fat, or cortisol to economic resources like income and wealth (Mirowsky and Ross 2005).

Furthermore, the very people who need education most to cope with the stressors of disadvantages like low income are the least likely to have a good education. Poorly educated people are least likely to have adequate household incomes, but household income is more important to the health of the poorly educated than of the well educated (Mirowsky and Hu 1996: Schnittker 2004). In support of resource substitution, education matters most to the health and well-being of people who are otherwise disadvantaged (Ross and Mirowsky 2006). This makes educational opportunities as the key to closing health disparities doubly important.

Educational attainment is a root cause of good health. Education gives people the resources to control and shape their own lives in a way that protects and fosters health. Apart from benefits to their own health, well-educated parents transmit resources to their children, including habits such as walking regularly and not smoking, which ultimately improve adult health status. Yet health policy makers typically do not view improved access to education as a way to improve the health of the U.S. population. Instead they usually view improved access to medical care as the way to decrease inequality in health (Davis and Rowland 1990), despite the fact that countries with universal access to medical care have large social inequalities in health (Marmot et al. 1987). Perhaps policy makers should invest in educators and schools, not just doctors and hospitals, for better health. Unfortunately, money for health (which goes to hospitals, physicians, pharmaceutical companies, and so on) often competes directly with money for schools, especially at the state level. In addition to the obvious benefits of education to knowledge, skills, jobs, wages, economic well-being, and living conditions, broadening educational opportunities for all Americans could also improve health.

Note

1. Feldman et al. 1989; Fox, Goldblatt, and Jones 1985; Guralnik et al. 1993; Kitagawa and Hauser 1973; Kunst and Mackenbach 1994; Leigh 1983; Lynch 2003; Matthews et al. 1989; Pappas et al. 1993; Regidor et al. 2003; Ross and Wu 1995, 1996; Steeland, Henley, and Thun 2002; Williams 1990; Winkleby et al. 1992.

References

Angell, M. 1993. "Privilege and Health: What Is the Connection?" *New England Journal of Medicine* 329:126–27.

Bailar, John C. 1976. "Mammography: A Contrary View." *Annals of Internal Medicine* 84:77–84.

Becker, Gary S. 1964. *Human Capital.* New York: Columbia University Press.

Best, Latrica E., Mark D. Hayward, and Mira M. Hidajat. 2005. "Life Course Pathways to Adult Onset Diabetes." *Social Biology* 52:94–106.

Billings, J., and N. Teicholz. 1990. "Uninsured Patients in District of Columbia Hospitals." *Health Affairs* 9:158–65.

Bird, Chloe E., and Catherine E. Ross. 1993. "Houseworkers and Paid Workers: Qualities of the Work and Effects on Personal Control." *Journal of Marriage and the Family* 55:913–25.

Blaxter, Mildred. 1987. "Evidence on Inequality in Health from a National Survey." *Lancet* 2:30–33.

Burstin, H. R., S. R. Lipsitz, and T. A. Brennan. 1992. "Socioeconomic Status and Risk for Substandard Medical Care." *Journal of the American Medical Association* 268(17): 2383–87.

Cairns, J. 1985. "The Treatment of Diseases and the War against Cancer." *Scientific American* 253(3): 51–59.

Canadian Task Force on the Periodic Health Examination. 1988. "The Periodic Health Examination." *Canadian Medical Association Journal* 121:1194–1254.

Cheng, Yawne, Ichiro Kawachi, Eugenie H. Coakley, Joel Schwartz, and Graham Colditz. 2000. "Association between Psychosocial Work Characteristics and Health Functioning in American Women: Prospective Study." *British Medical Journal* 320:1432–36.

Cutler, David, and Grant Miller. 2005. "The Role of Public Health Improvements in Health Advances: The Twentieth Century United States." *Demography* 42:1–22.

Davis, K., and D. Rowland. 1990. "Uninsured and Underserved: Inequalities in Health Care in the United States." In *The Sociology of Health and Illness Critical Perspectives*, ed. Peter Conrad and Rochelle Kern, 249–65. New York: St. Martin's Press.

Deyo, R. A. 1998. "Low–Back Pain." *Scientific American* 279(2): 48–53.

Deyo, R. A., D. Cherkin, D. Conrad and E. Volinn. 1991. "Cost, Controversy, Crisis: Low Back Pain and the Health of the Public." *Annual Review of Public Health* 12:141–56.

Diderichsen, F. 1990. "Health and Social Inequalities in Sweden." *Social Science and Medicine* 31:359–67.

Doornbos G., and D. Kromhout. 1990. "Educational Level and Mortality in a 32-Year Follow-Up Study of 18-Year-Old Men in the Netherlands." *International Journal of Epidemiology* 19:374–79.

Elder, Glen H., and Jeffrey K. Liker. 1982. "Hard Times in Women's Lives: Historical Influences across Forty Years." *American Journal of Sociology* 88:241–69.

Elo, Irma T., and Samuel H. Preston. 1992. "Effects of Early-Life Conditions on Adult Mortality: A Review." *Population Index* 58(2): 186–212.

———. 1996. "Educational Differentials in Mortality: United States, 1979–85." *Social Science and Medicine* 42(1): 47–57.

Epel, Elissa S., Bruce S. McEwen, and Jeannette R. Ickovics. 1998. "Embodying Psychological Thriving: Physical Thriving in Response to Stress." *Journal of Social Issues* 54:301–22.

Epstein, A. M. 1996. "Use of Diagnostic Tests and Therapeutic Procedures in a Changing Health Care Environment." *Journal of the American Medical Association* 275:1197–98.

Evans, Robert G. 1994. Introduction to *Why Are Some People Healthy and Others Not?* ed. Robert G. Evans, Morris L. Barer, and Theodore R. Marmor, 3–16. New York: Aldine de Gruyter.

Evans, Robert G., Matthew Hodge, and I. Barry Pless. 1994. "If Not Genetics, Then What? Biological Pathways and Population Health." In *Why are Some People Healthy and Others Not?* ed. Robert G. Evans, Morris L. Barer, and Theodore R. Marmor, 161–88. New York: Aldine de Gruyter.

Feldman, Jacob J., Diane M. Makuc, Joel C. Kleinman, and Joan Cornoni-Huntley. 1989. "National Trends in Educational Differentials in Mortality." *American Journal of Epidemiology* 129:919–33.

Fox, A. J., P. O. Goldblatt, and D. R. Jones. 1985. "Social Class Mortality Differentials: Artefact, Selection, or Life Circumstances?" *Journal of Epidemiology and Community Health* 39:1–8.

Fremont, Allen M., and Chloe E. Bird. 2000. "Social and Psychological Factors, Physiological Processes, and Physical Health." In *The Handbook of Medical Sociology*, 5th ed., ed. Chloe E. Bird, Peter Conrad, and Allen M. Fremont, 334–52. Upper Saddle River, N.J.: Prentice Hall.

Gecas, Viktor. 1989. "The Social Psychology of Self-Efficacy." *Annual Review of Sociology* 15:291–316.

Grembowski, David, Donald Patrick, Paula Diehr, Mary Durham, Shirley Beresford, Erica Kay, and Julia Hecht. 1993. "Self-Efficacy and Health Behavior among Older Adults." *Journal of Health and Social Behavior* 34:89–104.

Guralnik, Jack M., Kenneth C. Land, Gerda G. Fillenbaum, and Lauren G. Branch. 1993. "Educational Status and Active Life Expectancy among Older Blacks and Whites." *New England Journal of Medicine* 329:110–16.

Haas, Steven A., and Nathan Edward Fosse. 2008. "Health and the Educational Attainment of Adolescents: Evidence from the NLSY." *Journal of Health and Social Behavior* 49:178–92.

Hadley, J., E. P. Steinberg, and J. Feder. 1991. "Comparison of Uninsured and Privately Insured Hospital Patients: Condition on Admission, Resource Use and Outcome." *Journal of the American Medical Association* 265(3): 374–79.

Hahn, B., and A. B. Flood. 1995. "No Insurance, Public Insurance, and Private Insurance: Do These Options Contribute to Differences in General Health?" *Journal of Health Care for the Poor and Underserved* 691:41–59.

Hayes, Diane, and Catherine E. Ross. 1986. "Body and Mind: The Effect of Exercise, Overweight, and Physical Health on Psychological Well-Being." *Journal of Health and Social Behavior* 27(4): 387–400.

———. 1987. "Concern with Appearance, Health Beliefs, and Eating Habits." *Journal of Health and Social Behavior* 28(2): 120–30.

Hayward, Mark D., and Bridget K. Gorman. 2004. "The Long Arm of Childhood: The Influence of Early-Life Social Conditions on Men's Mortality." *Demography* 41:87–107.

Herd, Pamela, and James S. House. 2004. "Convergence or Divergence: Functional Status Decline among the 1931 to 1941 Birth Cohort." Paper presented at the American Sociological Association Meeting, San Francisco, August.

Hertzman, Clyde, John Frank, and Robert G. Evans. 1994. "Heterogeneities in Health Status and the Determinants of Population Health." In *Why Are Some People Healthy and Others Not?* ed. Robert G. Evans, Morris L. Barer, and Theodore R. Marmor, 67–92. New York: Aldine de Gruyter.

Hill, Terrence D., Catherine E. Ross, and Ronald J. Angel. 2005. "Neighborhood Disorder, Psychophysiological Distress, and Health" *Journal of Health and Social Behavior* 46:170–86.

Hollingsworth, J. R. 1981. "Inequality in Levels of Health in England and Wales, 1971–1981." *Journal of Health and Social Behavior* 22:268–83.

House, J. S., J. M. Lepkowski, A. M. Kinney, R. P. Mero, R. C. Kessler, and A. R Herzog. 1994. "The Social Stratification of Aging and Health." *Journal of Health and Social Behavior* 35:213–34.

Hyman, Herbert H., and Charles R. Wright. 1979. *Education's Lasting Influence on Values.* Chicago: University of Chicago Press.

Kaiser Foundation Health Plan. 1976. "Health Examinations." *Planning for Health* 19:2–3.

Karasek, Robert A., R. Russell, and Tores Theorell. 1982. "Physiology of Stress and Regeneration in Job Related Cardiovascular Illness." *Journal of Human Stress* 8:29–42.

Karasek, Robert A., and Tores Theorell. 1990. *Healthy Work, Stress, Productivity, and the Reconstruction of Working Life.* New York: Basic Books.

Kawachi, I., and B. P. Kennedy. 1997. "Socioeconomic Determinants of Health: Health and Social Cohesion: Why Care about Income Inequality?" *British Journal of Medicine* 314(5): 1037–40.

Kim, K. K., and P. M. Moody. 1992. "More Resources, Better Health: A Cross National Perspective." *Social Science and Medicine* 34(8): 837–42.

Kingston, Paul W., Ryan Hubbard, Brent Lapp, Paul Schroeder, and Julia Wilson. 2003. "Why Education Matters." *Sociology of Education* 76:53–70.

Kitagawa, Evelyn M., and Philip M. Hauser. 1973. *Differential Mortality in the United States: A Study in Socioeconomic Epidemiology.* Cambridge, Mass.: Harvard University Press.

Knowles, John H. 1977. "The Responsibility of the Individual." In *Doing Better and Feeling Worse: Health in the U.S.*, ed. J. H. Knowles, 57–80. New York: W. W. Norton.

Kohn, Melvin, and Carmi Schooler. 1982. "Job Conditions and Personality: A Longitudinal Assessment of Their Reciprocal Effects." *American Journal of Sociology* 87:1257–86.

Kreindel, S., R. Rosetti, R. Goldberg, J. Savageau, J. Yarzebski, J. Gore, A. Russo, and C. Bigelow. 1997. "Health Insurance Coverage and Outcomes Following Acute Myocardial Infarction." *Archives of Internal Medicine* 157:758–62.

Kunst, A. E., C. W. Looman, and J. P. Mackenbach. 1990. "Socio-economic Mortality Differences in the Netherlands in 1950–1984: A Regional Study of Cause-Specific Mortality." *Social Science and Medicine* 31:141–52.

Kunst, A. E., and J. P. Mackenbach. 1994. "The Size of Mortality Differences Associated with Educational Level in Nine Industrialized Countries." *American Journal of Public Health* 84(6): 932–37.

Lagasse, R., P. C. Humblet, A. Lenaerts, I. Godin, and G. F. Moens. 1990. "Health and Social Inequities in Belgium." *Social Science and Medicine* 31:237–48.

Lahelma E., and T. Valkonen. 1990. "Health and Social Inequities in Finland and Elsewhere." *Social Science and Medicine* 31:257–65.

Lauderdale, Diane S. 2001. "Education and Survival: Birth Cohort, Period, and Age Effects." *Demography* 38:551–61.

LaVecchia, C., E. Negri, R. Pagano, and A. Decarli. 1987. "Education, Prevalence of Disease and Frequency of Health Care Utilization: The 1983 Italian National Health Survey." *Journal of Epidemiology and Community Health* 41:161–65.

Lee, P., and D. Paxman. 1997. "Reinventing Public Health." *Annual Review of Public Health* 18:1–35.

Leigh, J. Paul. 1983. "Direct and Indirect Effects of Education on Health." *Social Science and Medicine* 17:227–34.

Lleras-Muney, A. 2005. "The Relationship between Education and Adult Mortality in the United States." *Review of Economic Studies* 72:189–221.

Lynch, Scott M. 2003. "Cohort and Life-Course Patterns in the Relationship between Education and Health: A Hierarchical Approach." *Demography* 42(2): 309–31.

———. 2006. "Explaining Life Course and Cohort Variation in the Relationship between Education and Health: The Role of Income." *Journal of Health and Social Behavior* 47:324–38.

MacDonald, L. A., R. A. Karasek, L. Punnett, and T. Scharf. 2001. "Covariation between Workplace Physical and Psychosocial Stressors: Evidence and Implications for Occupational Health Research and Prevention." *Ergonomics* 44(7): 696–718.

MacIntyre, Sally. 1997. "The Black Report and Beyond: What Are the Issues?" *Social Science and Medicine* 44(6): 723–45.

Marmor, Theodore R., Morris L. Barer, and Robert G. Evans. 1994. "The Determinants of Population Health: What Can Be Done to Improve a Democratic Nation's Health Status?" In *Why Are Some People Healthy and Others Not?* ed. Robert G. Evans, Morris L. Barer, and Theodore R. Marmor, 217–32. New York: Aldine de Gruyter.

Marmot, M. G., M. Kogevinas, and M. A. Elston. 1987. "Social/Economic Status and Disease." *Annual Review of Public Health* 8:111–35.

Marmot, Michael G., and J. Fraser Mustard. 1994. "Coronary Heart Disease from a Population Perspective." In *Why Are Some People Healthy and Others Not?* ed. Robert G. Evans, Morris L. Barer, and Theodore R. Marmor, 189–214. New York: Aldine de Gruyter.

Matthews, K. A., S. F. Kelsey, E. N. Meilahn, L. H. Kuller, and R. R. Wing. 1989. "Educational Attainment and Behavioral and Biological Risk Factors for Coronary Heart Disease in Middle-Aged Women." *American Journal of Epidemiology* 129:1132–44.

Mayer, Susan E. 1997. *What Money Can't Buy: Family Income and Children's Life Chances.* Cambridge, Mass.: Harvard University Press.

McKinlay, J., and S. McKinlay. 1977. "The Questionable Contribution of Medical Measures to the Decline of Mortality in the Twentieth Century." *Milbank Memorial Fund Quarterly* 55:405–28.

Mirowsky, John, and P. N. Hu. 1996. "Physical Impairment and the Diminishing Effects of Income." *Social Forces* 74(3): 1073–96.

Mirowsky, John, and Catherine E. Ross. 1989. *Social*

Causes of Psychological Distress. 2nd ed. New York: Aldine de Gruyter.

———. 1991. "Eliminating Defense and Agreement Bias from Measures of Sense of Control: A 2x2 Index." *Social Psychology Quarterly* 54:127–45.

———. 1998. "Education, Personal Control, Lifestyle and Health: A Human Capital Hypothesis." *Research on Aging* 20(4): 415–49.

———. 2003. *Education, Social Status, and Health.* Piscataway, N.J: Aldine Transaction.

———. 2005. "Education, Learned Effectiveness, and Health." *London Review of Education* 3:205–20.

———. 2007a. "Creative Work and Health." *Journal of Health and Social Behavior* 48:385–403.

———. 2007b. "Life Course Trajectories of Perceived Control and Their Relationship to Education." *American Journal of Sociology* 112:1339–82.

———. 2008. "Education and Self-Rated Health: Cumulative Advantage and Its Rising Importance." *Research on Aging* 30:93–122.

Morris, J. N. 1990. "Inequalities in Health: Ten Years and Little Further On." *Lancet* 336:491–93.

Pampel, Fred C., and Richard G. Rogers. 2004. "Socioeconomic Status, Smoking, and Health: A Test of Competing Theories of Cumulative Advantage." *Journal of Health and Social Behavior* 45:306–21.

Pamuk, Elsie R. 1985. "Social Class Inequality in Mortality from 1912–1972 in England and Wales." *Population Studies* 39:17–31.

———. 1988. "Social-Class Inequality in Infant Mortality in England and Wales from 1921 to 1980." *European Journal of Population* 4:1–21.

Pappas, Gregory, Susan Queen, Wilbur Hadden, and Gail Fisher. 1993. "The Increasing Disparity between Socioeconomic Groups in the United States, 1960 and 1986." *New England Journal of Medicine* 329:103–9.

Parchment, Winsome, Gerson Weiss, and M. R. Passannante. 1996. "Is the Lack of Health Insurance the Major Barrier to Early Prenatal care at an Inner-City Hospital?" *Women's Health Issues* 6:97–105.

Pascarella, Ernest T., and Patrick T. Terenzini. 1991. *How College Affects Students.* San Francisco: Jossey-Bass.

Pearce, N. E., P. B. Davis, A. H. Smith, and F. H. Foster. 1985. "Social Class, Ethnic Group, and Male Mortality in New Zealand, 1974–78." *Journal of Epidemiology and Community Health* 39:9–14.

Pearlin, Leonard I., Morton A. Lieberman, Elizabeth G. Menaghan, and Joseph T. Mullan. 1981. "The Stress Process." *Journal of Health and Social Behavior* 22:337–56.

Pincus, E. 1998. "Social Conditions and Self-Management Are More Powerful Determinants of Health Than Access to Care." *Annals of Internal Medicine* 129:406–11.

Pincus, T., and L. F. Callahan. 1985. "Formal Education as a Marker for Increased Mortality and Morbidity in Rheumatoid Arthritis." *Journal of Chronic Disease* 38:973–84.

Pincus, T., R. Esther, D. A. DeWalt, and L. F. Callahan. 1998. "Social Conditions and Self-Management Are More Powerful Determinants of Health Than Access to Care." *Annals of Internal Medicine* 129:406–11.

Regidor, E., M. E. Calle, P. Navarro, and V. Dominiquez. 2003. "The Size of Educational Differences in Mortality from Specific Causes of Death in Men and Women." *European Journal of Epidemiology* 18:395–400.

Reynolds, J. R., and C. E. Ross. 1998. "Social Stratification and Health: Education's Benefit beyond Economic Status and Social Origins." *Social Problems* 45:221–47.

Rodin, Judith. 1986. "Aging and Health: Effects of the Sense of Control." *Science* 233:1271–76.

Rogers, Richard G. 1992. "Living and Dying in the U.S.A.: Sociodemographic Determinants of Death among Blacks and Whites." *Demography* 29:287–304.

Rogers, Richard G., Robert A. Hummer, and Charles B. Nam. 2000. *Living and Dying in the USA.* New York: Academic Press.

Rogot, E., P. Sorlie, and N. J. Johnson. 1992. "Life Expectancy by Employment Status, Income and Education in the National Longitudinal Mortality Study." *Public Health Reports* 107:457–61.

Roos, Noralou P., and Leslie L. Roos. 1994. "Small Area Variations, Practice Style, and Quality of Care." In *Why Are Some People Healthy and Others Not?* ed. Robert G. Evans, Morris L. Barer, and Theodore R. Marmor, 231–52. New York: Aldine de Gruyter.

Ross, Catherine E. 2000. "Occupations, Jobs and the Sense of Control." *Sociological Focus* 33:409–20.

Ross, Catherine E., and Chloe E. Bird. 1994. "Sex Stratification and Health Lifestyle: Consequences for Men's and Women's Perceived Health." *Journal of Health and Social Behavior* 35:161–78.

Ross, Catherine E., and John Mirowsky. 1989. "Explaining the Social Patterns of Depression: Control and Problem-Solving—or Support and Talking." *Journal of Health and Social Behavior* 30(2): 206–19.

———. 1992. "Households, Employment, and the Sense of Control." *Social Psychology Quarterly* 55:217–35.

———. 1996. "Economic and Interpersonal Work Rewards: Subjective Utilities of Men's and Women's Compensation." *Social Forces* 75:223–46.

———. 1999. "Refining the Association between Education and Health: Effects of Quantity, Credential, and Selectivity." *Demography* 36:445–60.

———. 2000. "Does Medical Insurance Contribute to Socioeconomic Differentials in Health?" *Milbank Quarterly* 78:291–321.

———. 2006. "Sex Differences in the Effect of Education on Depression: Resource Multiplication or Resource Substitution?" *Social Science and Medicine* 63:1400–1413.

Ross, Catherine E., and Marieke Van Willigen. 1997. "Education and the Subjective Quality of Life." *Journal of Health and Social Behavior* 38:275–97.

Ross, Catherine E., and Marylyn P. Wright. 1998. "Women's Work, Men's Work and the Sense of Control." *Work and Occupations* 25:33–55.

Ross, Catherine E., and Chia-ling Wu. 1995. "The Links between Education and Health." *American Sociological Review* 60:719–45.

———. 1996. "Education, Age, and the Cumulative Advantage in Health." *Journal of Health and Social Behavior* 37:104–20.

Rotter, Julian B. 1966. "Generalized Expectancies for Internal vs. External Control of Reinforcements." *Psychological Monographs* 80:1–28.

Sagan, Leonard A. 1987. *The Health of Nations: True Causes of Sickness and Well-Being.* New York: Basic.

Schnittker, Jason. 2004. "Education and the Changing Shape of the Income Gradient in Health." *Journal of Health and Social Behavior* 45:286–305.

Schultz, Theodore. 1962. "Reflections on Investment in Man." *Journal of Political Economy* 70:1–8.

Seeman, Melvin. 1983. "Alienation Motifs in Contemporary Theorizing: The Hidden Continuity of Classic Themes." *Social Psychology Quarterly* 46:171–84.

Seeman, Melvin, and Susan Lewis. 1995. "Powerlessness, Health and Mortality: A Longitudinal Study of Older Men and Mature Women." *Social Science and Medicine* 41(4): 517–26.

Seeman, Melvin, Alice Z. Seeman, and Art Budros. 1988. "Powerlessness, Work, and Community: A Longitudinal Study of Alienation and Alcohol Use." *Journal of Health and Social Behavior* 29:185–98.

Seeman, Melvin, and Teresa E. Seeman. 1983. "Health Behavior and Personal Autonomy: A Longitudinal Study of the Sense of Control in Illness." *Journal of Health and Social Behavior* 24:144–60.

Sen, Amartya. 1997. "Human Capital and Human Capability." *World Development* 25:1959–61.

———. 1999. *Development as Freedom.* New York: Knopf.

Short, P. F., and T. J. Lair. 1994. "Health Insurance and Health Status: Implications for Financing Health Care Reform." *Inquiry: The Journal of Health Care Organization Provision and Financing* 31:425–37.

Siskind, V., R. Copeman, and J. M. Najman. 1987. "Socioeconomic Status and Mortality: A Brisbane Area Analysis." *Community Health Studies* 11:15–23.

Sorlie, P. D., N. J. Johnson, E. Backlund, and D. D. Bradham. 1994. "Mortality in the Uninsured Compared with that in Persons with Public and Private Health Insurance." *Archives of Internal Medicine* 154:2409–16.

Sorlie, Paul D., Eric Backlund, and Jacob B Keller. 1995. "U.S. Mortality by Economic, Demographic, and Social Characteristics: The National Longitudinal Mortality Study." *American Journal of Public Health* 85:949–57.

Steenland, K. S., J. Henley, and M. J. Thun. 2002. "All-Cause and Cause-Specific Death Rates by Educational Status for Two Million People in Two American Cancer Society Cohorts, 1959–1996." *American Journal of Epidemiology* 156:11–21.

Townsend, P., N. Davidson, and M. Whitehead. 1992. *Inequalities in Health and the Health Divide.* London: Penguin.

U.S. Congress, Office of Technology Assessment. 1992. "Does Health Insurance Make a Difference?" OTA-BP-H-99. Washington, D.C.: U.S. Government Printing Office.

U.S. Preventive Services Task Force. 1989. *Guide to Clinical Preventive Services.* Baltimore, Md.: Williams and Wilkins.

Verrilli, D., and H. G. Welch. 1996. "The Impact of Diagnostic Testing on Therapeutic Interventions." *Journal of the American Medical Association* 275:1189–91.

Wagstaff, A., P. Paci, and E. van Doorslaer. 1991. "On the Measurement of Inequalities in Health." *Social Science and Medicine* 3:545–57.

Wennberg, J., E. Davis, M. A. Kellett, J. D. Dickens Jr., D. J. Malenka, L. M. Keilson, and R. B. Keller. 1996. "The Association between Local Diagnostic Testing Intensity and Invasive Cardiac Procedures." *Journal of the American Medical Association* 275:1161–64.

Wheaton, Blair. 1980. "The Sociogenesis of Psychological Disorder: An Attributional Theory." *Journal of Health and Social Behavior* 21:100–124.

Wickrama, K. A. S., Frederick O. Lorenz, Rand D. Conger, Lisa Matthews, and Glen H. Elder. 1997. "Linking Occupational Conditions to Physical Health through Marital, Social, and Intrapersonal Processes." *Journal of Health and Social Behavior* 38:363–75.

Wilkinson, R. G. 1986. *Class and Health: Research and Longitudinal Data.* London: Tavistock.

———. 1997. "Socioeconomic Determinants of Health: Health Inequalities—Relative or Absolute Material Standards?" *British Medical Journal* 314:591–98.

Williams, David R. 1990. "Socioeconomic Differentials in Health: A Review and Redirection." *Social Psychology Quarterly* 53:81–99.

Williams, David R., and Chiquita Collins. 1995. "U.S. Socioeconomic and Racial Differences in Health: Patterns and Explanations." *Annual Review of Sociology* 21:349–86.

Winkleby, Marilyn A., Darius E. Jatulis, Erica Frank, and Stephen P. Fortmann. 1992. "Socioeconomic Status and Health: How Education, Income, and Occupation Contribute to Risk Factors for Cardiovascular Disease." *American Journal of Public Health* 82:816–20.

4

Understanding Gender and Health
Old Patterns, New Trends, and Future Directions

Patricia P. Rieker, Boston University and Harvard Medical School

Chloe E. Bird, RAND Corporation

Martha E. Lang, Guilford College

A central feature of mortality trends throughout the twentieth century is the sex/gender difference in life expectancy: in the United States, women live on average 5.2 years longer than men do (NCHS 2009). Women have not always held a mortality advantage (Berin, Stolnitz, and Tenenbein 1990) and it may not continue. In fact, the age-adjusted gender gap in longevity appears to widen and narrow due to environmental/behavioral risk and protective factors, as well as genetic, biological, and hormonal processes (Annandale 2009). Biomedical and social science researchers who have pursued the causes of men's and women's differential mortality seldom agree on explanations, partly because, as Nathanson (1984, 196) stated in her discussion of the literature on differences in men's and women's health, "investigators' disciplinary orientations are reflected in specification of what is to be explained . . . in their choice of potential explanatory variables, and in the methods they employ; . . . the biologist sees hormones; the epidemiologist, risk factors; and the sociologist, social roles and structural constraints."

Even sociologists' understanding of the differences and similarities in men's and women's physical and mental health has changed dramatically over the past twenty-five years. Reviews of this literature indicate that researchers have often asked the wrong questions. For example, "Which is the weaker sex?" is framed in the binary language of biological advantage of one sex over the other and "Which gender is more advantaged?" assumes social advantage of one gender over the other. Even if there are real circumstances where biological superiority and social inequality can be observed, the framing of such questions implies that biological differences or social positions and roles can be summed up to determine which sex is the fittest or which gender is the most privileged. At best, this approach produces oversimplified models of the complex patterns of gender differences in health with little thought given to similarities.

A binary approach has the additional limitation of treating men and women as distinct homogenous groups, whereas gender differences in health vary substantially by age, race/ethnicity, and socioeconomic status. The dichotomy also ignores the wide array of gender identities and sexualities. Although men and women do seem to have on average some unique biological advantages and disadvantages over each other, substantial variation occurs among women and among men, and these differences seem to vary with certain social conditions (Fausto-Sterling 2005, 2008). It is still the case that much of clinical research tends to minimize or ignore the social and environmental processes that can influence health differentially and to reify biomedical models that portray men's and women's health disparities as inherently biological or genetic.

In recent years, a growing number of clinical researchers has come to recognize that social and biological factors interact in complex ways, and that this explains not only health or illness at the individual level but also population health and the observed patterns of men's and women's health and longevity in general. Yet relatively few biomedical or sociological studies examine both sets of factors (Institute of Medicine 2001a, b), highlighting the need to move beyond the binary in thinking and research, as ultimately integrating them will contribute to better science. Biological "sex" and social "gender" processes can interact and may be confounded. In acknowledgement of this, we use the term "gender" to refer to observed differences in men's and women's lives, morbidity, and mortality.

In this chapter, we briefly review gender differences in longevity and health in the United States and cross nationally, examine U.S. disease patterns for four specific conditions to illustrate gender disparities, review recent findings on the relationship between mental and physical health and its possible connection to gender differences in health, and consider limitations of current approaches to understanding men's and women's health. We suggest that in contrast to prevailing models of inequality, our integrative framework of constrained choice describes how decisions made and actions taken at the levels of family, work, community, and government shape men's and women's opportunities to pursue health and contribute to observed disparities. The constrained-choice model and gender-based analysis provide a new direction for discourse, research, and policy. We close with suggestions of interesting questions and issues for researchers to consider.

Gender Gaps in Health and Longevity: Puzzle or Paradox?

For decades differences in men's and women's longevity and physical health have been considered paradoxical, although some challenge the conception of a "gender paradox" (Hunt and Annandale 1999). In the United States, as in most industrialized countries, men live shorter lives than women do, yet women have higher morbidity rates and in later years a diminished quality of life. The gender gap in longevity in the United States has been decreasing, from 7.8 years in 1970 to 5.2 years in 2006 (NCHS 2009). U.S. women's life expectancy has exceeded that of men since 1900, with women experiencing lower mortality rates in every age group and for most causes of death. Even though the female advantage is persistent and life expectancy has been increasing for both men and women, the gender gap in longevity has been closing in the United States and other countries. For example, Annandale (2009, 128) shows that between 1969 and 2007 in the United Kingdom men gained 9.0 years compared to women's 6.7 years. The same decreasing gender gap prevails in most industrialized countries, including Sweden, Finland, and Australia.

This female longevity advantage pattern holds worldwide except in the poorest countries, where life expectancy is low for both men and women (WHO 2006). However, the causes of death and gender difference in mortality rates vary substantially across age groups, as do the leading contributing factors (WHO 2008). For example, the higher infant mortality rates among boys compared to girls in the United States and other developed countries may have largely biological causes, such as congenital abnormalities and X-chromosome immune-related disorders (Abramowicz and Barnett 1970; Waldron 1998), while the gender gap among young adults between the ages of nineteen and twenty-two years may have primarily behavioral causes, such as motor vehicle accidents and homicide. Similarly, the gender gap in mental health is both age- and disorder-specific, with women experiencing higher rates of depression and anxiety, and men experiencing higher rates of alcoholism, other substance abuse, and antisocial behaviors (Bird and Rieker 2008; Kessler, Barker, et al. 2003; Kessler, Berglund, et al. 2003).

Life Expectancy Cross-Nationally

When we consider data on cross-national gender differences in life expectancy, the paradox becomes even greater. The comparative life expectancy rates listed in Table 4.1 help capture these differences, showing that both the size of the gender gap and the pattern of longevity vary considerably by country and by national wealth (United Nations 2005). As one would expect, the gap in life expectancy at birth between the thirty countries with the highest life expectancy and the thirty with the lowest life expectancy is dramatic, ranging from 82.3 years in Japan to 40.5 years in Zambia and 40.9 years in Zimbabwe.

The countries with the lowest life expectancy, with few exceptions, are mainly poor countries in Southeast Asia and sub-Saharan Africa. However, a country's wealth does not necessarily guarantee higher average longevity. For example, Japan ranks first in overall life expectancy (82.3) but sixteenth in its gross domestic product (GDP) per capita ($31,267). Luxembourg ranks first in GDP per capita ($60,228) but twenty-fourth in life expectancy (78.4 years). In fact, none of the four wealthiest countries (Ireland, United States, Luxembourg, and Norway) rank among the top five countries in terms of overall life expectancy.

Another interesting aspect of the information in Table 4.1 is that the variation in the gender gap in life expectancy itself is greater in the thirty wealthier countries (with higher overall life expectancy) than in the thirty poor countries (with lower life expectancy). The gap ranges from 3.2 to 7.5 years in the wealthier countries and −1.8 to 4 years in the poorer countries, with some exceptions. Pinnelli (1997), a demographer, has discussed "male supermortality" and suggests that a five-year life-expectancy gender gap favoring women might be normal. She also contends that a greater difference indicates that men may be disadvantaged, in part because of their aggressive and risky health behaviors, while a smaller gap indicates that women may be disadvantaged regarding access to medical care, diet, and restricted labor-force participation. One clear example of this is the overall decline in life expectancy in the Russian Federation (not shown in the table) with a thirteen-year gap between men and women (fifty-nine vs. seventy-two), which generally is attributed to men's excessive alcohol use and greater smoking, suicide, and homicide rates (Kalben 2002). While it is debatable whether a five-year gap reflects a normal or biologically driven gender difference in life expectancy, changing environmental hazards, such as pandemics or civil wars, might alter this interpretation by shifting the balance one way or the other. However, we generally agree that the current data tend to support Pinnelli's interpretation.

In contrast to the worldwide pattern of women outliving men, the difference disappears and is even reversed in several of the poorer countries, with women outliving men by one year or less, if at all (e.g., Zimbabwe, Zambia, and Malawi). The lower overall life span and the minimal gender gap in these countries illustrates the extent to which extreme poverty, political disruption, and disease-specific mortality patterns (such as AIDS, malaria, and other infectious diseases) diminish life expectancy for both men and women (Andoh et al. 2006; Rao, Lopez, and Hemed 2006). These data also suggest that if women do indeed have some biological advantages that contribute to greater life expectancy, they can be attenuated by harsh social conditions and restrictive gender roles. Although a country's wealth (as measured by GDP) can contribute to population health, it does not appear to be the main factor affecting the gender gap in life expectancy among relatively wealthy countries; but a specific wealth threshold may be more critical in poor countries.

The variability in the gender gap highlights the impact of differences in life circumstances overall, as well as between men and women. Having considered the variation in life expectancy across countries, we need also to consider how the causes of death differ geographically and by gender. In some parts of the world, adults typically die relatively young and most often from infectious disease (particularly Southeast Asia and sub-Saharan Africa). Yet even in these societies, the factors that contribute to early mortality differ somewhat for men and women. And the variation is not only by gender. For example, in countries with high rates of abject poverty such as Zambia and Zimbabwe, there are also geographic patterns to the leading causes of death both among men and among women. In Zambia (40.3 vs. 40.6) and Zimbabwe (41.4 vs. 40.2) there is little gender difference in life expectancy, which has been declining for both men and women due in large

Table 4.1. Countries with highest and lowest life expectancy, with GDP per capita

| Countries with highest life expectancy | | | | | | Countries with lowest life expectancy | | | | | |
Country	Life expectancy at birth	Women	Men	Difference	GDP per capita	Country	Life expectancy at birth	Women	Men	Difference	GDP per capita
Japan	82.3	85.7	78.7	7.0	31,267	Senegal	62.3	64.4	60.4	4.0	1,792
Hong Kong, China (SAR)	81.9	84.9	79.1	5.8	34,833	Yemen	61.5	63.1	60.0	3.1	930
Iceland	81.5	83.1	79.9	3.2	36,510	Timor-Leste	59.7	60.5	58.9	1.6	N/A
Switzerland	81.3	83.7	78.5	5.2	35,633	Gambia	58.8	59.9	57.7	2.2	1,921
Australia	80.9	83.3	78.5	4.8	31,794	Togo	57.8	59.6	56.0	3.6	1,506
Sweden	80.5	82.7	78.3	4.4	32,525	Eritrea	56.6	59.0	54.0	5.0	1,109
Spain	80.5	83.8	77.2	6.6	27,169	Niger	55.8	54.9	56.7	-1.8	781
Canada	80.3	82.6	77.9	4.7	33,375	Benin	55.4	56.5	54.1	2.4	1,141
Italy	80.3	83.2	77.2	6.0	28,529	Guinea	54.8	56.4	53.2	3.2	2,316
Israel	80.3	82.3	78.1	4.2	25,864	Djibouti	53.9	55.2	52.6	2.6	2,178
France	80.2	83.7	76.6	7.1	30,386	Mali	53.1	55.3	50.8	4.5	1,033
Norway	79.8	82.2	77.3	4.9	41,420	Kenya	52.1	53.1	51.1	2.0	1,240
New Zealand	79.8	81.8	77.7	4.1	24,996	Ethiopia	51.8	53.1	50.5	2.6	1,055
Austria	79.4	82.2	76.5	5.7	33,700	Burkina Faso	51.4	52.9	49.8	3.1	1,213
Singapore	79.4	81.4	77.5	3.9	29,663	Tanzania	51.0	52.0	50.0	2.0	744
Netherlands	79.2	81.4	76.9	4.5	32,684	Chad	50.4	51.8	49.0	2.8	1,427
Germany	79.1	81.8	76.2	5.6	29,461	Uganda	49.7	50.2	49.1	1.1	1,454
United Kingdom	79.0	81.2	76.7	4.5	33,238	Burundi	48.5	49.8	47.1	2.7	699
Cyprus	79.0	81.5	76.6	4.9	22,699	Cote d'Ivoire	47.4	48.3	46.5	1.8	1,648
Finland	78.9	82.0	75.6	6.4	32,153	Nigeria	46.5	47.1	46.0	1.1	1,128
Greece	78.9	80.9	76.7	4.2	23,381	Malawi	46.3	46.7	46.0	0.7	667
Belgium	78.8	81.8	75.8	6.0	32,119	Congo	45.8	47.1	44.4	2.7	714
Ireland	78.4	80.9	76.0	4.9	38,505	Guinea-Bissau	45.8	47.5	44.2	3.3	827
Luxembourg	78.4	81.4	75.4	6.0	60,228	Rwanda	45.2	46.7	43.6	3.1	1,206
United States	77.9	80.4	75.2	5.2	41,890	Central African Republic	43.7	45.0	42.3	2.7	1,224
Denmark	77.9	80.1	75.5	4.6	33,973	Mozambique	42.8	43.6	42.0	1.6	1,242
Korea (Republic of)	77.9	81.5	74.3	7.2	22,029	Sierra Leone	41.8	43.4	40.2	3.2	806
Portugal	77.7	80.9	74.5	6.4	20,410	Angola	41.7	43.3	40.1	3.2	2,335
Slovenia	77.4	81.1	73.6	7.5	22,273	Zimbabwe	40.9	40.2	41.4	-1.2	2,038
Brunei Darussalam	76.7	79.3	74.6	4.7	28,161	Zambia	40.5	40.6	40.3	0.3	1,023

Source: United Nations 2005

part to political turmoil and the countries' inability to control infectious diseases. In fact, a review of the data on the ten countries with the highest seropositivity rates over the past fifteen years shows that the female gender advantage decreases as HIV prevalence increases, a further reminder that neither the trends nor the gaps in life expectancy will remain constant over time, particularly as the leading causes of death vary with changing social and environmental circumstances (Velkoff and Kowal 2007).

Thus, it is clear that biological sex differences between men and women are not equally advantageous (or disadvantageous) in all circumstances; consequently the gender differences in mortality are dynamic. This insight is not new. Kalben (2002, 2) quotes a 1974 report by the Committee on Ordinary Issuance and Annuities that noted that differences in the leading causes of death "strongly suggest that sex differentials in mortality are due to biological as well as environmental factors and that the relative importance of the biological components varies by sex and social circumstances."

There is little precise understanding of the biological and social factors or pathways between them that can or do widen or narrow the gender gap in both longevity and general health. Although many reasons for the variation have been identified, biological or social factors alone are not considered a sufficient explanation for the cross-national gender differences (Kalben 2002; Krieger 2003; Yin 2007). Some social scientists argue that health status differences among individuals and groups within a country are due to income inequalities or other fundamental social causes (Phelan et al. 2004), while others contend it is the status syndrome associated with positions in the social hierarchy that explains such phenomena (Marmot 2004, 2005). Cross-national differences in life expectancy are often linked to a country's wealth (Kawachi and Kennedy 2006) or to the distribution of income within a country (Wilkinson 1996). Moreover, when Krieger and colleagues (2008) examined inequities in premature mortality rates in the United States between 1960 and 2002, they found that as population health improves the magnitude of health inequalities can either rise or fall, and the reasons for the observed trends are largely unknown. For the most part, the general explanations of population health disparities are not focused on gender differences or the gender gap, so they don't provide a comprehensive understanding of these complexities.

However, some evidence of what contributes to the gender gap is provided by biomedical studies of sex-related changes in mortality rates in cardiovascular diseases and other specific diseases. In an influential article, Verbrugge and Wingard (1987) explained the paradox of men's higher mortality and lower morbidity compared to women's on the basis of gender differences in the patterns of disease. Unlike others who advanced the prevailing paradigm of focusing on men's premature mortality, Verbrugge and Wingard also called for researchers and clinicians to move beyond the focus on men's higher cardiovascular disease (CVD) mortality toward a more nuanced view of the gender differences in disease patterns over the life course. They also offered more complex explanations of the implications of gender differences in disease prevalence, including women's increased risk for CVD after menopause and their greater morbidity from debilitating illnesses such as rheumatoid arthritis. But a knowledge gap remains in understanding the sex-specific differences in the epidemiology of many specific diseases, and most notably cardiovascular diseases.

Disease Patterns in the United States

Our examination here of four conditions that vary considerably by gender—CVD and immune function disorders for physical health, and depression and substance abuse for mental health—is not intended to be exhaustive; rather we seek to provide a more complex portrait of specific patterns of gender difference in mental and physical health that extends beyond the life expectancy and mortality difference. We contend that this more nuanced picture also requires more multifaceted explanations than are typically articulated in a summary of gender differences in health.

CARDIOVASCULAR DISEASE (CVD)

CVD is the world's leading cause of death, causing one-third of all deaths globally, and the single largest cause of death among both men and women worldwide. In the United States, 8.4 percent of men and 5.6 percent of women report a diagnosis of CVD (Thom et al. 2006). Historically, men have greater prevalence and age-adjusted CVD mortality rates than women, a consistent finding across most developed countries (WHO 2006). While men outnumber women three or four to one in mortality from coronary heart disease (CHD) before age seventy-five, the gender difference in prevalence and incidence narrows at older ages (Verbrugge and Wingard 1987). A growing body of research indicates that despite later onset in women, risk factors such as smoking, family history, depression, diabetes, and inflammation (measured using C-reactive protein) may have a more negative influence on CVD in women than in men (Bassuk and Manson 2004; Pai et al. 2004; Thorand et al. 2007).

Due in part to earlier onset among men than among women, CVD also contributes substantially to gender differences in the number of years lived with and without CVD and related conditions (Crimmins, Kim, and Hagedorn 2002). For example, Crimmins and colleagues indicate that a cohort of women in the United States will experience 70 percent more years of life after age sixty-five with hypertension than a similar-sized birth cohort of men. Today, the patient undergoing treatment for CVD and hypertension is likely to be a woman beyond middle age. Yet until recently, scientists and clinicians focused on explaining and addressing the earlier onset of CVD in men, whereas the role of biological mechanisms in women's greater lifetime risk remained largely unexplored.[1] Ultimately women's increased inclusion in research led to a dramatic shift in knowledge and understanding regarding women's CVD risk (see Bird and Rieker 2008 for details on the Women's Health Initiative and this shift in research). However, this shift is only beginning to produce insights into the antecedents of gender differences in risk and life expectancy differences. For example, Shetty and colleagues (2009) took advantage of the sharp drop in women's use of Hormone Replacement Therapy (HRT) following the negative findings reported in 2002 regarding HRT and CVD to conduct an observational study of the relationship between HRT use and cardiovascular outcomes in the entire U.S. population. They found that the decreased use of HRT was associated with a decreased acute myocardial infarction rate among women but not with a reduced stroke rate.

IMMUNE FUNCTION AND DISORDERS

Researchers and clinicians are challenged and perplexed by the sex-linked patterns of immune function and disorders. The sex ratios in immune function also contribute to substantial differences in men's and women's disease risks and longevity. Although men and women tend to develop different disorders, women still have a greater risk than men of autoimmune rheumatic disorders and a higher risk of genetic immune suppression disorders (Jacobson et al. 1997; Lockshin 2001; Walsh and Rau 2000). Although the incidence of female/male ratios varies, the severity of the disease does not. For example, the female-to-male ratio of lupus, Graves', and Sjögren's is 7–10:1; that of rheumatoid arthritis, scleroderma, and multiple sclerosis is 2–3:1; while Type 1 diabetes and inflammatory bowel disease have equal sex frequencies (Lockshin 2006). Much of the disability men and women experience from rheumatologic and thyroid disorders, especially from middle age on, can be attributed to autoimmune disease. However, the differences in incidence in the most common disorders contribute to women's greater morbidity.

Since Selye's original work (1956) delineating physiological responses to stress, transdisciplinary research has greatly expanded our knowledge of human physiology and the ways that it can be influenced by social psychological phenomena (see Dedovic et al. 2009 for a review of gender socialization and stress reactivity). A growing body of evidence indicates that a variety of psychosocial factors can affect physiologic processes with implications for immune function. Researchers have described various possible pathways through which psychological factors impact immune function (Kiecolt-Glaser et al. 2002a, b). For example, some researchers and physicians argue that gender differences in men's and women's exposure to environmental substances and experiences of stress also contribute to gender differences in autoimmune disease incidence and severity

(Legato 2002; Lockshin et al. 1999). Moreover, there is considerable debate about whether sex hormones, including estrogen and testosterone, affect inflammatory and immune responses (Begg and Taylor 2006; Lockshin 2006; Lockshin, forthcoming).

MENTAL HEALTH

Although the overall rate of mental health disorders in the United States is similar for men and women, researchers, clinicians, and even women's rights advocates believed until the early 1990s that women suffer from higher rates of mental illness than do men (Chodorow 1978; Cleary, Mechanic, and Greenly 1982; Dohrenwend and Dohrenwend 1976, 1977; Gove and Tudor 1973). This assumption was based largely on the higher prevalence of depression among women and the fact that more women than men sought care for mental health problems. In addition, clinical studies suggested that the gender differences in depression had a hormonal basis and were at least partly biological, while sociologists contended that the differences were due to gender inequalities and restricted social roles.

However, findings based on the 1991 Epidemiologic Catchment Area Data (ECA) revealed that there are no large gender differences in the overall prevalence of major psychological disorders, whether one compares prevalence rates for one month, six months, a year, or a lifetime (Kessler, McGonagle, Zhao, et al. 1994; Regier and Robins 1991; Regier et al. 1993). Ten years later, the first nationally representative mental health study, the National Comorbidity Survey (NCS 1), confirmed these findings (Kessler and Walters 2002; Narrow et al. 2002).

The discrepancy with respect to prior findings is partly the result of the development of more rigorous research methods and of previous studies' focus on rates of depressive and anxiety disorders, which are higher among women; the ECA and the NCS included substance abuse, which is more common among men. The interpretation of the overall gender differences in mental health changed radically in light of new information on the full range of mental health disorders from these population-based studies. The new insights into men's and women's mental health reflected a typical pattern of scientific progress resulting from challenges to prior findings along with the application of more rigorous methods to answer both old and new questions.

In our discussion of gender differences in mental health, we focus on depression and substance abuse because they represent disorders with substantially different prevalence rates among men and women and because they create an enormous health burden (Kessler, Barker, et al. 2003). The World Health Organization (WHO) ranks major depression and substance abuse among the most burdensome diseases in the world (WHO 2002). Moreover, a growing body of research links depression and serious psychological distress with physical health (Pratt 2009; Whang et al. 2009), further illustrating the need to consider the interaction between physical and mental health in unraveling the puzzle of gender differences in health.

DEPRESSIVE DISORDERS

Women's rates of depressive disorders are 50 to 100 percent higher than men's (Gove and Tudor 1973; Kessler, Barker, et al. 2003; Kessler, Berglund, et al. 2003; Mirowsky and Ross 2003). Until the recent men's health movement, women's disproportionately high depression rates generated the erroneous impression that men were comparatively immune to depression (Courtenay 2000a, b). Clinicians' underdiagnosis of men's depression has been linked to a combination of gender differences in the causes and symptoms of depression, men's unwillingness to seek help for such feelings, as well as men's tendency to cope with sadness and loss through drinking and drug use and through acting-out and risk-taking behaviors (Bird and Rieker 2008; Chino and Funabaki 1984; Courtenay 2000a, b; Nolen-Hoeksema 1987, 1990). When symptoms of depression are acknowledged and diagnosed, men as well as women appear to seek treatment (Nazroo, Edwards, and Brown 1998; Rhodes et al. 2002).

Although men and women do differ in the age and rates of onset of depression (young males have higher rates until early adolescence), the gender gap appears to be greatest during the reproductive years (Bebbington 1996; Piccinelli and Wilkinson 2000). Moreover, while cross-sectional studies indicate that once major depression develops, the course is similar for both genders (Kessler, McGonagle, Swartz et al. 1993; Wilhelm, Parker, and Hadzi-Pavlovic 1997), several longitudinal studies have reported that girls and women have longer episodes and higher rates of recurrent and chronic depression (Aneshensel 1985; Ernst and Angst 1992; Keitner et al. 1991; Kornstein et al. 2000; Sargeant et al. 1990; Winokur et al. 1993). What is clear is that women have consistently higher lifetime prevalence rates for depression, and that depressed women are more likely than are men to have comorbid anxiety (Gregory and Endicott 1999; Kessler, Berglund et al. 2003), while men are more likely to have comorbid substance abuse or dependence (Endicott 1998; Kessler, Berglund et al. 2003). However the determinants of these gender differences and how they are related to substance abuse and other mental health disorders is unclear (Piccinelli and Wilkinson 2000).

SUBSTANCE ABUSE DISORDERS

Men have significantly higher rates of alcohol and drug use, abuse, and dependence, as well as antisocial behavior disorders, than do women (Kessler, McGonagle, Zhao et al. 1994; Regier et al. 1993). In fact, the prevalence of substance abuse disorders in men and women is the reverse of that seen for depression. The gender difference in prevalence of substance use is smallest among adolescents, increases with age, and varies by type and level of drug use (Kandel, Warner, and Kessler 1998).

Although those who initiate substance use earlier in life are more likely to continue using and to become dependent, not all users in any age group become dependent (even with highly addictive substances). With the exception of tobacco, lifetime dependence rates are considerably higher for men than for women (Kessler, Crum et al. 1997; Kessler, McGonagle, Zhao et al. 1994; Kessler, Nelson et al. 1996). It is unclear whether the gendered patterns in dependence among users are due to greater use of alcohol by men and of psychotherapeutics by women, or to other biological and environmental factors that vary by drug type (see Pescosolido et al. 2008 for a detailed and nuanced analysis of the pathway

to alcohol dependence in men and women and the complex interplay between social and genetic influences). However, extensive comorbidity exists between drug and alcohol disorders, as well as with other psychiatric disorders in both men and women, especially in those with a major depressive disorder (Kessler, Berglund et al. 2003; Kessler, Nelson et al. 1996).

The emerging field of men's studies recognizes that while gender roles advantage men in some ways, they disadvantage them in others, and that not all men are equally advantaged nor are all women equally disadvantaged (Cameron and Bernardes 1998; Harrison 1978; Kimmel and Messner 1993; Pleck 1983, 1984; Pleck and Brannon 1978; Rieker and Bird 2000, 2005; Sabo and Gordon 1995). Work by Courtenay (2000a, b) and others has also begun to reexamine the role of masculine identities in the development of men's unhealthy and risky behaviors and subsequent mental and physical health problems. Other research has focused on stressors to which men are either more exposed or potentially more vulnerable, such as those in the workplace and in the military (Connell 1987; Jaycox 2008; Levant and Pollack 1995; Sabo and Gordon 1995). For instance, combat duty, which continues to be more common for men, puts soldiers at risk for post-traumatic stress disorder (PTSD), whereas physical and sexual abuse remains the most likely PTSD risk factor for women (Rieker and Carmen 1984).[2] In contrast, the stress associated with being unemployed can differ depending on one's options and constraints: unemployed women frequently have access to more socially acceptable roles than men do, including caregiver and housewife, which are more highly stigmatized for men and may therefore lead to greater stress or simply deter men from considering or accepting these roles (Lennon 2006). The high rates of combat duty in recent and ongoing wars and conflicts, along with the high current rates of unemployment, provide an important opportunity for much-needed research to better understand vulnerability to depression and PTSD and to learn more about how to provide better care to men and women afflicted with these debilitating disorders. Such research can also inform theories that explain both male and female psychological health and illness and the ways these gender patterns vary across race, class, and ethnicity.

Pathways and Mechanisms Underlying Gender Differences

Although social and biological pathways to illness and the mechanisms connecting them with gender differences in health are relatively unexplored, we would like to suggest some topics that warrant attention. For example, a growing body of research demonstrates that mental and physical health are deeply intertwined. Thus, not only can physical health problems cause symptoms that appear to be attributable to one's mental health or current mental state (such as fatigue, hopelessness), but also mental health conditions can exacerbate physical health problems, and serious or chronic physical health problems can lead to depression or anxiety. Understanding relationships between physical and mental health is relevant to researching and explaining health trajectories, identifying opportunities for intervention, and recognizing the full benefits of such interventions in terms of reduced morbidity and mortality.

Impact of Health Behaviors on Physical and Mental Health

Health behaviors are a primary pathway through which psychological distress and depression impact health. For example, a longitudinal study of patients with stable cardiovascular disease found that the association between depressive symptoms and subsequent cardiovascular events was explained in part by differences in health behaviors, including smoking, alcohol use, and level of physical activity (Whooley et al. 2008). Individuals with more depressive symptoms at baseline engaged in fewer positive and more negative health behaviors and consequently faced an increased risk of cardiovascular events.

Gender differences in both mental health and self-care may exacerbate the problem of negative effects of psychological distress and depression on specific health behaviors. In particular, although women engage more often in self-care behaviors than men do, they are somewhat less likely to engage in regular physical activity. Moreover, depressed mood may reduce any female advantage in health behaviors, as women typically begin to drop self-care behaviors before decreasing their caring for others (Rosenfield 1999). Depressed mood and other mental health problems may similarly affect men and women by reducing positive health behaviors, even though men and women engage on average in somewhat different positive behaviors (Reeves and Rafferty 2005; Whooley et al. 2008).

Recent research also suggests that some negative health behaviors play a central role in gender differences in health. For example, Grundtvig and colleagues (2009) examined data from 1,784 patients admitted for a first heart attack at a hospital in Lillehammer, Norway. Their retrospective study found that on average men had their first heart attack at age seventy-two if they didn't smoke, and at sixty-four if they did. In contrast, women in the study had their first heart attack at age eighty-one if they didn't smoke, and at age sixty-six if they did. If supported by prospective studies, their data suggest that smoking drastically reduces gender differences in age at first heart attack, narrowing women's advantage from nine to merely two years. Grundtvig speculated that smoking may lead to earlier onset of menopause in women, reducing the length of women's premenopausal protection from heart disease. Thus smoking represents a negative health behavior that is frequently used in part as a means of coping with stress, but that also interacts differently with men's and women's biology to increase their health risks. Other health conditions related to health behavior and cardiovascular disease have also been found to have a greater negative effect on women's health than men's. For example, diabetes in particular has been found to outweigh (and even eliminate) women's otherwise lower cardiovascular risk prior to menopause (Kannel and Wilson 1995; Sowers 1998). In regard to diabetes, Lutfey and Freese (2005) use ethnographic data to provide an in-depth analysis of the mechanisms that perpetuate disparities in diabetes treatment regimens, including some differences between men and women.

As West and Zimmerman (1987) argued, a cost and consequence of living in a social world is the ongoing process of *doing gender*. Specifically, individuals are expected in innumerable social circumstances to express themselves in gender-appropriate ways (Ridgeway and Smith-Lovin 1999; Taylor et al. 2000). While gender roles have become far less circumscribed over time, gender scripts remain and are obvious even in fitness recommendations (Dworkin and Wachs 2009). Moreover, behaving and communicating in ways that are seen as gender appropriate are rewarded in subtle ways.

Recent work suggests that men and women also have some physiologic differences that may complement the social norms to behave in gender-appropriate ways. Partly in response to the extensive literature on the fight-or-flight response, most of which was theorized and studied in males (including animal studies), Taylor and colleagues (2000) began to study and write about the "tend or befriend" stress response, which they contend is supported by a hormonal response present only in females. They do not suggest that males are prevented from responding to stress with the same hypervigilance aimed at protecting and caring for others they found in females, but that in females, oxytocin encourages these specific behaviors. Compared to men, women tend to engage in more nurturant activities designed to protect the self and others that in turn promote safety and reduce distress. Women also tend to create and maintain social networks that may aid in this process. This gendered response to stress is encouraged and supported both socially and biologically (Ridgeway and Smith-Lovin 1999; Taylor et al. 2000). Unlike the fight-or-flight response, which is hormonally present in both men and women, oxytocin in conjunction with female reproductive hormones and endogenous opioid peptide mechanisms supports the "tend and befriend" stress regulatory mechanism. Taylor and colleagues proposed that the attachment-caregiving system forms the biobehavioral underpinnings of tending and befriending in response to stress. These in turn may contribute to differences in men's and women's CVD risk and mortality.

Pescosolido and colleagues (2008) provide another example in their study of how gendered stress reactions become part of the pathway to alcohol dependence. In their provocative findings, they explicate the causal pathway through which the gene GABRA2 interacts with social factors to produce gender differences in alcohol dependence. Specifically, they conclude that "genetic predisposition to alcohol dependence on GABRA2 is operative in men but not in women" (S192). The genetic inheritance of GABRA2 can become triggered or suppressed through social patterns. Daily hassles, past stressors, and the coping response differentiate men and women regarding their propensity to engage in "escapist drinking." The researchers contend that drinking to excess in public is also more acceptable for men and that such behavior sets men up for greater alcohol dependence, which then can be attenuated or exacerbated by early childhood deprivation and family-based social support.

Thus social processes and biological mechanisms can interact in complex ways to produce observed differences in men's and women's health. Earlier explanations of women's higher morbidity hinged largely or exclusively on the negative consequences of female social and economic disadvantages (for a review, see Wingard 1984), whereas the explanations of women's greater longevity focused solely on the hypothesized biological advantages of hormones (see Ramey 1982). Yet each explanation applied to only a narrow portion of the complex differences in men's and women's health. As we have argued elsewhere, what is needed to advance research and understanding of gender differences in morbidity and mortality is a synthesis of social and biological theories and evidence. To begin to address this conundrum, we introduced a model of constrained choice as a promising direction for understanding and researching gender differences and other health disparities (Rieker and Bird 2005).

Constrained Choice: A Different Way to View Health Disparities

Much of the recent work on health disparities focuses primarily on the contribution of socioeconomic status. We take a broader perspective on the range of factors that pattern individual lives. In so doing, we identify additional potential levers for addressing gender, racial/ethnic, and socioeconomic disparities in health. While population health and the health of disadvantaged subgroups are in part functions of the income distribution in a society, it does not necessarily follow that income redistribution is the most feasible and effective way to address such disparities. Nor is it clear that such efforts would address gender differences in health or effectively resolve disparities among men and among women (James et al. 2009; Murray et al. 2006). While other countries (notably, the Nordic countries) have instituted a multifaceted series of policies affecting the distribution of income, such policies are unlikely in the United States in the foreseeable future.

We offer constrained choice as an alternative framework that recognizes a wider range of contributing factors and thus identifies additional research foci and intervention points for improving individual and population health. Our approach is not intended to minimize the role of social inequalities in health or to emphasize individual behaviors over structural factors. To the contrary, we developed a framework that shows how structural constraints narrow the opportunities and choices available to individuals in both absolute and relative ways. In the extreme case, structural inequalities socially pattern health, creating or exacerbating particular gender, racial/ethnic, and socioeconomic disparities in health; for example, when discrimination creates differential opportunities for specific groups, it enhances or protects the range of opportunities for some while constraining them for others. But discrimination is not the only factor that socially patterns the constraints that men and women (as a group or individually) experience in their everyday lives and that also affect their health. While the impact of gender roles may be obvious —including differences in the distribution and nature of caregiving and other relationships at the level of family—the indirect health impact of decisions at the levels of community and social policy have received far less attention in research to date.

In *Gender and Health* (Bird and Rieker 2008), we presented the constrained-choice model to address these gaps. The multilevel model explains how decisions made and actions taken at the family, work, community, and government levels contribute to differences in individuals' opportunities to incorporate health into a broad array of everyday choices. We argue that the unintentional and cumulative consequences of constrained choice socially pattern women's and men's lives in differential ways that impact their exposure to stressors, their health behaviors, and their physiology. Therefore, we conclude that health is not only an individual responsibility but one shared by decision makers at multiple levels.

Levels and Processes of Constrained Choice

Individuals make everyday choices that create health outcomes. Furthermore, they make these choices in the context of family, employment settings, and community. For example, many young families must negotiate ongoing decisions on where to live, how to balance career with family life, child rearing, child care, and financial management. When attempting to meet these explicit priorities every day, young families may make immediate choices that are not health promoting. Consider a dual income family: over the course of a day a parent may choose to skip breakfast to ensure being able to drop a child off at daycare and get to work on time. A parent may bring home a fast-food dinner in order to spend time with family rather than spend time cooking, or simply to get food on the table quickly to feed a hungry family. Similarly, a parent may choose to sleep less in order to spend time with children, manage the household, or complete work-related tasks. None of these actions are necessarily gender-specific nor may any of them as discreet, individual actions result in major health consequences. Yet when the wider context shapes and constrains opportunities and choices, as it does in everyone's life to varying degrees, such trade-offs can have cumulative effects on health. These choices occur and play out in gendered ways, as men's and women's everyday decisions and priorities differ somewhat on average, due in part to differences in their social roles. Moreover, the consequences of such everyday actions cumulatively affect health, and their impact depends in part on innate and acquired differences in men's and women's biology or genetic predisposition.

Our model of constrained choice includes three levels of organizational context that can influence men's and women's health outcomes: social policy, community actions, and work and family (see Figure 4.1). The model demonstrates how decisions made within these organizational contexts can limit the opportunities that individuals have to choose healthy behaviors. Two recent reports on racial and ethnic disparities in women's health across the United States demonstrate clearly such constraints (James et al. 2009; Rustgi, Doty, and Collins 2009). The model also acknowledges how the interplay between gendered health choices and sex-specific biological patterns and responses can shape morbidity and mortality outcomes.

WORK AND FAMILY

Many of the differences in men's and women's lives are rooted in their work and family roles. Men and women are exposed to different kinds of work, as well as differences in pay and other benefits. Occupations and social roles carry expectations, create routines of daily life, and establish norms of social interaction, all of which contribute to stress levels, health-related behaviors, and coping styles. For example, a role such as single parent or caregiver to aging parents or to children with special health-care needs can be time consuming and stressful, and these roles are more often performed by women. Moreover, both work and family roles include flexible or inflexible demands (such as urgent situations that require immediate attention) or routines that may not easily be combined with other obligations. Even for those who do not work from home, the boundaries between work and home life have become increasingly blurred as technology makes us always available. While in theory this flexibility increases the possibilities for managing conflicting demands, it also reduces the physical and temporal boundaries between work and home life for both singles and couples.

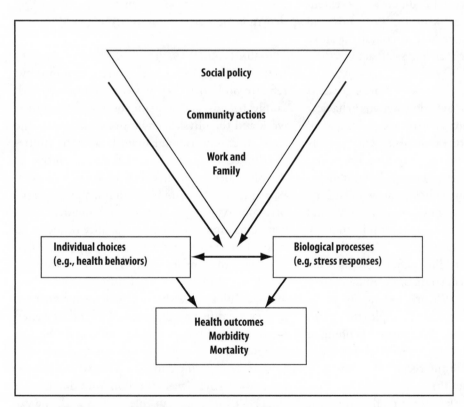

Figure 4.1. Conceptualization of Constrained Choice
Source: Bird, C.E., & Rieker, P.P. (2008). *Gender and health: The effects of constrained choices and social policies.* New York: Cambridge University Press.

Even though differences in men's and women's roles have diminished over time, the lingering differences have cumulative effects on health and on the ways in which family decisions impact health. For example, compared to men, women typically acquire more health information and take a larger role in the health of their families. Clearly men and women continue to be differentially distributed across industries and workplaces, with more women in service occupations and men more concentrated in manufacturing, transportation, and military work. Occupations and work environments differ substantially in both the demands placed on workers and the level of control individuals have over the speed and content of their work. Whereas some occupations and work environments provide manageable demands and healthy and supportive environments, others place substantial physical or emotional demands on employees. High-demand and low-control work has been shown to be particularly stressful in ways that impact health (Theorell and Karasek 1996). Workplaces also differ in the extent to which they provide work-life programs and policies that facilitate or even encourage positive health behaviors such as physical activity and healthy eating.

Some workplaces or work arrangements may indirectly promote destructive behaviors such as smoking, poor diet, or even excess alcohol consumption. For example, a British study demonstrated that working very long hours was negatively associated with women's, but not men's, health behaviors; among those who worked long hours, the women consumed more high-fat and high-sugar snacks, exercised less, and, if smokers, smoked more (O'Connor et al. 2005). There is generally less understanding about how men experience structural constraints, formulate their priorities, or respond to work and family stress, or about when and how, for example, they learn to turn to alcohol and drugs as forms of coping or self-care. Such information is essential to designing gender-appropriate interventions to improve men's and women's health.

Norms of long work hours can affect the costs and consequences of achieving success at work by reducing the possibility of balancing work, family, and time for exercise and other positive self-care

activities. In their insightful critique of the media's role in selling the desire for perfect bodies rather than health and healthy behaviors, Dworkin and Wachs (2009) describe the different priorities and time constraints on men's and women's health behavior and self-care. In describing the barriers women face after pregnancy and childbirth, they characterize paid work as the first shift, work in the home (child care, feeding oneself and the family, paying bills, and otherwise maintaining a household) as the second shift, and the time spent pursuing health and fitness regimens that allow for adherence to the latest bodily requirements as promoted in the media as the third shift (see also Dworkin 2001; Dworkin and Messner 1999). Individuals, particularly those with long work hours or family caregiving responsibilities, typically fit exercise and other activities they view as health promoting into their schedules after addressing these other tasks and responsibilities. Thus, both theory and evidence suggest that women are more likely than men to minimize or forgo such self-care in response to the competing demands on their time and energy.

COMMUNITY ACTIONS

In the constrained-choice model, "community" refers to both social networks of relationships with family, friends, and acquaintances at home and at work and the physical environment in which one lives. Thus one can imagine these communities distributed on a continuum from supportive to draining, negating the effects of stress or exacerbating them or enlarging or diminishing options of many types. These social and physical environments affect the ease or difficulty of men and women in meeting the demands of specific roles. However, the impact of living in a community at a given point along this continuum would on average differ somewhat for men versus women, as they are differentially exposed to and impacted by available resources and stressors. For example, as noted earlier, men and women differ in their exposure to specific daily stressors, which in turn affect their stress levels and responses due in part to gender differences in role activity and role expectations. At the community level, gender roles and responsibilities interact with resources and barriers such as employment opportunities or security, the provision of child care and elder care (both as givers and recipients of each), mass transit, and public safety.

The study of the impact of community or neighborhood on health is a rapidly growing transdisciplinary field of research. Yet research focused on assessing and explaining gender differences in the links between neighborhood factors and mortality is just emerging. For example, Grafova and colleagues (2008) found that economic and social environment aspects were important for men's risk of obesity, whereas aspects of the built environment were more important for women's. Similarly, Anderson and colleagues (1997) reported that the relationship between neighborhood socioeconomic status and mortality varied by age, gender, and race/ethnicity. Men and women typically live in the same neighborhoods, so unlike workplace effect, residential place effects are not related to gender segregation. Also, many studies have found gender differences in the link between neighborhood deprivation—an index generally based on unemployment, income, educational attainment, and utilization of public assistance—and health and mortality (Berke et al. 2007; Ross et al. 2007). Winkleby, Sundquist, and Cubbin (2007) found an association between higher neighborhood-level deprivation and both incident coronary heart disease and one-year case fatality for Swedish adults, with slightly stronger effects among women.

While such studies show that neighborhood effects contribute to gender differences in health, it remains unclear how neighborhood effects get under the skin. Men and women may differ in their physiological responses to particular neighborhood features partly through the possible impact on health behaviors. For example, Ross and colleagues (2007) found metropolitan sprawl was associated with higher body mass index (BMI) for men, but the effect was not significant for women. This finding may be explained by research showing that men and women use neighborhood features such as parks differently and that neighborhood walkability is more strongly associated with men's walking (Cohen et al. 2006; Morenoff and Sampson 1997). Other research has shown gender differences in how men and women incorporate social support and social

networks. For men, such influences are often more place based. For women, place of residence may not be as strong an influence as work, family, and other social and role-related influences in their lives. Taken together, this work suggests that men's health behaviors may be more strongly affected by characteristics of their residential environment.

SOCIAL POLICY

Finally, the constrained-choice framework includes the impact of social policy, including federal, state, and local government decisions and policies. To illustrate this at the federal level, we explored the proposition that different types of policy regimes formulate policies and regulations that directly and indirectly affect gender differences in health. We used cross-national differences in longevity and the gender gap in health behaviors to show how these policies could differentially increase the options and opportunities to for men and women to pursue health (see Bird and Rieker 2008, chapters 3 and 6). Obvious examples of social policies that affect health are universal day care, universal access to education, and retirement benefits not tied to employment or retirement benefits that affect continued employment. Such policies provide an economic safety net through a variety of public and private mechanisms and assure at least a minimum level of income and health-care access for a country's citizens. In addition, for a more general discussion emphasizing the value of integrating and the need to integrate medical sociology and social welfare theory, see Olafsdottir and Beckfield 2009.

These policies can have intended and unintended differential effects on men's and women's lives regardless of whether policy makers assume the genders are the same or different. However, the more critical issue is how much responsibility the state assumes for protective public health regulations and especially for family well-being and child care, and how much remains the responsibility of individuals and families. For example, in social democratic regimes such as the Nordic countries, where the state has more responsibility, both longevity and health status are better than in liberal regimes such as the United States and

Australia, where social policies rely on the market and where health care is tied to employment. Other examples concern antismoking and alcohol regulations enacted at the country or state level and the demonstrable effects these have had on declines in smoking rates and alcohol abuse (see Bird and Rieker 2008, chapter 6).

Consider also, for example, how in the United States the current recession has had a far greater effect on men's employment to date than on women's, due largely to the job losses in manufacturing (U.S. Department of Labor 2009a, b, c), resulting in the highest gender gap in unemployment in U.S. history (10 percent for men vs. 7.6 percent for women in April 2009). However, women are more highly represented in the part-time work force, which offers fewer benefits; thus a combination of recent economic trends and employment policies differentially affect men's and women's exposure to job and income loss and the related risk of loss of health insurance. Ironically perhaps, within families, higher rates of unemployment among men increase pressure on women to fill the role of breadwinner, despite their lower average incomes and differences in average work hours and benefits (Hartmann 2008; Lorber 1995; Risman 1998). Moreover as Heidi Hartmann (2008) noted in her congressional testimony on the impact of the current economic downturn on women: "A recession or weak job growth will only exacerbate the problems that face mothers who want and need to work but must find work that is compatible with their families' needs."

Loue (2008) notes that our cross-national comparison of health and economic indicators "underscores the irony of the position of the United States: even as we emphasize individual choice and responsibility for health, we fail as a nation to address and rectify the larger constraints that constitute barriers to opportunities and impediments to choice." Thus while our work to date has focused on the ways in which the social organization of men's and women's lives contributes to gender differences in health, our constrained-choice model clearly applies to racial/ethnic and socioeconomic health disparities as well. For example, differences in opportunities shape the trade-offs and choices made by racial and ethnic minorities—from where to live and what job to take, to who is responsible for caring for children and the elderly (Bird and Rieker 2008). Thus, we argue that the constrained-choice framework is also relevant to understanding and intervening on racial/ethnic disparities in health. An explanation of the complex link between gender and health behaviors cannot be complete without addressing the relationship of SES to healthy lifestyles and to health over the life course, but that broader discussion is beyond the scope of this chapter.

Future Research Questions and Issues to Consider

The idea that decisions and policies at multiple levels affect health is not new. Researchers, employers, public health officials, and policy makers use both implicit and explicit ecological models to understand and estimate the health effects of specific decisions and to identify individual, environmental, and population-based ways to reduce risk and unsafe behaviors. However, such models and health improvement efforts seldom focus on whether and how pathways and effects may differ by gender.

What do constrained-choice and gender-based analysis have to contribute to the study of health disparities and ultimately to population health? They can provide an understanding of how decisions made and actions taken at the family, work, community, and government levels differentially shape women's and men's health-related priorities, opportunities, and choices. This is not to suggest that individual health and behavior are fully determined by external forces, but that priorities and decisions beyond the level of the individual can reduce the latitude or sense of agency individuals have and the options they perceive in everyday life to pursue health. Clearly, many regulatory measures such as protecting and improving air quality and assuring a clean water supply or the safety of food and other products are largely beyond the reach of most individuals. Thus, we view constrained choice as a platform for prevention where the intention is to create a different kind of health consciousness, one that recognizes the role of differential gender constraints as an additional means for improving population health, both among individuals and decision makers at all levels. Moreover this model includes consideration of how racial/ethnic and socioeconomic constraints interact with sex and gender to produce health disparities among men and among women. As a research framework, it calls for transdisciplinary and comparative approaches at a variety of levels, and for studies that take into account the longer-term costs of policies that damage or undermine health, as well as the benefits of policies that foster health.

Recognizing the contributions to both individual and population health and to health disparities of decisions made at multiple levels beyond the individual raises key questions for researchers, clinicians, and policy makers. For example: Whose responsibility is health? Are protective measures, preventive behaviors, and the costs and consequences of poor health practices the province of individuals, families, the workplace, communities, states, or some combination of these? How such questions are answered has ramifications for improving population health and studying gender and health (see for example Walter and Neumann 2009 on how advances in gender sensitivity and analysis can affect health).

Other key questions seldom raised are: How can we measure the contribution of social, political, and economic policies to gender differences in health? How important are nonhealth policies for improving population health and preventing illness? How do we account for health-care access and quality within a constrained-choice framework (see Banks et al. 2006 and Schoeni et al. 2008 for an elaboration of some of these issues)? How do such policies interact with advances in biomedical science and technology to produce health? Although not focused on gender, others have been thinking about these topics as well. For example, Phelan and Link (2005) address the bidirectionality of biomedical processes and social phenomena in a way that resonates with our model. They argue that over the past century biomedical science and technology advances have made it possible for individuals to avoid some diseases and live longer, thereby transforming disease patterns and increasing human control over health. The added

control makes understanding social factors even more important for improving population health through a "social shaping" approach (Link 2008). Link also notes that "when humans have control, it is their policies, their knowledge, and their behaviors that shape the consequences of biomedical accomplishments and thereby extant patterns of disease and death" (36).

We contend that constrained choice along with gender-based research can lead to better science. This approach provides an opportunity to explore biological and social pathways and mechanisms together as gender opens a window into biological processes, which is not the case with race/ethnicity and SES. However, if we start with gender and examine the intersectionalities with race/ethnicity and SES, then constrained choice can provide a glimpse of the pathways and mechanisms that create gendered health behaviors and outcomes (see Loue 2006 for a discussion of methods and measurement issues in such sex/gender research). Moreover there are a variety of ways and levels at which gender differences can be addressed. Briefly, research can be focused on: disease patterns; a specific disease or biological and genetic predispositions; health behaviors; comparative social regimes and health status; employment patterns; differential stress exposure and responses; and social networks. These topics can be studied as variations within a country, as cross-national comparisons, or as some combination of these.

Research such as what we are advocating is already under way. There is considerable momentum to include both biological and social factors in health studies, a trend observable in both research and policy domains where gender-based analysis is promoted (see for example Fausto-Sterling 2008, 2005; Johnson, Greaves, and Repta 2007, 2009; Klinge 2007; Lohan 2007; Spitzer 2005). These efforts will substantially advance understanding of the biological and social circumstances and identify pathways and mechanisms that expose men and women to harmful stress levels or that place them at risk for adopting unsafe health behaviors that contribute to differential outcomes. Pescosolido and colleagues' (2008) analysis of the intersecting biological and social pathways to gender differences in alcohol dependence provides one very promising example. These authors not only examine the genetic and social interaction empirically but also address the implications of the findings for sociological theories. Extending this thinking to gender-based analysis and theories would advance our knowledge of these phenomena.

If sociologists seek to improve population health and reduce health disparities by influencing the broad range of decisions that occur beyond the level of the individual but affect opportunities to pursue a healthy life, there is much work to be done. The next phase of gender and health comparison work should include the application of the constrained-choice framework to various research agendas. Decision makers at all levels need actionable evidence from gender-focused, generalizable studies on the health benefits or costs of specific choices and policies. This approach requires analyses of the health effects of particular policies that provide clear directives for action beyond the provision of and access to health care. For example, where work to date has typically sought to capture the short-term, and in some cases longer-term, economic costs of policies as diverse as education, employment, and transportation, constrained choice suggests that assessing and reporting the probable health impacts would allow policy makers to take population health effects into account and to value health in considering the trade-offs among policy options (Schoeni et al. 2008). In a society where future prosperity depends on the health and well-being of the population, researchers have tremendous new opportunities to inform policy decisions and a responsibility to take into account whether and how specific policies will affect population health. Attention to the differences in men's and women's lives can further assure that policies will not inadvertently exacerbate these differences or contribute to health disparities among men or among women.

Notes

1. The *Canadian Medical Association Journal* devoted a special issue (March 13, 2007) to the knowledge gap in understanding the sex-specific differences in the epidemiology of CVD. For example, in one article Pilote and colleagues (2007) conclude that the knowledge gap might explain why cardiovascular health is not improving as rapidly among women as it is in men, and that the regional/country gender differences in CVD incidence may result from an interaction between sex- and gender-related factors.

2. Although both combat duty and exposure to sexual abuse are PTSD risk factors for both men and women, their exposure rates differ by gender. However, women's increasing presence in combat roles and a growing recognition of the prevalence of sexual abuse of boys by clergy members may be narrowing these long-standing differences.

References

Abramowicz, Mark, and Henry L. Barnett. 1970. "Sex Ratio of Infant Mortality." *American Journal of Diseases of Children* 119(4): 314–15.

Anderson, Roger T., Paul Sorlie, Eric Backlund, Norman Johnson, and George A. Kaplan. 1997. "Mortality Effects of Community Socioeconomic Status." *Epidemiology* 8(1): 42–47.

Andoh, S. Y., M. Umezaki, K. Nakamura, M. Kizuki, and Takehito Takano. 2006. "Correlation between National Income, HIV/AIDS and Political Status and Mortalities in African Countries." *Public Health* 120(7): 624–33.

Aneshensel, Carol S. 1985. "The Natural History of Depressive Symptoms." *Research in Community and Mental Health* 5:45–74.

Annandale, Ellen. 2009. *Women's Health and Social Change*. London: Routledge.

Banks, James, Michael Marmot, Zoe Oldfield, and James P. Smith. 2006. "Disease and Disadvantage in the United States and in England." *Journal of the American Medical Association* 295(17): 2037–45.

Bassuk, Shari S., and JoAnn E. Manson. 2004. "Gender and Its Impact on Risk Factors for Cardiovascular Disease." In *Principles of Gender Specific Medicine*, ed. M. J. Legato, 193–213. London: Elsevier Academic Press.

Bebbington, Paul. 1996. "The Origins of Sex Differences in Depressive Disorder: Bridging the Gap." *International Review of Psychiatry* 8(4): 295–332.

Begg, Lisa, and Christopher E. Taylor. 2006. "Regulation of Inflammatory Responses: Influence of Sex and Gender: Workshop Summary." In *NIH Workshop: Regulation of Inflammatory Responses: Influence of Sex and Gender*. Bethesda, Md.: Office of Research on Women's Health.

Berin, Barnet N., George L. Stolnitz, and Aaron Tenenbein. 1989. "Mortality Trends of Males and Females over the Ages." *Transactions of Society of Actuaries* 41(1): 9–32.

Berke, Ethan M., Laura M. Gottlieb, Anne V. Moudon,

and Eric B. Larson. 2007. "Protective Association between Neighborhood Walkability and Depression in Older Men." *Journal of the American Geriatrics Society* 55(4): 526–33.

Bird, Chloe E., and Patricia P. Rieker. 2008. *Gender and Health: The Effects of Constrained Choices and Social Policies*. New York: Cambridge University Press.

Cameron, Elaine, and Jon Bernardes. 1998. "Gender and Disadvantage in Health: Men's Health for a Change." *Sociology of Health and Illness* 20(5): 673–93.

Chino, Allan F., and Dean Funabaki. 1984. "A Cross-Validation of Sex Differences in the Expression of Depression." *Sex Roles* 11(3–4): 175–87.

Chodorow, Nancy J. 1978. *The Reproduction of Mothering*. Berkeley: University of California Press.

Cleary, Paul D., David Mechanic, and James R. Greenly. 1982. "Sex Differences in Medical Care Utilization: An Empirical Investigation." *Journal of Health and Social Behavior* 23(2): 106–19.

Cohen, Deborah A.; Amber Sehgal, Stephanie Williamson, Ronald Sturm, Thomas L. McKenzie, Rosa Lara, and Nicole Lurie. 2006. "Park Use and Physical Activity in a Sample of Public Parks in the City of Los Angeles." Santa Monica, Calif.: RAND Corporation.

Connell, Robert W. 1987. *Gender and Power*. Stanford, Calif.: Stanford University Press.

Courtenay, Will H. 2000a. "Behavioral Factors Associated with Disease, Injury, and Death among Men: Evidence and Implications for Prevention." *Journal of Men's Studies* 9(1): 81–142.

———. 2000b. "Constructions of Masculinity and Their Influence on Men's Well-Being: A Theory of Gender and Health." *Social Science and Medicine* 50(10): 1385–1401.

Crimmins, Eileen M., Jung K. Kim, and Aaron Hagedorn. 2002. "Life with and without Disease: Women Experience More of Both." *Journal of Women and Aging* 14(1–2): 47–59.

Dedovic, Katarina, Mehereen Wadiwalla, Veronica Engert, and Jens C. Pruessner. 2009. "The Role of Sex and Gender Socialization in Stress Reactivity." *Developmental Psychology* 45(1): 45–55.

Dohrenwend, Bruce P., and Barbara S. Dohrenwend. 1976. "Sex Differences and Psychiatric Disorders." *American Journal of Sociology* 81(6): 1147–54.

———. 1977. "Reply to Gove and Tudor's Comment on 'Sex Differences and Psychiatric Disorders.'" *American Journal of Sociology* 82(6): 1336–45.

Dworkin, Shari L. 2001. "'Holding Back': Negotiating a Glass Ceiling on Women's Strength." *Sociological Perspectives* 44(3): 333–50.

Dworkin, Shari L., and Michael A. Messner. 1999. "Just Do What? Sport, Bodies, Gender." In *Revisioning Gender*, ed. M. M. Ferree, J. Lorber, and B. B. Hess, 341–61. Thousand Oaks, Calif.: Sage Publications.

Dworkin, Shari L., and Faye L. Wachs. 2009. *Body Panic: Gender, Health, and the Selling of Fitness*. New York: New York University Press.

Endicott, Jean. 1998. "Gender Similarities and Differences in the Course of Depression." *Journal of Gender-Specific Medicine* 1(3): 40–43.

Ernst, Cecille, and Jules Angst. 1992. "The Zurich Study, XII: Sex Differences in Depression: Evidence from Longitudinal Epidemiological Data." *European Archives of Psychiatry and Clinical Neuroscience* 241(4): 222–30.

Fausto-Sterling, Anne. 2005. "The Bare Bones of Sex: Part 1—Sex and Gender." *Signs* 30(5): 1491–1526.

———. 2008. "The Bare Bones of Race." *Social Studies of Science* 38(5): 657–94.

Gove, Walter R., and Jeannette F. Tudor. 1973. "Adult Sex Roles and Mental Illness." *American Journal of Sociology* 78(4): 812–35.

Grafova, Irina B., Vicki A. Freedman, Rizie Kumar, and Jeannette Rogowski. 2008. "Neighborhoods and Obesity in Later Life." *American Journal of Public Health* 98(11): 2065–71.

Gregory, Tanya, and Jean Endicott. 1999. "Understanding Depression in Women." *Patient Care* 33(19): 19–20.

Grundtvig, Morten, Terje P. Hagen, Mikael German, and Asmund Reikvam. 2009. "Sex-Based Differences in Premature First Myocardial Infarction Caused by Smoking: Twice as Many Years Lost by Women as Men." *European Journal of Cardiovascular Prevention and Rehabilitation* 16(2): 174–79.

Harrison, James. 1978. "Warning: The Male Sex Role May Be Dangerous to Your Health." *Journal of Social Issues* 34(1): 65–86.

Hartmann, Heidi. 2008. "The Impact of the Current Economic Downturn on Women (Testimony Presented to the Joint Economic Committee)." Washington, D.C.: Institute for Women's Policy Research.

Hunt, Kate, and Ellen Annandale. 1999. "Relocating Gender and Morbidity: Examining Men's and Women's Health in Contemporary Western Societies. Introduction to Special Issue on Gender and Health." *Social Science and Medicine* 48(1): 1–5.

Institute of Medicine. 2001a. *Exploring the Biological Contributions to Human Health: Does Sex Matter?* ed. T. M. Wizemann and M. L. Pardue. Washington, D.C.: National Academies Press.

———. 2001b. *Health and Behavior: The Interplay of Biological, Behavioral and Societal Influences*. Washington, D.C.: National Academies Press.

Jacobson, Denise L., Stephen J. Gange, Noel R. Rose,

and Neil M. Graham. 1997. "Epidemiology and Estimated Population Burden of Selected Autoimmune Diseases in the United States." *Clinical Immunology and Immunopathology* 84(3): 223–43.

James, Cara V., Alina Salganicoff, Megan Thomas, Usha Ranji, Marsha Lillie-Blanton, and Roberta Wyn. 2009. *Putting Women's Health Care Disparities on the Map: Examining Racial and Ethnic Disparities at the State Level.* Menlo Park, Calif.: Henry J. Kaiser Family Foundation.

Jaycox, Lisa H. 2008. "Invisible Wounds of War: Summary of Key Findings on Psychological and Cognitive Injuries." Santa Monica, Calif.: RAND Corporation.

Johnson, Joy L., Lorraine Greaves, and Robin Repta. 2007. *Better Science with Sex and Gender: A Primer for Health Research.* Vancouver, B.C.: Women's Health Research Network.

———. 2009. "Better Science with Sex and Gender: Facilitating the Use of a Sex and Gender-Based Analysis in Health Research." *International Journal for Equity in Health* 8(1): 14.

Kalben, Barbara B. 2002. *Why Men Die Younger: Causes of Mortality Differences by Sex.* SOA Monograph M-L101–1. Schamburg, Ill.: Society of Actuaries.

Kandel, Denise B., Lynn A. Warner, and Ronald C. Kessler. 1998. "The Epidemiology of Substance Use and Dependence among Women." In *Drug Addiction Research and the Health of Women*, ed. C. L. Wetherington and A. B. Roman, 105–30. NIDA Research Monograph. Rockville, Md.: National Institute of Drug Abuse.

Kannel, William B., and Peter W. Wilson. 1995. "Risk Factors That Attenuate the Female Coronary Disease Advantage." *Archives of Internal Medicine* 155(1): 57–61.

Kawachi, Ichiro, and Bruce Kennedy. 2006. *The Health of Nations: Why Inequality Is Harmful to Your Health.* New York: New Press.

Keitner, Gabor I., Christine E. Ryan, Ivan W. Miller, Robert Kohn, and Nathan B. Epstein. 1991. "12-Month Outcome of Patients with Major Depression and Comorbid Psychiatric or Medical Illness (Compound Depression)." *American Journal of Psychiatry* 148(3): 345–50.

Kessler, Ronald C., Peggy R. Barker, Lisa J. Colpe, Joan F. Epstein, Joseph C. Gfroerer, Eva Hiripi, Mary J. Howes, Sharon-Lise T. Normand, Ronald W. Manderscheid, Ellen E. Walters, and Alan M. Zaslavsky. 2003. "Screening for Serious Mental Illness in the General Population." *Archives of General Psychiatry* 60(2): 184–89.

Kessler, Ronald C., Patricia Berglund, Olga Demler, Robert Jin, Doreen Koretz, Kathleen R. Merikangas, A. John Rush, Ellen E. Walters, and Philip Wang. 2003. "The Epidemiology of Major Depressive Disorder: Results from the National Comorbidity Survey Replication (Ncs-R)." *Journal of the American Medical Association* 289(23): 3095–3105.

Kessler, Ronald C., Rosa M. Crum, Lynn A. Warner, Christopher B. Nelson, John Schulenberg, and James C. Anthony. 1997. "Lifetime Co-Occurrence of DSM-III-R Alcohol Abuse and Dependence with Other Psychiatric Disorders in the National Comorbidity Survey." *Archives of General Psychiatry* 54(4): 313–21.

Kessler, Ronald C., Katherine A. McGonagle, Marvin Swartz, Dan G. Blazer, and Christopher B. Nelson. 1993. "Sex and Depression in the National Comorbidity Survey 1: Lifetime Prevalence, Chronicity and Recurrence." *Journal of Affective Disorders* 29(2–3): 85–96.

Kessler, Ronald C., Katherine A. McGonagle, Shanyang Zhao, Christopher B. Nelson, Michael Hughes, Suzann Eshleman, Hans-Ulrich Wittchen, and Kenneth S. Kendler. 1994. "Lifetime and 12-Month Prevalence of DSM-III-R Psychiatric Disorders in the United States: Results from the National Comorbidity Survey." *Archives of General Psychiatry* 51(1): 8–19.

Kessler, Ronald C., Christopher B. Nelson, Katherine A. McGonagle, J. Liu, Marvin Swartz, and Dan G. Blazer. 1996. "Comorbidity of DSM-III-R Major Depressive Disorder in the General Population: Results from the U.S. National Comorbidity Survey." *British Journal of Psychiatry* 168, suppl. 30:17–30.

Kessler, Ronald C., and Ellen E. Walters. 2002. "The National Comorbidity Survey." In *Textbook in Psychiatric Epidemiology*, ed. M. T. Tsuang and M. Tohen, 243–62. New York: John Wiley and Sons.

Kiecolt-Glaser, Janice K., Lynanne McGuire, Theodore F. Robles, and Ronald Glaser. 2002a. "Emotions, Morbidity, and Mortality: New Perspectives from Psychoneuroimmunology." *Annual Review of Psychology* 53:83–107.

———. 2002b. "Psychoneuroimmunology: Psychological Influences on Immune Function and Health." *Journal of Consulting and Clinical Psychology* 70(3): 537–47.

Kimmel, Michael S., and Michael A. Messner. 1993. *Men's Lives.* New York: Macmillan.

Klinge, Ineke. 2007. "Bringing Gender Expertise to Biomedical and Health-Related Research." *Gender Medicine* 4, suppl. 2:S59–63.

Kornstein, Susan G., Alan F. Schatzberg, Michael E. Thase, Kimberly A. Yonkers, James P. McCullough, Gabor I. Keitner, Alan J. Gelenberg, C. E. Ryan, A. L. Hess, Wilma Harrison, Sonia M. Davis, and

Martin B. Keller. 2000. "Gender Differences in Chronic Major and Double Depression." *Journal of Affective Disorders* 60(1): 1–11.

Krieger, Nancy. 2003. "Genders, Sexes, and Health: What Are the Connections—and Why Does It Matter?" *International Journal of Epidemiology* 32(4): 652–57.

Krieger, Nancy, David H. Rehkopf, Jarvis T. Chen, Pamela D. Waterman, Enrico Marcelli, and Malinda Kennedy. 2008. "The Fall and Rise of U.S. Inequalities in Premature Mortality: 1960–2002." *PLoS Medicine* 5(2): e46.

Legato, Marianne J. 2002. *Eve's Rib: The Groundbreaking Guide to Women's Health*. New York: Three Rivers Press.

Lennon, Mary C. 2006. "Women, Work and Depression: Conceptual and Policy Issues." In *The Handbook for the Study of Women and Depression*, ed. C. L. M. Keyes and S. H. Goodman, 309–27. New York: Cambridge University Press.

Levant, Ronald F. and William S. Pollack. 1995. *A New Psychology of Men*. New York: Basic Books.

Link, Bruce G. 2008. "Epidemiological Sociology and the Social Shaping of Population Health." *Journal of Health and Social Behavior* 49(4): 367–84.

Lockshin, Michael D. 2001. "Genome and Hormones: Gender Differences in Physiology: Invited Review: Sex Ratio and Rheumatic Disease." *Journal of Applied Physiology* 91(5): 2366–73.

———. 2006. "Sex Differences in Autoimmune Disease." *Lupus* 15(11): 753–56.

———. Forthcoming. "Non-Hormonal Explanations for Sex Discrepancy in Human Illness."

Lockshin, Michael D., Sherine Gabriel, Zahra Zakeri, and Richard A. Lockshin. 1999. "Gender, Biology and Human Disease: Report of a Conference." *Lupus* 8(5): 335–38.

Lohan, Maria. 2007. "How Might We Understand Men's Health Better? Integrating Explanations from Critical Studies on Men and Inequalities in Health." *Social Science and Medicine* 65(3): 495–504.

Lorber, Judith. 1995. *Paradoxes of Gender*. New Haven, Conn.: Yale University Press.

Loue, Sana. 2006. *Assessing Race, Ethnicity and Gender in Health*. New York: Springer.

———. 2008. "Gender and Health: The Effects of Constrained Choices and Social Policies." *New England Journal of Medicine* 359(11): 1187.

Lutfey, Karen, and Jeremy Freese. 2005. "Toward Some Fundamentals of Fundamental Causality: Socioeconomic Status and Health in the Routine Clinic Visit for Diabetes." *American Journal of Sociology* 110(5): 1326–72.

Marmot, Michael. 2004. *The Status Syndrome: How Social Standing Affects Our Health and Longevity*. New York: Henry Holt.

———. 2005. "Social Determinants of Health Inequalities." *Lancet* 365(9464): 1099–1104.

Mirowsky, J., and K. Ross. 2003. *Education, Social Status, and Health*. Hawthorne, N.Y.: Aldine De Gruyter.

Morenoff, Jeffrey D., and Robert J. Sampson. 1997. "Violent Crime and the Spatial Dynamics of Neighborhood Transition: Chicago, 1970–1990." *Social Forces* 76(1): 31–64.

Murray, Christopher J., Sandeep C. Kulkarni, Catherine Michaud, Niels Tomijima, Maria T. Bulzacchelli, Terrell J. Iandiorio, and Majid Ezzati. 2006. "Eight Americas: Investigating Mortality Disparities across Races, Counties and Race-Counties in the United States." *PLoS Medicine* 3(9): e260.

Narrow, William E., Donald S. Rae, Lee N. Robins, and Darrel A. Regier. 2002. "Revised Prevalence Estimates of Mental Disorders in the United States." *Archives of General Psychiatry* 59(2): 115–130.

Nathanson, Constance A. 1984. "Sex Differences in Mortality." *Annual Review of Sociology* 10:191–213.

National Center for Health Statistics (NCHS). 2009. *Health, United States, 2008, with Chartbook*. Hyattsville, Md.: NCHS.

Nazroo, James Y., Angela C. Edwards, and George W. Brown. 1998. "Gender Differences in the Prevalence of Depression: Artefact, Alternative Disorders, Biology or Roles?" *Sociology of Health and Illness* 20(3): 312–30.

Nolen-Hoeksema, Susan. 1987. "Sex Differences in Unipolar Depression: Evidence and Theory." *Psychological Bulletin* 101(2): 259–82.

———. 1990. *Sex Differences in Depression*. Stanford, Calif.: Stanford University Press.

O'Connor, Daryl B., Mark T. Conner, and Fiona Jones. 2005. "Effects of Stress on Eating Behaviour: An Integrated Approach." Swindon, UK: Economic and Social Research Council.

Olafsdottir, Sigrun, and Jason Beckfield. 2009. "Health and the Social Rights of Citizenship: Integrating Welfare State Theory and Medical Sociology." In *Handbook of Sociology of Health, Illness, and Healing*, ed. B. A. Pescosolido, J. K. Martin, J. D. McLeod, and A. Rogers. New York: Springer.

Pai, Jennifer K., Tobias Pischon, Jing Ma, JoAnn E. Manson, Susan E. Hankinson, Kaumudi Joshipura, Gary C. Curhan, Nader Rifai, Carolyn C. Cannuscio, Meir J. Stampfer, and Eric B. Rimm. 2004. "Inflammatory Markers and the Risk of Coronary Heart Disease in Men and Women." *New England Journal of Medicine* 351(25): 2599–2610.

Pescosolido, Bernice A., Brea L. Perry, J. Scott Long, Jack K. Martin, John I. Nurnberger Jr., and

Victor Hesselbrock. 2008. "Under the Influence of Genetics: How Transdisciplinarity Leads Us to Rethink Social Pathways to Illness." *American Journal of Sociology* 114, suppl. 1:S171–201.

Phelan, Jo C., Bruce G. Link, Ana Diez-Roux, Ichiro Kawachi, and Bruce Levin. 2004. "'Fundamental Causes' of Social Inequalities in Mortality: A Test of the Theory." *Journal of Health and Social Behavior* 45(3): 265–85.

Phelan, Jo C., and Bruce G. Link. 2005. "Controlling Disease and Creating Disparities: A Fundamental Cause Perspective." *The Journals of Gerontology Series B: Psychological Sciences and Social Sciences* 60(2): S27–33.

Piccinelli, Marco, and Greg Wilkinson. 2000. "Gender Differences in Depression: Critical Review." *British Journal of Psychiatry* 177:486–92.

Pilote, Louise, Kaberi Dasgupta, Veena Guru, Karin H. Humphries, Jennifer McGrath, Colleen Norris, Doreen Rabi, Johanne Tremblay, Arsham Alamian, Tracie Barnett, Jafna Cox, William A. Ghali, Sherry Grace, Pavel Hamet, Teresa Ho, Susan Kirkland, Marie Lambert, Danielle Libersan, Jennifer O'Loughlin, Gilles Paradis, Milan Petrovich, and Vicky Tagalakis. 2007. "A Comprehensive View of Sex-Specific Issues Related to Cardiovascular Disease." *Canadian Medical Association Journal* 176(6): S1–44.

Pinnelli, Antonella. 1997. "Gender and Demography." In *Démographie: Analyse et synthèse: Causes et conséquences des évolutions démographiques: Actes du Séminaire "Population et démographie: Problèmes et politiques."* San Miniato. Vol 1. Rome: Universita' La Sapienza, Dipartimento di Scienze.

Pleck, Joseph H. 1983. *The Myth of Masculinity.* Cambridge, Mass.: MIT Press.

———. 1984. "Men's Power with Women, Other Men, and Society: A Men's Movement Analysis." In *The Gender Gap in Psychotherapy: Social Realities in Psychological Processes*, ed. P. P. Rieker and E. H. Carmen, 79–90. New York: Plenum Press.

Pleck, Joseph H., and Robert Brannon. 1978. "Male Roles and the Male Experience: Introduction." *Journal of Social Issues* 34(1): 1–4.

Pratt, Laura A. 2009. "Serious Psychological Distress, as Measured by the K6, and Mortality." *Annals of Epidemiology* 19(3): 202–9.

Ramey, Estelle R. 1982. "The Natural Capacity for Health in Women." In *Women: A Developmental Perspective*, ed. P. W. Berman and E. R. Ramey, 3–12. NIH Publication No. 82–2298. Washington, D.C.: U.S. Department of Health and Human Services.

Rao, Chalapati, Alan D. Lopez, and Yusuf Hemed. 2006. "Causes of Death." In *Disease and Mortality in Sub-Saharan Africa*, 2d ed., ed. D. T. Jamison, R. G. Feachem, M. W. Makgoba, E. R. Bos, F. K. Bainganan, K. J. Hofman, and K. O. Rogo, 43–58. Washington, D.C.: World Bank Publications.

Reeves, Mathew J., and Ann P. Rafferty. 2005. "Healthy Lifestyle Characteristics among Adults in the United States, 2000." *Archives of Internal Medicine* 165(8): 854–57.

Regier, Darrel A., William E. Narrow, Donald S. Rae, Ronald W. Manderscheid, B. Z. Locke, and F. K. Goodwin. 1993. "The De Facto U.S. Mental and Addictive Disorders Service System: Epidemiological Catchment Area 1-Year Prevalence Rates of Disorders and Services." *Archives of General Psychiatry* 50(2): 85–94.

Regier, Darrel A., and Lee N. Robins. 1991. *Psychiatric Disorders in America: The Epidemiologic Catchment Area Study.* New York: Free Press.

Rhodes, Anne E., Paula N. Goering, Teresa To, and J. Ivan Williams. 2002. "Gender and Outpatient Mental Health Service Use." *Social Science and Medicine* 54(1): 1–10.

Ridgeway, Cecilia L., and Lynn Smith-Lovin. 1999. "The Gender System and Interaction." *Annual Review of Sociology* 25:191–216.

Rieker, Patricia P., and Chloe E. Bird. 2000. "Sociological Explanations of Gender Differences in Mental and Physical Health." In *The Handbook of Medical Sociology*, 5th ed., ed. C. E. Bird, P. Conrad, and A. M. Fremont, 98–113. Englewood Cliffs, N.J.: Prentice Hall.

———. 2005. "Rethinking Gender Differences in Health: Why We Need to Integrate Social and Biological Perspectives." *Journals of Gerontology Series B: Psychological Sciences and Social Sciences* 60(2): S40–47.

Rieker, Patricia P., and Elaine H. Carmen. 1984. *The Gender Gap in Psychotherapy: Social Realities in Psychological Processes.* New York: Plenum Press.

Risman, Barbara J. 1998. *Gender Vertigo: American Families in Transition.* New Haven, Conn.: Yale University Press.

Rosenfield, Sarah. 1999. "Gender and Mental Health: Do Women Have More Psychopathology, Men More, or Both the Same (and Why)?" In *The Sociology of Mental Health and Illness*, ed. A. Horwitz and T. Sheid, 348–60. New York: Cambridge University Press.

Ross, Nancy A., Stephane Tremblay, Saeeda Khan, Daniel Crouse, Mark Tremblay, and Jean-Marie Berthelot. 2007. "Body Mass Index in Urban Canada: Neighborhood and Metropolitan Area Effects." *American Journal of Public Health* 97(3): 500–508.

Rustgi, Sheila D., Michelle M. Doty, and Sara R.

Collins. 2009. *Women at Risk: Why Many Women Are Forgoing Needed Health Care—Analysis from the Commonwealth Fund 2007; Biennial Health Insurance Survey*. New York: Commonwealth Fund.

Sabo, Don, and David F. Gordon. 1995. "Rethinking Men's Health and Illness." In *Men's Health and Illness: Gender, Power and the Body*, ed. D. Sabo and D. F. Gordon, 1–21. Thousand Oaks, Calif.: Sage.

Sargeant, J. Kent, Martha L. Bruce, Louis P. Florio, and Myrna M. Weissman. 1990. "Factors Associated with 1-Year Outcome of Major Depression in the Community." *Archives of General Psychiatry* 47(6): 519–26.

Schoeni, Robert F., James S. House, George A. Kaplan, and Harold Pollack. 2008. *Making Americans Healthier: Social and Economic Policy as Health Policy*. New York: Russell Sage Foundation.

Selye, Hans. 1956. *The Stress of Life*. New York: McGraw-Hall.

Shetty, Kanaka D., William B. Vogt, and Jayanta Bhattacharya. 2009. "Hormone Replacement Therapy and Cardiovascular Health in the United States." *Medical Care* 47(5): 600–606.

Sowers, James R. 1998. "Diabetes Mellitus and Cardiovascular Disease in Women." *Archives of Internal Medicine* 158(6): 617–21.

Spitzer, Denise. 2005. "Engendering Health Disparities (Commentary)." *Canadian Journal of Public Health* 96, suppl. 2: S78–S96.

Taylor, Shelley E., Laura C. Klein, Brian P. Lewis, Tara L. Gruenewald, Regan A. Gurung, and John A. Updegraff. 2000. "Biobehavioral Responses to Stress in Females: Tend-and-Befriend, Not Fight-or-Flight." *Psychological Review* 107(3): 411–29.

Theorell, Tores, and Robert A. Karasek. 1996. "Current Issues Relating to Psychosocial Job Strain and Cardiovascular Disease Research." *Journal of Occupational Health Psychology* 1(1): 9–26.

Thom, Thomas, Nancy Haase, Wayne Rosamond, Virginia J. Howard, John Rumsfeld, Teri Manolio, Zhi-Jie Zheng, Katherine Flegal, Christopher O'Donnell, Steven Kittner, Donald Lloyd-Jones, David C. Goff Jr., Yuling Hong, Robert Adams, Gary Friday, Karen Furie, Philip Gorelick, Brett Kissela, John Marler, James Meigs, Veronique Roger, Stephen Sidney, Paul Sorlie, Julia Steinberger, Sylvia Wasserthiel-Smoller, Matthew Wilson, Philip Wolf, and American Heart Association Statistics Committee and Stroke Statistics Subcommittee. 2006. "Heart Disease and Stroke Statistics—2006 Update: A Report from the American Heart Association Statistics Committee and Stroke Statistics Subcommittee." *Circulation* 113(6): e85–151.

Thorand, Barbara, Jens Baumert, Hubert Kolb, Christa Meisinger, Lloyd Chambless, Wolfgang Koenig, and Christian Herder. 2007. "Sex Differences in the Prediction of Type 2 Diabetes by Inflammatory Markers: Results from the Monica/Kora Augsburg Case-Cohort Study, 1984–2002." *Diabetes Care* 30(4): 854–60.

United Nations. 2005. "The World's Women 2005: Trends and Statistics." New York: United Nations.

U.S. Department of Labor. Bureau of Labor Statistics. 2009a. "Employed Persons by Occupation, Sex, and Age." May 29. bls.gov/cps/cpsaat9.pdf.

———. 2009b. "Extended Mass Layoffs." May 29. bls.gov/news.release/pdf/mslo.pdf.

———. 2009c. "News: The Employment Situation; April 2009." May 29. bls.gov/news.release/pdf/empsit.pdf.

Velkoff, Victoria A., and Paul R. Kowal. 2007. *Current Population Reports, P95/07–1 Population Aging in Sub-Saharan Africa: Demographic Dimensions 2006*. Washington, D.C.: U.S. Department of Health and Human Services, U.S. Department of Commerce.

Verbrugge, Lois M., and Deborah L. Wingard. 1987. "Sex Differentials in Health and Mortality." *Women and Health* 12(2): 103–45.

Waldron, Ingrid. 1998. "Sex Differences in Infant and Early Childhood Mortality: Major Causes of Death and Possible Biological Causes." In *Too Young to Die: Genes or Gender?* Department of Economic and Social Affairs, Population Division, 64–83. New York: United Nations.

Walsh, Stephen J., and Laurie M. Rau. 2000. "Autoimmune Diseases: A Leading Cause of Death among Young and Middle-Aged Women in the United States." *American Journal of Public Health* 90(9): 1463–66.

Walter, Ulla, and Brigitte Neumann. 2009. *Gender in Prevention and Health Promotion: Policy Research Practice*. New York: Springer.

West, Candace, and Don H. Zimmerman. 1987. "Doing Gender." *Gender and Society* 1(2): 125–51.

Whang, William, Laura D. Kubzansky, Ichiro Kawachi, Kathryn M. Rexrode, Candyce H. Kroenke, Robert J. Glynn, Hasan Garan, and Christine M. Albert. 2009. "Depression and Risk of Sudden Cardiac Death and Coronary Heart Disease in Women: Results from the Nurses' Health Study." *Journal of the American College of Cardiology* 53(11): 950–58.

Whooley, Mary A., Peter de Jonge, Eric Vittinghoff, Christian Otte, Rudolf Moos, Robert M. Carney, Sadia Ali, Sunaina Dowray, Beeya Na, Mitchell D. Feldman, Nelson B. Schiller, and Warren S. Browner. 2008. "Depressive Symptoms, Health Behaviors, and Risk of Cardiovascular Events in Patients with Coronary Heart Disease." *Journal of the American Medical Association* 300(20): 2379–88.

Wilhelm, Kay, Gordon Parker, and Dusan Hadzi-Pavlovic. 1997. "Fifteen Years On: Evolving Ideas in Researching Sex Differences in Depression." *Psychological Medicine* 27(4): 875–83.

Wilkinson, Richard. 1996. *Unhealthy Societies: The Afflictions of Inequality.* London: Routledge.

Wingard, Deborah L. 1984. "The Sex Differential in Morbidity, Mortality, and Lifestyle." *Annual Review of Public Health* 5:433–58.

Winkleby, Marilyn, Kristina Sundquist, and Catherine Cubbin. 2007. "Inequities in CHD Incidence and Case Fatality by Neighborhood Deprivation." *American Journal of Preventive Medicine* 32(2): 97–106.

Winokur, George, William Coryell, Martin Keller, Jean Endicott, and Hagop Akiskal. 1993. "A Prospective Follow-Up of Patients with Bipolar and Primary Unipolar Affective Disorder." *Archives of General Psychiatry* 50(6): 457–65.

WHO [World Health Organization]. 2002. "The World Health Report: Reducing Risks, Promoting Healthy Life." Geneva: World Health Organization.

———. 2006. "World Health Statistics 2006." February 18. who.int/whosis/whostat2006.pdf.

———. 2008. "Primary Health Care: Now More Than Ever." May 29. who.int/whr/2008/summary/en/index.html.

Yin, Sandra. 2007. "Gender Disparities in Health and Mortality 2007. Population Reference Bureau." February 16. prb.org/Articles/2007/genderdisparities.aspx?p=1.

5

Social Support, Sex, and Food
Social Networks and Health

Gina S. Lovasi, Columbia University Mailman School of Public Health

jimi adams, Arizona State University

Peter S. Bearman, Columbia University

Patterns of social connection are essential to human health and well-being. Researchers are increasingly taking note of the importance of networks, exploring how social networks shape health and health behaviors, and examining how health contributes to the formation, dissolution, and maintenance of social relationships. While several resources are broadly devoted to describing social networks and health (Levy and Pescosolido 2002; Luke and Harris 2007; Smith and Christakis 2008), here we focus on a subset of the ways that networks affect health through their influence on social support, sex, and food consumption—topics both relevant to health and inherently social. In summarizing research in these areas, we highlight how three primary conceptualizations of networks shape what questions are addressed, how studies are designed, what researchers find, and the implications of those findings. (For a more systematic or historically oriented review of the literature on social networks and health, we recommend Hawe, Webster, and Shiell 2004; Luke and Harris 2007; Smith and Christakis 2008.)

Framing Networks and Health Research

The key components of social networks are actors and the social ties between them (Hawe, Webster, and Shiell 2004). Although actors of interest are usually individual people, actors in a social network could also be organizations such as hospitals or community groups. Ties within social networks can include an array of potential relationships; here we follow Borgatti's classification strategy (2008). Some ties are based on direct interpersonal interactions. The social interactions that delineate social ties may include behaviors with direct health ramifications, such as sex, smoking, drinking, dining, and exercise. Another type of interpersonal interaction tie that has relevance for health is based on the transfer of material goods or information. The most commonly measured personal network tie is based on discussion of important matters (Bearman and Parigi 2004; Marsden 1987; McPherson, Smith-Lovin and Brashears 2006); discussion partners are an important source of social support and of health-relevant information. Other common ties are role based, including kin relationships, friendships, and cognitive relations based on whom an actor knows, likes/dislikes, and so on. Finally, ties may be purely association based, such as those that arise through shared memberships in organizations or shared participation in events. The diverse social ties that can exist between any two individuals are not mutually exclusive, and the overlaps between different tie types or different shared activities may themselves be of interest (Rothenberg, Woodhouse et al. 1995).

An Epidemic of Networks Research

Social networks were used as a metaphor in the social sciences, and even in literature, long before they became prominent in public health research (Luke and Harris 2007). Studies of social networks have increased markedly since the creation of International Network for Social Network Analysis in 1977, as evidenced by the growing number of journal articles on the subject. Informal searches of Medline and the Social Sciences Citation Index (SSCI) found parallel increases in the number of entries listing "social network" or "network analysis" (Figure 5.1). These sources listed 3,574 and 5,514 abstracts from 1977 to 2007, respectively, of which approximately two-thirds have been published in the last decade. Medline and SSCI are not mutually exclusive, so some manuscripts may appear in both databases. Of the social network abstracts identified in Medline, the most common subject categories

were behavioral sciences, psychology, and sociology; the most common subject categories for social network abstracts on SSCI were sociology, psychiatry, and public, environmental, and occupational health. Although fewer listings included the specific term "social network analysis" (99 and 313 in Medline and SSCI, respectively), these exhibited a similar increasing trend. In short, an enormous amount of research now considers network impacts on health.

Pathways Connecting Social Networks to Health

While individuals exert some control over their access to social support, sexual experiences, and diet, their choices are constrained and contingent on the behavior of others, on local norms, and in some cases on commercial distribution networks. Specific examples in the balance of this chapter highlight three ways that social networks are likely to affect health (see Figure 5.2).

First, an individual's health may be affected by connectivity to or isolation from others, and by the individual's position within a broader network

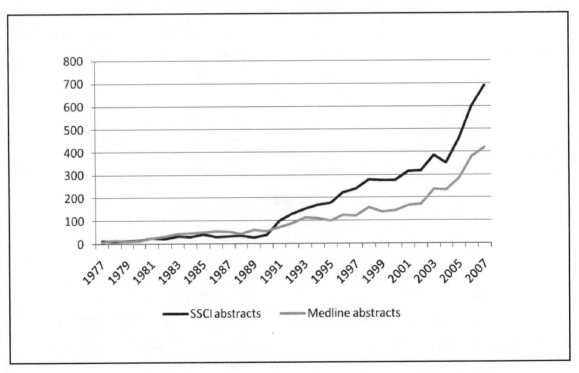

Figure 5.1. Temporal trend in the number of studies about social networks published annually

(Figure 5.2a). Second, the qualities of the social network in which an individual is embedded may influence the individual's health-related behaviors (Figure 5.2b). And third, health-promoting or harmful substances may flow through networks in ways that protect health or increase risk (Figure 5.2c). Each potential pathway has important implications for the ways that research on social networks and health can be conducted.

These three ways that social networks affect health are shown schematically in Figure 5.2, using the convention that actors or nodes are connected by lines that represent social ties. Shading of the nodes can indicate actor characteristics, such as gender or disease status. Although in this simple representation relationships are either present or absent, more sophisticated characterizations of social ties may include information on their strength or direction. For example, if asked

who individuals go to for advice, A may say she turns to B for advice, while B says she goes to C for advice. Such "directed ties" are usually displayed as an arrow rather than a line. In such directed networks, a double-headed arrow indicates a reciprocal relationship, such as where A turns to B for advice and B also turns to A. Similarly, lines could be assigned values to represent the strength of a relationship or the frequency of contact between two actors.

Suppose we want to characterize social networks in order to understand the health of a specific individual; such a focal individual is usually labeled "ego." Study participants may be asked about their social ties in order to generate "egocentric" social network data. Individuals with a social tie to ego are usually labeled ego's "alters." In some cases it may be sufficient to characterize only the immediate social environment of each

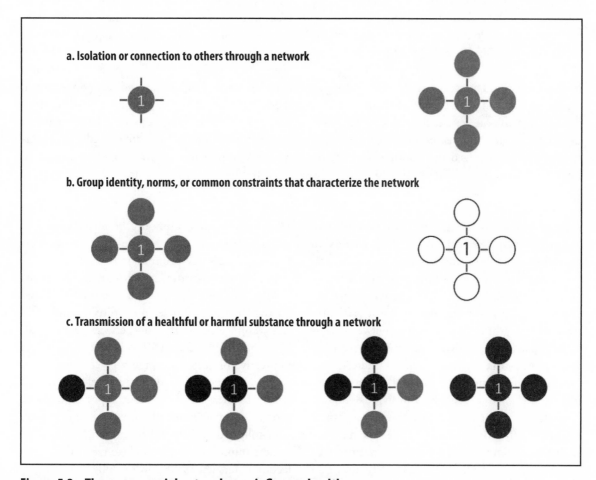

Figure 5.2. Three ways social networks can influence health

study participant by asking that individual about alters of particular types, such as family, friends, sex partners, or other social ties. Those with no alters of a particular type would be classified as isolates without any further investigation. That they have zero such contacts would sufficiently characterize their position within the broader social network.

For certain health-related questions, the number of alters an ego has may be less important than who those alters are. The characteristics of alters may be collected by asking ego questions, but these characteristics may be reported with error or bias since ego may not know, or may not wish to report, the alters' characteristics or behavior patterns (Marsden 1990). Studies in which social environments are reported by a single focal individual provide an incomplete view of their social network but may be sufficient for some research questions, especially those in which ego's perceptions of alters' characteristics are seen to influence health-relevant behaviors.

Partial network designs not only collect information from index respondents about their alters but also subsequently recruit those alters into the study and ask about their relationships—a process that can be repeated as many times as desired. On the one hand, the value of such additional information must be weighed against the risks and costs involved in obtaining identifying information on alters (Klovdahl 2005). On the other hand, interviews with alters, or other corroboration of ego reports, may help address concerns about self-reported data. For example, an individual may falsely perceive their friends to have similar attitudes and beliefs (Baldassarri and Bearman 2007), while an interview with some or all of those friends would reveal new information about heterogeneity within the local network. Beyond confirming information between ego-alter pairs, partial network designs also provide some sense of the wider networks of interest. This extension of the network data collection can allow researchers to observe how individual characteristics, tie characteristics, and the patterning of those ties differ (or are similar) across the network as distance from the initially sampled respondents increases. In addition to the characteristics of an

ego and its alters, we may also be interested in the arrangement of relationships among an interacting population of actors. Unfortunately, in the absence of population data, the position of an individual within their larger network must be estimated (Marsden 1990; Morris 2004).

A researcher may be interested in describing the overall network structure or in characterizing the social position of all individuals within a tangible social network. Characterization of an entire network, while often desirable, is difficult and costly and may be impossible. The boundaries of such a sociocentric network may be clear-cut if the primary interest is in members of an organization or students within a school, but the relevant population boundaries are not always apparent. Sampling from a network may be an efficient strategy when measurement of the entire network is not feasible (Marsden 1990).

A range of structural characteristics may be relevant to the spread of pathogens, resources, or ideas through a population (Marsden 1990). Network structure can be characterized in terms of cohesion, distance, reachability, or density (Hawe, Webster, and Shiell 2004). Two actors within a network are said to have an indirect connection if there is a connected chain of actors leading from one to the other. Subgroups of a larger network may also be of interest, and are typically characterized as "components" (a group of actors connected to each other directly or indirectly) or "cliques" (a group of actors in which every pair of actors is directly connected). An individual's position within a network would commonly be characterized in terms of "centrality," which captures various estimates of network prominence or influence: for example, degree centrality is based simply on the number of direct ties, closeness centrality is based on the shortest distance to all directly and indirectly connected actors, and betweenness centrality is based on how many other actor pairs are indirectly connected through a given actor (Freeman 1979; Hawe, Webster, and Shiell 2004). The ability to measure the various types of network properties is constrained by the nature of network data collected and should be carefully considered in determining what approach to take in data collection (Marsden 1990; Morris 2004).

Social Support and the Risks of Isolation

Social isolation, the complete absence of social support, has been linked to psychological disturbances and increased mortality (Cacioppo et al. 2000; Cacioppo and Hawkley 2003; Hawkley and Cacioppo 2003; Seeman 1996). In fact, enforced social isolation in the form of exile or solitary confinement is occasionally used as a powerful punishment. Much of the health research on social support is based on samples of presumably independent individuals who report on the presence of relationships or the level of social support received. Other innovative approaches have considered ways that the health benefits of support might be deliberately cultivated or inadvertently undermined.

Connections to Healthful Behavior, Stress Buffering, and Illness Recovery

Moderate amounts of social support, socially cohesive networks, and social contacts seem to be health enhancing across a range of health outcomes. In a large population of French employees, for example, an index of social integration was calculated based on several types of social ties (marital status/cohabitation, contacts with close friends and family, and affiliation with voluntary associations) and used to predict mortality (Berkman et al. 2004). A graded trend was seen across the four social integration groups, and for age-adjusted models, the mortality risk in the least integrated group was about three to four times higher than that of the most integrated group.

Some of the health benefits of social integration and social support may be mediated by healthful behavior patterns. Isolation, in contrast, has been linked to adolescent smoking (Ennett and Bauman 1994) and sedentary lifestyles (Mac-Dougall et al. 1997). However, health behaviors do not fully explain the detrimental effects of social isolation (Cacioppo and Hawkley 2003; Hawkley and Cacioppo 2003).

Alternative explanations for the benefits of social support include a direct effect on the biological systems involved in repair and maintenance

(S. Cohen 1988). Supportive social ties may also serve to reduce stress, or to counteract and buffer stressful or otherwise hazardous environments. The ways that individuals obtain support, resources, and ideas from the other people in their lives has been discussed as potentially buffering the harmful effects of stress (Wheaton 1985) or deprivation (Bobak et al. 1998). Such buffering may occur either because a harmful exposure is less harmful in the presence of social support, or because social support is mobilized in response to the harmful exposure (Wheaton 1985). These explanations are not mutually exclusive; social support may play a buffering role and also have a direct effect on health.

Social support may be particularly helpful to those who need to manage chronic health conditions (Gallant 2003) and is an important determinant of survival after a major health event such as a myocardial infarction (Mookadam and Arthur 2004). However, two careful attempts to improve social support for secondary prevention, the Enhancing Recovery in Coronary Heart Disease Patients (ENRICHD) trial and the Families in Recovery from Stroke Trial (FIRST), were unable to reduce mortality (Writing Committee 2003; Glass et al. 2004). Each of these trials randomized isolated or depressed individuals recovering from myocardial infarction or stroke to receive either standard care or additional psychosocial support. The intervention to address isolation developed for the ENRICHD trial employed cognitive behavior therapy techniques to address social skill deficits, cognitive factors contributing to low social support, and social outreach and network development (Writing Committee 2003). The FIRST intervention went a step further, by conducting the sessions at the participants' home and integrating participants' close alters, including family, friends, and caregivers, whenever possible (Glass et al. 2004). The psychosocial intervention did successfully decrease depression and isolation in the ENRICHD trial but did not significantly improve the primary health endpoints in either trial. These results raise the possibility that the beneficial effects of social support may accumulate across the life course such that new connections (or newly activated connections) late in life do not benefit otherwise isolated individuals. The trial findings also call into question the numerous observational studies of social support, which may have been biased by confounding or reverse causation.

Relationship Quality and Support Satisfaction

The heterogeneity of relationships and interpersonal interactions may also help reconcile the observational and experimental literatures. One's interpretation of social support and evaluation of the supportive person may matter for determining behavior beyond the mere presence of social support. In a study by Tang and colleagues (2008), individuals with diabetes were asked about their experiences of positive and negative support, and these had different effects on diabetes self-care behaviors. Support perceived as negative was associated with poor medication adherence, while positive support predicted healthy physical activity and eating patterns. Future research may further elucidate the network characteristics, alter characteristics, behaviors, or communication patterns that contribute to the perception of support as positive or negative.

In a different setting, the potential benefits of so-called invisible support have been contrasted with the possible harms of receiving conspicuous help in a time of stress (Bolger, Zuckerman, and Kessler 2000). In a study of couples, Bolger and colleagues collected daily diary data on social support received and given during preparation for a difficult exam. Partners' reports of supportiveness were not necessarily associated with better health outcomes; only those who did not notice the support benefited from it. The authors suggest that acts of conspicuous support may increase distress by reminding stressed individuals about the source of stress, or a failure to adequately cope with the stress on their own. This contrary response to support may be evident even as the less salient acts of support reduce distress and depression. Notably, the advantages of invisible support could not be studied if only the support recipient were interviewed; obtaining information from an alter was necessary to reveal a nuanced effect of social support on short-term health and well-being.

Support Flows

Social support may provide benefits through specific and relatively intense interpersonal interactions, but the benefits may also accrue over time through a variety of more mundane experiences and exchanges. Supportive social networks can serve as a flexible infrastructure through which resources and services flow, though the benefits an individual receives may differ by relationship type or intensity, gender, and geographic proximity (Wellman and Wortley 1990).

Geographic variations in social connectedness, measured as social capital or social cohesion, may indicate differential potential for the exchange of goods and information, and these group-level measures have been correlated with geographic variations in health (Browning and Cagney 2002; Kawachi, Kennedy, and Wilkinson 1999; Sampson, Morenoff, and Gannon-Rowley 2002). In line with the literature on social support as a buffer against stress at the individual level, authors have suggested that the health effects of economic deprivation (D. Cohen, Farley, and Mason 2003) or inequalities (Wilkinson 1999) may be mediated or modified by the level of social cohesion within the local community.

Thus, social support may be thought of as the presence or abundance of interaction-based and role-based social connections, the quality of those connections, or the potential for such connections to serve as conduits for health-promoting resources and information. Although social isolation seems clearly linked to worse health, there is not a complete understanding of which types of social connections are most beneficial to health.

Sex: Numbers, Norms, and Webs of Contacts

Scholars of sexual health and behavior, along with public health practitioners, have played a central role in developing methods for gathering data on and analyzing interpersonal networks. Many network studies have focused on HIV/AIDS and other sexually transmitted infections (STIs) or on sexual and reproductive health in general. Given this research area's integral role in the history of social network analysis, investigations of sexual activity and networks are prime examples of the different conceptualizations of how networks can affect health.

Partner Acquisition

Researchers across the social and behavioral sciences have examined when people start engaging in sexual activity, as well as how often and with whom they continue to do so. This focus stems in part from the presumption that sexual activity itself is an important outcome for adolescent development (Laumann et al. 1994; Udry and Billy 1987), with researchers particularly interested in explaining differences in the timing of sexual debut across eras and societies (Cavanagh 2004; Mensch, Grant, and Blanc 2006; Zaba et al. 2004) or subcultures of societies (Browning, Leventhal, and Brooks-Gunn 2004, 2005). Sexual debut is also a predictor of individual life trajectories and behaviors, for example, delinquency (Armour and Haynie 2007); as well as of later sexual behavior, for example, condom use or "risky" sexual behaviors (Brückner and Bearman 2005; Uecker, Angotti, and Regnerus 2008). Individuals' involvement in a wide range of activities can substantially alter these trends, for example, research finds mixed effects of education attainment or religious participation on timing of sexual debut (DeRose, Dodoo, and Patil 2002; Rostosky, Regnerus, and Wright 2003).

The number of sexual partners individuals accumulate across their lifetime may also be important for health (Laumann et al. 1994), in part because it may be an important predictor of their risk of contracting an STI. For adult populations, the distribution of the number of partners individuals have can inform epidemic potential and inform intervention targets, for example, highlighting actors with numerous partners as targets for behavior change (Liljeros, Edling, and Nunes Amaral 2003; Liljeros, Edling, Stanley et al. 2003). Additionally, individuals who have multiple concurrent partnerships—overlapping in time—are epidemiologically important (Adimora et al. 2002; Adimora, Schoenbach, and Doherty 2007) especially for the spread of STIs (Morris and Kretzchmar 1997).

Patterning of Partnership Selection

Social networks play an important role in shaping the nature, timing, and extent of individuals' sexual behavior, along with the patterning of those relationships among potential partners. Peer groups frequently exhibit similarity or homophily across a range of sexual behavioral patterns, such that friends and other closely connected peers are alike in the timing of their sexual debuts (Cavanagh 2004; Kinsman et al. 1998), the number of lifetime sexual partners they accumulate (Santelli et al. 1998), and the types of behavior they engage in within those partnerships (Behrman, Kohler, and Watkins 2002; Morris et al. 1995).

In addition to controlling the extent and types of sexual behavior individuals engage in, social networks also encourage or discourage particular patterns of partner selection. Bearman and colleagues (2004) demonstrate that romantic relationships in a U.S. high school are relatively strictly patterned. Within studies of general relationship formation patterns, it is well known that local networks exhibit high probability of local closure—that is the notion of "a friend of a friend is a friend" (Holland and Leinhardt 1971). This finding applies across a wide range of tie types and is among the most common theoretical concepts and empirical findings cited in social network research. For sexual partnering the same pattern does not hold. Bearman and colleagues in fact demonstrate that local closure is virtually forbidden among romantic relationships. Specifically, they find that teens avoid partnering with their former partners' current partners' former partners (Bearman et al. 2004). This local relationship pattern has strong implications for overall network structure within the school, in this instance producing a partnership chain within the romantic network that directly or indirectly links 52 percent of those involved in a romantic relationship.

Networks as Conduits for the Spread of STIs

Studies of the spread and containment of infectious diseases have explicitly leaned on network insights and analytic strategies for decades, with

STIs in particular receiving much of the attention. While questions about how often and with whom individuals have sex may scratch the surface of describing the potential spread of a pathogen within a population, fully mapping the structure of relevant contact networks provides an opportunity for more precise estimation. Sexual network structure both describes epidemic risk for entire populations (Helleringer and Kohler 2007; Morris 2007; Potterat et al. 1999, 2002; Woodhouse et al. 1994) and can improve estimations of the risk to individuals, based on their position within the network (Bell, Atkinson, and Carlson 1999; Rothenberg, Potterat et al. 1995).

Insights from network structure can usefully inform recommendations for preventing the spread of STIs. Individuals who have multiple sexual partners are a common prevention target, with the implication that reducing their numbers can substantially alter their personal risk of contracting or transmitting an STI. However, individual characteristics and simple social network summaries (e.g., number of partners) can misestimate a population's epidemic potential (Hamilton, Handcock, and Morris 2008; Handcock, Jones, and Morris 2003). Network structures with the same population distribution of partner numbers can plausibly generate a wide range of population-level epidemic outcomes (Handcock, Jones, and Morris 2003). Simulations show that reducing the number of high-risk actors in particular sets of conditions can actually *increase* population-level risk (Moody et al. 2007). In the best-case scenario, intervention efforts should make use of known network properties where available (Neaigus 1998; Ward 2007) or should target entire populations. One such example, for human papillomavirus (HPV) vaccination, is provided by Everett, Bearman, and Moody (2009).

Food Consumption and Body Weight

Eating has a rich history as a social activity; in fact, the word "companion" is derived from the Latin words for "with bread." Meal sharing has been used to define social ties in some studies where other shared activities are of primary interest (Klovdahl et al. 1994). Shared meals mark moments of cele-bration and cement the social bonds within families, between romantic partners, and among friends. Lévi-Strauss (1969) discusses the roles of food and cuisine in delimiting culture and society, and modern groups and individuals also define and distinguish themselves by their culinary choices.

Nutritional epidemiologists and others interested in the health consequences of dietary intake face the difficulty of separating the role food plays in shaping social connections and identities from the more direct health effects of food. For example, although some research indicates that a vegetarian diet may be healthful (Appel 2003), vegetarians differ in other ways that may matter for their health. Back and Glasgow (1981) highlight the value vegetarians place on having other vegetarians in their social network, as well as the distinct socioeconomic correlates of a vegetarian lifestyle. They note also that discretionary food preferences like vegetarianism are more feasible for those with more resources: vegetarians tend to be middle class and from a metropolitan background. Thus a study reporting a health benefit of vegetarian diets or diet components may be confounded by class, geography, social context, or other aspects of the environment that influence both discretionary food choices and health.

While socially anchored, dietary patterns have long been linked to weight and health (Schwartz 1986). Excess calorie intake has become an increasingly prominent concern, and the production, distribution, and promotion of food have changed in ways that contribute to dietary excess and overweight (Nesse and Williams 1994; Nestle 2002; Pollan 2006). Socially enforced boundaries on when to eat have also been changing (Astrup et al. 2006). Against this backdrop of an obesigenic environment, social networks help explain some variations among individuals.

Integration vs. Isolation

Isolation from important peer networks can influence dietary patterns. Social isolation itself is associated with elevated hunger (Martin et al. 2004) and a higher risk of being overweight (Lemeshow et al. 2008). Isolation among the elderly, by contrast, is associated with insufficient food intake

(Donini, Savina, and Cannella 2003). As with the evidence on individual isolation, the lack of collective efficacy within neighborhoods is also associated with obesity risk (D. Cohen et al. 2006). Social networks similarly affect other behavior patterns critical to energy balance and health, such as breastfeeding (Fonseca-Becker and Valente 2006; Wutich and McCarty 2008) and physical activity (McNeill, Kreuter, and Subramanian 2006).

Relational Constraints on Food Consumption

Predictable patterns of food selection within social networks provide avenues for understanding and changing patterns of excess caloric intake and dietary composition at a population level. In a partial network study by Feunekes and colleagues (1998), for example, fatty food intake was correlated within households but less so among friends. This study involved recruiting adolescents and their parents and then interviewing each of them plus their best friend, so that each mini-network included up to six individuals. These individuals were interviewed about their food consumption patterns, and correlation analyses were used to consider the similarities among pairs of individuals: matched friends, spouses, or parents and their children. For each pair type, the intake of some specific foods were correlated. In this study, friendship pairs, whether adult or adolescent, are likely to have similar intakes of snack foods and alcoholic beverages. Fat intake, however, was most correlated for child-parent pairs and between spouses. This suggests that adolescent friends share snacks and have influence on each other's overall calorie intake, while the consumption of fats is mainly determined by food-preparation decisions made at the household level. In this population, which was based in the Netherlands, a public health promotion effort aimed at reducing snacking among adolescents would likely be most successful if it includes friends and family, while an effort aimed at changing the types or amounts of fat consumed might do well to focus on the household food-preparation patterns. These conclusions suggest that the most relevant social leverage points for dietary interventions could depend on the type of dietary change sought.

Along with the social influence on intake of specific food items, there is evidence that body image responds to peer influence (Hutchinson and Rapee 2007). Such influence may contribute to both healthy and extreme weight-loss behavior. Paxton and colleagues (1999), for example, find that friendship cliques among adolescent girls are relatively homogenous with regard to body-image concern, eating behaviors, and the use of such extreme weight-loss strategies as fasting, crash dieting, or vomiting, and using laxatives, appetite suppressants, or diuretics. The role of social influence may deserve further consideration in the design of eating-disorder prevention programs, so that such interventions effectively discourage risky behaviors; previous evaluations suggest that effectiveness is limited when participants fail to identify with the information presented (Rosenvinge and Westjordet 2004), or identify with it so much that the risky behavior is inadvertently increased by the intervention (Mann et al. 1997).

As in much observational research, a study asserting that social influences cause dietary and weight changes may not be able to rule out the possibility that such an association is explained by reverse causation. Body weight may affect how future social interactions unfold (Janssen et al. 2004; Strauss and Pollack 2003), and the psychosocial effects of obesity among children are of particular concern (Wabitsch 2000). This does not exclude the possibility that social induction is also occurring and reinforcing the general tendency toward homophily within networks, but such a reciprocal relationship makes the effects difficult to disentangle. An individual who is both isolated and overweight may have gained weight in response to isolation, become isolated because of weight status, or had a combination of these two reinforcing processes. Likewise, friends who have similar weight status may have influenced each other to become more similar, chosen to be friends because of their similarity, or both.

Contagious Consumption

Another recent study takes advantage of social network data collected incidentally within a long-term prospective cohort study and finds that weight changes are correlated within social networks over time (Christakis and Fowler 2007). At each study examination, participants identified their first-order relatives and at least one close friend, and many of these alters were themselves enrolled as study participants. During the study period, 1971 to 2003, U.S. obesity rates increased dramatically, and the study participants were also at risk for becoming obese (as defined by a body mass index of thirty or more). A direct social tie to an individual who became obese was associated with about a 45 percent increased risk of obesity. That is to say, if an alter recently became obese, then ego was likely to become obese in this same time period. If an alter's alter became obese, ego was about 20 percent more likely to become obese, and if an alter's alter's alter became obese, ego was about 10 percent more likely to become obese. Thus, the association remained significant up to three degrees of separation but decayed with social distance. The observed pattern also suggests that the type of social tie may determine the strength of the association, with spouse, same-sex sibling, and same-sex friend being especially influential. The authors consider three explanations for the observed associations: direct influence or "induction," shared behaviors, and bias due to confounding or selection. They interpret the observed pattern in which alter's sex mattered but geographic proximity did not to support the induction-based explanation of why obesity appears to flow through social networks. This suggests that changes in body size within one's social network may act through changing body-size norms and subsequent attention (or inattention) to dietary or physical activity choices.

Although we focus on networks of individuals, individuals' food choices are also constrained by the upstream networks within which food production and distribution take place (Sage 2003). A range of social policies and economic incentives influences the choices one faces at the market or in a restaurant (Nestle 2002; Pollan 2006). Further, the production networks may be important for their effect on the safety of the food supply. Cattle markets, for example, may be relevant to tracing the spread of illness among cattle (Ortiz-Pelaez et al. 2006; Robinson and Christley 2007) and its transmission to humans. Thus, consideration of social networks at multiple scales and across types of actors and ties may increase our understanding of the dietary choices individuals make.

Using Networks to Promote Health

In general, strategies to use what we know about social networks to improve health can be classified as efforts to change the network structure or as efforts to strategically use the network or leverage points within the network. A classic epidemiologic strategy might use contact tracing and quarantine to disrupt social contacts and halt the spread of illness through a network (Eichner 2003). Social network interventions can also be designed to enhance network activation and social integration (Israel 1985), although caution is warranted on the basis of the experience of social support intervention trials (e.g., Berkman et al. 2003; Glass et al. 2004). Another type of social network enhancement relevant to health could involve building coalitions of groups with a common interest in health promotion (Feinberg, Riggs, and Greenberg 2005; Schulz et al. 2005).

The strategic use of social networks to influence behavior change or the spread of information may involve targeting influential or otherwise strategically positioned individuals (Cross and Prusak 2002). Such social network strategies have been used in the implementation of interventions, for example, to encourage dietary change (Foley and Pollard 1998), smoking cessation (Valente et al. 2003), and STI prevention efforts (Amirkhanian et al. 2003). Social networks can also be used to find high-risk or difficult-to-recruit individuals for screening or targeted interventions (Salganik and Heckathorn 2004).

Another way that social network studies can support health promotion efforts is by explaining how population-level health changes occur. Changes to the structure of the social network, or the level of social support, could mediate some public health interventions, and understanding this may help justify strategic improvements or draw attention to other considerations. As an example, Fuemmeler and colleagues (2006) evaluated a church-based intervention to promote the consumption of fruits and vegetables and found that it works in part through increased social support and self-efficacy. Some researchers have also suggested that improvements to the physical environment could be mediated by social network changes (D. Cohen, Inagami, and Finch 2008), and these hypotheses warrant further testing. If social network changes mediate the effects of health promotion interventions, the health benefits may be contingent on a particular process of implementation that does not undermine the existing social networks (Fullilove 2004).

Common Challenges and Convergent Mechanisms

Our examination of how networks affect social support, sex, and food consumption and subsequent health raises a number of common research challenges. While each of these is important to an individual's health, the effects are difficult to isolate. Social ties form and dissolve in ways that respond to health or health behaviors, even as the ties themselves influence health. Endogeneity and complexity are commonplace in social network research, perhaps even more than in other observational research. Yet face validity makes the possibility of strong social induction difficult to dismiss: we all feel how people influence us, and that we can attempt to influence them in turn.

While social network data have sometimes been measured using individual questionnaires, any single person has a limited ability to report on the full social context that may be relevant to their health. In their work with social networks, Bolger, Zuckerman, and Kessler (2000) highlight a situation in which the discordance between reports of social support is itself informative, a finding that would have been overlooked in a study reliant upon the reports of only one member of the dyad. Likewise, studies of STIs have indicated that the number of sex ties one has is less important for an ego's contracting an STI than is the number of sex ties their alters have, or the temporal ordering or concurrency of such relationships (Morris 2007). Finally, in considering the social network influences on weight, Christakis and Fowler (2007) found that direct ties are the most

influential, but that persons two and three degrees of separation away may also be important. Thus, there is reason to believe that a complete picture of the health-relevant social environment can best be attained in studies with multiple informants, despite the challenges inherent in doing so (Klovdahl 2005).

Studies of social networks are particularly valuable for the topics we have highlighted because individuals have limited ability to change the level of social support they receive, the amount and type of sex they have, and the foods they consume. Our choices are contingent on the choices of others around us, and on the broader cultural contexts and production networks that shape our options.

Social connections are cemented through shared conversations, sex acts, and meals, so while each come with risks, they also deliver a benefit to individuals who thus avoid isolation (Berkman and Syme 1979), and the meaning and importance of such activities may overshadow their health implications. Studies have documented a possible biological basis for the perceived benefits of these social behaviors and of avoiding isolation (Cacioppo and Hawkley 2003). The neuroendocrine consequences of social connections, sex, and food consumption are noteworthy, with oxytocin and dopamine apparently playing critical roles (Spanagel and Weiss 1999).

Even if beneficial effects overlap, the nature of the risks can vary greatly. Low levels of social support may leave a person vulnerable to chronic stress or sudden hardship. While the transmission of pathogens across networks has been particularly salient in the literature on sex ties and sexual networks, the gradual accumulation of harms has been the focus of the research on nutritional excess.

Linking to Other Contexts for Health Behavior

While most sampling and statistical analysis techniques are based on studying independent samples from a population, individuals are not autonomous or randomly affiliated. Social networks tend to be homophilous (McPherson, Smith-Lovin, and Cook 2001). As a result, individuals sampled from a small population should not necessarily be assumed to be "independent" in the statistical sense—characteristics will be more highly correlated for socially connected individuals. But social networks overlap importantly with, and are complemented by, other types of context. Since further information on the surrounding social environment may be crucial for understanding an individual's access to resources and exposures to risk, we briefly consider these other contexts.

Institutional settings such as schools or workplaces define groups with potentially similar risks and exposures, and provide opportunities for health promotion interventions. These can also serve as settings for social network studies, as was the case for the Add Health study (Bearman, Jones, and Udry 1997). Characteristics of the physical environment or of geographically defined communities also determine exposure to risk and access to resources. The spatial proximity of individuals influences the probability of a social connection between them and may also affect opportunities for shared activities. A parallel between associations across spatial and social "distance" was explicitly drawn by Christakis and Fowler in their paper on obesity (2007). In fact, the social and physical environments of geographic areas may interact to determine the health of area residents. The degree to which physical environments predict obesity, for example, varies with social context (Lovasi et al. 2009). Several studies have explicitly considered how social networks overlap with physical or geographic settings to predict behavior and the spread of illness, but the data and analytic methods to capture these multiple layers of context simultaneously are not widely available (Schensul, Levy, and Disch 2003; Wylie, Cabral, and Jolly 2005; Wylie, Shah, and Jolly 2007).

Social network analysis is one of an interrelated set of tools that are useful for understanding the contexts in which individuals live. To capture spatial or other hierarchical patterns, geographic information systems, cluster analysis, generalized estimating equations, and multilevel modeling can be employed, as each of these is useful for accommodating the similarities among individuals with a shared group identity or physical space (Luke 2005).

Although social networks are only one of the contexts that shape health and health behavior, their effects are pervasive. The study of social networks is especially complex because of the need to protect human subjects and their confidentiality and the potential for bidirectional causation, that is, social networks affect health and health in turn affects social networks. The need to consider social networks at multiple scales—from interpersonal to organizational—further complicates the picture. Nonetheless, the potential for increased understanding and enhanced health promotion makes the incorporation of social networks into health research worthwhile.

References

Adimora, Adaora A., Victor J. Schoenbach, Dana M. Bonas, Francis E. A. Martinson, Kathryn H. Donaldson, and Tonya R. Stancil. 2002. "Concurrent Sexual Partnerships among Women in the United States." *Epidemiology* 13(3): 320–327.

Adimora, Adaora A., Victor J. Schoenbach, and Irene A. Doherty. 2007. "Concurrent Sexual Partnerships among Men in the United States." *American Journal of Public Health* 97(12): 2230–237.

Amirkhanian, Yuri A., Jeffrey A. Kelly, Elena Kabakchieva, Timothy L. McAuliffe, and Sylvia Vassileva. 2003. "Evaluation of a Social Network HIV Prevention Intervention Program for Young Men Who Have Sex with Men in Russia and Bulgaria." *Aids Education and Prevention* 15(3): 205–20.

Appel, Lawrence J. 2003. "Lifestyle Modification as a Means to Prevent and Treat High Blood Pressure." *Journal of the American Society of Nephrology* 14, 7 Suppl. 2: S99–102.

Armour, Stacy, and Dana L. Haynie. 2007. "Adolescent Sexual Debut and Later Delinquency." *Journal of Youth and Adolescence* 36(2): 141–52.

Astrup, A., M. W. Bovy, K. Nackenhorst, and A. E. Popova. 2006. "Food for Thought or Thought for Food? A Stakeholder Dialogue around the Role of the Snacking Industry in Addressing the Obesity Epidemic." *Obesity Reviews* 7(3): 303–12.

Back, Kurt W., and Margaret Glasgow. 1981. "Social Networks and Psychological Conditions in Diet Preferences: Gourmets and Vegetarians." *Basic and Applied Social Psychology* 2(1): 1–9.

Baldassarri, Delia, and Peter Bearman. 2007. "Dynamics of Political Polarization." *American Sociological Review* 72(5): 784.

Bearman, Peter S., Jo Jones, and J. Richard Udry. 1997.

"The National Longitudinal Study of Adolescent Health: Research Design." Chapel Hill: University of North Carolina at Chapel Hill, Carolina Population Center.

Bearman, Peter S., James Moody, and Katherine Stovel. 2004. "Chains of Affection: The Structure of Adolescent Romantic and Sexual Networks." *American Journal of Sociology* 110(1): 44–91.

Bearman, Peter S., and Paolo Parigi. 2004. "Cloning Headless Frogs and Other Important Matters: Conversation Topics and Network Structure." *Social Forces* 83(2): 535–57.

Behrman, Jere R., Hans-Peter Kohler, and Susan Cotts Watkins. 2002. "Social Networks and Changes in Contraceptive Use over Time: Evidence from a Longitudinal Study in Rural Kenya." *Demography* 39(4): 713–38.

Bell, David C., John S. Atkinson, and Jerry W. Carlson. 1999. "Centrality Measures for Disease Transmission Networks." *Social Networks* 21(1): 1–21.

Berkman, L. F., J. Blumenthal, M. Burg, R. M. Carney, D. Catellier, M. J. Cowan, S. M. Czajkowski, R. DeBusk, J. Hosking, A. Jaffe, P. G. Kaufmann, P. Mitchell, J. Norman, L. H. Powell, J. M. Raczynski, and N. Schneiderman. 2003. "Effects of Treating Depression and Low Perceived Social Support on Clinical Events after Myocardial Infarction: The Enhancing Recovery in Coronary Heart Disease Patients (ENRICHD) Randomized Trial." *Journal of the American Medical Association* 289:3106–16.

Berkman, Lisa F., Maria Melchior, Jean-François Chastang, Isabelle Niedhammer, Annette Leclerc, and Marcel Goldberg. 2004. "Social Integration and Mortality: A Prospective Study of French Employees of Electricity of France-Gas of France: The GAZEL Cohort." *American Journal of Epidemiology* 159(2): 167–74.

Berkman, Lisa F., and S. Leonard Syme. 1979. "Social Networks, Host Resistance, and Mortality: A Nine-Year Follow-Up Study of Alameda County Residents." *American Journal of Epidemiology* 109(2): 186–204.

Bobak, Martin, Hynek Pikhart, Clyde Hertzman, Richard Rose, and Michael Marmot. 1998. "Socioeconomic Factors, Perceived Control and Self-Reported Health in Russia. A Cross-Sectional Survey." *Social Science and Medicine* 47(2): 269–79.

Bolger, Niall, Adam Zuckerman, and Ronald C. Kessler. 2000. "Invisible Support and Adjustment to Stress." *Journal of Personality and Social Psychology* 79(6): 953–61.

Borgatti, Steve. 2008. "Network Reasoning: Keynote Address." Paper presented at Sunbelt XXVIII, annual meetings of the International Network for Social Network Analysis, St. Petersburg, Fla.

Browning, Christopher R., and Kathleen A. Cagney. 2002. "Neighborhood Structural Disadvantage, Collective Efficacy, and Self-Rated Physical Health in an Urban Setting." *Journal of Health and Social Behavior* 43(4): 383–99.

Browning, Christopher R., Tama Leventhal, and Jeanne Brooks-Gunn. 2004. "Neighborhood Context and Racial Differences in Early Adolescent Sexual Activity." *Demography* 41(4): 697–720.

———. 2005. "Sexual Initiation in Early Adolescence: The Nexus of Parental and Community Control." *American Sociological Review* 70(5): 758–78.

Brückner, Hannah, and Peter Bearman. 2005. "After the Promise: The STD Consequences of Adolescent Virginity Pledges." *Journal of Adolescent Health* 36(4): 271–78.

Cacioppo, John T., John M. Ernst, Mary H. Burleson, Martha K. McClintock, William B. Malarkey, Louise C. Hawkley, Ray B. Kowalewski, Alisa Paulsen, J. Allan Hobson, Kenneth Hugdahl, David Spiegel, and Gary G. Berntson. 2000. "Lonely Traits and Concomitant Physiological Processes: The MacArthur Social Neuroscience Studies." *International Journal of Psychophysiology* 35(2–3): 143–54.

Cacioppo, John T., and Louise C. Hawkley. 2003. "Social Isolation and Health, with an Emphasis on Underlying Mechanisms." *Perspectives in Biology and Medicine* 46, 3 Suppl.: S39–52.

Cavanagh, Shannon E. 2004. "The Sexual Debut of Girls in Early Adolescence: The Intersection of Race, Pubertal Timing, and Friendship Group Characteristics." *Journal of Research on Adolescence* 14(3): 285–312.

Christakis, Nicholas A., and James H. Fowler. 2007. "The Spread of Obesity in a Large Social Network over 32 Years." *New England Journal of Medicine* 357(4): 370–79.

Cohen, Deborah A., Thomas A. Farley, and Karen Mason. 2003. "Why Is Poverty Unhealthy? Social and Physical Mediators." *Social Science and Medicine* 57(9): 1631–41.

Cohen, Deborah A., Brian K. Finch, Aimee Bower, and Narayan Sastry. 2006. "Collective Efficacy and Obesity: The Potential Influence of Social Factors on Health." *Social Science and Medicine* 62(3): 769–78.

Cohen, Deborah A., Sanae Inagami, and Brian K. Finch. 2008. "The Built Environment and Collective Efficacy." *Health and Place* 14(2): 198–208.

Cohen, Sheldon. 1988. "Psychosocial Models of the Role of Social Support in the Etiology of Physical Disease." *Health Psychology* 7(3): 269–97.

Cross, Rob, and Laurence Prusak. 2002. "The People Who Make Organizations Go—Or Stop." *Harvard Business Review* 80(6): 104–12.

DeRose, Laurie F., F. Nii-Amoo Dodoo, and Vrushali Patil. 2002. "Schooling and Attitudes on Reproductive-Related Behavior in Ghana." *International Journal of Sociology of the Family* 30(1): 50–65.

Donini, Lorenzo M., Claudia Savina, and Carlo Cannella. 2003. "Eating Habits and Appetite Control in the Elderly: The Anorexia of Aging." *International Psychogeriatrics* 15(1): 73–87.

Eichner, Martin. 2003. "Case Isolation and Contact Tracing Can Prevent the Spread of Smallpox." *American Journal of Epidemiology* 158(2): 118.

Ennett, Susan T., and Karl E. Bauman. 1994. "The Contribution of Influence and Selection to Adolescent Peer Group Homogeneity: The Case of Adolescent Cigarette Smoking." *Journal of Personality and Social Psychology* 67(4): 653–63.

Everett, Katie, Peter Bearman, and James Moody. 2009. "Chain of Infection: A Sexual-Network-Based Model Evaluating the Impact of Human Papilloma Virus Vaccination on Infection Prevalence in an Adolescent Population." Unpublished paper.

Feinberg, Mark E., Nathaniel R. Riggs, and Mark T. Greenberg. 2005. "Social Networks and Community Prevention Coalitions." *Journal of Primary Prevention* 26(4): 279–98.

Feunekes, Gerda I. J., Cees de Graaf, Saskia Meyboom, and Wija A. van Staveren. 1998. "Food Choice and Fat Intake of Adolescents and Adults: Associations of Intakes within Social Networks." *Preventive Medicine* 27(5): 645–56.

Foley, Ruth M., and Christina M. Pollard. 1998. "Food Cent$: Implementing and Evaluating a Nutrition Education Project Focusing on Value for Money." *Australian and New Zealand Journal of Public Health* 22(4): 494–501.

Fonseca-Becker, Fannie, and Thomas W. Valente. 2006. "Promoting Breastfeeding in Bolivia: Do Social Networks Add to the Predictive Value of Traditional Socioeconomic Characteristics?" *Journal of Health, Population and Nutrition* 24(1): 71–80.

Freeman, Linton C. 1979. "Centrality in Social Networks: Conceptual Clarification." *Social Networks* 1(3): 215–39.

Fuemmeler, Bernard F., Louise C. Mâsse, Amy L. Yaroch, Ken Resnicow, Marci Kramish Campbell, Carol Carr, Terry Wang, and Alexis Williams. 2006. "Psychosocial Mediation of Fruit and Vegetable Consumption in the Body and Soul Effectiveness Trial." *Health Psychology* 25(4): 474–83.

Fullilove, Mindy T. 2004. *Root Shock: How Tearing Up City Neighborhoods Hurts America, and What We Can Do About It.* New York: Ballantine Books.

Gallant, Mary P. 2003. "The Influence of Social Support on Chronic Illness Self-Management: A Review and Directions for Research." *Health Education and Behavior* 30(2): 170–95.

Glass, Thomas A., Lisa F. Berkman, Elizabeth F. Hiltunen, Karen Furie, Maria M. Glymour, Marta E. Fay, and James Ware. 2004. "The Families in Recovery from Stroke Trial (FIRST): Primary Study Results." *Psychosomatic Medicine* 66(6): 889–97.

Hamilton, Deven T., Mark S. Handcock, and Martina Morris. 2008. "Degree Distributions in Sexual Networks: A Framework for Evaluating Evidence." *Sexually Transmitted Diseases* 35(1): 30–40.

Handcock, Mark S., James Holland Jones, and Martina Morris. 2003. "On 'Sexual Contacts and Epidemic Thresholds,' Models and Inference for Sexual Partnership Distributions." CSS Working Paper No. 31. Seattle: University of Washington, Center for Statistics and the Social Sciences.

Hawe, Penelope, Cynthia Webster, and Alan Shiell. 2004. "A Glossary of Terms for Navigating the Field of Social Network Analysis." *Journal of Epidemiology and Community Health* 58(12): 971–75.

Hawkley, Louise C., and John T. Cacioppo. 2003. "Loneliness and Pathways to Disease." *Brain Behavior and Immunity* 17, 1 Suppl.: S98–105.

Helleringer, Stephane, and Hans-Peter Kohler. 2007. "Sexual Network Structure and the Spread of HIV in Africa: Evidence from Likoma Island, Malawi." *AIDS* 21(17): 2323–32.

Holland, Paul W., and Samuel Leinhardt. 1971. "Transitivity in Structural Models of Small Groups." *Comparative Groups Studies* 2(2): 107–24.

Hutchinson, Delyse M., and Ronald M. Rapee. 2007. "Do Friends Share Similar Body Image and Eating Problems? The Role of Social Networks and Peer Influences in Early Adolescence." *Behavioral Research and Therapy* 45(7): 1557–77.

Israel, Barbara A. 1985. "Social Networks and Social Support: Implications for Natural Helper and Community Level Interventions." *Health Education and Behavior* 12(1): 65.

Janssen, Ian, Wendy M. Craig, William F. Boyce, and William Pickett. 2004. "Associations between Overweight and Obesity with Bullying Behaviors in School-Aged Children." *Pediatrics* 113(5): 1187–94.

Kawachi, Ichiro, Bruce P. Kennedy, and Richard G. Wilkinson. 1999. "Crime: Social Disorganization and Relative Deprivation." *Social Science and Medicine* 48(6): 719–31.

Kinsman, Sara B., Daniel Romer, Frank F. Furstenberg, and Donald F. Schwarz. 1998. "Early Sexual Initiation: The Role of Peer Norms." *Pediatrics* 102(5): 1185–92.

Klovdahl, Alden S. 2005. "Social Network Research and Human Subjects Protection: Towards More Effective

Infectious Disease Control." *Social Networks* 27(2): 119–37.

Klovdahl, Alden S., John J. Potterat, Donald E. Woodhouse, John B. Muth, Stephen Q. Muth, and William W. Darrow. 1994. "Social Networks and Infectious Disease: The Colorado Springs Study." *Social Science and Medicine* 38(1): 79–88.

Laumann, Edward O., John H. Gagnon, Robert T. Michael, and Stuart Michaels. 1994. *The Social Organization of Sexuality: Sexual Practices in the United States*. Chicago: University of Chicago Press.

Lemeshow, Adina R., Laurie Fisher, Elizabeth Goodman, Ichiro Kawachi, Catherine S. Berkey, and Graham A. Colditz. 2008. "Subjective Social Status in the School and Change in Adiposity in Female Adolescents: Findings from a Prospective Cohort Study." *Archives of Pediatric and Adolescent Medicine* 162(1): 23–28.

Lévi-Strauss, Claude. 1969. *The Raw and the Cooked*. New York: Harper and Row.

Levy, Judith A., and Bernice A. Pescosolido, eds. 2002. *Social Networks and Health*. Vol. 8 of *Advances in Medical Sociology*. New York: Elsevier Science.

Liljeros, Fredrik, Christofer R. Edling, and Luis A. Nunes Amaral. 2003. "Sexual Networks: Implications for the Transmission of Sexually Transmitted Infections." *Microbes and Infection* 5(2): 189–96.

Liljeros, Fredrik, Christofer R. Edling, H. Eugene Stanley, Y. Åberg, and Luis A. Nunes Amaral. 2003. "Distributions of Number of Sexual Partnerships Have Power Law Decaying Tails and Finite Variance." arXiv:cond-mat/0305528v1.

Lovasi, Gina S., Kathryn M. Neckerman, James W. Quinn, Christopher C. Weiss, and Andrew Rundle. 2009. "Individual or Neighborhood Disadvantage Modifies the Association between Neighborhood Walkability and Body Mass Index." *American Journal of Public Health* 99(2): 279–84.

Luke, Douglas A. 2005. "Getting the Big Picture in Community Science: Methods That Capture Context." *American Journal of Community Psychology* 35(3–4): 185–200.

Luke, Douglas A., and Jenine K. Harris. 2007. "Network Analysis in Public Health: History, Methods and Applications." *Annual Review of Public Health* 28:69–93.

MacDougall, Colin, Richard Cooke, Neville Owen, Kristyn Willson, and Adrian Bauman. 1997. "Relating Physical Activity to Health Status, Social Connections and Community Facilities." *Australian and New Zealand Journal of Public Health* 21(6): 631–37.

Mann, Traci, Susuan Nolen-Hoeksema, Karen Huang, Debora Burgard, Alexi Wright, and Kaaren Hanson. 1997. "Are Two Interventions Worse Than None? Joint Primary and Secondary Prevention of Eating Disorders in College Females." *Health Psychology* 16(3): 215–25.

Marsden, Peter V. 1987. "Core Discussion Networks of Americans." *American Sociological Review* 52(1): 122–31.

———. 1990. "Network Data and Measurement." *Annual Review of Sociology* 16(1): 435–63.

Martin, Katie S., Beatrice L. Rogers, John T. Cook, and Hugh M. Joseph. 2004. "Social Capital Is Associated with Decreased Risk of Hunger." *Social Science and Medicine* 58(12): 2645.

McNeill, Lorna H., Matthew W. Kreuter, and S. V. Subramanian. 2006. "Social Environment and Physical Activity: A Review of Concepts and Evidence." *Social Science and Medicine* 63(4): 1011–22.

McPherson, Miller, Lynn Smith-Lovin, and James M. Cook. 2001. "Birds of a Feather: Homophily in Social Networks." *Annual Reviews in Sociology* 27(1): 415–44.

McPherson, Miller, Lynn Smith-Lovin, and Matthews E. Brashears. 2006. "Social Isolation in America: Changes in Core Discussion Networks over Two Decades." *American Sociological Review* 71(3): 353–75.

Mensch, Barbara S., Monica J. Grant, and Ann K. Blanc. 2006. "The Changing Context of Sexual Initiation in sub-Saharan Africa." *Population and Development Review* 32(4): 699–727.

Moody, James, Martina Morris, jimi adams, and Mark Handcock. 2007. "Epidemic Potential in Low Degree Networks." Word document. Author files.

Mookadam, Farouk, and Heather M. Arthur. 2004. "Social Support and Its Relationship to Morbidity and Mortality after Acute Myocardial Infarction: Systematic Overview." *Archives of Internal Medicine* 164(14): 1514–18.

Morris, Martina. 2004. *Network Epidemiology: A Handbook for Survey Design and Data Collection*. London: Oxford University Press.

———. 2007. "Local Acts, Global Consequences: Networks and the Spread of HIV." Paper presented at NIH Director's Wednesday Afternooon Lecture Series. Washington, D.C. csde.washington.edu/news/spotlight/docs/wals042507.rm.

Morris, Martina, and Mirjam Kretzchmar. 1997. "Concurrent Partnerships and the Spread of HIV." *AIDS* 11(5): 641–48.

Morris, Martina, Anthony Pramualratana, Chai Podhisita, and Maria J. Wawer. 1995. "The Relational Determinants of Condom Use with Commercial Sex Partners in Thailand." *AIDS* 9(5): 507–15.

Neaigus, Alan. 1998. "The Network Approach and Interventions to Prevent HIV among Injection Drug Users." *Public Health Reports* 113, 1 Suppl.: 140–50.

Nesse, Randolph M., and George C. Williams. 1994. "Diseases of Civilization." In *Why We Get Sick: The New Science of Darwinian Medicine*, 143–57. New York: Random House.

Nestle, Marion. 2002. *Food Politics: How the Food Industry Influences Nutrition and Health*. Los Angeles: University of California Press.

Ortiz-Pelaez, A., D. U. Pfeiffer, R. J. Soares-Magalhaes, and F. J. Guitian. 2006. "Use of Social Network Analysis to Characterize the Pattern of Animal Movements in the Initial Phases of the 2001 Foot and Mouth Disease (FMD) Epidemic in the UK." *Preventive Veterinary Medicine* 76(1–2): 40–55.

Paxton, Susan J., Helena K. Schutz, Eleanor H. Wertheim, and Sharry L. Muir. 1999. "Friendship Clique and Peer Influences on Body Image Concerns, Dietary Restraint, Extreme Weight-Loss Behaviors, and Binge Eating in Adolescent Girls." *Journal of Abnormal Psychology* 108(2): 255–66.

Pollan, Michael. 2006. *The Omnivore's Dilemma: A Natural History of Four Meals*. New York: Penguin Press.

Potterat, John J., Helen Zimmerman-Rogers, Stephen Q. Muth, Richard B. Rothenberg, David L. Green, Jerry E. Taylor, Mandy S. Bonney, and Helen A. White. 1999. "Chlamydia Transmission: Concurrency, Reproduction Number and the Epidemic Trajectory." *American Journal of Epidemiology* 150:1331–39.

Potterat, John J., Richard B. Rothenberg, Helen Zimmerman-Rogers, David L. Green, Jerry E. Taylor, Mandy S. Bonney, and Helen A. White. 2002. "Sexual Network Structure as an Indicator of Epidemic Phase." *Sexually Transmitted Infections* 78: i152–58.

Robinson, S. E., and R. M. Christley. 2007. "Exploring the Role of Auction Markets in Cattle Movements within Great Britain." *Preventive Veterinary Medicine* 81(1–3): 21–37.

Rosenvinge, Jan H., and Marthe O. Westjordet. 2004. "Is Information about Eating Disorders Experienced as Harmful? A Consumer Perspective on Primary Prevention." *Eating Disorders* 12(1): 11–20.

Rostosky, Sharon S., Mark D. Regnerus, and Margaret L. C. Wright. 2003. "Coital Debut: The Role of Religiosity and Sex Attitudes in the Add Health Survey." *Journal of Sex Research* 40(4): 358–67.

Rothenberg, Richard B., John J. Potterat, Donald E. Woodhouse, William W. Darrow, Stephen Q. Muth, and Alden S. Klovdahl. 1995. "Choosing a Centrality Measure: Epidemiologic Correlates in the Colorado Springs Study of Social Networks." *Social Networks: Special Edition on Social Networks and Infectious Disease: HIV/AIDS* 17:273–97.

Rothenberg, Richard B., Donald E. Woodhouse, John J. Potterat, Stephen Q. Muth, William W. Darrow, and Alden S. Klovdahl. 1995. "Social Networks in Disease Transmission: The Colorado Springs Study." *NIDA Research Monographs* 151:3–19.

Sage, Colin. 2003. "Social Embeddedness and Relations of Regard: Alternative 'Good Food' Networks in South-West Ireland." *Journal of Rural Studies* 19(1): 47–60.

Salganik, Matthew J., and Douglas D. Heckathorn. 2004. "Sampling and Estimation in Hidden Populations using Respondent Driven Sampling." *Sociological Methodology* 34:193–240.

Sampson, Robert. J., Jeffrey D. Morenoff, and Thomas Gannon-Rowley. 2002. "Assessing 'Neighborhood Effects': Social Processes and New Directions in Research." *Annual Review of Sociology* 28:443–78.

Santelli, John S., Nancy D. Brener, Richard Lowry, Amita Bhatt, and Laurie S. Zabin. 1998. "Multiple Sexual Partners among U.S. Adolescents and Young Adults." *Family Planning Perspectives* 30(6): 271–75.

Schensul, Jean J., Judith A. Levy, and William B. Disch. 2003. "Individual, Contextual, and Social Network Factors Affecting Exposure to HIV/AIDS Risk among Older Residents Living in Low-Income Senior Housing Complexes." *Journal of Acquired Immune Deficiency Syndrome* 33, 2 Suppl.: S138–52.

Schulz, Amy J., Srimathi Kannan, J. Timothy Dvonch, Barbara A. Israel, Alex Allen III, Sherman A. James, James S. House, and James Lepkowski. 2005. "Social and Physical Environments and Disparities in Risk for Cardiovascular Disease: The Healthy Environments Partnership Conceptual Model." *Environmental Health Perspectives* 113(12): 1817–25.

Schwartz, Hillel. 1986. *Never Satisfied: A Cultural History of Diets, Fantasies, and Fat*. New York: Doubleday.

Seeman, Teresa E. 1996. "Social Ties and Health: The Benefits of Social Integration." *Annals of Epidemiology* 6(5): 442–51.

Smith, Kirsten P., and Nicholas A. Christakis. 2008. "Social Networks and Health." *Annual Review of Sociology* 34(1): 405–29.

Spanagel, Rainer, and F. Weiss. 1999. "The Dopamine Hypothesis of Reward: Past and Current Status." *Trends in Neuroscience* 22(11): 521–27.

Strauss, Richard S., and Harold A. Pollack. 2003. "Social Marginalization of Overweight Children." *Archives of Pediatric and Adolescent Medicine* 157(8): 746–52.

Tang, Tricia S., Morton B. Brown, Martha M. Funnell, and Robert M. Anderson. 2008. "Social Support, Quality of Life, and Self-Care Behaviors among African Americans with Type 2 Diabetes." *Diabetes Educator* 34(2): 266–76.

Udry, J. Richard, and John O. G. Billy. 1987. "Initiation of Coitus in Early Adolescence." *American Sociological Review* 52(6): 841–55.

Uecker, Jeremy E., Nicole Angotti, and Mark D. Regnerus. 2008. "Going Most of the Way: 'Technical Virginity' among American Adolescents." *Social Science Research* 37:1200–1215.

Valente, Thomas W., Beth R. Hoffman, Annamara Ritt-Olson, Kara Lichtman, and C. Anderson Johnson. 2003. "Effects of a Social-Network Method for Group Assignment Strategies on Peer-Led Tobacco Prevention Programs in Schools." *American Journal of Public Health* 93(11): 1837–43.

Wabitsch, Martin. 2000. "Overweight and Obesity in European Children: Definition and Diagnostic Procedures, Risk Factors and Consequences for Later Health Outcome." *European Journal of Pediatrics* 159(1 Supplement): S8–13.

Ward, Helen. 2007. "Prevention Strategies for Sexually Transmitted Infections: Importance of Sexual Network Structure and Epidemic Phase." *Sexually Transmitted Infections* 83: i43–49.

Wellman, Barry, and Scot Wortley. 1990. "Different Strokes from Different Folks: Community Ties and Social Support." *American Journal of Sociology* 96(3): 558.

Wheaton, Blair. 1985. "Models for the Stress-Buffering Functions of Coping Resources." *Journal of Health and Social Behavior* 26(4): 352–64.

Wilkinson, Richard G. 1999. "Health, Hierarchy, and Social Anxiety." *Annals of the New York Academy of Science* 896:48–63.

Woodhouse, Donald E., Richard B. Rothenberg, John J. Potterat, William W. Darrow, Stephen Q. Muth, Alden S. Klovdahl, Helen P. Zimmerman, Helen L. Rogers, Tammy S. Maldonado, John B. Muth, and Judith U. Reynolds. 1994. "Mapping a Social Network of Heterosexuals at High Risk for HIV infection." *AIDS* 8(9): 1331–36.

Writing Committee for the ENRICHD Investigators. 2003. "Effects of Treating Depression and Low Perceived Social Support on Clinical Events after Myocardial Infarction: The Enhancing Recovery in Coronary Heart Disease Patients (ENRICHD) Randomized Trial." *Journal of the American Medical Association* 289(23): 3106–16.

Wutich, Amber, and Christopher McCarty. 2008. "Social Networks and Infant Feeding in Oaxaca, Mexico." *Maternal and Child Nutrition* 4(2): 15.

Wylie, John L., Teresa Cabral, and Ann M. Jolly. 2005. "Identification of Networks of Sexually Transmitted Infection: A Molecular, Geographic, and Social Network Analysis." *Journal of Infectious Diseases* 191(6): 899–906.

Wylie, John L., Lena Shah, and Ann Jolly. 2007. "Incorporating Geographic Settings into a Social Network Analysis of Injection Drug Use and Bloodborne Pathogen Prevalence." *Health and Place* 13(3): 617–28.

Zaba, Basia, Elizabeth Pisani, E. Slaymaker, and J. Ties Boerma. 2004. "Age at First Sex: Understanding Recent Trends in African Demographic Surveys." *Sexually Transmitted Infections* 80: ii28–35.

6

Race, Social Contexts, and Health
Examining Geographic Spaces and Places

David T. Takeuchi, University of Washington

Emily Walton, University of Washington

ManChui Leung, University of Washington

Race continues to have a strong association with health outcomes. African Americans, for example, have a higher incidence, greater prevalence, and longer duration of hypertension than do whites. These higher rates are a major risk factor for heart disease, kidney disease, and stroke (CDC 2007; Morenoff et al. 2007). The age-adjusted death rates for African Americans exceed those of whites by 46 percent for stroke, 32 percent for heart disease, 23 percent for cancer, and 787 percent for HIV disease (CDC 2007). Among Latinos, Puerto Rican Americans have the highest rate of lifetime asthma prevalence (196 per 1,000) making them almost 80 percent more likely to be diagnosed with asthma. Mexican American adults are 100 percent more likely than white adults to have been diagnosed with diabetes by a physician. Cancer incidence and death rates are higher for Native Hawaiians and Pacific Islanders (549 per 100,000) than for whites (448.5 per 100,000) due to higher rates for cancers of the prostate, lung, liver, stomach, and colorectum among men, and cancers of the breast and lung among women (CDC 2007; Miller et al. 2008). Native Americans, especially males ages fifteen to twenty-four, have substantially higher death rates (232 percent) for motor vehicle-related injuries and for suicide (194 percent) than other racial and ethnic groups (CDC 2007). Asian Americans are 20 percent more likely to have hepatitis B than whites and comprise almost 50 percent of chronic hepatitis B infections; these rates are related to a higher incidence and mortality of liver cancer among Asians (CDC 2006; Miller et al. 2008).

While racial variations in diseases are observed, the meaning and measurement of race is frequently contested. An early explanation for racial differences, which continues into the present but with less scientific support, attributes these variations to genetic differences. Essentialism, or biological determinism, sees racial categories as fixed, distinct, and constant over time. Essentialism suggests that some racial groups are less healthy and more apt to become ill and to die prematurely because they have physical, moral, or mental deficiencies based on their genetic or biological makeup. Genetic theories for explaining racial differences in health status are not widely supported in the contemporary scientific literature. Few genetic differences exist across racial groups, and social scientists challenge essentialist notions of race by arguing that people make attributions about groups based on stereotypes and prejudices that are tied to some physical traits (Omi and Winant 1994; Rosenberg et al. 2002).

Despite the ambiguities and complexities of racial categories, race still matters in many quality-of-life indicators (Smelser, Wilson, and Mitchell 2001). Sociologists consider race categories to be socially created boundaries that change in meaning and importance depending on the social and political climate of the time. Racial categories carry with them implicit and explicit images and beliefs about racial groups that provide rationales for treatment of group members (Takeuchi and Gage 2003). Race is particularly critical and meaningful when individuals have difficulty obtaining desired goods and resources because of their group membership (Williams and Williams-Morris 2000).

While the social science debate about the relative merits of different conceptualizations and measurements of race continues, it is clear by most measures that the population of the United States has become increasingly diverse and complex. Demographers predict that there will be significantly more changes over the next fifty years. Through the 1950s, African Americans comprised the primary racial minority group, with about 10 percent of the adult and 12 percent of the children's population (U.S. Bureau of the Census 2002). In the 2000 census, Latinos were identified as the largest minority group (U.S. Bureau of the Census 2001a); the 281,421,906 people living in the United States reflected the following racial representation: white (75 percent), Latino (13 percent), black or African American (12 percent), American Indian and Alaska Native (1 percent), Asian (4 percent), Native Hawaiian and Pacific Islander (0.1 percent), and other racial groups (6 percent). The complexity of race is magnified when mixed-race individuals are included in the picture. In 2000, when the U.S. census gave respondents the opportunity to check more than one racial group, 6.8 million people (2 percent of the population) identified themselves with two or more races.

Given the increased racial diversity in society and the move away from biological and genetic explanations, how is race linked to health? Scholars have provided a discussion of the possible social, cultural, and psychological factors that help answer this question, such as socioeconomic status, discrimination, coping styles, social support,

and stress (Reskin 2003; Williams and Collins 1995). Rather than cover similar ground, this chapter focuses on some of the social and geographic spaces that help frame empirical examinations of race and health.In the United States, race and space are historically intertwined. Racial and ethnic segregation sorts individuals and groups of comparable socioeconomic status into different neighborhood environments and have been primary mechanisms by which discrimination has operated (Massey and Denton 1993). The organization of racially and ethnically segregated neighborhoods reinforces inequality, concentrates poverty, and limits the socioeconomic mobility of residents. These neighborhoods are characterized by inferior schools, lack of employment opportunities, poor housing, smaller returns on real estate investments, unequal access to a broad range of public and private services, and neglect of the physical environment (e.g., landfills, deserted factories, vacant lots). These socioeconomic factors produced by residential segregation have been found to have a significant impact on health outcomes and mortality (Acevedo-Garcia and Lochner 2003; Collins and Williams 1999; Robert 1998).

Geographic Distribution of Racial and Ethnic Groups

The most recent U.S. census estimates show that racial and ethnic diversity is geographically expanding into metropolitan central cities, suburbs, and rural areas (U.S. Bureau of the Census 2008). The United States continues to be a predominately urbanized country, with 81 percent of the population residing in metropolitan central cities and suburbs and with racial and ethnic minorities accounting for 50 percent of residents in some of the largest cities such as Los Angeles and New York City. The urban decline among whites and the increase in racial and ethnic minorities is mirrored in the suburbs, where the white population has decreased from 76 to 72 percent over the past decade (U.S. Bureau of the Census 2008). Reversing trends, nonmetropolitan or rural areas received a substantial net-migration gain from metropolitan areas between 1995 and 2000 as a result of racial and ethnic minority migration from abroad and from other regions. In rural areas, white and African American populations remained stable but the migration of Latinos, Asians, Native Hawaiians, and Pacific Islanders increased the racial minority population to almost 20 percent, with a growth rate eight times faster than that of whites (U.S. Bureau of the Census 2003b).

Racial and ethnic minorities have significant populations in all four regions of the country but are unevenly distributed across these areas. Table 6.1 shows the regional distribution of racial and ethnic groups and their percentage change in the U.S. census from 1990 to 2000. The South experienced the most growth among Asians, Africans Americans, Latinos, and whites, while the Northeast increased for American Indians and Alaskan Natives, and Native Hawaiians and Pacific Islanders. Table 6.2 further shows the five states with the highest proportion of each racial/ethnic group. While California and Texas are in the top five states for all groups and New York is in the top five states for four groups, these three states represent larger or smaller proportions depending on the group being examined. An overall trend, especially among Asians, Latinos, Native Hawaiians, and Pacific Islanders, is migration to states not in the top five as well as to suburban and rural counties, with Latinos the most geographically dispersed. Of note, the 2000 census recorded a very high state-level net-migration rate (563.1 percent) of Native Hawaiians and Pacific Island-

ers to Nevada, which points to a steeper trend of high population growth outside the top five states (U.S. Bureau of the Census 2001b).

According to the 2000 census, primary and secondary migration of the foreign born helped offset domestic migration loss in many areas, especially the Northeast and West. In terms of population distribution, immigrants can have tremendous impact on an area's racial and ethnic makeup. Historically, immigrants settled in central cities in gateway states such as California and New York in their primary migration. A secondary migration may then ensue, often to suburbs or other states, leading to a wider spread of immigrant populations (U.S. Bureau of the Census 2003a). The 2000 census shows a new trend. While the majority of immigrants (49 percent) still migrated to the metropolitan central cities, more immigrants than in earlier censuses moved to suburbs, smaller cities, and rural areas in their primary migration. In the secondary migration of immigrants, Nevada had the highest rates of net migration (276 percent), followed by North Carolina (187 percent), Georgia (178 percent), and Arkansas (155 percent) (U.S. Bureau of the Census 2003a).

Place Stratification

Sociology has long focused on the problems associated with the geographic concentration of racial

Table 6.1. Population distribution and percentage change by racial/ethnic group and region

	Northeast		Midwest		South		West	
	% in 2000*	% change 1990–2000	% in 2000	% change 1990–2000	% in 2000	% change 1990–2000	% in 2000	% change 1990–2000
American Indians and Alaska Natives	9.08	2.69	17.35	0.11	30.57	1.85	43.00	−4.65
Asians	19.90	0.73	11.71	0.77	19.05	3.22	49.34	−4.71
Blacks or African Americans	18.00	−2.43	18.78	−5.21	53.62	19.26	9.60	−11.63
Hispanics or Latinos	14.88	−1.91	8.85	1.13	32.82	2.55	43.45	−1.76
Native Hawaiians and Pacific Islanders	7.31	4.43	6.33	2.86	13.49	5.80	72.87	−13.09
Whites	19.54	−1.52	25.22	−0.83	34.25	1.41	20.98	0.94

Source: U.S. Bureau of the Census 2000

* Number based on Racial/Ethnic Group Alone or In Combination Population Count

Table 6.2. Percentages of racial/ethnic groups in states with highest racial/ethnic proportions

American Indians and Alaska Natives		Asians		Blacks or African Americans		Hispanics or Latinos		Native Hawaiians and Pacific Islanders		Whites	
California	15.23	California	34.93	New York	8.88	California	31.06	Hawaii	32.33	California	9.91
Oklahoma	9.51	New York	4.41	California	6.90	Texas	18.89	California	25.33	Oklahoma	7.03
Arizona	7.10	Hawaii	5.91	Texas	6.85	New York	8.12	Washington	4.89	Arizona	6.12
Texas	5.23	Texas	5.41	Florida	6.79	Florida	7.60	Texas	3.33	Texas	5.87
New Mexico	4.65	New Jersey	4.41	Georgia	6.57	Illinois	4.33	New York	3.27	New Mexico	4.88
Total	41.73	Total	55.06	Total	35.98	Total	70.01	Total	69.14	Total	33.81

Source: U.S. Bureau of the Census 2000

and ethnic groups in selected states and in certain locations within states. Geographic areas that include neighborhoods, residences, businesses, waste dumps, and environmental hazards become prized or devalued depending on their historic importance, proximity to power and influence, and quality of natural or manufactured environmental resources (e.g., forests, buildings, parks). The differential value placed on residential areas creates and fosters a spatial stratification system that often intersects with race. At various points in history, some racial groups were allowed to work but not live in select residential areas. Immigrants often began residing in certain areas of cities before they could move to other locations. It is this critical melding of space and race that still operates and has important consequences for the study of health and illness.

What Is the Meaning of Residential Segregation?

One form of place stratification, residential segregation, like socioeconomic status and gender, can be considered a fundamental cause of racial disparities in health because it structures opportunities and resources that facilitate or constrain access to power, social and psychological resources, and economic capital that are linked to health and illness (Link and Phelan 1995; Schulz et al. 2002; Williams and Collins 2001). Residential segregation is far from being a problem of the past; most racial and ethnic minority groups today experience high levels of segregation from whites in cities across the United States (Iceland 2004). Residential segregation can be measured

in multiple ways (Massey and Denton 1988) but generally includes: (1) unevenness or dissimilarity in the distribution of groups across an area; (2) degree of potential contact or interaction between members of different groups; (3) concentration, or the relative amount of physical space occupied by groups; (4) degree of centralization, or location near the central city; and (5) spatial clustering of group neighborhoods. These five dimensions of segregation, and the indexes commonly used to measure them, are summarized in Table 6.3. Table 6.3 also provides a comparison of the indexes for racial and ethnic groups in different regions.

African American–white segregation has declined only modestly over the past two decades, while Asian and Latino segregation from whites has increased, largely due to sustained immigration. A recent investigation into the decline in segregation among African Americans could not attribute it to any of the hypothesized sources, such as attitudinal changes on the part of whites regarding integration, the growth of the African American middle class, population shifts of African Americans to regions in the West and South with lower overall segregation, or the increase of multiethnic metropolises (Logan, Stults, and Farley 2004). Segregation is likely to persist because of the continued immigration of Asians and Latinos to the United States and few substantive changes in racial attitudes. Accordingly, segregation may continue to be an important setting in predicting the life chances of racial and ethnic minority group members well into the future. As the racial and ethnic minority population in the United States continues to be shaped by immigration trends in the twenty-first century, theoretical models underlying residential segregation as a fundamental cause of health and disease outcomes must account for the ways in which this phenomenon differs among racial and ethnic groups.

The literature on racial residential segregation typically rests on the premise that disadvantaged segregated neighborhood conditions explain poorer health outcomes among African Americans living in segregated neighborhoods. In place stratification theory, majority group preferences and active discrimination constrain the social and spatial mobility of minority group members, resulting in their residential concentration in poor,

Table 6.3. Residential segregation indexes (weighted averages) by racial/ethnic group and region

	Number of Metropolitan Areas	Dissimilarity Index[b]	Isolation Index[c]	Delta Index[d]	Absolute Centralization Index[e]	Spatial Proximity Index[f]
American Indians and Alaska Natives						
Northeast	0	(X)	(X)	(X)	(X)	(X)
Midwest	1	0.384	0.177	0.885	0.871	1.050
South	4	0.253	0.144	0.587	0.561	1.053
West	8	0.465	0.239	0.755	0.706	1.228
Asians and Pacific Islanders[a]						
Northeast	6	0.461	0.320	0.720	0.699	1.089
Midwest	2	0.431	0.175	0.719	0.725	1.074
South	3	0.418	0.221	0.780	0.776	1.088
West	19	0.426	0.467	0.735	0.644	1.146
Blacks or African Americans						
Northeast	31	0.739	0.679	0.819	0.717	1.465
Midwest	53	0.741	0.651	0.859	0.788	1.526
South	114	0.581	0.581	0.748	0.695	1.303
West	22	0.559	0.435	0.823	0.740	1.283
Hispanics or Latinos						
Northeast	22	0.615	0.578	0.757	0.666	1.290
Midwest	13	0.567	0.449	0.765	0.710	1.328
South	38	0.461	0.601	0.736	0.706	1.182
West	50	0.514	0.597	0.791	0.695	1.261

Source: U.S. Bureau of the Census 2000, Summary File 1.

a. Asian and Pacific Islanders are grouped together to facilitate comparison with earlier versions of the census.

b. Dissimilarity Index: Measures the percentage of a group's population that would have to change residence for each neighborhood to have the same percentage of that group as the metropolitan area overall. The index ranges from 0.0 (complete integration) to 1.0 (complete segregation).

c. Isolation Index: Measures "the extent to which minority members are exposed only to one another" (Massey and Denton 1993, 288) and is computed as the minority-weighted average of the minority proportion in each area. Higher values of isolation indicate higher segregation.

d. Delta Index: "Computes the proportion of [minority] members residing in areal units with above average density of [minority] members" (Massey and Denton 1993, 290). The index gives the proportion of a group's population that would have to move across areal units to achieve a uniform density.

e. Absolute Centralization Index: Examines the distribution of the minority group around the center and varies between -1.0 and 1.0. "Positive values indicate a tendency for [minority] group members to reside close to the city center, while negative values indicate a tendency to live in outlying areas. A score of 0 means that a group has a uniform distribution throughout the metropolitan area" (Massey and Denton 1993, 293).

f. Spatial Proximity Index: Average of intragroup proximities for the minority and majority populations, weighted by the proportion each group represents of the total population. Spatial proximity equals 1.0 if there is no differential clustering between minority and majority group members. It is greater than 1.0 when members of each group live nearer to one another than to members of the other group, and is less than 1.0 if minority and majority members live nearer to members of the other group than to members of their own group.

inner-city ghettos with limited resources. Massey and Denton (1993) contend that "white society is deeply implicated in the ghetto. White institutions created it, white institutions maintain it, and white society condones it." White preferences historically took the form of de jure discrimination in housing markets, mortgage lending, racial steering, and exclusionary zoning practices that restricted racial and ethnic minority groups to certain neighborhoods (Cutler, Glaeser, and Vigdor 1999). While legally enforced discrimination ended with the civil rights legislation in the 1960s, de facto discrimination has taken its place in the form of white preferences for white neighbors (Charles 2000) and high housing prices that effectively keep economically disadvantaged racial and ethnic minority individuals out of certain areas.

Recent evidence suggests that the reasons for and experiences of residential segregation among other minority groups, especially those containing large immigrant populations, differ from those of African Americans along important dimensions (Zhou and Logan 1991; Zhou 1992). Asian and Latino Americans have unique residential experiences that may relate more to factors associated with recent immigration than to active discrimination by whites, suggesting that place stratification theory does not universally explain the effects of residential segregation on health status among members of these diverse racial and ethnic minority groups. Among racial and ethnic groups with large proportions of immigrants, classic spatial assimilation theory and segmented assimilation theory may be more applicable for understanding the ways in which structural and social resources are distributed and function to affect health in different types of neighborhoods.

Viewed through a classic spatial assimilation lens, recent immigrants settle in immigrant enclaves located near the inner city that can concentrate social resources but that often lack structural resources (K. Wilson and Portes 1980). These neighborhoods ease individuals' transition into the U.S. labor market and provide them with social support as they adapt to a new culture. The spatial assimilation model predicts that as individuals acculturate, become more fluent in English, and gain economic security, they and subsequent generations will assimilate with mainstream society by moving into white, suburban, and affluent neighborhoods. This decreased segregation is hypothesized to lead to better health status as individuals utilize resources located in residentially integrated neighborhoods. Socioeconomic diversity among contemporary immigrants, however, suggests that the trajectory defined by classic spatial assimilation may not apply uniformly across individuals and groups.

Segmented assimilation theory offers an alternative hypothesis (Portes and Zhou 1993). Individual attributes and group social position predict divergent patterns of spatial incorporation among immigrants and subsequent generations. If, upon settling in the United States, personal human capital attributes are low, immigrants and subsequent generations are less likely to assimilate into white, middle-class neighborhoods, instead cultivating ties within poorer, native-born coethnic or African American communities (South, Crowder, and Chavez 2005). In this case, the health effects of living in segregated neighborhoods are more likely to represent those described by a place stratification perspective.

An alternative application of segmented assimilation theory predicts that immigrants who come to the United States with high levels of human capital have more options in terms of choosing to live in communities that are not based on socioeconomic or linguistic necessity. It is plausible that groups entering the United States with many highly educated individuals who speak English well and have corresponding occupational prestige have little to gain by spatially assimilating and thus have some choice in forming residentially segregated ethnic communities (Alba et al. 1999; Logan, Alba, and Zhang 2002). Instead of being areas of concentrated poverty and structural deprivation, these racial and ethnic communities may, in fact, concentrate structural resources like supplemental education institutions that likely exert a positive effect on health status (Zhou 2007).

In summary, because of the differences in the way residentially segregated neighborhoods in which racial and ethnic minorities live are formed, the direction of association between segregation and health outcomes is likely also diverse. In the following sections, we consider the existing evidence on the relationship of residential segregation to health outcomes and the pathways through which segregation affects health status, while taking into account the complexity underlying the formation and maintenance of racially and ethnically segregated neighborhoods.

Segregation and Health Outcomes

Research on the effects of geographic context on individual health outcomes commonly conceives of residential segregation as exposing individuals to poverty and social deprivation. A burgeoning literature demonstrates that this model works well when exploring the differences among African Americans and whites. Measured by the various segregation indexes, most evidence suggests that residential segregation contributes to inferior health status among African Americans. The effects vary depending on the dimension of segregation analyzed, however, hinting that some aspects of segregation may be beneficial to health outcomes, even among African Americans.

In a study of mortality, Jackson and colleagues (2000) found that African American men living in highly segregated neighborhoods have three times the mortality risk of African American men living in the least segregated areas. Among African American women in this study, the mortality risk for living in areas of high segregation was twice that of African American women living in areas of low segregation. Using the index of dissimilarity, LaVeist (1993) found that living in more segregated cities is associated with a rise in the African American infant mortality rate, while the rate for whites declined in such cities. In a similar analysis examining infant mortality in thirty-eight major U.S. metropolitan areas, Polednak (1991) established that the index of dissimilarity is the most important predictor of African American–white differences and that this effect is independent of socioeconomic factors. Employing a measure of spatial isolation at the census-tract level, Grady (2006) demonstrated that residential segregation predicts low birth weight for African American infants in New York City, after controlling for individual risk factors and neighborhood poverty.

Concentration of African Americans in central cities is associated with increased incidence of low birth weight, somewhat influenced by exposure to older housing and less-educated neighbors (Ellen 2000). Subramanian, Acevedo-Garcia, and Osypuk (2005) established that residential isolation of African Americans from whites across U.S. metropolitan areas is associated with increased odds of their reporting poor self-rated health. In agreement with this, higher residential isolation is also associated with higher body mass index and greater odds of being overweight among African Americans (Chang 2006). One study discovered opposing effects of segregation on birth outcomes among African Americans: higher metropolitan area isolation was associated with worse birth outcomes, while higher clustering was associated with more optimal birth outcomes among African American women (Bell et al. 2006). The high contiguity between racial and ethnic minority neighborhoods may be a correlate of community attributes that are health promoting through the pathways of political empowerment, social cohesion, and protection from discrimination.

While a considerable body of research demonstrates that many aspects of residential segregation are harmful to the health status of African Americans, the findings of the limited number of studies of residential segregation and well-being among Asians and Latinos are not consistent. Among Latinos, one study showed that segregation increases the risk of tuberculosis infection (Acevedo-Garcia 2001), while others reported beneficial health effects from increased segregation: better self-rated health (Patel et al. 2003), lower disease prevalence (Eschbach et al. 2004), and lower mortality rates (LeClere, Rogers, and Peters 1997). A recent investigation reported mixed results based on the Latino ethnic subgroup under consideration, with segregation increasing the number of health problems among Puerto Rican Americans but not Mexican Americans; further, among Mexican Americans, generational status conditioned the effect: second and later generations had better health than immigrant Mexican Americans in segregated neighborhoods (M. Lee and Ferraro 2007). In the only study on residential segregation and well-being conducted among Asian Americans, Gee (2002) found that Chinese Americans living in redlined areas of Los Angeles (areas in which banks were biased against racial and ethnic minorities in their lending practices) reported better physical and mental health compared to those living in other areas of the city. In the same study, segregation, as measured by the index of dissimilarity, did not predict health status. In sum, a complicated picture emerges: most studies show beneficial effects of segregation on the well-being of Latinos and Asian Americans, but this finding varies according to the health outcome being assessed, the racial or ethnic group under consideration, the nativity status of the respondent, and the dimension of segregation analyzed.

How Does Segregation Affect Health?

While a majority of the current research on the health effects of residential segregation has documented that a relationship exists, by examining neighborhood effects in a broad way we note that an emerging literature has also begun to explore the underlying pathways through which this relationship may operate. Residential segregation shapes access to important structural and social resources, typically measured by aggregating individual characteristics such as socioeconomic status that are seen as markers of neighborhood institutional structures and social conditions—levels of crime, community infrastructure and services, educational and employment opportunities, social integration, and exposure to discrimination. Relying largely on a place stratification perspective, a bulk of the evidence suggests that segregation is harmful to racial and ethnic minorities because features of disadvantage are clustered in segregated neighborhoods. Alternatively, the spatial and segmented assimilation perspectives suggest that aspects of segregation may be beneficial to certain minorities because structural and social resources are concentrated in the areas in which they live.

Residential segregation is often marked by institutional abandonment that has created a uniquely disadvantaged physical and infrastructure environment. Lack of political power among residentially segregated neighborhoods leads to disinvestment of economic resources and services

provided by the city, such as police and fire protection, and increased exposure to higher levels of air pollution, traffic noise, and industrial contaminants (Brown 1994; LaVeist 1993). Individuals in disadvantaged neighborhoods have less access to health care and grocery stores, which can affect health outcomes directly through poor nutritional and health behavior choices (Cheadle et al. 1991). While there is increasing interest in the health impacts of aspects of the neighborhood built environment, such as housing quality, street design, and the availability of parks and recreation (Rao et al. 2007), comprehensive investigation of these pathways is still forthcoming.

Residential segregation shapes access to educational and employment opportunities, leading to limited socioeconomic attainment and corresponding poor health among racial and ethnic minorities living in disadvantaged neighborhoods (Adler et al. 1994). In most cities in the United States, residence determines which public schools students attend, and community resources determine the quality of neighborhood schools. Compared to schools in nonsegregated neighborhoods, schools that serve segregated areas tend to have lower test scores, less-qualified teachers, fewer connections with colleges and employers, more structural decay, and higher dropout rates (Orfield and Eaton 1996). Residential segregation can also systematically separate the residents of certain neighborhoods from jobs. The spatial mismatch hypothesis posits that as businesses move away from metropolitan centers and toward the suburbs, low-skilled minorities are less able to find employment due to their residential concentration in the inner city (W. Wilson 1996). Further, Tilly and colleagues (2001) find that potential employers discriminate based on the residences of job applicants. Employers were found to associate inner-city applicants with family problems, drug use, and low reading, writing, communication, and motivational skills. Lack of infrastructure, physical decay, and socioeconomic disadvantage create stressful conditions that may be expressed in terms of poor health behaviors and create unsupportive social relationships among residents in segregated communities.

Stressful social conditions in residentially segregated neighborhoods have also been linked to poorer health outcomes. Shaw and McKay (1969) argue that socially disorganized neighborhoods have fewer formal and informal types of social control and monitoring. Segregation concentrates conditions such as drug use, joblessness, welfare dependency, and unwed teenage childbearing, producing a social context where these conditions are not only common but also the norm (Massey and Denton 1993). Neighborhood safety and levels of crime may affect whether individuals engage in physical activity (Stahl et al. 2001). The perception of disorder and the resulting fear among residents in disadvantaged neighborhoods have also been shown to correlate with increases in stress and poor health (Ross and Mirowsky 2001). Disadvantaged and unstable neighborhoods may also be less able to sustain cohesive social networks and positive social norms, which have been consistently shown to be protective of health and to increase the likelihood that healthy behaviors will be adopted (Berkman 1995; House, Landis, and Umberson 1988).

While residentially segregated neighborhoods can exhibit disadvantaged structural and social characteristics, some unique features of immigrant enclaves and racial and ethnic communities may mitigate or reverse the destructive effects of residential segregation. More specifically, immigrant enclaves and ethnic communities may concentrate educational and economic resources and increase social integration and support, all of which are beneficial to health outcomes. Structural features such as educational and economic resources may be protective of health for members of these communities. Immigrant enclaves and ethnic communities often house a highly sophisticated system of education that supplements public schooling, including language schools and after-school education (Zhou 2007). These educational institutions facilitate social mobility by providing access to quality education and as settings for social support, network building, and formation of social capital for immigrant and U.S.-born children alike. Increased educational participation may be complemented by higher economic returns among participants in the enclave economy. Though controversial, some evidence suggests that returns to human capital are significantly greater among individuals employed in enclave enterprises than among those employed in businesses tied to the traditional labor market (K. Wilson and Portes 1980; Portes and Bach 1985).

Community structure can also influence social processes that are important to health status. Individuals living among others of the same ethnicity may be more likely to receive instrumental social support, be influenced by shared norms relating to health behaviors, and be more socially engaged than those living among neighbors they consider to be different from them. Strong ethnic networks can work instrumentally by providing assistance with financial needs, aid in getting to appointments, help with decision making, and informal health care (Berkman and Glass 2000; Weiss et al. 2005). For example, the receipt of mental health care is facilitated for refugees being welcomed by a strong ethnic community, which works directly by improving knowledge of the location of services and indirectly through referral to services (Portes, Kyle, and Eaton 1992). The presence of similar racial and ethnic neighbors can also influence health behaviors (e.g., exercise, alcohol and cigarette use, and dietary patterns) through shared norms (Marsden and Friedkin 1994). Residents of racial and ethnic neighborhoods may also be more likely to have opportunities for social engagement—for example, getting together with family and friends, and participating in recreational or religious activities. Such social engagement can provide a sense of belonging, meaning, and attachment to others, which have salubrious health effects. Individuals feel that having supportive people to care for them when they are sick will increase their ability to survive health crises, and they may also feel obligated to care for themselves so they can be the provider of support for others (Ross and Mirowsky 2002).

There is some evidence that living in more ethnically dense, isolated neighborhoods reduces exposure to prejudice and discrimination. Perceptions of everyday discrimination, routine practices that infuse the daily lives of racial and ethnic minorities (e.g., being treated as if one does not speak English, is in this country illegally, or is untrustworthy), have repeatedly been shown to relate negatively to health and well-being (Forman, Williams, and Jackson 1997; Gee et al.

2007; Kessler, Mickelson, and Williams 1999). The ethnic density hypothesis suggests that living primarily among coethnic neighbors may structurally reduce the opportunities for negative encounters with whites, and thus reduce the social stress felt by minorities living in these neighborhoods by limiting their exposure to everyday discrimination (Halpern and Nazroo 1999; Hunt et al. 2007).

Conceptual and Measurement Issues

The past two decades have shown an enormous increase in research that examines the effects of residential areas and health. The statistical and computer software innovations in spatial analyses have especially been useful in providing accurate means for characterizing residential areas. Despite the increase in empirical work and the solid contributions of past studies, several problems have impeded the field from making even more impressive gains. First, there is a lack of uniformity about the conceptualization of place. Several notable scholars argue that place is more than a geographic location and should be conceptualized as a socioecological force that has detectable and independent effects on social life (Gieryn 2000; Habraken 1998; Werlen 1993). If this area of study is to advance, more serious work on the conceptualization of place is needed (Macintyre, Ellaway, and Cummins 2002). Second, studies have often used different measures of place such as cities, counties, census tracts, and zip codes. When researchers show divergent findings, it is often not clear whether the differences are real or whether they are artifacts of the different measures used in the studies. Third, many studies that investigate contextual effects are actually based on the aggregated characteristics of individuals rather than of geographic areas. While the aggregate of individuals in a geographic area is important, it does not fully describe the attributes of the resources and built environment within places. Making distinctions between the compositional and true contextual effects will more clearly identify the factors that best explain how race is associated with health (Ellen, Mijanovich, and Dillman 2001).

Social environments help contextualize how race is associated with health outcomes. The current research on residential areas builds on the early work of sociologists, especially the Chicago school, who developed theories and methods to study the growth of the city and its attendant strengths and challenges. One overlooked facet of the Chicago school, especially when it comes to investigating residential areas and neighborhoods, is the social psychology of place. The social psychology of place concerns itself with how people establish connections or become disengaged with a location. Since much of the history of race and place centers on how racial groups are excluded from some geographic spaces, the social psychology of place can provide keen insights about how race is linked to health and illness.

Much of what we know about race, place, and health comes from cross-sectional studies, and longitudinal studies about place and health are essential. We lack information about how mobility, stability, and frequent moves to and from neighborhoods influence health. Studies over time can also provide insights about reverse causality; people with illnesses may move to neighborhoods that provide them with more comfort and support. It has long been suspected that immigrants who suffer from an illness, for example, may move from a predominantly white neighborhood to a racial or ethnic enclave because it provides them with social support and resources. Longitudinal designs can provide the data that can examine these types of hypotheses, which are not possible to test with cross-sectional data.

Future studies will also do well to investigate place effects in nonconventional settings. Much of the work on residential areas has focused on urban areas, and we are absent a large body of data on place and health in other geographic areas such as suburbs and rural regions. We are also absent much data on whether and how virtual places may influence health. It is possible to visit areas or to create residential areas without leaving one's computer. Since racial and ethnic groups may vary in their use of computers, and we do not know whether these virtual places have any salutary effects, this area opens up a potential area of inquiry.

In sum, the effect of place on health and health behaviors is far from uniform across population groups and health outcomes. The need, at this time, is to move toward more nuanced theorizing about the effects of place on health, and toward creating and testing hypotheses about the specific pathways by which place influences health. Accordingly, there is compelling scholarly need to make major theoretical, methodological, and empirical contributions toward understanding specifically how places promote social engagement or social estrangement, stress or security, and health or illness within and across racial and ethnic minority groups.

Note

This chapter is supported by the National Institutes of Health grants R01HD049142, U01 MH62209, U01 MH62207, and P50MH073511.

References

Acevedo-Garcia, Dolores. 2001. "Zip Code–Level Risk Factors for Tuberculosis: Neighborhood Environment and Residential Segregation in New Jersey, 1985–1992." *American Journal of Public Health* 91:734–41.

Acevedo-Garcia, Dolores, and Kimberley K. Lochner. 2003. "Residential Segregation and Health." In *Neighborhoods and Health*, ed. Ichiro Kawachi and Lisa F. Berkman, 265–87. New York: Oxford University Press.

Adler, Nancy E., Thomas Boyce, Margaret A. Chesney, Sheldon Cohen, Susan Folkman, Robert L. Kahn, and S. Leonard Syme. 1994. "Socioeconomic Status and Health: The Challenge of the Gradient." *American Psychologist* 49:15–24.

Alba, Richard D., John R. Logan, Brian J. Stults, Gilbert Marzan, and Wenquan Zhang. 1999. "Immigrant Groups in the Suburbs: A Reexamination of Suburbanization and Spatial Assimilation." *American Sociological Review* 64:446–60.

Bell, Janice F., Frederick J. Zimmerman, Gunnar R. Almgren, Jonathan D. Mayer, and Colleen E. Huebner. 2006. "Birth Outcomes among Urban African-American Women: A Multilevel Analysis of the Role of Racial Residential Segregation." *Social Science and Medicine* 63:3030–45.

Berkman, Lisa F. 1995. "The Role of Social Relations in Health Promotion." *Psychosomatic Medicine* 57:245–54.

Berkman, Lisa F., and Thomas Glass. 2000. "Social Integration, Social Networks, Social Support, and Health." In *Social Epidemiology*, ed. L. F. Berkman and I. Kawachi, 137–73. New York: Oxford University Press.

Brown, Phil. 1994. "Race, Class, and Environmental Health: A Review and Systematization of the Literature." *Environmental Research* 69:15–30.

Centers for Disease Control (CDC). 2006. "Screening for Chronic Hepatitis B among Asian/Pacific Islander Populations—New York City, 2005." *Morbidity and Mortality Weekly Report* 55:18, www.cdc.gov/mmwr/preview/mmwrhtml/mm5518a2.htm.

———. 2007. *Health United States, 2007 with Chartbook on Trends in the Health of Americans.* Hyattsville, Md.: National Center for Health Statistics.

Chang, Virginia W. 2006. "Racial Residential Segregation and Weight Status among U.S. Adults." *Social Science and Medicine* 63:1289–1303.

Charles, Camille Zubrinsky. 2000. "Residential Segregation in Los Angeles." In *Prismatic Metropolis: Inequality in Los Angeles*, ed. L. D. Bobo, M. L. Oliver, J. H. Johnston Jr., and A. Valenzuela Jr., 167–219. New York: Russell Sage Foundation.

Cheadle, Allen, Bruce M. Psaty, Susan Curry, Edward Wagner, Paula Diehr, Thomas Koepsell, and Alan Kristal. 1991. "Community-Level Comparisons between the Grocery Store Environment and Individual Dietary Practices." *Preventive Medicine* 20:250–61.

Collins, Chiquita, and David Williams. 1999. "Segregation and Mortality: The Deadly Effects of Racism." *Sociological Forum* 14(3): 495–532.

Cutler, David M., Edward L. Glaeser, and Jacob L. Vigdor. 1999. "The Rise and Decline of the American Ghetto." *Journal of Political Economy* 107:455–506.

Ellen, Ingrid Gould. 2000. "Is Segregation Bad for Your Health? The Case of Low Birth Weight." *Brookings-Wharton Papers on Urban Affairs* 2000:203–29.

Ellen, Ingrid Gould, Tod Mijanovich, and Keri-Nicole Dillman. 2001. "Neighborhood Effects on Health: Exploring the Links and Assessing the Evidence." *Journal of Urban Affairs* 23:391–408.

Eschbach, Karl, Glenn V. Ostir, Kushang V. Patel, Kyriakos S. Markides, and James S. Goodwin. 2004. "Neighborhood Context and Mortality among Older Mexican Americans: Is There a Barrio Advantage?" *American Journal of Public Health* 94:1807–12.

Forman, Tyrone A., David R. Williams, and James S. Jackson. 1997. "Race, Place, and Discrimination." In *Perspectives on Social Problems*, ed. C. Gardner, 237–61. Greenwich, Conn.: JAI Press.

Gee, Gilbert C. 2002. "A Multilevel Analysis of the Relationship between Institutional and Individual Racial Discrimination and Health Status." *American Journal of Public Health* 92:615–23.

Gee, Gilbert C., Michael S. Spencer, Juan Chen, and

David Takeuchi. 2007. "A Nationwide Study of Discrimination and Chronic Health Conditions among Asian Americans." *American Journal of Public Health* 97:1275–82.

Gieryn, Thomas F. 2000. "A Space for Place in Sociology." *Annual Review of Sociology* 26:463–96.

Grady, Sue C. 2006. "Racial Disparities in Low Birthweight and the Contribution of Residential Segregation: A Multilevel Analysis." *Social Science and Medicine* 63:3013–29.

Habraken, Nicolaas John. 1998. *The Structure of the Ordinary: Form and Control in the Built Environment.* Cambridge, Mass.: MIT Press.

Halpern, David, and James Nazroo. 1999. "The Ethnic Density Effect: Results from a National Community Study of England and Wales." *International Journal of Social Psychiatry* 46:34–46.

House, James, Karl Landis, and Debra Umberson. 1988. "Social Relationships and Health." *Science* 241:540–45.

Hunt, Matthew O., Lauren A. Wise, Marie-Claude Jipguep, Yvette C. Cozier, and Lynn Rosenberg. 2007. "Neighborhood Racial Composition and Perceptions of Racial Discrimination: Evidence from the Black Women's Health Study." *Social Psychology Quarterly* 70:272–89.

Iceland, John. 2004. "Beyond Black and White: Metropolitan Residential Segregation in Multi-Ethnic America." *Social Science Research* 33:248–71.

Jackson, Sharon A., Roger T. Anderson, Norman J. Johnson, and Paul D. Sorlie. 2000. "The Relation of Residential Segregation to All-Cause Mortality: A Study in Black and White." *American Journal of Public Health* 90:615–17.

Kessler, Ronald C., Kristin D. Mickelson, and David R. Williams. 1999. "The Prevalence, Distribution, and Mental Health Correlates of Perceived Discrimination in the United States." *Journal of Health and Social Behavior* 40:208–30.

LaVeist, Thomas A. 1993. "Segregation, Poverty, and Empowerment: Health Consequences for African Americans." *Milbank Quarterly* 71:41–64.

LeClere, Felicia B., Richard G. Rogers, and Kimberley D. Peters. 1997. "Ethnicity and Mortality in the United States: Individual and Community Correlates." *Social Forces* 76:169–98.

Lee, Barrett A., Sean F. Reardon, Glenn Firebaugh, Chad R. Farrell, Stephen A. Matthews, and David O'Sullivan. 2008. "Beyond the Census Tract: Patterns and Determinants of Racial Segregation at Multiple Geographic Scales." *American Sociological Review* 73:766–91.

Lee, Min-Ah, and Kenneth F. Ferraro. 2007. "Neighborhood Residential Segregation and Physical Health among Hispanic Americans: Good, Bad, or Benign?" *Journal of Health and Social Behavior* 48:131–48.

Link, Bruce G., and Jo Phelan. 1995. "Social Conditions as Fundamental Causes of Disease." *Journal of Health and Social Behavior*, extra issue: 80–94.

Logan, John R., Richard D. Alba, and Wenquan Zhang. 2002. "Immigrant Enclaves and Ethnic Communities in New York and Los Angeles." *American Sociological Review* 67:299–322.

Logan, John R., Brian J. Stults, and Reynolds Farley. 2004. "Segregation of Minorities in the Metropolis: Two Decades of Change." *Demography* 41:1–22.

Macintyre, Sally, Anne Ellaway, and Steven Cummins. 2002. "Place Effects on Health: How Can We Conceptualise, Operationalise, and Measure Them?" *Social Science and Medicine* 55:125–39.

Marsden, Peter V., and Noah E. Friedkin. 1994. "Network Studies of Social Influence." In *Advances in Social Network Analysis*, ed. S. Wasserman and J. Galaskiewicz, 127–51. Thousand Oaks, Calif.: Sage Publications.

Massey, Douglas S. and Nancy A. Denton. 1988. "The Dimensions of Residential Segregation." *Social Forces* 67:281–315.

———. 1993. *American Apartheid: Segregation and the Making of the Underclass.* Cambridge, Mass.: Harvard University Press.

Miller, Barry A., Kenneth C. Chu, Benjamin F. Hankey, and Lyn A. G. Ries. 2008. "Cancer Incidence and Mortality Patterns among Specific Asian and Pacific Islander Populations in the U.S." *Cancer Causes Control* 19(3): 227–56.

Morenoff, Jeffrey, James House, Ben B. Hansen, David Williams, George A. Kaplan, and Haslyn E. Hunte. 2007. "Understanding Social Disparities in Hypertension Prevalence, Awareness, Treatment, and Control: The Role of Neighborhood Context." *Social Science and Medicine* 65:1853–66.

Omi, Michael, and Howard Winant. 1994. *Racial Formation in the United States: From the 1960s to the 1990s.* New York: Routledge.

Orfield, Gary, and Susan E. Eaton. 1996. *Dismantling Desegregation: The Quiet Reversal of Brown v. Board of Education.* New York: New Press.

Patel, Kushang V., Karl Eschbach, Laura L. Rudkin, M. Kristen Peek, and Kyriakos S. Markides. 2003. "Neighborhood Context and Self-Rated Health in Older Mexican Americans." *Annals of Epidemiology* 13:620–28.

Polednak, Anthony P. 1991. "Black-White Differences in Infant Mortality in 38 Standard Metropolitan Statistical Areas." *American Journal of Public Health* 81:1480–82.

Portes, Alejandro, and Robert L. Bach. 1985. *The Latin Journey: Cuban and Mexican Immigrants in the*

United States. Berkeley: University of California Press.

Portes, Alejandro, David Kyle, and William W. Eaton. 1992. "Mental Illness and Help-Seeking Behavior among Mariel Cuban and Haitian Refugees in South Florida." *Journal of Health and Social Behavior* 33:283–98.

Portes, Alejandro, and Min Zhou. 1993. "The New Second Generation: Segmented Assimilation and Its Variants." *Annals of the American Academy* 530:74–96.

Rao, Mala, Sunand Prasad, Fiona Adshead, and Hasitha Tissera. 2007. "The Built Environment and Health." *Lancet* 370:1111–13.

Reskin, Barbara F. 2003. "Including Mechanisms in Our Models of Ascriptive Inequality: 2002 Presidential Address." *American Sociological Review* 68:1–21.

Robert, Stephanie A. 1998. "Community-Level Socioeconomic Status Effects on Adult Health." *Journal of Health and Social Behavior* 39:18–37.

Rosenberg, Noah A., Jonathan K. Pritchard, James L. Weber, Howard M. Cann, Kenneth K. Kidd, Lev A. Zhivotovsky, and Marcus W. Feldman. 2002. "Genetic Structure of Human Populations." *Science* 298:2381–85.

Ross, Catherine E., and John Mirowsky. 2001. "Neighborhood Disadvantage, Disorder, and Health." *Journal of Health and Social Behavior* 42:258–76.

Ross, Catherine E., and John Mirowsky. 2002. "Family Relationships, Social Support and Subjective Life Expectancy." *Journal of Health and Social Behavior* 43:469–89.

Schulz, Amy J., David R. Williams, Barbara A. Israel, and Lora Bex Lempert. 2002. "Racial and Spatial Relations as Fundamental Determinants of Health in Detroit." *Milbank Quarterly* 80:677–707.

Shaw, Clifford R., and Henry D. McKay. 1969. *Juvenile Delinquency and Urban Areas*. Chicago: University of Chicago Press.

Smelser, Neil J., William J. Wilson, and Faith Mitchell. 2001. *America Becoming: Racial Trends and Their Consequences*. Washington, D.C.: National Academy Press.

South, Scott J., Kyle Crowder, and Erick Chavez. 2005. "Migration and Spatial Assimilation among U.S. Latinos: Classical versus Segmented Trajectories." *Demography* 42:497–521.

Stahl, T., A. Rutten, D. Nutbeam, A. Bauman, L. Kannas, T. Abel, G. Luschen, J. A. Diaz-Rodriguez, J. Vinck, and J. Vanderzee. 2001. "The Importance of the Social Environment for Physically Active Lifestyle: Results from an International Study." *Social Science and Medicine* 52:1–10.

Subramanian, S. V., Dolores Acevedo-Garcia, and

Theresa L. Osypuk. 2005. "Racial Residential Segregation and Geographic Heterogeneity in Black/White Disparity in Poor Self-Rated Health in the U.S.: A Multilevel Statistical Analysis." *Social Science and Medicine* 60:1667–79.

Takeuchi, David T., and Sue-Je L. Gage. 2003. "What to Do with Race? Changing Notions of Race in the Social Sciences." *Culture, Medicine and Psychiatry* 27:435–45.

Tilly, Chris, Philip Moss, Joleen Kirschenman, and Ivy Kennelly. 2001. "Space as a Signal: How Employers Perceive Neighborhoods in Four Metropolitan Labor Markets." In *Urban Inequality: Evidence from Four Cities*, ed. A. O'Connor, C. Tilly, and L. Bobo, 304–40. New York: Russell Sage Foundation.

U.S. Bureau of the Census. 2001a. "The Hispanic Population: Census 2000 Brief." Washington, D.C.: GPO.

———. 2001b. "The Native Hawaiian and Other Pacific Islander Population: Census 2000 Brief." Washington, D.C.: GPO.

———. 2002. "Historical Census Statistics on Population Totals by Race, 1790 to 1990, and by Hispanic Origin, 1970 to 1990, for the United States, Regions, Divisions, and States." Washington, D.C.: GPO.

———. 2003a. "Migration by Native and the Foreign Born: 1995 to 2000." Washington, D.C.: GPO.

———. 2003b. "Migration by Race and Hispanic Origin: 1995 to 2000." Washington, D.C.: GPO.

———. 2008. "Housing and Household Economic Statistics Division, Journey-to-Work and Migration Statistics Branch." Washington, D.C.: GPO.

Weiss, Carlos O., Hector M. Gonzalez, Mohammed U. Kabeto, and Kenneth M. Langa. 2005. "Differences in Amount of Informal Care Received by Non-Hispanic Whites and Latinos in a Nationally Representative Sample of Older Americans." *Journal of the American Geriatrics Society* 53:146–51.

Werlen, Benno. 1993. *Society, Action and Space: An Alternative Human Geography*. London: Routledge.

Williams, David R., and Chiquita Collins. 1995. "U.S. Socioeconomic and Racial Differences in Health: Patterns and Explanations." *Annual Review of Sociology* 21:349–86.

———. 2001. "Racial Residential Segregation: A Fundamental Cause of Racial Disparities in Health." *Public Health Reports* 116:404–16.

Williams, David R., and R. Williams-Morris. 2000. "Racism and Mental Health: The African American Experience." *Ethnicity and Health* 5:243–68.

Wilson, Kenneth L., and Alejandro Portes. 1980. "Immigrant Enclaves: An Analysis of the Labor Market Experiences of Cubans in Miami." *American Journal of Sociology* 86:295–319.

Wilson, William Julius. 1987. *The Truly Disadvantaged*. Chicago: University of Chicago Press.

———. 1996. *When Work Disappears: The World of the New Urban Poor*. New York: Vintage Books.

Zhou, Min. 1992. *Chinatown: The Socioeconomic Potential of an Urban Enclave*. Philadelphia: Temple University Press.

———. 2007. "The Ethnic System of Supplementary Education: Non-profit and For-profit Institutions in Los Angeles Chinese Immigrant Community." In *Toward Positive Youth Development: Transforming Schools and Community Programs*, ed. B. S. a. H. Yoshikawa, 229–51. New York: Oxford University Press.

Zhou, Min, and John R. Logan. 1991. "In and Out of Chinatown: Residential Mobility and Segregation of New York City's Chinese." *Social Forces* 70:387–407.

7

The Latino Health Paradox
Looking at the Intersection of Sociology and Health

Tamara Dubowitz, RAND Corporation

Lisa M. Bates, Columbia University Mailman School of Public Health

Dolores Acevedo-Garcia, Bouve College of Health Sciences, Northeastern University

The link between socioeconomic disadvantage and poor health has been observed consistently and over time (Berkman and Kawachi 2000). According to U.S. census statistics, in 2007, 21.5 percent of Hispanics/Latinos were living in poverty, compared with 8.2 percent of non-Hispanic whites, 24.5 percent of blacks, and 10.2 percent of Asians.[1] In spite of their disproportionate representation among the poor, Hispanics/Latinos have demonstrated lower all-cause mortality and higher life expectancy than we otherwise might expect (Falcon, Molina, and Molina 2001; Hummer et al. 2000; Lin et al. 2003; Singh and Siahpush 2002; Sorlie et al. 1993). The growing domain of health research on Hispanics/Latinos has identified a Latino immigrant health paradox: foreign-born Hispanics/Latinos overall have better health outcomes than we might expect, given their lower socioeconomic standing (Markides and Coreil 1986).

For many researchers, the health advantage that Hispanics/Latinos appear to have may be rooted in their "cultural orientation" (presumably related to engagement in healthy behaviors) and strong social networks. Others argue that the so-called paradoxes are the result of immigrant selection processes because U.S. Hispanic/Latino immigrants are healthier than their nonimmigrant co-nationals. According to this school of thought, these paradoxes are, after all, not paradoxical. In this chapter, we address conceptual issues related to Latino and immigrant health research and discuss some policy implications. We contend that an integration of the sociology of immigration and social epidemiology of health is critical to understanding health paradoxes. By understanding the social and political context of Hispanic/Latino immigration in the United States, including processes of immigrant adaptation as well as the Latin American sending countries, Hispanic/Latino health can become an interdisciplinary dialogue between sociologists of immigrant adaptation and public-health researchers. This may allow for a more effective means of tending to health and health-care concerns of immigrants and specifically of Hispanics/Latinos.

Migration Patterns, Demographics, and Socioeconomic Status of the U.S. Latino Population

Legal immigration to the United States has increased steadily from 250,000 in the 1930s, 2.5 million in the 1950s, 4.5 million in the 1970s, and 7.3 million in the 1980s to about 10 million in the 1990s. Following this history, new immigrants (those born outside the United States, or first generation) and their descendants are projected to account for 82 percent of the population increase through the year 2050 (Passel and Cohn 2008). Today, immigrants in the United States are more diverse than ever before in terms of race, ethnicity, language, religion, education, social class, and reasons for and process of immigration. Mexican-born immigrants accounted for 30.8 percent of all foreign born residing in the United States in 2007, by far the largest immigrant group in the United States. Among the remaining countries of origin, the Philippines accounted for 4.5 percent of all foreign born, followed by India and China (excluding Hong Kong and Taiwan) with 3.9 percent and 3.6 percent, respectively. These four countries—together with El Salvador (2.9 percent), Vietnam (2.9 percent), Korea (2.7 percent), Cuba (2.6 percent), Canada (2.2 percent), and the Dominican Republic (2.0 percent)—made up 58.1 percent of all foreign born residing in the United States in 2007 (Terrazas and Batalova 2008).

"Generation status" differentiates between individuals who were born outside the United States, those whose *parents* were born outside the United States, and those who have lived in the United States for two or more generations. In general, studies have demonstrated that as generation status increases, health behaviors and outcomes decline. Traditionally, the term "first-generation immigrants" defines immigrants born outside the United States; "second-generation immigrants" describes individuals born in the United States, one or both of whose parents are first-generation immigrants. Often, each subsequent generation born in the United States is numbered sequentially (second generation are the U.S.-born children of at least one first-generation parent; later generations are the children of U.S.-born parents). "Generation status" can also include categories such as "mixed parentage" to refer to those who have both foreign-born and U.S.-born parents or "1.5 generation" to refer to foreign-born who arrived in the United States as children or adolescents (Portes and Rumbaut 2001). Using this classification, approximately 39 percent of Latinos in the United States are first generation,

29 percent are second generation, and the remaining 32 percent are later generations (U.S. Census Bureau 2002).

Between 1970 and 2000, first-generation Latino immigrants contributed 45 percent of the growth of the Latino population, while second-generation Latinos contributed 25 percent. In contrast, from 2000 to 2020, the second generation is anticipated to contribute 47 percent of the growth of the Latino population, while the first generation is projected to contribute only 28 percent, which means the second generation will surpass the first in size by 2020 (Suro and Passel 2003). Given that foreign-born Latinos appear to have a health advantage over U.S.-born Latinos, the increase in the second generation may have implications for the health status of Latinos.

Hispanics in the United States until relatively recently had been heavily concentrated in long-established areas of Hispanic settlement. In 1990, almost three-quarters of the Hispanic population resided in 65 of the nation's 3,141 counties. However, beginning in the 1990s, the Hispanic population began to disperse across the United States, increasing Hispanic populations in counties that previously had relatively small Hispanic populations. Most notable perhaps are some of the settling points in many counties in the South and Midwest that historically had few Hispanics residents. Since 2000, many Latinos have settled in counties in the West and the Northeast that once had few Latinos, continuing a pattern that began in the previous decade. Yet, although the increase in the Hispanic population between 2000 and 2007 was relatively widespread across the United States, just 40 counties accounted for half of the 10.2 million increase in the nation's Hispanics.

Despite the geographic dispersal of Hispanics in the United States, the Hispanic population is more geographically concentrated than the non-Hispanic population. In 2007, the hundred counties with the largest Hispanic populations proportionate to the county population were home to 73 percent of the total U.S. Latino population. In contrast to this, the hundred counties with the lowest Hispanic populations proportionate to the county population were home to 39 percent of the nation's non-Hispanics. Accordingly, across the United States, Hispanics are more geographically concentrated than the nation's black population; 59 percent of the non-Hispanic black population lives in the nation's hundred largest non-Hispanic black counties (Fry 2008).

The majority (64.1 percent) of Hispanics in the United States are Mexican; the remaining percentages are Puerto Ricans (9), Cubans (3.4), Salvadorans (3.1), Dominicans (2.7), Guatemalans (2), Colombians (1.8), Hondurans (1.1), Ecuadorians (1.1), Peruvians (1), and other Spanish/Hispanic/Latino groups (6.9) (Suro and Passel 2003). While approximately 40 percent of the Mexican population is foreign-born (i.e., born outside the United States), other Hispanic groups reflect a greater percentage of foreign born: Cubans, 61.1; Salvadorans, 67.1; Dominicans, 60.1; Guatemalans, 71.3; and Colombians, 68.4 (Ruggles et al. 2008).

Overall, Latinos experience low socioeconomic status (SES) (Ramirez and de la Cruz 2003). In 2002, among those aged twenty-five or older, 27 percent of Latinos had not completed ninth grade, compared to only 4 percent of non-Hispanic whites. The Mexican-origin population is more likely to be of low SES than are other Latino subgroups. Of the total U.S. Hispanic population, 21.7 percent live in poverty (for a family of four, an annual income of $17,184 or less) (IPUMS United States 2009). When broken down by nativity, 28 percent of native born and 36.5 percent of foreign born make up this statistic. In comparison, 9.3 percent of non-Hispanic whites, 25.3 percent of non-Hispanic blacks, and 10.7 percent of Asians live in poverty.

Latino Health Paradoxes: Definition and Empirical Evidence

Some patterns in Latino health have received attention because they appear to contradict our expectations based on the well-documented social gradient in health that individuals of higher SES have better health than those of lower SES (Berkman and Kawachi 2000), and the pervasive patterns of poor health among African Americans vis-à-vis whites (Williams 2001). However, the issue of Latino health paradoxes is still ambiguous in its definitions of paradox, limited comparable empirical evidence, limited testing of explanations, and limited discussion of policy and intervention applications (Franzini, Ribble, and Keddie 2001; Jasso et al. 2004; Palloni and Arias 2004; Palloni and Morenoff 2001).

Toward a Working Definition of Latino Health Paradoxes

The term health or epidemiologic "paradox" typically refers to a pattern of morbidity or mortality for a particular group (e.g., Latinos, immigrants) that is at odds with what would be expected given the group's socioeconomic profile. However, definitions and reference groups are often not made explicit and may vary from study to study. For example, epidemiologic paradoxes are sometimes defined in relation to the *average* SES of a population group, for example, it is paradoxical that Latinos have low rates of low birth weight given that, on average, they have low SES. In other cases, the term "paradox" denotes a *residual protective effect* of Latino (or foreign-born) status that cannot be accounted for by measured demographic, socioeconomic, behavioral, or medical risk factors.

Since the notion of a health paradox presumes a socioeconomic gradient in health, an important first step should entail examining whether the association between SES and health is different among Latinos than among other racial/ethnic groups. Ideally, understanding Latino health paradoxes requires addressing the combined effects of race/ethnicity, immigrant status (i.e., nativity), and SES on health outcomes.

Research has documented that Latino immigrants often exhibit a health advantage over non-Latinos and their U.S.-born counterparts, but the protective effect of immigrant status is not exclusive to Latinos. For some outcomes, immigrants of other racial/ethnic groups have also been shown to exhibit better health than their U.S.-born counterparts. A central research question is the extent to which Latino health paradoxes are related to Latino ethnicity versus immigration. Given that Latino health paradoxes are often attributed to cultural or social factors presumed to be specific to Latinos, the comparison with other immigrant groups may help clarify the role of such factors vis-à-vis immigrant health selectivity.

Empirical Evidence

Most studies that have examined differences in all-cause mortality have found that Hispanics have lower mortality rates than whites (Elo et al. 2004; Franzini, Ribble, and Keddie 2001; Hummer, Benjamins, and Rogers 2004; Liao et al. 1998; Markides and Eschbach 2005). Results on Latino health paradoxes have differed depending on the health outcome and specific population examined. Evidence for a Hispanic mortality advantage has been found among men, persons of advanced age, and those born in Mexico (Markides and Eschbach 2005). Yet some studies have found no difference in mortality between Hispanics and whites (Hunt et al. 2003). Still other studies have looked at health paradoxes in terms of nativity (born in or outside the United States). Based on the National Longitudinal Mortality Study (1979–1989), Singh and Siahpush (2001) found all-cause mortality significantly lower among immigrants than among the U.S. born (18 percent lower for men and 13 percent lower for women) after adjusting for age, race/ethnicity, marital status, urban/rural residence, education, occupation, and family income. More recent work by Turra and Goldman (2007) showed a mortality advantage for Hispanics concentrated at lower levels of socioeconomic status, with little or no advantage at higher levels.

Several studies have documented that infants born to Latino immigrant women tend to have lower rates of low birth weight (birth weight <2,500 grams = LBW) and of infant mortality (death during the first year of life) than do infants of U.S.-born Latino women (Acevedo-Garcia, Pan et al. 2005). In the 2004 Pediatric Nutrition Surveillance System, the crude prevalence of LBW was highest among black infants (13.1 percent) and lowest among Latinos (7.6 percent), with white (8.8 percent) and Asian/Pacific Islander (8.3 percent) infants falling in the middle. The authors also reported, based on data

from 1998 U.S. vital statistics, that immigrant status was not protective against LBW among whites and increased the risk among Asians by 24 percent, but it reduced the risk by about 25 percent among blacks and by about 19 percent among Latinos, after adjusting for maternal age, prenatal care, health behaviors and medical risk factors during pregnancy, and education. By educational attainment, for whites, blacks, and Latinos, the protective effect of foreign-born status was stronger among women with low education (zero to eleven years) than among women with more education. The association between maternal education and LBW was less pronounced among foreign-born white, black, and Hispanic women than among their U.S.-born counterparts. While there was a clear negative education gradient among U.S.-born women in these three racial/ethnic groups (i.e., low birth weight rates decreased as education level increased), the gradient was less pronounced among foreign-born whites and blacks, and nearly flat among foreign-born Hispanics.

This research illustrates again that the health advantage of immigrants vis-à-vis the U.S. born is not confined to Latinos. Here, the immigrant health advantage was strongest among blacks. Also, instead of merely controlling for SES, this research examined whether the effect of SES on health is different among immigrants than among the U.S. born. It appears that low SES increases the risk of low birth weight among U.S.-born Latinos but not among Latino immigrants. Additionally, the research on infant health outcomes has shown that there are variations across Latino subgroups: immigrant status is associated with a reduced risk of low birth weight among Mexicans of about 20 percent but does not seem to be protective against low birth weight among other Latino subgroups—Puerto Ricans, Cubans, and Central/South Americans (Acevedo-Garcia, Soobader, and Berkman 2005).

Some studies suggest that Latinos and immigrants have more positive health behaviors, particularly related to substance use, than do their non-Latino and U.S.-born counterparts. For example, compared to non-Latino whites, Latinos are less likely to use cigarettes or alcohol, independent of SES (Abraído-Lanza et al. 2005). Foreign nativity has also been found to be protective for illicit drug use among Mexican Americans, particularly women (Vega and Amaro 1994). Data from the 1995–1996 Tobacco Use Supplement of the Current Population Survey indicated that for all racial/ethnic groups, smoking rates were lower among first-generation immigrants and second-generation Latinos than among the third generation (Acevedo-Garcia, Pan et al. 2005).

The protective effect of being second-generation or of being foreign born varied across racial/ethnic groups. For whites, Asians, and Latinos, being second-generation and being foreign-born were similarly protective against smoking. In contrast, for blacks, while being foreign-born was highly protective, being second-generation was not. The protective effect of foreign-born status was highest for blacks (Odds Ratio [OR] = 0.32) and lowest for whites (OR = 0.77), while Asians (OR = 0.45) and Latinos (OR = 0.42) fell in the middle.

National and community-based studies have documented dietary behavior advantages of being foreign born (compared to U.S. born), a phenomenon that seems to erode the longer an immigrant lives in the United States In a sample of U.S.-born non-Hispanic white and first- and second-generation Hispanic women (immigrants and those with an immigrant parent), first-generation Mexican American women had a higher average intake of protein and of vitamins A, C, and folic acid, despite lower socioeconomic status, compared to second-generation or non-Hispanic white women (Abrams and Guendelman 1995). Other studies have shown lower fruit and vegetable intake with longer residence in the United States and greater acculturation (Gordon-Larsen et al. 2003; Lin et al. 2003; Neuhouser et al. 2004; Winkleby et al. 1994). Among immigrants, increasing number of years of residence in the United States is associated with higher body mass index or obesity (Gordon-Larsen et al. 2003; Lin et al. 2003; Winkleby et al. 1994).

Research also suggests that Latino ethnicity and foreign nativity may be protective against psychiatric disorders. In broad racial/ethnic comparisons, "Hispanics" as well as non-Hispanic blacks were at lower risk than non-Hispanic whites for disorders such as depression, generalized anxiety disorder, and social phobia (Breslau et al. 2005). In national estimates, foreign-born Mexicans were at lower risk than their U.S.-born counterparts for substance use and for mood and anxiety disorders, and U.S.-born Mexican Americans were in turn at lower risk than U.S.-born non-Hispanic whites (Grant et al. 2004). Once again, however, it is not clear that this relative advantage extends to all Latinos (Ortega et al. 2000) or, conversely, that it is unique to Mexican Americans; foreign nativity has also been shown to be protective for non-Hispanic whites (Grant et al. 2004).

Challenges to Latino Health

In spite of many examples of Latino health paradoxes, there are health conditions for which Latinos either do not exhibit a health advantage or appear to have a disadvantage. In 2002–2003, the prevalence of obesity among Latinos overall was 29.1 percent compared to 9.4 percent among Asian Americans (Acevedo-Garcia, Soobader, and Berkman et al. 2007). These data also reveal dramatic increases in obesity among Latinos with each generation in the United States, ranging from 25.4 percent among the foreign born to 35.7 percent in the third generation (U.S.-born with two U.S.-born parents) (Bates et al. 2008). A similar pattern is suggested by analyses showing that obesity appears to increase among immigrants the longer they live in the United States (Antecol and Bedard 2006; Goel et al. 2004).

National data indicate that 36.8 percent of Mexican Americans are obese (BMI at the 95th percentile) compared to 30 percent of non-Hispanic white adults (Ogden et al. 2006), with Latino adults demonstrating nearly an 80 percent increase in obesity prevalence from 1991 to 1998 (Freedman et al. 2002). The latest data from the 2003–2004 National Health and Nutrition Examination Survey (NHANES) show a higher prevalence of Latino children (37 percent) considered at risk for overweight (BMI for age at 85th percentile) compared to non-Hispanic black (35.1 percent) and non-Hispanic white children (33.5 percent); among six- to eleven-year-olds, the prevalence of Latino children at risk of overweight is as high as 42.9 percent (Ogden et al. 2006). Recent research suggests that such disparities may begin at an early age. A study of a New York City WIC population found Latino preschoolers more than twice as likely to be at risk for overweight than other groups (Nelson, Chiasson, and Ford 2004). Similarly, in a recent cross-sectional study of preschool children from twenty U.S. cities, the highest prevalence of obesity was found among Latino children (25.8 percent) compared to blacks (16.2 percent) or whites (14.8 percent), controlling for sociodemographic factors (Whitaker and Orzol 2006).

There are also health conditions for which some Latino subgroups show a disadvantage, while other Latino subgroups show an advantage. For instance, while Puerto Ricans are the U.S. racial/ethnic group with the highest adult asthma rate (17 percent versus a national average of 8.9 percent), Mexicans have the lowest rate (3.9 percent) (Rose, Mannino, and Leaderer 2006). Compared with black children (16 percent) and white children (13 percent), Puerto Rican children have the highest prevalence of lifetime asthma (26 percent) and Mexican children have the lowest (10 percent) (Lara et al. 2006).

The attention paid toward Latino health paradoxes should not blind us to the considerable barriers facing the Latino population, including the highest number of individuals without health insurance (Brown and Yu 2004); large numbers of individuals with undocumented immigrant status; and limited access to social benefits for immigrants who entered the United States after the 1996 Welfare Reform Act (Fix and Passel 2002). Among individuals under sixty-five, Mexicans have the lowest rate of health insurance (less than 60 percent) compared to other Latino subgroups such as Cubans (75 percent) and Puerto Ricans (85 percent), and to non-Hispanic whites (87 percent) (NCHS 2002). Certain Latino subpopulations such as migrant farmworkers (Villarejo 2003) and residents of *colonias* along the Mexico-U.S. border (Weinberg et al. 2004) are at high risk for dangerous occupational and environmental exposures such as musculoskeletal disorders, infectious diseases, and injuries.

A related challenge in Latino health paradox research is that the measures used to gauge La-

tino health have been largely based on measures of acculturation. While measures of acculturation are themselves debated, such sociocultural explanations are often invoked without theoretically nuanced propositions concerning the interplay among culture, social structure, and well-being (Viruell-Fuentes 2007). That acculturation has become central to sociocultural explanations for immigrant health diverts attention from the historical, political, and economic contexts of migration, and how they impinge on immigrant health (Arcia et al. 2001; Hunt et al. 2002; Rogler, Cortes, and Malgady 1991).

Limitations of Research on Latino Health

For the most part, the explanations for Latino health paradoxes have not been empirically tested due to the interplay of conceptual and data limitations. Palloni and Morenoff 2001 argued that testing these hypotheses may be precluded by a tendency to prematurely dismiss selection and data artifacts as possible mechanisms. A tendency in some studies is to exclude the possibility that several mechanisms may be operating simultaneously, or to acknowledge that with the data at hand, the ability to test for competing explanations is limited.

Other conceptual issues seem to prevent a more comprehensive examination of Latino health paradoxes. The notion of acculturation has been used in health research with limited attention to its conceptualization. Often, immigrant health outcomes are examined with a focus on demographic variables or English use as markers for acculturation, without considering the broader concept of immigrant adaptation (i.e., social integration) as postulated, for example, in the segmented assimilation theory (Portes and Rumbaut 2001). Encouragingly, though, health studies have begun to address socioeconomic factors, contextual factors, and discrimination in the host society along with acculturation (Arcia et al. 2001). For instance, Finch, Kolody, and Vega (2000) showed that perceived discrimination and acculturative stress had independent effects on depression among Mexican-origin adults in California.

Another conceptual limitation, strongly influenced by lack of relevant data, is the limited attention paid to the country of origin background and influence, although some studies have begun to examine Latino health in this light. Using health data for Mexico and the United States, Soldo, Wong, and Palloni (2002) compared the health of Mexican immigrants in the United States to that of their nonimmigrant counterparts in Mexico and of immigrants to the United States who returned to Mexico. Increasingly, health researchers realize that a meaningful examination of immigrant health requires health data on the origin and destination countries.

Problematic Conceptual Issues in Latino Health Paradox Literature

Defining Acculturation and Theories of Assimilation

Many studies have captured acculturation through immigrant-generation status, which is often more readily measured, but the concept of acculturation is multidimensional and involves simultaneous maintenance and adaptation of cultural characteristics (Abraido-Lanza et al. 2006). Although definitions vary, acculturation has commonly been defined as the process of change that occurs within populations or societies because of interaction with other populations or societies, specifically with respect to evolution of cultural traditions, customs, beliefs, or artifacts. In contrast to the "immigrant health paradox," the acculturation hypothesis posits an overall disadvantage in health outcomes for Latino immigrants over time spent living in the United States, suggesting that any protective cultural buffering offered by immigrant status may dramatically diminish with acculturation, approaching the U.S. norm (Singh and Siahpush 2002; Vega and Amaro 1994).

Importantly, we know there is diversity among Latino groups in the United States in terms of history of their country of origin, impact on patterns on of migration, reception to the United States (e.g., qualifications for safety net programs), and specific communities of settlement

in the United States. Yet acculturation traditionally has been conceptualized as a group process of assimilation, assuming a minority group adopts a majority group's cultural norms over time. In assimilation, rather than a blending of values, the tendency is for the dominant cultural group to force the minority group to adopt its values.

Recent work has called for explanations of acculturation to take a contextual and process-oriented approach to understanding the impacts of culture change (Alegria et al. 2004). The scales developed for measuring acculturation, particularly in the case of Latinos, have been critiqued for their focus predominantly on Mexican Americans. Further, most scales have focused on a unidirectional process of acculturation, implying that the more Latinos adopted U.S. cultural attributes, the more they lost their Latino culture. Thus, recognition of the diversity among the Latino population has by and large been a challenge. Exceptions to this include the work of Rumbaut and Portes (Portes and Rumbaut 2001; Rumbaut 1997). In their Children of Immigrants Longitudinal Study (CILS) of diverse immigrant youth in San Diego and Miami, Portes and Rumbaut assessed a range of specific social and cultural factors. Their work paid attention to the differing contexts and cultures of the groups to identify their impacts on a range of important outcomes.

Despite the common use of immigrant-generation status as a proxy for acculturation, Rogler, Cortes, and Malgady (1991) caution that other factors such as SES may be associated with immigrant-generation status. Rumbaut and Portes (2001) note that contextual and demographic characteristics such as socioeconomic status associated with a particular immigrant cohort can affect the life opportunities or level of discrimination immigrants encounter in the United States. Acculturation, seen as a complex multidimensional process, can occur unevenly across immigrant generations and does not exclude the possibility of biculturalism (Chun, Organista, and Marín 2003). Nonetheless, generation status has come to be acknowledged as one of the more important variables related to acculturation (Escobar and Vega 2000).

A growing body of work has embraced a segmented assimilation perspective, which understands Latino assimilation as nonlinear (South, Crowder, and Chavez 2005). Spatial assimilation and residential integration, from the segmented assimilation perspective, are contingent on macroeconomic trends, national origin, race, and place, as well as other factors that collectively generate a diverse set of residential trajectories among Latinos. This perspective contends that prejudice and discrimination limit the spatial assimilation of many darker-skinned Hispanics, thus bringing race into the question of ethnicity. Thus, compared to other Latinos, for Puerto Ricans and other "black" Hispanics, racial bias together with high poverty rates have resulted in a level of segregation more comparable to that facing African Americans (Alba and Nee 1997; Massey and Bitterman 1985; Santiago and Galster 1995). Some scholars have projected that Puerto Rican segregation is not influenced by increase in SES, while others contend that the returns on education and income are lower for Puerto Ricans than for other Latinos, making it more difficult to move from ethnic enclaves to other neighborhoods (Massey and Bitterman 1985; Rosenberg and Lake 1976).

Nativity versus Ethnicity

A significant issue in the study of health paradoxes is the appropriate choice of reference group. Some studies have compared immigrants with the majority (U.S.-born non-Hispanic white) population, while others have compared immigrants to their U.S.-born racial/ethnic counterparts (foreign-born Mexicans to U.S.-born Mexicans or to other U.S.-born racial/ethnic minorities such as African Americans). Social science and health research on immigrant adaptation suggest that all these comparisons may be important, since Latino immigrants follow multiple adaptation pathways, including assimilation into the majority culture, and preservation of an ethnic identity and assimilation into a U.S.-born ethnic minority group (Portes and Rumbaut 2001). Additionally, intergenerational comparisons within a given national-origin group allow us to test whether there is intergenerational advancement in health (or other) outcomes (Smith 2003).

According to census data from 2000, 47.9 percent of individuals who identified themselves as Latino or of Hispanic origin also identified themselves as white; 42.2 percent of individuals identifying as Latino also identified as being "some other race" (not white, black or African American, American Indian and Alaska Native, Asian and Native Hawaiian or Other Pacific Islander); and 6.3 percent of Latinos identified themselves as belonging to two or more races.

Variation across Health Outcomes and Latino Subgroups

Because in so many situations "Hispanic" implies one general group, the differences in ethnic subgroups and immigration cohorts and the potential variation in health outcome are not always documented. In 2006, the largest subgroups by percentage of the total U.S. Hispanic population, by country/territory of origin were Mexican (66.9), Puerto Rican (8.6), and Cuban (3.7); other more heterogeneous Hispanic census classification groups include Central (8.2) and South (6.0) American and "Other" Hispanic (8), which includes Dominicans (U.S. Census Bureau 2006).

Because Mexicans comprise 66.9 percent of the U.S. Latino population (25.1 million) and 8.9 percent of the total U.S. population, discussions of Latino immigration and health often focus on this Latino subgroup. In other cases, Latinos are not disaggregated by national origin, which may conceal important variations across Latino subgroups.

There are health conditions for which Latinos do not exhibit a health advantage, as mentioned earlier, including obesity and asthma. While asthma varies by subgroup, obesity is an example of a health condition contrary to the paradox. Other research has documented variation by outcome, for example, self-reported health has been found to vary by subgroup. Recent work found that Mexicans had significantly higher scores in self-reported mental and physical health status than either whites or other Hispanics (controlling for language and nativity), although the absolute differences were somewhat smaller for physical health than for mental health. For Cubans, Dominicans, and Puerto Ricans, mental and physical health scores were generally lower than those of whites (Jerant, Arellanes, and Franks 2008).

Other work has reinforced findings that Mexicans having health advantages over whites, and Puerto Ricans have poorer health outcomes. Other subgroups such as Cubans and Dominicans have demonstrated a mix of health disparities and health advantages, both reporting poorer subjective health ratings and each indicating a health advantage on one of the objective health measures.

Explanations and Issues Related to Latino Health and Paradoxes

There are least three types of explanation for Latino health paradoxes. First, some studies maintain that paradoxes are due to *cultural or social protective factors* (Hayes-Bautista 2002), such as social support, familism, religion, and norms related to diet and substance use. This hypothesis is often presented in association with an acculturation hypothesis that posits an erosion of such protective factors with time spent in the United States (within one generation) and across generations, which results in a deterioration of health outcomes. Some studies have shown that the initial health advantage that Latino immigrants have over their U.S.-born counterparts declines with length of residence or in subsequent generations. However, acculturation is often poorly defined and is operationalized through demographic or English-language use proxy indicators (L. Hunt, Schneider, and Comer 2004). Some health research also tends to romanticize the Latino immigrant by speculating about (but rarely measuring) the role that social networks and families may play in protecting health, while ignoring the socioeconomic hardship and tenuous immigration status that may severely compromise the effectiveness of these social supports (Menjívar 2000).

A second type of explanation includes authors who contend that health paradoxes arise from a process of *healthy immigrant selection*. According to this view, some patterns in Latino health indeed run against our expectations based on social epidemiologic regularities observed in other populations, but we should not interpret them as paradoxical because they reflect this selection effect (Palloni and Morenoff 2001). A parallel selection process may also yield an "unhealthy remigration effect." There is evidence that the likelihood of staying in the destination country or reemigrating occurs selectively (Lindstrom 1996) in ways that may similarly correspond to health status.

In the third type of explanation, researchers suggest that paradoxical patterns may be due to *data artifacts*, including undercounting of Latino deaths, inconsistent definitions of Latino identity (e.g., self-identification vs. Latino surnames), and underreporting of health problems (Franzini, Ribble, and Keddie 2001; Jasso et al. 2004; Palloni and Morenoff 2001). Additionally, some nonhealth studies of Mexican intergenerational performance suggest that inappropriate cross-sectional comparisons may create the impression of deterioration in health outcomes across generations (Jasso et al. 2004).

Immigration Status

Legal status may play a large role both in access to services and in general health and wellbeing. Undocumented Latino immigrants may experience multiple stresses and concerns about their legal status, and preoccupation with disclosure and deportation have been shown to heighten the risk for emotional distress and impaired quality of health (Cavazos-Rehg, Zayas, and Spitznagel 2007). Legal status is also the entry to various services, which include employment with benefits such as health insurance. Although health insurance by no means guarantees access to health care, 45 percent of noncitizen immigrants in the United States lack health insurance. Noncoverage for naturalized citizens is closer to that of the U.S. born (15–20 percent), while 65 percent of undocumented immigrants and 32 percent of permanent residents lack health insurance. Such differences may also manifest in other measures of access, such as having a regular source of care, having had a physician or dental visit in the past year, and having fewer visits, even after adjusting for health insurance and health status (Jackson et al. 2006; Lucas, Barr-Anderson, and Kington 2003).

English Proficiency

Although language is one measure of acculturation and increased acculturation has been shown to correlate with deterioration of health outcomes and behaviors, lack of proficiency in English may limit many immigrants' ability to take full advantage of education and programs that could protect and improve their health. English proficiency has also been demonstrated to play a role in access to care. Adults with limited English proficiency and their children have been shown less likely to have insurance and a usual source of care, to have fewer physician visits, and to receive less preventive care than those who speak only English (Derose and Baker 2000; Yu et al. 2006). Further, quality of care has been demonstrated to be associated with English proficiency; immigrants with limited English proficiency have reported lower satisfaction with care and lower understanding of their medical situation. Interpretation and quality have been shown to be important, although in spite of national standards for culturally and linguistically appropriate services, trained interpreters are also found to be rare in many settings. Patient safety is also an important issue related to English proficiency, as problems in understanding instructions can lead to medication misuse.

Testing Possible Explanations for Latino Health Paradoxes

Although it appears that for various health outcomes, Latino or foreign-born Latino status confers a protective effect, new research designs are needed to test explanations. For instance, on average immigrants may have better health than those in their country of origin who do not migrate, and than immigrants who return to their country of origin. Ideally, to explore the issue of selection, we would compare health outcomes among the foreign born from a given country of origin with their U.S.-born ethnic counterparts, as well as with comparable individuals in their country of origin, including those who have never migrated and return migrants. If we are interested in testing the effect of immigrant adaptation on health outcomes, we need longitudinal study designs that al-

low long-term follow-up of immigrant trajectories since arrival in the United States. The New Immigrant Survey (Jasso et al. 2000) will allow such analyses for several cohorts of documented immigrant (sampled from green card recipients).

Research has suggested intriguing patterns in Latino health, but the findings are open to interpretation. In our research, we have found that education gradients in low birth weight are considerably attenuated among immigrant women (Latino and non-Latino) compared to their U.S.-born counterparts (Acevedo-Garcia, Soobader, and Berkman 2005, 2007). This pattern leaves room for several explanations. If immigrant women are indeed more likely to be healthier or to have better health behaviors across education levels compared to women who do not immigrate, for example, such patterns may be due to selection. If, as suggested by Jasso and colleagues (2004), there is a minimum health level that would make migration worthwhile, selection may limit the dispersion in health outcomes among immigrants, thus flattening SES gradients. Alternatively, if present across SES levels, protective cultural factors may attenuate SES gradients.

Studies that have integrated data from multiple sources with the development of migration models of health selectivity (Jasso et al. 2004) or simulation exercises (Palloni and Morenoff 2001) strongly suggest that paradoxical patterns in Latino health could result from migrant health selection. Some data presented to support this view are suggestive but not conclusive. Jasso and colleagues (2004) have shown that foreign-born Latinos (and Asians) in the United States have higher life expectancy than their U.S.-born counterparts and than those in their sending regions. Although compelling, these data do not prove that the health advantage among the foreign born is driven entirely or even primarily by immigrant selection.

Disentangling the potential effects on health of selection processes, immigration, and long-term adaptation in the receiving country is at best only approximated by existing study designs. Currently available data do not allow definitive determination of the causal role of any of these factors; theory would suggest that all three play a role to some degree, and that the relative influence of each may vary by immigrant subgroup. For example, the selection hypothesis suggests that, other factors equal, health selection would be stronger among immigrant groups that have to overcome greater obstacles, such as longer distances, to migrate to the United States. The evidence of health paradoxes among Mexicans may not be consistent with this logic. Until the mid-1980s, border controls along the Mexico-U.S. border were relatively loose, and Mexican immigration was dominated by a largely male-initiated, *circular* migration flow based on seeking work in the United States during a specific season (Massey, Durand, and Malone 2003). Despite the relative smoothness that characterized Mexican migration to the United States prior to 1986, there is empirical evidence of health paradoxes among Mexicans. In fact, the articulation of the Latino health paradox has been based largely on the Mexican case.

Where Does the Health-Care System Fit?

The 2002 National Survey of Latinos found that almost three in four Latino adults are either without health insurance or personally know someone without coverage. In addition, a substantial minority of Latinos reports health-care challenges, such as problems paying medical bills, delays seeking care because of costs, and not getting needed health-care services. Furthermore, some Latinos report having problems communicating with health-care providers due to language barriers, or having difficulty getting care due to their race and ethnic background.

Derose, Escarce, and Lurie (2007) in their work on immigrants and health care, have highlighted four policy suggestions: (1) expanding health-insurance coverage; (2) more broadly implementing cultural and linguistic standards for health-care providers; (3) addressing immigrant populations in the U.S. safety net; and (4) revising the Personal Responsibility and Work Opportunity Reconciliation Act (PRWORA).

Health Insurance

We know that there are relatively low rates of health insurance among immigrants, documented and undocumented. Understanding the importance of immigrant health could be addressed through programs such as employer-based health insurance, expansion of programs such as the states' Children's Health Insurance Program (CHIP), which has proven effective in maintaining coverage among immigrant children and their families post-PRWORA.

English Proficiency

Although Culturally and Linguistically Appropriate Services (CLAS) are federally mandated in the United States, implementation and enforcement is lacking. Further, Medicaid benefits that cover interpreter services, for example, exist in only twelve states; the effective expansion of these benefits has been demonstrated in California. Similarly, investment in medical education of bilingual individuals, or the offering of financial incentives for bilingual staff, could encourage and expand access to linguistically appropriate care.

Addressing Immigrant Populations in the U.S. Safety Net

Immigrant populations moving to new destinations across the United States are finding that some places don't have the resources typical of larger urban centers. In fact, compared to urban centers, many of the new destinations for immigrants are in states with more restrictive Medicaid policies, fewer interpreters and language-concordant providers, and weaker public-health systems. Many communities view immigration as a national, not a local, issue; a federal incentive to improve services for immigrants may go far in such places.

PRWORA

Immigrant provisions of PRWORA restrict immigrants to government-sponsored or subsidized health insurance. Such policies were put in place to discourage immigrants from coming to the United States to gain benefits. However, research has shown that the availability of jobs, not of health and social services, drives immigration. Current policies that allow access to Medicaid for emergency services (and not for primary care) have the potential to create incentives for patients and providers alike to use emergency services unnecessarily.

Policies of Reception

In addition to the foregoing policy suggestions, the social and political environment of the receiving country may play a role in the health effects on immigrants. For example, prior to PRWORA, most persons who were legal immigrants and permanent U.S. residents were entitled to full Medicaid coverage. Coverage for undocumented persons was restricted to emergency coverage only. After PRWORA, however, legal permanent residents and others who entered the country after August 22, 1996, were barred from receiving federal funding for Medicaid and CHIP for five years. After the five years, the sponsor's income was evaluated before determining eligibility. States could choose to deny Medicaid or CHIP to these immigrants after the five-year ban. Coverage for undocumented persons was restricted to emergency coverage only. Lastly, refugees were exempt from these provisions for seven years after receiving their status. Policies such as these can affect both physical and mental health. On a broader level, Reitz (2002) suggests major dimensions of society which affect health: (1) the state of preexisting ethnic or race relations within the host population; (2) differences in labor markets and related institutions; and (3) the impact of government policies and programs, including immigration policy, policies of immigrant integration, and policies for the regulation of social institutions (Reitz 2002).

Latino Immigrants and Their Adaptation: Research Designs

Health researchers should more proactively incorporate theories and research designs that have proven fruitful in the study of Latino-immigrant adaptation. Only recently, new health surveys have begun to incorporate such information. The National Latino and Asian American Study (NLAAS) is a representative study of psychiatric morbidity and mental health service use among Latino and Asian American adults that samples eight ethnic subgroups (Puerto Ricans, Cubans, Mexicans, other Latinos, Chinese, Filipinos, Vietnamese, and other Asians). The survey was administered in five languages and provides extensive data on immigration parameters (e.g., generation status, length of time in the United States, citizenship), acculturation processes, SES, and important aspects of immigrants' experience of the social context (e.g., social capital and support, and perceptions of discrimination and neighborhood safety) (Alegria et al. 2004). Similarly, studies of immigrant adaptation such as the New Immigrant Survey (Jasso et al. 2000), a longitudinal study of several documented immigrant cohorts, have begun to include extensive questions on health status, health behaviors, and access to health care before and after immigration to the United States.

Previous research, as noted, has highlighted heterogeneity in health outcomes among Hispanics/Latinos, showing, for example, a higher burden of asthma, low birth weight, and self-reported physical limitations among Puerto Ricans on the U.S. mainland (Hajat, Lucas, and Kington 2000; Mendoza et al. 1991; Rose, Mannino, and Leaderer 2006) and higher levels of obesity among U.S.-born Mexican Americans (Bates et al. 2008). However, nationally representative prevalence data accounting for the full heterogeneity of Latinos are rare, and sample size limitations almost always preclude analyses of subgroup differences in health determinants. The ideal study design allows comparisons across various national-origin groups, and among immigrants with varying tenure in the United States, their U.S.-born ethnic counterparts (including the second generation), their nonmigrant counterparts in the country of origin, and return migrants. Due to the large size of the Mexican origin population, any distinct pattern among Mexicans is likely to dominate patterns among Latinos overall. Differences across Latino subgroups may reflect differences in country of origin background factors, migration experiences, and incorporation into U.S. society. Puerto Ricans constitute an important subgroup both because they often have unfavorable health outcomes compared to other Latino groups, and because they can serve as a reference group to test the selection hypothesis. As U.S. citizens, Puerto Ricans face relatively lower obstacles to migration to the mainland and therefore may be less health selected—or selected differently—than other Latino subgroups.

There is also need for studies that address the issue of immigration broadly and allow us to compare Latino health paradoxes for different outcomes to the health profiles and trajectories of other immigrant groups, and to examine what individual and contextual factors account for any differences. The National Latino and Asian American Study (Alegria et al. 2004) and the New Immigrant Survey (Jasso et al. 2000) constitute important steps in this direction.

Longitudinal versus Cross-Sectional Studies

The lack of longitudinal data on immigrant health is a significant limitation. Important developments in sociological research on immigrant adaptation have relied on longitudinal surveys that collect information from immigrant parents and their children on domains of life such as family relations, employment, and school performance (Portes and Rumbaut 2001; Suarez-Orozco and Suárez-Orozco 2001). In addition, using sound analytic methods to make proper intergenerational comparisons may lead to reassessment of the deterioration of health and other outcomes across generations (Alba et al. 2004; Jasso et al. 2004). Studying intergenerational health patterns in light of differences in the context of immigration may help us assess the role of selection. For example, Mexicans who migrated to the United States after stricter border controls were implemented in 1986 (Massey, Durand, and Malone 2003) may be more health selected than those who migrated earlier.

Latino Health Paradoxes in the Context of Demographic Change

Why should we pay attention to Latino health paradoxes? Given the growing demographic significance of the Latino population, the apparent resilience of Latinos in relation to some health outcomes may imply that the health of the overall U.S. population is considerably better than it would have been if Latinos did not have paradoxical health outcomes. Consider, for example, the relatively low rates of low birth weight among Latino women with less than high-school education (Acevedo-Garcia, Soobader, and Berkman 2005). Given that 43 percent of U.S. Hispanic women have less than high school education (U.S. Census Bureau 2003), what would be the implications if Latino women with limited education had the high rates of low birth weight of U.S.-born white women or African American women with the same educational attainment?

Since it appears that Latinos in the first generation have a better health profile than Latinos born in the United States, the rapid growth in the second generation may imply that the health profile of the total U.S. Latino population may worsen over time, assuming no persistence of health paradoxes from the first into the second generation. Neither the selection nor the acculturation hypothesis explicitly negates the possibility of preserving the foreign-born health advantage into the second generation and beyond. The presumed bases for health selection are not well specified in the literature, but genes and behaviors consistent with good health can be passed on to subsequent generations. However, empirical evidence to date, though limited, is not consistent with this scenario. Further research should clarify whether this apparent deterioration in health across generations is real and inevitable, or whether the health advantages of the foreign born could be sustained through immigration policies and programs that facilitate successful immigrant adaptation, for example, by strengthening immigrant families (Portes and Rumbaut 2001).

Research on Latino health paradoxes may benefit from better explicit definitions of what is meant by "health paradox," including the variables involved (e.g., race/ethnicity, immigrant status, SES), the group of interest, and the reference group (Palloni and Morenoff 2001). Research questions should address both the verification of Latino health paradoxes and their possible explanations. Ideally, studies should simultaneously and rigorously address the three types of explanations discussed earlier, and allow for the possibility that more than one explanation may account for the observed patterns. Exploring explanations for Latino health paradoxes should involve explicit definitions (and sound operationalization) of concepts such as acculturation, protective cultural factors, and social support. Qualitative study designs may allow a better conceptualization and measurement of protective factors at the individual level, as well as at various contextual levels (e.g., family, neighborhood). For example, although it is often assumed that social networks are supportive, under economic hardship and unfavorable contexts of reception, immigrant social networks may offer limited support (Menjivar 2000). Therefore, examining the role of social factors in Latino health paradoxes may require measuring the structure of social networks, the content of their exchanges in different contexts, and specifically how these exchanges affect health.

The Latino population, at more than thirty-one million, is the largest minority group in the United States—and growing (National Population Estimates 2004). The tremendous variability within the Latino population has been difficult to capture on a population level. Future research in the field could definitely benefit from incorporating information around country of origin, consideration of the complex construct of acculturation (using multidisciplinary approaches), and examination of the influence of the residential environment's impact on the immigrant experience. The ability to effectively incorporate these diverse domains calls for a transdisciplinary approach that brings together demography, sociology, anthropology, epidemiology, and public health. Without looking at Latino health issues through all these lenses, understanding the paradoxical health outcomes and the mechanisms that drive these findings will continue to be a challenge.

Note

1. Throughout this chapter, we use "Hispanic" and "Latino" interchangeably. The category term of "Hispanic" was first used in the 1980 census but has remained controversial. Many Hispanics/Latinos would still identify by their country of origin, such as Puerto Rican, Mexican, Colombian, Brazilian, and so on, rather than either "Hispanic" or "Latino."

Because both terms are used in the literature in various contexts, we have decided to use both in this chapter.

References

Abraido-Lanza, Ana F., Adria N. Armbrister, Karen R. Florez, and Alejandra N. Aguirre. 2006. "Toward a Theory-Driven Model of Acculturation in Public Health Research." *American Journal of Public Health* 96:1342.

Abraído-Lanza, Ana F., Maria T. Chao, and Karen R. Flórez. 2005. "Do Healthy Behaviors Decline with Greater Acculturation? Implications for the Latino Mortality Paradox." *Social Science and Medicine* 61:1243–55.

Abrams, Barbara, and Sylvia Guendelman. 1995. "Nutrient Intake of Mexican-American and Non-Hispanic White Women by Reproductive Status Results of Two National Studies." *Journal of the American Dietetic Association* 95:916–18.

Acevedo-Garcia, Dolores, Jocelyn Pan, Hee-Jin Jun, Theresa L. Osypuk, and Karen M. Emmons. 2005. "The Effect of Immigrant Generation on Smoking." *Social Science and Medicine* 61:1223–42.

Acevedo-Garcia, Dolores, Mah-J. Soobader, and Lisa F. Berkman. 2005. "The Differential Effect of Foreign-Born Status on Low Birth Weight by Race/Ethnicity and Education." *American Academy of Pediatrics* 115: e20–30.

———. 2007. "Low Birthweight among US Hispanic/Latino Subgroups: The Effect of Maternal Foreign-Born Status and Education." *Social Science and Medicine* 65:2503–16.

Alba, Richard, D. Abdel-Hady, T. Islam, and K. Marotz. Forthcoming. "Downward Assimilation and Mexican Americans: An Examination of Intergenerational Advance and Stagnation in Educational Attainment." In *New Dimensions of Diversity: The Children of Immigrants in North America and Western Europe*, ed. M. C. Waters and R. Alba.

Alba, Richard, and Victor Nee. 1997. "Rethinking Assimilation Theory for a New Era of Immigration." *International Migration Review* 31(4): 826–74.

Alegria, Margarita, David Takeuchi, Glorisa Canino, Naihua Duan, Patrick Shrout, Xiao-Li Meng, William Vega, Nolan Zane, Doryliz Vila, Meghan Woo, Mildred Vera, Peter Guarnaccia, Sergio Aguilar-Gaxiola, Stanley Sue, Javier Escobar, Keh-Ming Lin, and Fong Gong. 2004. "Considering Context, Place and Culture: The National Latino and Asian American Study." *International Journal of Methods in Psychiatric Research* 13:208–20.

Antecol, Heather, and Kelly Bedard. 2006. "Unhealthy Assimilation: Why Do Immigrants Converge to

American Health Status Levels?" *Demography* 43(2): 337–60.

Arcia, Emily, Martie Skinner, Donald Bailey, and Vivian Correa. 2001. "Models of Acculturation and Health Behaviors among Latino Immigrants to the U.S." *Social Science and Medicine* 53:41–53.

Bates, Lisa M., Dolores Acevedo-Garcia, Margarita Alegria, and Nancy Krieger. 2008. "Immigration and Generational Trends in Body Mass Index and Obesity in the United States: Results of the National Latino and Asian American Survey, 2002–2003." *American Journal of Public Health* 98:70.

Berkman, Lisa F., and Ichiro Kawachi. 2000. *Social Epidemiology.* Oxford: Oxford University Press.

Breslau, Joshua, Sergio Aguilar-Gaxiola, Kenneth S. Kendler, Maxwell Su, David Williams, and Ronald C. Kessler. 2005. "Specifying Race-Ethnic Differences in Risk for Psychiatric Disorder in a United States National Sample." *Psychological Medicine* 36:57–68.

Brown, E. Richard, and Hongjian Yu. 2004. "Latinos' Access to Employment-Based Health Insurance." In *Understanding Society: An Introductory Reader*, ed. Margaret L. Andersen, Kim A. Logio, and Howard Francis Taylor. Belmont, Calif.: Wadsworth.

Cavazos-Rehg, Patricia A., Luis H. Zayas, and Edward L. Spitznagel. 2007. "Legal Status, Emotional Well-Being and Subjective Health Status of Latino Immigrants." *Journal of the National Medical Association* 99:126–31.

Chun, Kevin M., Pamela B. Organista, and Gerardo Marín. 2003. *Acculturation: Advances in Theory, Measurement, and Applied Research.* Washington, D.C.: American Psychological Association.

Derose, Kathryn Pitkin, and David W. Baker. 2000. "Limited English Proficiency and Latinos' Use of Physician Services." *Medical Care Research and Review* 57:76–91.

Derose, Kathryn Pitkin, Jose J. Escarce, and Nicole Lurie. 2007. "Immigrants and Health Care: Sources of Vulnerability," *Health Affairs* 26(5): 1258–68.

Elo, Irma T., Cassio M. Turra, Bert Kestenbaum, and B. Renee Ferguson. 2004. "Mortality among Elderly Hispanics in the United States: Past Evidence and New Results." *Demography* 41(1): 109–28.

Escobar, Javier, and William K. Vega. 2000. "Mental Health and Immigration's AAAs: Where Are We and Where Do We Go from Here?" *Journal of Nervous and Mental Disease* 188(11): 736–40.

Falcon, Angelo, Marilyn Aguirre-Molina, and Carlos W. Molina. 2001. "Latino Health Policy: Beyond Demographic Determinism." In *Health Issues in the Latino Community*, ed. Marilyn Aguirre-Molina, Carlos W. Molina, and Ruth Enid Zambrana, 3–22. San Francisco: Jossey Bass.

Finch, Brian K., Bohdan Kolody, and William A. Vega. 2000. "Perceived Discrimination and Depression among Mexican-Origin Adults in California." *Journal of Health and Social Behavior* 41:295–313.

Fix, Michael, and Jeffrey S. Passel. 2002. "Assessing Welfare Reform's Immigrant Provisions." In *Welfare Reform: The Next Act*, ed. Alan Weil and Kenneth Finegold, 179–202. Washington, D.C.: Urban Institute Press.

Franzini, Luis, John C. Ribble, and Arlene M. Keddie. 2001. "Understanding the Hispanic Paradox." *Ethnicity and Disease* 11:496–518.

Freedman, David S., Laura Kettel Khan, Mary K. Serdula, Deborah A. Galuska, and William H. Dietz. 2002. "Trends and Correlates of Class 3 Obesity in the United States from 1990 through 2000." *Journal of the American Medical Association* 288:1758–61.

Fry, Richard. 2008. "Latino Settlement in the New Century." pewhispanic.org/files/reports/96.pdf. Accessed February 6, 2009.

Goel, Mita Sanghavi, Ellen P. McCarthy, Russell S. Phillips, and Christina C. Wee. 2004. "Obesity among U.S. Immigrant Subgroups by Duration of Residence." *Journal of the American Medical Association* 292:2860–67.

Gordon-Larsen, Penny, Kathleen Mullan Harris, Dianne S. Ward, and Barry M. Popkin. 2003. "Acculturation and Overweight-Related Behaviors among Hispanic Immigrants to the U.S.: the National Longitudinal Study of Adolescent Health." *Social Science and Medicine* 57:2023–34.

Grant, Bridget F., Frederick S. Stinson, Deborah S. Hasin, Deborah A. Dawson, S. Patricia Chou, and Karyn Anderson. 2004. "Immigration and Lifetime Prevalence of DSM-IV Psychiatric Disorders among Mexican Americans and Non-Hispanic Whites in the United States: Results from the National Epidemiologic Survey on Alcohol and Related Conditions." *Journal of the American Medical Association* 61:1226–33.

Hajat, Anjum, Jacqueline B. Lucas, and Raynard Kington. 2000. "Health Outcomes among Hispanic Subgroups: Data from the National Health Interview Survey, 1992–95." *Advance Data* 310:1–14.

Hayes-Bautista, David E. 2002. "The Latino Health Research Agenda for the Twenty-First Century." In *Latinos: Remaking America*, ed. Marcelo Suarez-Orozco and Mariela Páez, 215–35. Berkeley: University of California Press.

Hummer, Robert A., Maureen R. Benjamins, and Richard G. Rogers. 2004. "Racial and Ethnic Disparities in Health and Mortality among the U.S. Elderly Population." In *Critical Perspectives on Racial and Ethnic Differences in Health in Late Life*, ed. Norman B. Anderson, Randy A. Bulatao, and

Barney Cohen, 53–94. Washington, D.C.: National Academies Press.

Hummer, Robert A., Richard G. Rogers, Sarit H. Amir, Douglas Forbes, and W. Parker Frisbie. 2000. "Adult Mortality Differentials among Hispanic Subgroups and Non-Hispanic Whites." *Social Science Quarterly* 81:459–76.

Hunt, Kelly J., Roy G. Resendez, Ken Williams, Steve M. Haffner, Michael P. Stern, and Helen P. Hazuda. 2003. "All-Cause and Cardiovascular Mortality among Mexican-American and Non-Hispanic White Older Participants in the San Antonio Heart Study: Evidence against the Hispanic Paradox." *American Journal of Epidemiology* 158:1048–57.

Hunt, Kelly J., Ken Williams, Roy G. Resendez, Helen P. Hazuda, Steve M. Haffner, and Michael P. Stern. 2002. "All-Cause and Cardiovascular Mortality among Diabetic Participants in the San Antonio Heart Study: Evidence against the Hispanic Paradox." *Diabetes Care* 25:1557–63.

Hunt, Linda M., Suzanne Schneider, and Brendon Comer. 2004. "Should 'Acculturation' be a Variable in Health Research? A Critical Review of Research on U.S. Hispanics." *Social Science and Medicine* 59:973–86.

Integrated Public Use Microdata Series [IPUMS] United States. 2009. "Definition of Poverty in the IPUMS Samples." usa.ipums.org/usa/volii/poverty.shtml.

Jackson, James S., Harold W. Neighbors, Myriam Torres, Lisa A. Martin, David R. Williams, and Raymond Baser. 2006. "Use of Mental Health Services and Subjective Satisfaction with Treatment among Black Caribbean Immigrants: Results from the National Survey of American Life." *American Journal of Public Health* 97(1): 60–67.

Jasso, Guillermina, Douglas S. Massey, Mark R. Rosenzweig, and James P. Smith. 2000. "The New Immigrant Survey Pilot (NIS-P): Overview and New Findings about U.S. Legal Immigrants at Admission." *Demography* 37:127–38.

———. 2004. "Immigrant Health: Selectivity and Acculturation." *Critical Perspectives on Racial and Ethnic Differences in Health in Late Life*, ed. Norman B. Anderson, Randy A. Bulatao, and Barney Cohen, 227–66. Washington, D.C.: National Academies Press.

Jerant, Anthony F., Rose Arellanes, and Peter Franks. 2008. "Health Status among U.S. Hispanics: Ethnic Variation, Nativity, and Language Moderation." *Med Care* 46(7): 709–17.

Lara, Marielena, Lara Akinbami, Glenn Flores, and Hal Morgenstern. 2006. "Heterogeneity of Childhood Asthma among Hispanic Children: Puerto Rican Children Bear a Disproportionate Burden." *Pediatrics* 117:43–53.

Liao, Youlian, Richard S. Cooper, Guichan Cao, Ramon Durazo-Arvizu, Jay Kaufman, Amy Luke, and Daniel McGee. 1998. "Mortality Patterns among Adult Hispanics: Findings from the NHIS, 1986 to 1990." *American Journal of Public Health* 88:227–232.

Lin, Charles C., Eugene Rogot, Norman J. Johnson, Paul D. Sorlie, and Elizabeth Arias. 2003. "A Further Study of Life Expectancy by Socioeconomic Factors in the National Longitudinal Mortality Study." *Ethnicity and Disease* 13:240–47.

Lindstrom, David P. 1996. "Economic Opportunity in Mexico and Return Migration from the United States." *Demography* 33:357–74.

Lucas, Jacqueline W., Daheia J. Barr-Anderson, and Raynard S. Kington. 2003. "Health Status, Health Insurance, and Health Care Utilization Patterns of Immigrant Black Men." *American Journal of Public Health* 93:1740–47.

Markides, Kyriakos S., and Jeannine Coreil. 1986. "The Health of Southwestern Hispanics: An Epidemiologic Paradox." *Public Health Reports* 101:253–65.

Markides, Kyriakos S., and Karl Eschbach. 2005. "Aging, Migration, and Mortality: Current Status of Research on the Hispanic Paradox." *Journals of Gerontology Series B: Psychological Sciences and Social Sciences* 60:68–75.

Massey, Douglas S., and Brooks Bitterman. 1985. "Explaining the Paradox of Puerto Rican Segregation." *Social Forces* 64:306–31.

Massey, Douglas S., Jorge Durand, and Nolan J. Malone. 2003. *Beyond Smoke and Mirrors: Mexican Immigration in an Era of Economic Integration.* New York: Russell Sage Foundation.

Mendoza, Fernando S., Stephanie J. Ventura, R. Burciaga Valdez, Ricardo O. Castillo, Laura Escoto Saldivar, Katherine Baisden, and Reynaldo Martorell. 1991. "Selected Measures of Health Status for Mexican-American, Mainland Puerto Rican, and Cuban-American Children." *Journal of the American Medical Association* 265:227–32.

Menjivar, Cecilia. 2000. *Fragmented Ties: Salvadoran Immigrant Networks in America.* Berkeley: University of California Press.

National Population Estimates. 2004. "Characteristics, National Demographic Components of Change by Hispanic or Latino Origin, 2003." Washington, D.C.: U.S. Census Bureau. census.gov/popest/archives/2000s/vintage_2004/.

NCHS [National Centers for Health Statistics, Centers for Disease Control and Prevention, and Department of Health and Human Services]. 2002. "A Demographic and Health Snapshot of the U.S. Hispanic/Latino Population." CDC

website, cdc.gov/NCHS/data/hpdata2010/
chcsummit.pdf.

Nelson, Jennifer A., Mary Ann Chiasson, and Viola
Ford. 2004. "Childhood Overweight in a New York
City WIC Population." *American Journal of Public
Health* 94:458–62.

Neuhouser, Marian L., Beti Thompson, Gloria D.
Coronado, and Cam C. Solomon. 2004. "Higher
Fat Intake and Lower Fruit and Vegetables Intakes
Are Associated with Greater Acculturation among
Mexicans Living in Washington State." *Journal of the
American Dietetic Association* 104:51–57.

Ogden, Cynthia L., Margaret D. Carroll, Lester R.
Curtin, Margaret A. McDowell, Carolyn J. Tabak,
and Katherine M. Flegal. 2006. "Prevalence of
Overweight and Obesity in the United States,
1999–2004." *Journal of the American Medical
Association* 295:1549–55.

Ortega, Alexander, Robert Rosenheck, Margarita Alegría,
and Rani A. Desai. 2000. "Acculturation and the
Lifetime Risk of Psychiatric and Substance Use
Disorders among Hispanics." *Journal of Nervous and
Mental Disease* 188(11): 728–35.

Palloni, Alberto, and Elizabeth Arias. 2004. "Paradox
Lost: Explaining the Hispanic Adult Mortality
Advantage." *Demography* 41(3): 385–415.

Palloni, Alberto, and Jeffrey D. Morenoff. 2001.
"Interpreting the Paradoxical in the Hispanic
Paradox: Demographic and Epidemiologic
Approaches." *Annals of the New York Academy of
Sciences* 954:140–74.

Passel, Jeffrey S., and D'Vera Cohn. 2008. *U.S.
Population Projections, 2005–2050.* Washington,
D.C.: Pew Research Center.

Portes, Alejandro, and Ruben G. Rumbaut. 2001. *The
New Americans: An Overview.* Berkeley: University of
California Press, Russell Sage Foundation.

Ramirez, Roberto R., and G. Patricia de la Cruz. 2003.
*The Hispanic Population in the United States: March
2002.* Washington, D.C.: U.S. Department of
Commerce, Bureau of the Census, Economics and
Statistics Administration.

Reitz, Jeffrey. 2002. "Host Societies and the Reception
of Immigrants: Research Themes, Emerging Theories
and Methodological Issues." *International Migration
Review* 36(4): 1005–19.

Rogler, Lloyd H., Dharma E. Cortes, and Robert G.
Malgady. 1991. "Acculturation and Mental Health
Status among Hispanics: Convergence and New
Directions for Research." *American Psychologist*
46(6): 585–97.

Rose, Deborah, David M. Mannino, and Brian P.
Leaderer. 2006. "Asthma Prevalence among U.S.
Adults, 1998–2000: Role of Puerto Rican Ethnicity

and Behavioral and Geographic Factors." *American
Journal of Public Health* 96:880–88.

Rosenberg, Terry J., and Robert W. Lake. 1976.
"Toward a Revised Model of Residential
Segregation and Succession: Puerto Ricans in New
York, 1960–1970." *American Journal of Sociology*
81(5): 1142–50.

Ruggles, Steven, Matthew Sobek, Trent Alexander,
and Catherine Fitch. 2008. "Statistical Portrait of
the Foreign-Born Population in the United States,
2006." pewhispanic.org/factsheets/factsheet
.php?FactsheetID=36. Accessed January 23, 2008.

Rumbaut, Ruben G. 1997. "Assimilation and Its
Discontents: Between Rhetoric and Reality."
International Migration Review 31:923–60.

Rumbaut, Ruben G., and Alejandro Portes. 2001.
Ethnicities: Children of Immigrants in America.
Berkeley: University of California Press.

Santiago, Anna M., and George Galster. 1995. "Puerto
Rican Segregation in the United States: Cause or
Consequence of Economic Status?" *Social Problems*
42(3): 361–89.

Singh, Gopal K., and Mohammad Siahpush. 2001. "All-
Cause and Cause-Specific Mortality of Immigrants
and Native Born in the United States." *American
Journal of Public Health* 91:392–99.

———. 2002. "Ethnic-Immigrant Differentials in
Health Behaviors, Morbidity, and Cause-Specific
Mortality in the United States: An Analysis
of Two National Data Bases." *Human Biology*
74:83–110.

Smith, James P. 2003. "Assimilation across the Latino
Generations." *American Economic Review*
93:315–19.

Soldo, Beth, Rebecca Wong, and Alberto Palloni. 2002.
"Migrant Health Selection: Evidence from Mexico
and the U.S." Paper presented at the Population
Association of America Conference, Atlanta.
mhas.pop.upenn.edu/Papers/1.pdf.

Sorlie, Paul, Eric Backlund, Norman Johnson, and
Eugene Rogot. 1993. "Mortality by Hispanic Status
in the United States." *Journal of the American Medical
Association* 270:2464–68.

South, Scott J., Kyle Crowder, and Erick Chavez. 2005.
"Migration and Spatial Assimilation among U.S.
Latinos: Classical versus Segmented Trajectories."
Demography 42(3): 497–521.

Suárez-Orozco, Carola, and Marcelo M. Suárez-Orozco.
2001. *Children of Immigration.* Cambridge, Mass.:
Harvard University Press.

Suro, Roberto, and Jeffrey S. Passel. 2003. *The Rise of
the Second Generation: Changing Patterns in Hispanic
Population Growth.* Washington D.C.: Pew Hispanic
Center, Urban Institute.

Terrazas, Aaron, and Jeanne Batalova. 2008. "The Most Up-to-Date Frequently Requested Statistics on Immigrants in the United States." migrationinformation.org/USFocus/display .cfm?ID=714.

Turra, Cassio M., and Noreen Goldman. 2007. "Socioeconomic Differences in Mortality among U.S. Adults: Insights into the Hispanic Paradox." *Journals of Gerontology Series B: Psychological Sciences and Social Sciences* 62: S184.

U.S. Census Bureau. 2002. "Nativity and Parent Age for Selected Race and Hispanic-Origin Groups: 2000." census.gov/population/socdemo/foreign/ppl-145/ tab09-1A.pdf. Accessed January 21, 2009.

———. 2003. Current Population Survey, March 2002. Conducted by the Population Division of the Bureau of the Census for the Bureau of Labor Statistics. Washington, D.C.: U.S. Census Bureau. census.gov/ prod/2003pubs/p20–539.pdf.

———. 2006. "U.S. Hispanic Population Size and Composition." census.gov/population/socdemo/ hispanic/cps2006/CPS_Powerpoint_2006.pdf.

Vega, William A., and Hortensia Amaro. 1994. "Latino Outlook: Good Health, Uncertain Prognosis." *Annual Review of Public Health* 15:39–67.

Villarejo, Don. 2003. "The Health of U.S. Hired Farm Workers." *Annual Review of Public Health* 24:175–93.

Viruell-Fuentes, Edna A. 2007. "Beyond Acculturation: Immigration, Discrimination, and Health Research among Mexicans in the United States." *Social Science and Medicine* 65:1524–35.

Weinberg, Michelle, Jackie Hopkins, Leigh Farrington, Louise Gresham, Michele Ginsberg, and Beth P. Bell. 2004. "Hepatitis A in Hispanic Children Who Live along the United States–Mexico Border: The Role of International Travel and Food-Borne Exposures." *Pediatrics* 114(1): e68–73.

Whitaker, Robert C., and Sean M. Orzol. 2006. "Obesity among U.S. Urban Preschool Children: Relationships to Race, Ethnicity, and Socioeconomic Status." *Archives of Pediatrics and Adolescent Medicine* 160:578–84.

Williams, David R. 2001. "Racial Variations in Adult Health Status: Patterns, Paradoxes, and Prospects." In *America Becoming: Racial Trends and Their Consequences*, ed. Neil J. Smelser, William Julius Wilson, and Faith Mitchell, 371–410. Vol. 2. Washington, D.C.: National Academy Press.

Winkleby, Marilyn A., Cheryl L. Albright, Beth Howard-Pitney, Jennifer Lin, and Stephen P. Fortmann. 1994. "Hispanic/White Differences in Dietary Fat Intake among Low Educated Adults and Children." *American Journal of Preventive Medicine* 23:465–73.

Yu, Stella M., Z. Jennifer Huang, Renee H. Schwalberg, and Rebecca M. Nyman. 2006. "Parental English Proficiency and Children's Health Services Access." *American Journal of Public Health* 96(8): 1449–55.

8

A Life-Course Approach to the Study of Neighborhoods and Health

Stephanie A. Robert, University of Wisconsin–Madison

Kathleen A. Cagney, University of Chicago

Margaret M. Weden, RAND Corporation

Renewed attention to the importance of neighborhood context to health and well-being (Entwisle 2007; Sampson et al. 2002) has led to insight and innovation in health research over the last decade. While biomedical research has focused on how processes within our bodies affect health, and much social science and public health research has emphasized how the behavioral and psychosocial characteristics of individuals affect health, research on neighborhoods reminds us that individuals live in a variety of social and spatial contexts, and that these contexts are important to shaping health and well-being.

We argue that most research on neighborhoods and health has been hampered by considering individuals and neighborhoods as static entities. Little research has examined how neighborhoods affect the health of individuals over time, how neighborhoods themselves change over time, and how the life courses of individuals and neighborhoods interact to impact individual and population health.

A life-course approach "guides research on human lives within context" (Elder, Johnson, and Crosnoe 2004, 10) and is therefore a natural approach for studying the impact of neighborhoods on health. This approach highlights issues of age and time to pinpoint critical periods when neigh-

borhood might be most important to health in a person's life course, and which aspects of neighborhood might matter at different times. A life-course approach can also point to the dynamic nature of neighborhoods, and how neighborhood stability and change over time can contribute to the health and well-being of residents. While most life-course research examines the life course of *individuals*, we argue that studying the life course of *neighborhoods* might significantly expand our understanding of the impact of neighborhoods on health.

Five Principles of the Life Course Applied to Individuals

The life course is described variously as a theoretical orientation, a perspective, and a framework (Mortimer and Shanahan 2004). We highlight five general principles common to most life-course approaches: life-span development, place and time, timing, linked lives, and agency (for more thorough summaries, see, e.g., Elder, Johnson, and Crosnoe 2004; Mortimer and Shanahan 2004). We provide examples of how the principle has been applied to improve our understanding of how neighborhood context affects the health of individuals as they age, then describe how the principles might be applied to better understand the life course of *neighborhoods*, and how the neighborhood life course might affect health.

Life-Span Development

The principle of life-span development emphasizes taking a long-term perspective on individual development and how it is shaped by experiences throughout life (Elder, Johnson, and Crosnoe 2004). Although this principle suggests that the impact of neighborhoods on health should be examined over people's entire life span, much of the literature has examined the relationship between neighborhood context and health at one point in time. Although such cross-sectional analyses provide useful insights into the relationship between neighborhood context and health, they cannot test whether neighborhood context has contemporaneous, lagged, or cumulative effects on health.

As notable exceptions, several studies have simultaneously tested the relevance of lagged and contemporaneous influence of neighborhoods on health, exploring the influence of early life neighborhood exposures on health at different points later in the life course (Curtis et al. 2004; Wheaton and Clarke 2003; Naess et al. 2008). For example, Wheaton and Clarke (2003) found that childhood neighborhood socioeconomic disadvantage had a lagged effect on early adult mental health over and above the effects of adult neighborhood context.

Neighborhood context also may have a cumulative impact on health over time. Living in a disadvantaged neighborhood context may instigate a chain of risk (Kuh et al. 2003; Ferraro and Shippee 2008)—a sequence of events that accumulate over the life course to produce poor health. From this perspective, neighborhood context affects not only clusters of risk and protective factors, but chains of risk or protective factors that compound over time to produce cumulative advantage or disadvantage that affects health (Dannefer 2003; O'Rand 1996). For example, research examining an index of cumulative neighborhood disadvantage over decades finds that cumulative neighbor-

hood disadvantage is associated with subclinical atherosclerosis in women (Carson et al. 2007; Lemelin et al. 2009).

The principle of life-span development also suggests that we conceptualize how neighborhoods can have both direct and indirect effects on health over time. While much research demonstrates that neighborhood context has an *independent* impact on health over and above individual socioeconomic status (Robert 1999; Pickett and Pearl 2001; Kawachi and Berkman 2003), research has not sufficiently examined how neighborhood context indirectly affects health *through* its impact on individual SES—that is, by shaping individual educational, occupational, and economic achievement, which then have more proximal effects on health.

Scholars have tested various aspects of these relationships rather than considering entire pathways. For example, research demonstrates that neighborhoods impact schooling and educational achievement of children. Sampson, Sharkey, and Raudenbush (2008) showed that among black children in Chicago, living in severely disadvantaged neighborhoods very early in life had a lagged effect on lower verbal ability a number of years later. The magnitude of this relationship was approximately equal to missing a year or more of schooling. Theoretically, these neighborhood effects on verbal ability might subsequently impact health through a number of pathways, such as children's ability to succeed in school; to secure a good job, income, and health insurance in adulthood; and to make healthy lifestyle choices (Mirowsky and Ross 2003).

In sum, the principle of life-span development highlights the idea that neighborhoods may have lagged, cumulative, and contemporaneous effects on individual health over a person's life span. Longitudinal studies are needed to understand the complex pathways linking neighborhoods to health as people age.

Place and Time

The principle of place and time highlights the idea that both place and historical context matter to a person's health. Indeed, the primary strength of research on neighborhoods and health is that it emphasizes how one of the places we are exposed to in our daily lives—our neighborhood—shapes our health. Research on neighborhoods shifts our understanding of health from a state determined only by individual and family processes to one promoted or constrained by the physical, social, economic, and service environments of the neighborhoods in which we live and work.

Health outcomes have been linked to multiple aspects of neighborhood context—neighborhood socioeconomic status (Diez Roux et al. 2004; Pickett and Pearl 2001; Robert 1999), social capital (Cagney and Browning 2004; Carpiano 2007), age structure (Cagney 2006), the built environment (Freedman et al. 2008), and crime (Sundquist et al. 2006; Morenoff, Sampson, and Raudenbush 2001).

Aspects of larger place contexts have also been linked to health (Osypuk and Galea 2007)—county- or state-level income inequality (Lynch et al. 2001; Wen, Browning, and Cagney 2003; Kawachi, Kennedy, and Lochner 1997), county- or state-level policies and services (Kaplan et al. 1996), and racial residential segregation at metropolitan area, city, and county levels (Lee and Ferraro 2007; Robert and Ruel 2006; Subramanian, Acevedo-Garcia, and Osypuk 2005; Walton 2009).

Moreover, research has highlighted the importance of neighborhood context in understanding racial and ethnic disparities in health—disparities in hypertension (Morenoff et al. 2007), obesity (Robert and Reither 2004), self-rated health (Cagney, Browning, and Wen 2005; Browning, Cagney, and Wen 2003; Robert and Ruel 2006; Robert and Lee 2002; Subramanian, Acevedo-Garcia, and Osypuk 2005), asthma prevalence (Rosenbaum 2008; Cagney and Browning 2004), and mortality (Yao and Robert 2008).

An understanding of the importance of neighborhood to a range of economic and quality of life outcomes led to implementation of and research on the effects of housing relocation programs such as the Moving to Opportunity (MTO), Gautreaux, and Yonkers experiments. These housing mobility experiments are directly relevant to examining how changing a family's neighborhood place might effect changes in physical and mental

health outcomes over the life course. Research on these programs provides some evidence that moving out of high-poverty neighborhoods improves the mental health (Leventhal and Brooks-Gunn 2003) and physical health (Fauth, Leventhal, and Brooks-Gunn 2008) of movers compared to stayers, though these effects are modest and are generally stronger for adults than for children.

Although housing relocation experiments provide some evidence of the impact of neighborhoods on health and other outcomes, neighborhoods can impact health and well-being over the life course in ways that cannot be overcome by housing relocation alone (Ludwig et al. 2008; Sampson, Sharkey, and Raudenbush 2008; Sharkey 2008). For example, because childhood neighborhood context has a lagged effect on the mental health of young adults (Wheaton and Clarke 2003), moving young adults out of poor neighborhoods may not overcome the lagged impact of childhood poverty residence on their mental health. Similarly, if exposure to poor neighborhoods is particularly critical in childhood, then children in housing relocation programs have already been exposed to poor neighborhoods—exposures that a residential move may not easily overcome (Sampson, Sharkey, and Raudenbush 2008). However, the housing relocation too may produce either lagged or cumulative benefits to mental and physical health that will appear much later. For example, Fauth, Leventhal, and Brooks-Gunn (2008) find that adults randomly assigned to move to lower-poverty neighborhoods experienced improvements in self-reports of collective efficacy and safety and improvements in weak social ties, while maintaining strong social ties outside their neighborhood. These beneficial aspects of their new neighborhood may have a lagged or cumulative impact on the physical and mental health of these adults and their children over a longer period of time.

Although the literature on neighborhoods and health has emphasized well the place aspect of the life-course principle of place and time, less attention has been paid to time (cohort and period effects). Yet the cohort and period effects of historical events have been examined in some economic and demographic research to evaluate the influence of exposures at different points along the life course. For example, historical disasters like famine and pandemics have been used to study the long-lasting effects of early life exposures on later life health and longevity of the survivors of these events (Susser and Lin 1992; Preston, Hill, and Drevenstedt 1998; Almond 2006; O'Connor 2003).

Age, period, and cohort characteristics can also converge to produce different environments that affect health. For example, Small (2004) conducted ethnographic work in a low-income Puerto Rican enclave, documenting how residents resisted relocation efforts. He showed that the initial migratory generation was more invested than the younger generations in neighborhood-level social capital and in maintaining the enclave; younger generations did not feel the same sense of social ties or belonging. He illustrates how age and cohort converged to shape expectations about neighborhood.

Though clearly the life-course principle of place and time is the underpinning of most neighborhood research on health, almost all the recent research has focused on urban areas to the exclusion of rural areas, even though rural residents have worse health on a number of outcomes (Hartley 2004). Indeed, racial disparities in health are often more severe in rural areas (Probst et al. 2004), but get overlooked in the recent neighborhood research, including racial-segregation research, which focuses on urban and suburban areas (Robert and Ruel 2006).

Moreover, the recent resurgence of attention to neighborhoods and health has been predominantly quantitative in nature, building upon the strength of a number of large national and regional surveys. However, a number of qualitative approaches have been advanced to fill gaps in our understanding of the meaning that residents place on their neighborhoods, and to describe people's spatial and social interactions in their neighborhoods (Airey 2003; Altschuler, Somkin, and Adler 2004; Israel et al. 2005; Patillo 1999). For example, Carpiano (2009) utilized the "go-along" interview (Kusenbach 2003) to better understand the meaning people assign to the "action space" (Cummins et al. 2007) of the neighborhoods in which they interact. Dennis and colleagues (2008) introduced participatory

photo mapping (PPM) to study the implications of place for the health of children. They involved children living in a low-income neighborhood in a project in which children took photos of aspects of their neighborhood environments related to their health, provided narratives about the meaning of the photos, and participated in mapping their experiential data along with other existing neighborhood-level data using GIS mapping technologies. Such approaches are needed to help us better understand how people experience and interpret their spatial and social spaces, variations in these experiences and interpretations across residents, and the implications for individual and neighborhood health and well-being.

Timing

The life-course principle of timing suggests that the timing of an exposure or experience can be important in determining health, as Elder, Johnson, and Crosnoe explain: "The developmental antecedents and consequences of life transitions, events, and behavioral patterns vary according to their timing in a person's life" (2003, 12). For example, critical-period models in epidemiology emphasize the importance of the timing of health risks or exposures, often focusing on how exposures during particular biological or social developmental stages can have long-lasting health impacts (Lynch and Davey Smith 2005).

The principle of timing raises the question of whether neighborhood context is particularly important to health at specific ages, as some theory and evidence suggests may be true for childhood (Brooks-Gunn et al. 1993; Jelleyman and Spencer 2007) or for older adulthood (Robert and Li 2001; Glass and Balfour 2003). For example, young children and older adults may have greater physiological vulnerability to environmental exposures in poor neighborhoods than do young adults and adults in midlife. On the other hand, young and middle-aged adults may experience more immediate direct exposure to the stressful aspects of high unemployment in disadvantaged neighborhoods. Researchers studying the Chicago heat wave found that the higher mortality of older adults could be attributed not only to their greater physiological vulnerability to temperature, but also to their being the most likely to live in areas hardest hit by commercial decline (Browning et al. 2006). Further research is needed to explore which dimensions of neighborhoods are more or less important to people at specific ages or critical periods in their development.

Other aspects of timing can be explored to understand neighborhood effects on health. For example, Wen, Cagney, and Christakis (2005) studied older adults in Chicago who had experienced hospitalizations and examined the impact of neighborhood on their subsequent mortality. Their findings suggest that during a critical period of illness, older adults (or perhaps people of all ages) are more vulnerable to their neighborhood environments, with some neighborhoods being more facilitative of recovery than others.

Using a life-course approach to examine how timing of neighborhood exposure affects health also requires attention to how the timing of neighborhood exposure may have impacts on different measures of health. Naess and colleagues (2008) examined the relative contribution of neighborhoods on mortality risk along the life course of different cohorts for different causes of death. They found that for the youngest age group, area of residence close to death is most strongly related to mortality for psychiatric and violent causes of death. However, determinants of cardiovascular mortality included area of residence in both childhood and adulthood.

The principle of timing suggests that we explore whether exposures to neighborhood may be more or less salient at different points during an individual's development, or during critical events, such as illness or pregnancy, and whether such exposures affect different health outcomes at different ages.

Linked Lives

The life-course principle of linked lives, as conceived by Elder, suggests that "each generation is bound to fateful decisions and events in the other's life course" (1985, 40). This principle of linked lives is consistent with a body of research that examines social networks and social capital

as particularly important aspects of the neighborhood context that promote or constrain health (Wen, Cagney, and Christakis 2005). Although the social network and social capital literatures have developed separately, the combination of these theoretical approaches provides great promise for improving our understanding of how neighborhoods affect health over the life course.

Social network theory highlights the social structure of social networks, which can shape a range of outcomes, including health. Wellman and Frank (2001) conceptualize multiple levels in which networks take root, highlighting the interdependence of individual, dyadic, and larger network characteristics. Network analysis, then, provides a structure to which we can apply theoretical ideas regarding how individuals, network ties, and network properties might interact at different levels to produce health within and between neighborhoods (Berkman and Glass 2000; Smith and Christakis 2008; Luke and Harris 2007).

While social network theory focuses on the structure of social networks, social capital theory focuses on their function. Social capital is conceptualized either as the resources that result from social structure (Burt 2001; Bourdieu 1986) or as a function of social structure that is beneficial to those who hold it (Coleman 1990). Lin, Cook, and Burt (2001) define social capital as resources embedded in a social structure that are accessed, mobilized, or both in purposive actions.

To further understand how linked lives within neighborhoods affect health, we should consider neighborhood social networks and the social capital that flows through them in ways that promote and constrain health. Although dense social networks might protect health through social support mechanisms (Berkman and Glass 2000), they might simultaneously promote unhealthy behaviors. For example, Carpiano (2007) found that higher neighborhood-level social support was associated with greater odds of individual-level daily smoking and binge drinking, controlling for neighborhood socioeconomic conditions and social cohesion.

Indeed, social networks and the social capital that flows through them to affect health may function differently depending on other characteristics of the neighborhood context. As summarized by Berkman and Clark: "It would seem that one must differentiate between the existence of networks and their capacity to provide resources" (2003, 299). For example, although being socially isolated is generally detrimental to individual health (Berkman and Glass 2000), some suggest that social isolation might be protective when people live in hazardous neighborhood environments. Caughy, O'Campo, and Muntaner (2003) found that, in poor neighborhoods, children whose parents reported knowing few of their neighbors had lower levels of internalizing problems than those whose parents knew many of their neighbors. Being part of a dense social network can also place excess demands on network members (Portes and Sensenbrenner 1993). Schieman and Meersman (2004) found that the association between neighborhood problems and physical health problems among older men was exacerbated for men who contributed greater levels of support, suggesting that the demands of living in challenging neighborhoods may tap individual health resources.

The life-course principle of linked lives may be particularly relevant when examining the positive and negative health effects of living in neighborhood ethnic enclaves. Although most of the literature on racial segregation and health focuses on the negative impact, particularly economically, of living in neighborhoods with high concentrations of ethnic minorities, some research on ethnic enclaves suggests that their social networks can serve to constrain and promote positive health behaviors, distribution of health-system knowledge, and good health and well-being (Eschbach et al. 2004; Lee and Ferraro 2007). Studies have found that living in neighborhoods with a high proportion of Hispanic residents is protective of self-rated health and of depressive symptoms among older Mexican American adults (Patel et al. 2003; Ostir et al. 2003). Other research found that the health advantage of living in a high-density Mexican American neighborhood outweighed the health disadvantages of even high-poverty residence for Mexican American older adults (Eschbach et al. 2004).

Future research on neighborhoods and health would benefit from attention to the structure of social networks within and between neighborhoods, the social capital that flows through them in different types of neighborhoods, and the ways that these networks and capital support or constrain health over time.

The life-course principle of linked lives also draws on the vertical notion of the life course; that is, that our life trajectories are shaped by generations before and after us (O'Rand 1996). This leads us to ask about intergenerational characteristics, interactions, or relationships, and the extent to which they matter for the way in which neighborhood social context affects health over the individual life span. Sharkey (2008) recently demonstrated that neighborhood socioeconomic context has much continuity from one generation to the next. Indeed, his results suggest that although family income, education, and occupational status all contribute to a child's later neighborhood type, the characteristics of the child's neighborhood of origin have even stronger effects on later neighborhood type (see also Jackson and Mare 2007). Moreover, Sharkey (2008) found that this intergenerational transmission of neighborhood context was particularly strong for African Americans and that among children born in the poorest U.S. neighborhoods, 70 percent of African Americans were still living in poor neighborhoods as adults, compared to 40 percent of white adults born into the poorest neighborhoods—findings consistent with Crowder, South, and Chavez's (2006) determination that blacks have less locational return on their social, economic, and educational attainment.

Such intergenerational transmission of neighborhood context, and racial differences in this transmission, suggests that a cross-sectional estimate of adult neighborhood context is likely to be correlated with lifetime neighborhood context (Jackson and Mare 2007; Sharkey 2008), and that this correlation is likely stronger for African Americans (Sharkey 2008). Future research should consider the duration of exposure to neighborhoods over one's life span (Quillian 2002, 2003; Clampet-Lundquist and Massey 2008) as well as a measure of intergenerational transmission of neighborhood context (Sharkey 2008) when examining how neighborhood context might affect health. Such an approach may be particularly crucial to understanding racial disparities in health.

Agency

The life-course principle of agency suggests that individuals "construct their own life course through the choices and actions they take within the opportunities and constraints of history and social circumstance" (Elder, Johnson, and Crosnoe 2004, 11). This may be the life-course principle least attended to in contemporary research on neighborhoods and health (Entwisle 2007). Much of the recent neighborhood research has taken a primarily structuralist approach, examining how neighborhoods constrain individual opportunities in a fairly deterministic way, with less attention to how individuals impact neighborhoods in return.

One exception is research that examines residential mobility—how individuals sort into different neighborhoods based on their individual and neighborhood preferences and characteristics, thereby affecting the context of their neighborhoods (e.g., Charles 2001; Harris 1999; Krysan 2002; Moffit 2001; Quillian 2002). Yet mobility in and out of neighborhoods is only one way in which individuals can change their neighborhoods.

Almost no attention has been paid to variation in how individual residents make choices or react (other than moving), given the same neighborhood constraints, and the individual, family, and group characteristics that may buffer the impacts of neighborhood constraints on health. Research focusing on mean health effects of living in a disadvantaged neighborhood virtually ignores the variance in health among people in disadvantaged neighborhoods. Why do some residents of disadvantaged neighborhoods remain healthy in the face of neighborhood constraints and challenges?

Although directly improving the neighborhood context—reducing neighborhood constraints or shoring up neighborhood assets—might be the best long-term approach to reducing the detrimental impact of disadvantaged neighborhood environments on health (Osypuk and Galea 2007; Link and Phelan 1995; Schulz et al. 2002), steps could be taken to buffer the impacts of disadvantaged neighborhoods on poor health. Stress and coping theories (Pearlin 1999; Thoits 1995; Turner, Wheaton, and Lloyd 1995), as well as risk and resilience theories (Ryff et al. 1998; Rutter 1990), can be applied to examine how individual and neighborhood factors may buffer the effects of exposure to neighborhood stressors and risks. For example, Krause (1998) found that religious coping style buffered the association between living in dilapidated neighborhoods and self-rated health among older adults. Schieman and Meersman (2004) found that the relationship between neighborhood problems and depression among older women was buffered by the support that women received. Opportunities for future research include the exploration of individual and neighborhood characteristics that might buffer the impact of neighborhood disadvantage on poor health.

Public health interventions often attempt to support and encourage aspects of human agency that can be health enhancing, such as providing tools and resources for people to choose and implement healthy behaviors despite constrained resources (Bird and Rieker 2008). But there are few examples of theory applied to empirically examine the role of human agency in reciprocal exchange with the neighborhood—examining how individual agents attempt to actively change their environments through social organization, social networks, and social action in ways that promote health.

Yet sociology provides many theories about social movements (Della Porta and Diani 1999; McAdam, McCarthy, and Zald 1996; Meyer and Whittier 1994; Poletta and Jasper 2001) that could help us understand how individuals and groups interact with their neighborhoods in ways that might improve individual and neighborhood health. Small (2002) applied social organization theory to examine structure, culture, and neighborhood participation and change in a Puerto Rican housing project in Boston and found that how different cohorts frame the same neighborhood can affect their participation. While having a positive frame can sustain willingness to participate in the neighborhood, those who have less positive frames need mechanisms to incite neighborhood participation such as an exogenous threat or a momentary crisis, both of which can transform cultural perceptions of neighborhoods and reconfigure the conception of neighborhood participation as important. Other promising research examines the active role of community organizations as transformative agents in neighborhoods through which individuals can express agency and action, perpetuating or transforming the neighborhood environment (Swaroop and Morenoff 2006; Stoll 2001).

A view of human agency as a force of neighborhood change has been applied fruitfully in the social movements literature regarding environmental health movements and neighborhood reactions to environmental challenges (Brown and Mikkelsen 1990; Bullard 1994; Szasz 1994), but rarely regarding the social movements literature on health more generally. However, Brown and colleagues (2004) have presented a new theoretical conceptualization of "health social movements" with a framework that could be applied to social movements that occur within and across neighborhoods and that may improve individual and population health.

The growing attention to community-based participatory research is partly based on an understanding that individuals are active agents—they can come together to either respond to or proactively change their environments (e.g., Israel et al. 2005). Participatory research provides promise for generating knowledge that is deemed useful by communities and for instigating processes that may more effectively lead to the application of that knowledge to social change that could promote health.

Future research should build upon theories of social organization and social movements to expand our understanding of the role of individuals and community organizations in inciting participation and bringing about neighborhood change to improve individual and population health.

Five Principles of the Life Course Applied to Neighborhoods

Most theoretical approaches to the life course focus on the life course of individuals, not the life course of neighborhoods. Similarly, research on neighborhoods and health has been slow to examine how neighborhoods themselves change over time, and how their life course may affect residents (Sampson, Morenoff, and Gannon-Rowley 2002). Yet sociologists and other social scientists have a range of rich theories about neighborhood change, though such theories are not commonly applied to individual and population health outcomes.

Approaches to neighborhood change have been explored through research in sociology, human ecology, political science, population studies, and economics. Studies have considered various dimensions of neighborhood change, addressing the evolving U.S. landscape determined by industrialization, urbanization, and the patterns of migration and segregation. Here we highlight key approaches either that have been used to look at health outcomes, or that appear particularly fruitful in this regard.

Life-Span Development

The principle of life-span development encourages us to examine how neighborhoods themselves change over time, and how neighborhood trajectories impact the lives of residents. Theoretical models of neighborhood stability and change can be differentiated by whether they focus more on the role of the characteristics or interactions of individuals in shaping neighborhood change (the ecological and subcultural perspectives) or more on institutional factors external to the neighborhood that significantly shape its characteristics and processes (the political economy perspective) (Schwirian 1983; Temkin and Rowe 1996).

A dominant approach to thinking about neighborhood change over time is the ecological perspective, closely linked with the Chicago School of sociological theory, which emphasizes individual-environment interactions (Schwirian 1983; Temkin and Rowe 1996). A seminal example is Park's (1952) invasion-succession model of neighborhood change, in which neighborhoods are viewed as comprising "ecological niches" that are more or less favorable to habitation by different types of people. Essentially, individuals vote with their feet to determine where they will live, and the sum of these choices determines how neighborhoods take shape and change over time—affecting the life course of neighborhoods.

Duncan and Duncan (1957) and Taeuber and Taeuber (1965) derived racial residential succession models to explain the residential resettlement and segregation of blacks in the 1950s and 1960s. More recent iterations include locational attainment theory (Alba and Logan 1993) and spatial assimilation theory (South and Crowder 1997, 1998; South, Crowder, and Chavez 2005b), both focusing on how people determine whether to remain in or leave a neighborhood depending on their human capital and assessment of the neighborhood's suitability to their own social and economic characteristics. This approach highlights the life-span development of neighborhoods while integrating the life-course principle of individual agency, as individuals choose to select into or out of neighborhoods, though the constraints on these choices may be uneven.

An important focus in ecological perspectives on neighborhood change has been dimensions of neighborhood change and stability related to race and social class, particularly in the study of residential segregation, gentrification, and urban decline (Massey 1990; Alba and Logan 1993; South and Deane 1993; Jargowsky 1997; South and Crowder 1997; Gotham 1998; Iceland, Sharpe, and Steinmetz 2005; Scopilliti and Iceland 2008). Duncan and Duncan (1957) created neighborhood change typologies describing the succession of neighborhoods through economic and racial change. These typologies for neighborhood succession have been updated and applied to outcomes in health and social development (Massey, Condran, and Denton 1987; Ruel and Robert 2009).

For example, Massey, Condran, and Denton (1987) examined changes in neighborhood racial context over time and categorized neighborhood census tracts as either white, black entry, black transitioning, black established, or declining. They found that living in black transition or established black census tracts is associated with higher crime rates, high school dropout rates, infant mortality rates, and adult mortality rates. Ruel and Robert (2009) extended this work using a dynamic typology of neighborhood racial residential history

between 1970, 1980, and 1990. Using a national longitudinal survey of U.S. adults, they examined whether living in neighborhoods with different racial histories was associated with individual self-rated health and mortality. Results showed that racial disparities in health and mortality are explained by neighborhood racial residential history, neighborhood poverty level, and individual socioeconomic factors. Some results suggest that living in an established black neighborhood or in an established interracial neighborhood may actually be protective of health, once neighborhood poverty is controlled. They conclude that examining the dynamic nature of neighborhoods contributes to an understanding of health outcomes generally and racial health disparities more specifically.

Additional research is needed to examine how the life span of neighborhoods affects the health of residents. It may be important to understand not only how people's neighborhood experiences change when they move, but also how neighborhoods change around the people residing within them, and the effects on individual and population health.

Place and Time

Not only are neighborhoods places themselves but also they are located within larger places (cities, counties, states, countries) that shape their nature. Attention to the life-course principle of place attends to the dynamics of neighborhood change in the context of changes to surrounding neighborhoods. For example, Crowder and South (2008) demonstrate that individuals' mobility decisions were based not only on neighborhood racial composition, but also on the racial composition of surrounding areas, resulting in mobility that affected patterns of segregation. The literature on racial residential segregation considers the nesting of spatial residence, since racial segregation indices are created by comparing the racial composition among smaller residential units (i.e., census tracts) to create the racial-segregation index of a larger residential unit (e.g., city or county). But additional research should capitalize on recent innovations in geographic information systems

(GIS), mapping, and spatial statistics to relate changes in one neighborhood to those in others. This may be particularly important in light of current national trends in immigration, growth of the Latino population, and changing economic circumstances, which will all likely distribute people and resources unevenly across place, with unclear implications for individual and population health.

In contrast to ecological perspectives on neighborhood change, which focus on how individual residential mobility shapes neighborhood contexts, a political economy perspective focuses upstream on the political, economic, and social factors that produce or reinforce differences across neighborhoods in the first place (Navarro 2002). Such upstream factors affect the neighborhood conditions and resources that then have a more proximal impact on residents' health (Osypuk and Galea 2007; Link and Phelan 1995).

The political economy perspective places neighborhood change in the context of an overarching system in which economic, political, and social forces external to neighborhoods guide neighborhood dynamics (Schwirian 1983; Temkin and Rowe 1996). Central themes of the political economy approach are social conflict, power, and the role of macroeconomic forces in shaping local conditions (Logan and Molotch 1987). From a political economy perspective, the dynamics of neighborhood change and the distribution of individuals and resources across neighborhoods do not reflect only the attributes of individual residents who vote with their feet to change neighborhoods, but rather the interests of external power structures.

Neighborhood research consistent with this approach includes research on inequality that views cities and metropolitan areas as the context within which housing, employment, and education markets develop in ways that segregate people and resources into different neighborhoods (e.g., Jargowsky 1997; Wilson 1987). Galea, Freudenberg, and Vlahov (2006) suggest that three municipal-level factors are important determinants of health: government, markets (e.g., housing and labor), and civil society (e.g., community organizations). Altschuler, Somkin, and Adler (2004) find evidence that politicians may be more responsive to white and more afflu-

ent neighborhoods than to black and poor ones, potentially shaping the availability of health-producing resources in neighborhoods. LaVeist (1993) demonstrated that neighborhoods with greater black political empowerment had lower levels of infant mortality. Each of these examples highlights the embeddedness of neighborhoods in a larger social, political, and economic context that shapes them.

Again, the life-course principle of place and time encourages us to consider the importance of not only place but also historical time when examining the life course of neighborhoods. Here, it seems relevant to highlight the January 2009 volume of the *Annals of the American Academy of Political and Social Science* that addressed the relevance of the 1965 Moynihan report to our present-day understanding of urban neighborhoods and the persistence of racial and economic residential segregation in urban America. Clearly, historical circumstances that led to racial and economic residential segregation in the United States have been perpetuated rather than interrupted by more recent social, economic, and political periods (Sampson 2009). As we move to redress such segregation, an ecological approach to neighborhood change might suggest that we need to better understand how to create individual incentives and neighborhood environments that will promote a distribution of individuals across neighborhoods that might promote health for individuals and populations. A political economy perspective would suggest a focus on understanding the societal-level decisions and structures that need to change in order to distribute economic, social, political, and human resources more equitably across neighborhoods. Both approaches need to incorporate a more thorough understanding of how social networks within and across neighborhoods might facilitate either a different distribution of residential mobility or a different distribution and flow of resources through the networks.

Timing

Just as individuals may experience neighborhood characteristics as more salient to their health at different critical periods in their life, neighborhoods may be affected by events during critical periods of their development. Early work by Schelling (1978) examined thresholds or "tipping points" at which a neighborhood reaches a racial or ethnic composition that motivates residents to begin to leave. The event in this case is the outmigration of select residents during a tipping point stage of neighborhood racial/ethnic composition. Recent studies have provided further insight about the pace and progression of racial and economic neighborhood change, addressing the timing of neighborhood changes (Frankel and Pauzner 2002) and the potential role of threshold effects (Quercia and Galster 2000). However, most recent research demonstrates that despite much individual mobility in and out of neighborhoods, neighborhoods themselves remain fairly stable in their socioeconomic and racial characteristics over time—individual mobility serves only to replicate the economic and racial segregation of neighborhoods (Bruch and Mare 2006; Sampson and Sharkey 2008).

Although most of this research has not yet been applied to examining the role of individual or neighborhood health as either a determinant of individual moves or as a neighborhood-level outcome of the sum of individual moves, this line of research may be fruitful. In particular, agent-based models have been suggested as a promising approach to examining the dynamic nature of individuals, neighborhoods, and health (Entwisle 2007; Auchincloss and Diez Roux 2008). Agent-based models are an example of systems dynamics models that provide simulations of how microentities (i.e., people) change over time when interacting with other microentities and in response to characteristics of the environment (i.e., neighborhoods). Agent-based computer simulations might be used to produce representations of the individual-level and neighborhood-level health outcomes of these dynamic interactions between individuals and neighborhoods over time (Auchincloss and Diez Roux 2008; Entwisle 2007).

Also addressing the life-course principle of timing, the timing and geographic spread of public health programs, medical technology, and economic development have been used to identify the relative contribution of social, economic, medical, and public health factors in the timing and pace of

changes in the causes of mortality within a population—specifically, the declines in infant mortality and infectious disease in the United States and Western European countries (McKeown 1976; Szreter 2004; Fogel and Costa 1997).

Linked Lives

The principle of linked lives, highlighting that those before and after us shape our life trajectories (O'Rand 1996), can be applied to neighborhoods as well. Sampson and Sharkey (2008) demonstrated the durability of neighborhood characteristics over time in terms of neighborhood income and racial structure. Although there is much mobility on an individual level, with individuals moving into and out of neighborhoods for a variety of economic and racial preference reasons (Quillian 2002), an ecological approach to neighborhood change demonstrates that the resulting individual choices in residential mobility culminate in stunning stability of neighborhood characteristics over time, at least in terms of stable neighborhood income and racial structure (Sampson and Sharkey 2008; Sampson 2009).

One criticism of the ecological perspective on neighborhood change is that it overemphasizes economic competition for land and resources as the drivers of individual mobility and resulting neighborhood change (Temkin and Rowe 1996). Ecological models have also been criticized for their "value-free" assumptions regarding the nature of individual-environment interactions (Beatty 1988), and for emphasizing residential mobility as an efficient redistribution of people rather than as a cultural and social phenomenon.

One resolution offered for this criticism entails developing models with greater attention to the historical, cultural, and social exchange processes involved in neighborhood change and stability. "Subcultural models" are often seen as a type of ecological perspective that focuses on the role of cultural forms (like social networks and symbolism) in neighborhood dynamics. From this perspective, subcultural models more directly address the life-course principles of historical embeddedness and linked lives that are less developed in many ecological models.

Consistent with this approach, Logan, Alba, and Zhang (2002) find that, among immigrant groups in New York and Los Angeles, living in ethnic enclaves was a choice many made, unrelated to economic constraints. Similarly, Spilimbergo and Ubeda (2004) found that racial differences in residential mobility between whites and African Americans were explained by local ties to family members. Such research highlights noneconomic reasons for ties to place, consistent with theory on the social and psychological ties that connect people to neighborhoods (Altman and Low 1992; Gerson, Stueve, and Fischer 1977).

Subcultural models are also interested in residents' relationships with one another and how these relationships lead to neighborhood attachment and cohesion (Schwirian 1983; Temkin and Rowe 1996). This stickiness of relationships that can prevent residential mobility can affect health in both positive and negative ways. On the one hand, a subcultural approach is consistent with an active area of research on the role of neighborhood social and cultural capital and cohesion (Putnam 2000; Bourdieu and Wacquant 1992; Carpiano 2006; Sampson, Morenoff, and Gannon-Rowley 2002), usually seen as positive and protective of health, while their absence can lead to "social disorganization," increasing the risk of exposure to violence, of poor social well-being, and of death (Sampson, Morenoff, and Gannon-Rowley 2002). On the other hand, the presence of social capital and cohesion is not always positive for neighborhoods. Strong neighborhood social cohesion may inhibit neighborhood racial and ethnic change, and thereby be implicated in explicit or implicit neighborhood conditions that increase race- or class-based segregation and discriminatory housing policies or practices (Schwirian 1983). Examples include local efforts to block in-migration of minorities (Cutler, Glaeser, and Vigdor 1999). A subcultural model suggests that we examine how the social networks of neighborhoods can perpetuate or change neighborhoods over time. A political economy perspective would further suggest that we examine the political and economic social structures that might serve to preserve or change these networks, or to infuse resources through them in ways that may improve health and reduce health disparities within and between neighborhoods.

Agency

Despite the differences in focus between the subcultural and ecological perspectives, both recognize a role for individual agency, focusing on how individual factors interact with neighborhood factors to produce individual residential mobility that leads to neighborhood stability or change. However, this is a limited view of agency in the neighborhood context, as there may be other neighborhood characteristics that bring about neighborhood change and affect individual and population health.

When examining the dynamic nature of neighborhoods, we might consider variations in the resilience of neighborhoods to weather challenges. Although the concept of resilience is most often applied to the protective factors that individuals marshal to adapt to risk (Ryff et al. 1998; Rutter 1990), neighborhoods can be seen as resilient as well. The best theoretical and empirical work explicitly addressing neighborhood resilience has been conducted in the area of disaster readiness and response (Pais and Elliott 2008), examining the characteristics of neighborhoods that affect their ability to adapt in the face of a disaster (see Norris et al. 2008).

However, we can also view collective action supported by neighborhood social and cultural capital as providing an opportunity for neighborhood-level resilience—developing and employing neighborhood social capital which can be employed for advancing the health and social well-being of neighborhood residents even in the face of other neighborhood constraints and stressors. Swaroop and Morenoff (2006) demonstrate that neighborhoods both affect and are affected by neighborhood participation in complex ways. One of their important findings was that rates of participation in local social organizations for expressive purposes were higher in stable neighborhoods, but rates of participation in local social organizations for instrumental purposes were higher in disadvantaged neighborhoods. Neighborhoods produce conditions that create action and are in turn changed by the actions they invoked. More work is needed to examine the ways in which neighborhood participation and organization can buffer the impacts of neighborhood disadvantage on the health of individuals and populations.

Other theories of social capital and collective efficacy can also be invoked to examine neighborhood-level agency. Whereas social capital refers to the resources that result from social structure (Burt 2001; Bourdieu 1986), collective efficacy is about converting those relationships into beneficial action. In high collective-efficacy neighborhoods, residents are willing to intervene on each other's behalf, even if they do not know one another. Sampson, Raudenbush, and Earls's (1997) articulation of the collective-efficacy concept emphasizes neighborhood social capital in the form of mutual trust and solidarity (social cohesion) and expectations for action (informal social control) in explaining the impact of neighborhood context on residents' well-being. As applied to health, collective-efficacy theory suggests that neighborhoods vary in the density and size of their social networks and their associated levels of social cohesion and informal social control—the neighborhood's capacity to mobilize existing social resources (network ties and neighborhood attachments) toward beneficial ends (Cagney, Browning, and Wen 2005; Wen, Hawkley, and Cacioppo 2006). Interestingly, most of this work examines the individual-level outcomes of collective efficacy, not how collective efficacy changes other aspects of neighborhood context. In theory, collective efficacy should eventually lead to the mobilization of resources that benefit and change a neighborhood's social and economic context over time.

It is the very idea of creating change from within neighborhoods that has inspired much of the recent participatory approach to research on neighborhoods and health. Community-based participatory research (CBPR) projects are used to mobilize individual and neighborhood resources to produce both knowledge and social change (Israel et al. 2005). Therefore, they explicitly consider issues of agency, sometimes at the neighborhood level, and can be used to create neighborhood change and improve individual and population health. However, we know of no research that has systematically examined the cumulative impact of CBPR projects on changing the trajectories of neighborhoods over time.

Summary

This chapter offers the life-course perspective as a lens through which to view research on neighborhoods and health; its application can help us creatively integrate old and new theories and methods for their study, encouraging us to attend to not only the life course of individuals within their neighborhood context, but also to the life course of neighborhoods themselves—examining how the neighborhood contexts in which we live, work, and play change over time, and the implication of those changes for individual and population health.

Incorporating life-course principles can help us better understand the dynamic effects of neighborhoods on health over the individual life course. In particular, research is needed to examine the contemporaneous, lagged, and cumulative effects of neighborhoods on health over the individual life span. Research must distinguish age, period, and cohort effects, and attend to the timing of particular neighborhood exposures at specific ages or stages of development. The overlooked principle of agency can illuminate not only how neighborhoods affect individuals, but also how individuals interact with and change their neighborhoods in ways that affect individual and population health. A variety of research methods are needed to address these questions, including longitudinal analysis of individuals across diverse neighborhoods, qualitative analyses to understand people's experiences within and interpretations of their neighborhoods, and participatory approaches that help us both understand and support action to create change.

Understanding how neighborhood networks and social capital affect health over the life course requires a dynamic approach that goes beyond characterizing networks and social capital at one point in time to examining how they evolve over time within particular neighborhoods and historical periods. Research should examine how networks produce different types and amounts of social capital depending on the neighborhood context, and how this relates to individual health at different ages and developmental stages. Insight into how individuals engage with networks and neighborhoods to both draw on and produce social capital is needed to understand how these interactions can be either protective of or detrimental to health.

The limited body of health research that has examined neighborhood change has focused on how neighborhood contexts change when people move, but not on how neighborhoods change around residents. Ecological, subcultural, and political economy perspectives help us think about how future research might consider the life course of neighborhoods in conjunction with the life course of individuals. Recent research on neighborhood change has sought to integrate one or more of these theoretical perspectives to consider the demographic, cultural, and institutional forces at play in the temporal dynamics of neighborhoods. Integrated consideration of individual and neighborhood dynamics will be instructive to understanding the relevance of neighborhood change for individual and population health. Agent-based models may provide one method of examining the intersecting dynamics of individuals, neighborhoods, and health over time.

Given both the persistence of neighborhood income and racial segregation over time, and the intergenerational transmission of neighborhood context to individuals, it is imperative that we gain a better understanding of the individual- and neighborhood-level factors that continue to perpetuate racial and income inequality, and the mechanisms through which they affect individual and population health. Moreover, we need to understand not only the factors that have perpetuated social and economic inequalities and disparities in health, but to identify and understand the outliers. What are the individual- and neighborhood-level protective factors that have produced individual and neighborhood resilience in the face of adversity? What aspects of individual- and neighborhood-level agency could be promoted to bring about neighborhood change within and across neighborhoods in ways that promote and protect health? What aspects

of our political economy might be effectively changed to restructure the individual incentives and barriers to neighborhood selection and mobility, and what are the societal resources that could be redistributed across neighborhoods in ways that would promote heath? Addressing these questions will be crucial not only to improving mean health, but also to reducing health disparities along racial and economic dimensions.

References

Airey, Laura. 2003. "Nae as Nice a Scheme as It Used to Be: Lay Accounts of Neighbourhood Incivilities and Well-Being." *Health and Place* 9:129–37.

Alba, Richard D., and John R. Logan. 1993. "Minority Proximity to Whites in Suburbs: An Individual-Level Analysis of Segregation." *American Journal of Sociology* 98:1388–1427.

Almond, Douglas. 2006. "Is the 1918 Influenza Pandemic Over? Long-Term Effects of IN Utero Influenza Exposure in the Post-1940 U.S. Population." *Journal of Political Economy* 114(4): 672–712.

Altman, Irwin, and Setha M. Low, eds. 1992. *Place Attachment, Human Behavior, and Environment: Advances in Theory and Research*. Vol. 12. New York: Plenum.

Altschuler, Andrea, Carol P. Somkin, and Nancy E. Adler. 2004. "Local Services and Amenities, Neighborhood Social Capital, and Health." *Social Science and Medicine* 59:1219–29.

Auchincloss, Amy H., and Ana Diez Roux. 2008. "A New Tool for Epidemiology: The Usefulness of Dynamic-Agent Models in Understanding Place Effects on Health." *American Journal of Epidemiology* 168(1): 1–8.

Barber, Jennifer S., Lisa D. Pearce, Indra Chaudhury, and Susan Gurung. 2002. "Voluntary Associations and Fertility Limitation." *Social Forces* 80(4): 1369–1401.

Beatty, John. 1988. "Ecology and Evolutionary Biology in the War and Post-War Years." *Journal of Historical Biology* 21:245–63.

Berkman, Lisa F., and Cheryl Clark. 2003. "Neighborhoods and Networks: The Construction of Safe Places and Bridges." In *Neighborhoods and Health*, ed. Ichiro Kawachi and Lisa F. Berkman, 288–302. New York: Oxford University Press.

Berkman, Lisa F., and Thomas Glass. 2000. "Social Integration, Social Networks, Social Support, and Health." In *Social Epidemiology*, ed. Lisa F. Berkman and Ichiro Kawachi, 137–73. Oxford: Oxford University Press.

Bird, Chloe E., and Patricia R. Rieker. 2008. *Gender and Health: The Effects of Constrained Choices on Social Policies.* New York: Cambridge University Press.

Bourdieu, Pierre. 1986. "The Forms of Social Capital." In *Handbook of Theory and Research for the Sociology of Education,* ed. John G. Richardson, 241–58. New York: Macmillan.

Bourdieu, Pierre, and Loïc J. D. Wacquant. 1992. *An Invitation to Reflexive Sociology.* Chicago: University of Chicago Press.

Brooks-Gunn, Jeanne, Greg Duncan, Pamela Klebanov, and Naomi Sealand. 1993. "Do Neighborhoods Influence Child and Adolescent Development?" *American Journal of Sociology* 99:353–95.

Brown, Phil, and Edwin J. Mikkelsen. 1990. *No Safe Place: Toxic Waste, Leukemia, and Community Action.* Berkeley: University of California Press.

Brown, Phil, Stephen Zavestoski, Sabrina McCormick, Brian Mayer, Rachel Morello-Frosch, and Rebecca Gasior Altman. 2004. "Embodied Health Movements: New Approaches to Social Movements in Health." *Sociology of Health and Illness* 26(1): 50–80.

Browning, Christopher R., Kathleen A. Cagney, and Ming Wen. 2003. "Explaining Variation in Health Status across Space and Time: Implications for Racial and Ethnic Disparities in Self-Rated Health." *Social Science and Medicine* 57:1221–35.

Browning, Christopher R., Seth L. Feinberg, Danielle Wallace, and Kathleen A. Cagney. 2006. "Neighborhood Social Processes, Physical Conditions, and Disaster-Related Mortality: The Case of the 1995 Chicago Heat Wave." *American Sociological Review* 71:661–78.

Bruch, Elizabeth E., and Robert D. Mare. 2006. "Neighborhood Choice and Neighborhood Change." *American Journal of Sociology* 112(3): 667–709.

Bullard, Robert D., ed. 1994. *Confronting Environmental Racism: Voices from the Grassroots.* Boston: South End Press.

Burt, Ronald S. 2001. "Structural Holes versus Network Closure as Social Capital." In *Social Capital: Theory and Research,* ed. Nan Lin, Karen Cook, and Ronald S. Burt, 31–56. New York: Aldine de Gruyter.

Cagney, Kathleen A. 2006. "Neighborhood Age Structure and Its Implications for Health." *Journal of Urban Health* 83(5): 827–34.

Cagney, Kathleen A., and Christopher R. Browning. 2004. "Exploring Neighborhood-Level Variation in Asthma and Other Respiratory Diseases: The Contribution of Neighborhood Social Context." *Journal of General Internal Medicine* 19(3): 229–36.

Cagney, Kathleen A., Christopher R. Browning, and Ming Wen. 2005. "Racial Disparities in Self-Rated Health at Older Ages: What Difference Does the Neighborhood Make?" *Journal of Gerontology: Social Sciences* 60B: S181–90.

Carpiano, Richard M. 2006. "Toward a Neighborhood Resource-Based Theory of Social Capital for Health: Can Bourdieu and Sociology Help?" *Social Science and Medicine* 62(1): 165–75.

———. 2007. "Neighborhood Social Capital and Adult Health: An Empirical Test of a Bourdieu-Based Model." *Health and Place* 13(3): 639–55.

———. 2009. "Come Take a Walk with Me: The 'Go-Along' Interview as a Novel Method for Studying the Implications of Place for Health and Well-Being." *Health and Place* 15:263–72.

Carson, April P., Kathryn M. Rose, Diane J. Catellier, Jay S. Kaufman, Sharon B. Wyatt, Ana V. Diez-Roux, and Gerardo Heissl. 2007. "Cumulative Socioeconomic Status across the Life Course and Subclinical Atherosclerosis." *Annals of Epidemiology* 17(4): 296–303.

Caughy, Margaret, Patricia J. O'Campo, and Carles Muntaner. 2003. "When Being Alone Might be Better: Neighborhood Poverty, Social Capital, and Child Mental Health." *Social Science and Medicine* 57(2): 227–37.

Charles, Camille Zubrinsky. 2001. "Processes of Residential Segregation." In *Urban Inequality: Evidence from Four Cities,* ed. Alice O'Connor, Chris Tilly, and Lawrence Bobo, 217–71. New York: Russell Sage Foundation.

Clampet-Lundquist, Susan, and Douglas S. Massey. 2008. "Neighborhood Effects on Economic Self-Sufficiency: A Reconsideration of the Moving to Opportunity Experiment." *American Journal of Sociology* 114(1): 107–43.

Coleman, James S. 1990. *The Foundations of Social Theory.* Cambridge, Mass.: Belknap Press.

Cornwell, Benjamin, Edward O. Laumann, and L. Philip Schumm. 2008. "The Social Connectedness of Older Adults: A National Profile." *American Sociological Review* 73(2): 185–203.

Crowder, Kyle, and Scott J. South. 2008. "Spatial Dynamics of White Flight: The Effects of Local and Extralocal Racial Conditions on Outmigration." *American Sociological Review* 73(5): 792–812.

Crowder, Kyle, Scott J. South, and Erick Chavez. 2006. "Wealth, Race, and Inter-Neighborhood Migration." *American Sociological Review* 71:72–94.

Cummins, Steven, Sarah Curtis, Ana V. Diez-Roux, and Sally Macintyre. 2007. "Understanding and Representing 'Place' in Health Research: A Relational Approach." *Social Science and Medicine* 65(9): 1825–38.

Curtis, Sarah, H. Southall, P. Congdon, and B. Dodgeon. 2004. "Area Effects on Health Variation over the Life-Course: Analysis of the Longitudinal

Study Sample in England Using New Data on Area of Residence in Childhood." *Social Science and Medicine* 58:57–74.

Cutler, David M., Edward L. Glaeser, and Jacob L. Vigdor. 1999. "The Rise and Decline of the American Ghetto." *Journal of Political Economy* 107(3): 455–506.

Dannefer, Dale. 2003. "Cumulative Advantage/ Disadvantage and the Life Course: Cross Fertilizing Age and Social Science Theory." *Journal of Gerontology: Social Sciences* 58B: S327–37.

Della Porta, Donatella, and Mario Diani. 1999. *Social Movements: An Introduction*. Malden, Mass.: Blackwell.

Dennis, Samuel F., Suzanne Gaulocher, Richard M. Carpiano, and David Brown. 2008. "Participatory Photo Mapping (PPM): Exploring an Integrated Method for Health and Place Research with Young People." *Health and Place* 15(2): 466–73.

Diez Roux, A. V., L. N. Borrell, M. Haan, S. A. Jackson, and R. Schultz. 2004. "Neighbourhood Environments and Mortality in an Elderly Cohort: Results from the Cardiovascular Health Study." *Journal of Epidemiology and Community Health* 58(11): 917–23.

Duncan, Otis Dudley, and Beverly Duncan. 1957. *The Negro Population of Chicago*. Chicago: University Press.

Elder, Glen H., Jr. 1985. "Perspectives on the Life Course." In *Trajectories and Transitions, 1968–1980*, ed. Glen H. Elder Jr., 23–49. Ithaca, N.Y.: Cornell University Press.

Elder, Glen H., Jr., Monica Kirkpatrick Johnson, and Robert Crosnoe. 2004. "The Emergence and Development of Life Course Theory." In *Handbook of the Life Course*, ed. Jeylan T. Mortimer and Michael J. Shanahan, 3–22. New York: Springer.

Entwisle, Barbara. 2007. "Putting People into Place." *Demography* 44(4): 687–703.

Eschbach, Karl, Glenn V. Ostir, Kushang V. Patel, Kyriakos S. Markides, and James S. Goodwin. 2004. "Neighborhood Context and Mortality among Older Mexican Americans: Is There a Barrio Advantage?" *American Journal of Public Health* 94:1807–12.

Fauth, Rebecca C., Tama Leventhal, and Jeanne Brooks-Gunn. 2008. "Seven Years Later: Effects of a Neighborhood Mobility Program on Poor Black and Latino Adults' Well-Being." *Journal of Health and Social Behavior* 49:119–30.

Ferraro, Kenneth F., and Tetyana Pylypiv Shippee. 2008. "Black and White Chains of Risk for Hospitalization over 20 Years." *Journal of Health and Social Behavior* 49:193–207.

Fogel, Robert W., and Dora L. Costa. 1997. "A Theory of Technophysio Evolution, with Some Implications for Forecasting Population, Health Care Costs, and Pension Costs." *Demography* 34(1): 49–66.

Frankel, David M., and Ady Pauzner. 2002. "Expectations and the Timing of Neighborhood Change." *Journal of Urban Economics* 51(2): 295–314.

Freedman, Vicki A., Irina B. Grafova, Robert F. Schoeni, and Jeannette Rogowski. 2008. "Neighborhoods and Disability in Later Life." *Social Science and Medicine* 66:2253–67.

Galea, Sandro, Nicholas Freudenberg, and David Vlahov. 2006. "A Framework for the Study of Urban Health." In *Cities and the Health of the Public*, ed. Nicholas Freudenberg, Sandro Galea, and David Vlahov, 3–18. Nashville: Vanderbilt University Press.

Gerson, Kathleen, C. Ann Stueve, and Claude S. Fischer. 1977. "Attachment to Place." In *Networks and Places: Social Relations in the Urban Setting*, ed. Claude S. Fischer, Robert M. Jackson, C. Ann Stueve, Kathleen Gerson, Lynne McCallister Jones, and Mark Baldassare, 139–61. New York: Free Press.

Glass, Thomas A., and Jennifer L. Balfour. 2003. "Neighborhoods, Aging, and Functional Limitations." In *Neighborhoods and Health*, ed. Ichiro Kawachi and Lisa F. Berkman, 303–34. New York: Oxford University Press.

Gotham, Kevin Fox. 1998. "Blind Faith in the Free Market: Urban Poverty, Residential Segregation, and Federal Housing Retrenchment, 1970–1995." *Sociological Inquiry* 68(1): 1–31.

Harris, David R. 1999. "'Property Values Drop When Blacks Move in, Because . . .': Racial and Socioeconomic Determinants of Neighborhood Desirability." *American Sociological Review* 64:461–79.

Hartley, David. 2004. "Rural Health Disparities, Population Health, and Rural Culture." *American Journal of Public Health* 94(10): 1675–78.

Iceland, John, Cicely Sharpe, and Erika Steinmetz. 2005. "Class Differences in African American Residential Patterns in U.S. Metropolitan Areas: 1990–2000." *Social Science Research* 34(1): 252–66.

Israel, Barbara A., Eugenia Eng, Amy Schulz, and Edith A. Parker, eds. 2005. *Methods in Community-Based Participatory Research for Health*. San Francisco: Jossey Bass.

Jackson, Margot I., and Robert D. Mare. 2007. "Cross-Sectional and Longitudinal Measurements of Neighborhood Experience and Their Effects on Children." *Social Science Research* 36:590–610.

Jargowsky, Paul A. 1997. *Poverty and Place: Ghettos, Barrios, and the American City*. New York: Russell Sage Foundation.

Jelleyman, T., and N. Spencer. 2007. "Residential Mobility in Childhood and Health Outcomes: A

Systematic Review." *Journal of Epidemiology and Community Health* 62:584–92.

Kaplan, George A., Elsie R. Pamuk, John W. Lynch, R. D. Cohen, and Jennifer L. Balfour. 1996. "Inequality in Income and Mortality in the United States: Analysis of Mortality and Potential Pathways." *British Medical Journal* 312(7037): 999–1003.

Kawachi, Ichiro, and Lisa F. Berkman, eds. 2003. *Neighborhoods and Health*. New York: Oxford University Press.

Kawachi, Ichiro, Bruce P. Kennedy, and Kimberly Lochner. 1997. "Social Capital, Income Inequality, and Mortality." *American Journal of Public Health* 87(9): 1491–98.

Krause, Neil. 1998. "Neighborhood Deterioration, Religious Coping, and Changes in Health during Late Life. *Gerontologist* 38:653–64.

Krysan, Maria. 2002. "Community Undesirability in Black and White: Examining Racial Residential Preferences through Community Perceptions." *Social Problems* 49:521–43.

Kuh, D., Y. Ben-Shlomo, J. Lynch, J. Hallquvist, and C. Power. 2003. "Life Course Epidemiology." *Journal of Epidemiology and Community Health* 57:778–83.

Kusenbach, Margarethe. 2003. "Street Phenomenology: The Go-Along as Ethnographic Research Tool." *Ethnography* 4(3): 455–85.

LaVeist, Thomas A. 1993. "Segregation, Poverty and Empowerment: Health Consequences for African-Americans." *Milbank Quarterly* 71(1): 41–64.

Lee, Min-Ah, and Kenneth F. Ferraro. 2007. "Neighborhood Residential Segregation and Physical Health among Hispanic Americans: Good, Bad, or Benign?" *Journal of Health and Social Behavior* 48(2): 131–48.

Lemelin, Emily T., Ana V. Diez Roux, Tracy G. Franklin, Mercedes Carnethon, Pamela L. Lutsey, Hanyu Ni, Ellen O'Meara, and Sandi Shrager. 2009. "Life-Course Socioeconomic Positions and Subclinical Atherosclerosis in the Multi-Ethnic Study of Atherosclerosis." *Social Science and Medicine* 68:444–51.

Leventhal, Tama, and Jeanne Brooks-Gunn. 2003. "Moving to Opportunity: An Experimental Study of Neighborhood Effects on Mental Health." *American Journal of Public Health* 93:1576–82.

Lin, Nan, Karen S. Cook, and Ronald S. Burt. 2001. *Social Capital: Theory and Research*. New York: Aldine de Gruyter.

Link, Bruce G., and Jo C. Phelan. 1995. "Social Conditions as Fundamental Causes of Disease." *Journal of Health and Social Behavior*, extra issue: 80–94.

Logan, John R., Richard D. Alba, and Wenquan Zhang. 2002. "Immigrant Enclaves and Ethnic Communities in New York and Los Angeles." *American Sociological Review* 67:299–322.

Logan, John R., and Harvey L. Molotch 1987. *Urban Fortunes: The Political Economy of Place*. Los Angeles: University of California Press.

Ludwig, Jens, Jeffrey B. Liebman, Jeffrey R. Kling, Greg J. Duncan, Lawrence F. Katz, Ron C. Kessler, and Lisa Sanbonmatsu. 2008. "What Can We Learn about Neighborhood Effects from the Moving to Opportunity Experiment?" *American Journal of Sociology* 114(1): 144–88.

Luke, Douglas A., and Jennie K. Harris. 2007. "Network Analysis in Public Health: History, Methods, and Applications." *Annual Review of Public Health* 28:69–93.

Lynch, John, and George Davey Smith. 2005. "A Life Course Approach to Chronic Disease Epidemiology." *Annual Review of Public Health* 26:1–35.

Lynch, John, George Davey Smith, Marianne Hillemeier, Mary Shaw, Trivellore Raghunathan, and George Kaplan. 2001. "Income Inequality, the Psychosocial Environment, and Health: Comparisons of Wealthy Nations." *Lancet* 109(35): 194–200.

Massey, Douglas S. 1990. "American Apartheid: Segregation and the Making of the Underclass." *American Journal of Sociology* 96:329–58.

Massey, Douglas S., Gretchen A. Condran, and Nancy A. Denton. 1987. "The Effect of Residential Segregation on Black Social and Economic Well-Being." *Social Forces* 66(1): 29–56.

McAdam, Doug, John D. McCarthy, and Mayer N. Zald, eds. 1996. *Comparative Perspectives on Social Movements: Political Opportunities, Mobilizing Structures, and Cultural Framings*. Cambridge: Cambridge University Press.

McKeown, Thomas. 1976. *The Modern Rise of Population*. New York: Academic Press.

Meyer, David S., and Nancy Whittier. 1994. "Social Movement Spillover." *Social Problems* 41:277–98.

Mikolajczyk, Rafael T., and Mirjam Kretzschmar. 2008. "Collecting Social Contact Data in the Context of Disease Transmission: Prospective and Retrospective Study Designs." *Social Networks* 30(2): 127–35.

Mirowsky, John, and Catherine E. Ross. 2003. *Education, Social Status, and Health*. New York: Aldine de Gruyter.

Moffit, Robert. 2001. "Policy Interventions, Low-Level Equilibria, and Social Interaction." In *Social Dynamics*, ed. Steven N. Durlauf and H. Peyton Young, 45–82. Boston: MIT Press.

Morenoff, Jeffrey D., James S. House, Ben B. Hansen, David R. Williams, George A. Kaplan, and Haslyn E. Hunte. 2007. "Understanding Social Disparities in Hypertension Prevalence, Awareness, Treatment, and Control: The Role of Neighborhood Context." *Social Science and Medicine* 65(9): 1853–66.

Morenoff, Jeffrey D., Robert J. Sampson, and Stephen W. Raudenbush. 2001. "Neighborhood Inequality, Collective Efficacy, and the Spatial Dynamics of Urban Violence." *Criminology* 39(3): 17–60.

Mortimer, Jeylan T., and Michael J. Shanahan, eds. 2004. *Handbook of the Life Course.* New York: Springer.

Moynihan, Daniel P. 1965. *The Negro Family: The Case for National Action.* Washington, D.C.: Office of Policy Planning and Research, U.S. Department of Labor.

Naess, O., B. Claussen, G. Davey Smith, and A. H. Leyland. 2008. "Life Course Influence of Residential Area on Cause-Specific Mortality." *Journal of Epidemiology and Community Health* 62:29–34.

Navarro, Vincente. 2002. *The Political Economy of Social Inequalities.* Amityville, N.Y.: Baywood Publishing.

Norris, Fran H., Susan P. Stevens, Betty Pfefferbaum, Karen F. Wyche, and Rose L. Pfefferbaum. 2008. "Community Resilience as a Metaphor, Theory, Set of Capacities, and Strategy for Disaster Readiness." *American Journal of Community Psychology* 41:127–50.

O'Connor, Thomas G. 2003. "Natural Experiments to Study the Effects of Early Experience: Progress and Limitations." *Development and Psychopathology* 15(4): 837–52.

O'Rand, Angela M. 1996. "The Precious and the Precocious: Understanding Cumulative Disadvantage and Cumulative Advantage over the Life Course." *Gerontologist* 36(2): 230–38.

Ostir, Glenn V., Karl Eschbach, Kyriakos S. Markides, and James S. Goodwin. 2003. "Neighbourhood Composition and Depressive Symptoms among Older Mexican Americans." *Journal of Epidemiology and Community Health* 57:987–92.

Osypuk, Theresa L., and Sandro Galea. 2007. "What Level Macro? Choosing Appropriate Levels to Assess How Place Influences Population Health." In *Macrosocial Determinants of Population Health*, ed. Sandro Galea, 399–435. New York: Springer.

Pais, Jeremy F., and James R. Elliott. 2008. "Places as Recovery Machines: Vulnerability and Neighborhood Change after Major Hurricanes." *Social Forces* 86(4): 1415–53.

Park, Robert A. 1952. *Human Communities.* Glencoe, Ill.: Free Press.

Patel, Kushang V., Karl Eschbach, Laura L. Rudkin, M. Kristen Peek, and Kyriakos S. Markides. 2003. "Neighborhood Context and Self-Rated Health in Older Mexican Americans." *Annals of Epidemiology* 13(9): 620–28.

Pattillo, Mary E. 1999. *Black Picket Fences: Privilege and Peril among the Black Middle Class.* Chicago: University of Chicago Press.

Pearlin, Leonard I. 1999. "The Stress Process Revisited: Reflections on Concepts and Their Inter-Relationships" In *Handbook of the Sociology of Mental Health*, ed. Carol S. Aneshensel and Jo C. Phelan, 395–416. New York: Kluwer Academic/Plenum.

Pickett, K. E., and M. Pearl. 2001. "Multilevel Analysis of Neighbourhood Socioeconomic Context and Health Outcomes: A Critical Review." *Journal of Epidemiology and Community Health* 55:111–22.

Poletta, Francesca, and James M. Jasper. 2001. "Collective Identity and Social Movements." *Annual Review of Sociology* 27:283–305.

Portes, Alejandro, and Julia Sensenbrenner. 1993. "Embeddedness and Immigration: Notes on the Social Determinants of Economic Action." *American Journal of Sociology* 98:1320–50.

Preston, Samuel H., Martha E. Hill, and Gregory L. Drevenstedt. 1998. "Childhood Conditions That Predict Survival to Advanced Ages among African-Americans." *Social Science and Medicine* 47(9): 1231–46.

Probst, Janice C., Charity G. Moore, Sundra H. Glover, and Michael E. Samuels. 2004. "Person and Place: The Compounding Effects of Race/Ethnicity and Rurality on Health." *American Journal of Public Health* 94(10): 1695–1703.

Putnam, Robert D. 2000. *Bowling Alone: The Collapse and Revival of American Community.* New York: Simon and Schuster.

Quercia, Roberto G., and George C. Galster. 2000. "Threshold Effects and Neighborhood Change." *Journal of Planning Education and Research* 20:146–62.

Quillian, Lincoln. 2002. "Why Is Black-White Residential Segregation So Persistent? Evidence on Three Theories from Migration Data." *Social Science Quarterly* 31:197–229.

———. 2003. "How Long Are Exposures to Poor Neighborhoods? The Long-Term Dynamics of Entry and Exit from Poor Neighborhoods." *Population Research and Policy Review* 22:221–29.

Robert, Stephanie A. 1999. "Socioeconomic Position and Health: The Independent Contribution of Community Socioeconomic Context. *Annual Review of Sociology* 25:489–516.

Robert, Stephanie A., and Kum Yi Lee. 2002. "Explaining Race Differences in Health among Older Adults: The Contribution of Community Socioeconomic Context." *Research on Aging* 24:654–83.

Robert, Stephanie A., and Lydia W. Li. 2001. "Age Variation in the Relationship between Community

Socioeconomic Status and Adult Health." *Research on Aging* 23:233–58.

Robert, Stephanie A., and Eric N. Reither. 2004. "A Multilevel Analysis of Race, Community Disadvantage, and BMI." *Social Science and Medicine* 59(12): 2421–34.

Robert, Stephanie A., and Erin Ruel. 2006. "Racial Segregation and Health Disparities between Black and White Older Adults." *Journal of Gerontology: Social Sciences* 61B: S203–11.

Rosenbaum, Emily. 2008. "Racial/Ethnic Differences in Asthma Prevalence: The Role of Housing and Neighborhood Environments." *Journal of Health and Social Behavior* 49(2): 131–45.

Ruel, Erin, and Stephanie A. Robert. 2009. "A Model of Racial Residential History and Its Association with Self-Rated Health and Mortality among Black and White Adults in the U.S." *Sociological Spectrum* 29(4): 1–24.

Rutter, Michael. 1990. "Psychological Resilience and Protective Mechanisms." In *Risk and Protective Factors in the Development of Psychopathology*, ed. Jon Rolf, Ann S. Masten, Dante Cicchetti, Keith H. Nuechterlein, and Sheldon Weintraub, 181–214. Cambridge: Cambridge University Press.

Ryff, Carol D., Burt Singer, Gail D. Love, and Marilyn J. Essex. 1998. "Resilience in Adulthood and Later Life: Defining Features and Dynamic Processes." In *Handbook of Aging and Mental Health: An Integrative Approach*, ed. Jacob Lomranz, 69–100. New York: Plenum Press.

Sampson, Robert J. 2009. "Racial Stratification and the Durable Tangle of Neighborhood Inequality." *Annals of the American Academy of Political and Social Science* 621:243–59.

Sampson, Robert J., Jeffrey D. Morenoff, and Thomas Gannon-Rowley. 2002. "Assessing 'Neighborhood Effects': Social Processes and New Directions in Research." *Annual Review of Sociology* 28:443–78.

Sampson, Robert J., Stephen W. Raudenbush, and Felton Earls. 1997. "Neighborhoods and Violent Crime: A Multilevel Study of Collective Efficacy." *Science* 227:918–23.

Sampson, Robert J., and Patrick Sharkey. 2008. "Neighborhood Selection and the Social Reproduction of Concentrated Racial Inequality." *Demography* 45(1): 1–29.

Sampson, Robert J., Patrick Sharkey, and Stephen W. Raudenbush. 2008. "Durable Effects of Concentrated Disadvantage on Verbal Ability among African-American Children." *Proceedings of the National Academies of Science* 105:845–52.

Schelling, Thomas C. 1978. *Micromotives and Macrobehavior*. New York: W. W. Norton.

Schieman, Scott, and Stephen C. Meersman. 2004. "Neighborhood Problems and Health among Older Adults: Received and Donated Social Support and the Sense of Mastery as Effect Modifiers." *Journals of Gerontology: Psychological Sciences and Social Science* 59: S89–97.

Schulz, Amy J., David R. Williams, Barbara A. Israel, and Lora B. Lempert. 2002. "Racial and Spatial Relations as Fundamental Determinants of Health in Detroit." *Milbank Quarterly* 80:677–707.

Schwirian, Kent P. 1983. "Models of Neighborhood Change." *Annual Review of Sociology* 9:83–102.

Scopilliti, Melissa, and John Iceland. 2008. "Residential Patterns of Black Immigrants and Native-Born Blacks in the United States." *Social Science Quarterly* 89(3): 551–73.

Sharkey, Patrick. 2008. "The Intergenerational Transmission of Context." *American Journal of Sociology* 113(4): 931–69.

Small, Mario Luis. 2002. "Culture, Cohorts, and Social Organization Theory: Understanding Local Participation in a Latino Housing Project." *American Journal of Sociology* 1:1–54.

———. 2004. *Villa Victoria: The Transformation of Social Capital in a Boston Barrio*. Chicago: University of Chicago Press.

Smith, Kristin P., and Nicholas A. Christakis. 2008. "Social Networks and Health." *Annual Review of Sociology* 34:405–29.

South, Scott J., and Kyle D. Crowder. 1997. "Escaping Distressed Neighborhoods: Individual, Community, and Metropolitan Influences." *American Journal of Sociology* 102(4): 1040–84.

———. 1998. "Leaving the 'Hood: Residential Mobility between Black, White, and Integrated Neighborhoods." *American Sociological Review* 63:17–26.

South, Scott J., Kyle D. Crowder, and Erick Chavez. 2005a. "Exiting and Entering High-Poverty Neighborhoods: Latinos, Blacks, and Anglos Compared." *Social Forces* 84(2): 873–900.

———. 2005b. "Migration and Spatial Assimilation among U.S. Latinos: Classical versus Segmented Trajectories." *Demography* 42:497–521.

South, Scott J., and Glenn D. Deane. 1993. "Race and Residential Mobility: Individual Determinants and Structural Constraints." *Social Forces* 72:147–67.

Spilimbergo, Antonio, and Luis Ubeda. 2004. "Family Attachment and the Decision to Move by Race." *Journal of Urban Economics* 55:478–97.

Stoll, Michael A. 2001. "Race, Neighborhood Poverty, and Participation in Voluntary Associations." *Sociological Forum* 16:529–57.

Subramanian, S. V., Dolores Acevedo-Garcia, and Teresa

L. Osypuk. 2005. "Racial Residential Segregation and Geographic Heterogeneity in Black/White Disparity in Poor Self-Rated Health in the U.S.: A Multilevel Statistical Analysis." *Social Science and Medicine* 60:1667–79.

Sundquist, Kristina, Holger Theobald, Min Yang, Xinjun Li, Sven-Erik Johansson, and Jan Sundquist. 2006. "Neighborhood Violent Crime and Unemployment Increase the Risk of Coronary Heart Disease: A Multilevel Study in an Urban Setting." *Social Science and Medicine* 62(8): 2061–71.

Susser, Ezra S., and Shang P. Lin. 1992. "Schizophrenia after Prenatal Exposure to the Dutch Hunger Winter of 1944–1945." *Archives of General Psychiatry* 49(12): 983–88.

Swaroop, Sapna, and Jeffrey D. Morenoff. 2006. "Building Community: The Neighborhood Context of Social Organization." *Social Forces* 84(3): 1665–85.

Szasz, Andrew. 1994. *Ecopopulism: Toxic Waste and the Movement for Environmental Justice*. Minneapolis: University of Minnesota Press.

Szreter, Simon. 2004. "Industrialization and Health." *British Medical Bulletin* 69:75–86.

Taeuber, Karl E., and Alma R. Taeuber. 1965. *Negroes in Cities*. Chicago: Aldine.

Temkin, Kenneth, and William Rowe. 1996. "Neighborhood Change and Urban Policy." *Journal of Planning Education and Research* 15:159–70.

Thoits, Peggy A. 1995. "Stress, Coping, and Social Support Processes: Where Are We? What Next?" *Journal of Health and Social Behavior* 36, extra issue: 53–79.

Turner, R. Jay, Blair Wheaton, and Donald A. Lloyd. 1995. "The Epidemiology of Social Stress." *American Sociological Review* 60:104–25.

Walton, Emily. 2009. "Residential Segregation and Birth Weight among Racial and Ethnic Minorities in the United States." *Journal of Health and Social Behavior* 50:427–42.

Wasserman, Stanley, and Katherine Faust. 1994. *Social Network Analysis: Methods and Applications*. New York: Cambridge University Press.

Wellman, Barry, and Kenneth Frank. 2001. "Network Capital in a Multilevel World: Getting Support from Personal Communities." In *Social Capital: Theory and Research*, ed. Nan Lin, Karen S. Cook, and Ronald S. Burt, 233–73. New York: Walter de Gruyter.

Wen, Ming, Christopher R. Browning, and Kathleen A. Cagney. 2003. "Poverty, Affluence, and Income Inequality: Neighborhood Economic Structure and Its Implications for Health." *Social Science and Medicine* 57(5): 843–60.

Wen, Ming, Kathleen A. Cagney, and Nicholas A. Christakis. 2005. "Effect of Specific Aspects of Community Social Environment on the Mortality of Individuals Diagnosed with Serious Illness." *Social Science and Medicine* 61:119–34.

Wen, Ming, Louise C. Hawkley, and John T. Cacioppo. 2006. "Objective and Perceived Neighborhood Environment, Individual SES and Psychosocial Factors, and Self-Rated Health: An Analysis of Older Adults in Cook County, Illinois." *Social Science and Medicine* 63(10): 2575–90.

Wheaton, Blair, and Philippa Clarke. 2003. "Space Meets Time: Integrating Temporal and Contextual Influences on Mental Health in Early Adulthood." *American Sociological Review* 68:680–706.

Wilson, William Julius. 1987. *The Truly Disadvantaged*. Chicago: University of Chicago Press.

Yao, Li, and Stephanie A. Robert. 2008. "The Contributions of Race, Individual Socioeconomic Status, and Neighborhood Socioeconomic Context in the Self-Rated Health Trajectories and Mortality of Older Adults." *Research on Aging* 30(2): 251–73.

PART II

Health Trajectories and Experiences

9

The Social Construction of Illness
Medicalization and Contested Illness

Kristin K. Barker, Oregon State University

This chapter makes a case for the usefulness of a social constructionist approach to medical sociology, emphasizing the analytic potency of social constructionism for explaining a key cultural and historical trend of our time: medicalization (Clarke et al. 2003; Conrad 2007). It includes a detailed discussion of contested illnesses—illnesses where patients and their advocates struggle to have their medically unexplainable symptoms recognized in orthodox biomedical terms—and suggests that lay practices and knowledge, and the consumer demands they engender, are increasingly crucial in advancing medicalization in the twenty-first century.

Sociology of Knowledge and the Social Construction of Illness

Social constructionism is a diverse set of theories of knowledge developed and used by social scientists, historians, and cultural studies scholars. From a constructionist perspective, a social construct is an idea that appears to refer to some obvious, inevitable, or naturally given phenomenon, when in fact the phenomenon has been (in full or part) created by a particular society at a particular time. Pointing to the socially constructed character of an idea challenges its taken-for-granted nature and the social practices premised on it. As a case in point, feminists claim that gender is a social construction, meaning that our current ideas about gender (i.e., norms and standards concerning femininity and masculinity) are not biologically mandated; therefore, the ideas and the social practices they institutionalize are alterable. Social constructionism has been a centerpiece, theoretically and substantively, of the subfield of medical sociology. Stated in brief, its chief contribution has been to demonstrate just how complex the answers are to the seemingly straightforward questions, What is an illness? What is a disease? But before taking on these questions, it's useful to trace the intellectual origins that inform a sociological approach to social constructionism.

From its inception as a discipline, sociology has approached ideas as reflections of the specific historical and social environments in which they are produced. The founding sociological thinkers—Karl Marx (1818–1883), Max Weber (1864–1920), and Emile Durkheim (1858–1917)—each addressed the relationship between the ideas or beliefs of a society and the social and material conditions of that society. Published in 1936, Karl Manheim's *Ideology and Utopia* represented a significant advance in the sociology of ideas. Manheim urged sociology to study empirically how peoples' historical context and their station in life (i.e., class) condition their ideas. In the 1960s, Berger and Luckmann (1967) articulated the link between ideas, including taken-for-granted or commonsense knowledge about reality, and everyday social interaction. In more recent decades, feminist and postmodern sociologists have demonstrated the relationship between our ideas and our social locations in race, class, and gender hierarchies of power, and have built on Foucauldian views of knowledge as a type of discourse that arbitrarily gives some groups power over others (Collins 1991; Smith 1987). Finally, sociologists contributing to the interdisciplinary field of science studies claim that scientific knowledge, like other ideas, is the outcome of concrete social practices rather than of individual discoveries of truth that "carve nature at its joints" (Knorr Cetina 1997; Latour 1987; Timmerman 2007). This long and venerable tradition—often called the "sociology of knowledge"—studies ideas not as true or false expressions of the world per se, but as the realized expression of particular social interests within particular social systems and contexts (Merton 1973). In other words, from a sociology of knowledge perspective, our ideas are social constructions (Berger and Luckmann 1967).

Sociologists study the social construction of many different ideas, but of interest to us here are sociologists who study ideas about illness. Although perhaps not immediately obvious, the use of social constructionism in medical sociology can be traced to Talcott Parsons's (1951) concept of the *sick role*. The sick role describes illness as a form of medically sanctioned deviant behavior, and specifies the rights and obligations given a sick person to ensure that an episode of sickness doesn't disrupt social order and stability. Despite Parsons's social conservatism, his theoretical claims were premised on the conceptual distinction between the biophysical nature of disease and the social experience of sickness. Over the last fifty-plus years, medical sociologists have built on this distinction to make more radical and far-reaching claims concerning the social construction of illness and disease (Brumberg 2009; Conrad and Schneider 1992; Freidson 1971; Lorber and Moore 2002).

Social constructionist scholars emphasize the relationship between ideas about illness and the expression, perception, understanding, and response to illness at the individual, institutional, and societal level. Historical and cross-cultural comparisons are effective ways to illustrate social constructionists' claims. Imagine, for example,

two societies: one defines illness principally as the outcome of moral failings or spiritual transgressions (on the part of individuals or communities); the other defines illness principally as the result of organic disturbance within an individual human body. Who (or even what) is identified as "ill" in these two societies will differ dramatically, as will arrangements for how and by whom illness is to be treated. In addition, the subjective experience and meaning of being ill will be markedly dissimilar because the two societies provide very different interpretive frameworks of the illness experience. In one society, "the shamed" stand before a sacred figure who rights the wrong, cleanses the soul, or grants mercy; in the other, the individual victim of disease—"the patient"—seeks the physician's technical skills to restore or fix his or her wounded body.

Social constructionists also examine why some illnesses exist in one place and not another, or appear and then disappear in the same place. In many societies, for example, women do not suffer from premenstrual syndrome (PMS) or anorexia nervosa. Likewise, *susto* and *koro* are illnesses that exist only in certain cultures. A number of illnesses that were present in Western societies in the late nineteenth and early twentieth centuries—including fugue, hysteria, and neurasthenia—have now faded from view (Hacking 1998). These so-called culture-bound and transient illnesses effectively advance the social constructionist claim that illness and disease are something beyond fixed physical realities; they are also phenomena shaped by social experiences, shared cultural traditions, and shifting frameworks of knowledge.

From a social constructionist perspective, the task is not necessarily to determine which of the two societies has the *correct* ideas about illness, or which of the illnesses found only in certain places or certain times are *real*. Instead, the task is to determine how and why particular ideas about illness appear, change, or persist for reasons that are at least partly independent of their empirical adequacy vis-à-vis biomedicine. So, for example, social constructionists pay close attention to how and why particular definitions or ideas about illness became dominant in particular places and times and how they marginalize or silence alternative ideas (Conrad and Schneider 1992; Freidson 1971; Starr 1982; Tesh 1988). Additional questions follow: What factors help explain why one society defines illness in moral terms, whereas another eschews such ideas in favor of observable anatomic abnormality? What are the central consequences—for the society at large and for afflicted individuals—of one set of ideas versus another? What dynamics are at play in the appearance and disappearance of a certain illness or in the existence of an illness in one place but its absence elsewhere?

Although these are some archetypal social constructionist questions, questions about reality and truth inevitably arise: Don't some ideas about illness more accurately reflect the truth than others? Doesn't the scientific disease model better explain and treat illness than folkloric or religious approaches? Isn't death definitive proof that illness isn't simply a social construction? These questions arise because not everyone agrees what calling an illness "socially constructed" implies. This is largely because there is no single social constructionist perspective in general, or in medical sociology in particular (Brown 1995).[1] Instead there are several versions of social constructionism used by many different academic disciplines, each drawing on different intellectual assumptions about the relationship between ideas and the material world. The widespread use of several versions of social constructionism, by scholars from a host of disciplines, applied to an increasing array of phenomena (e.g., race, gender, sexuality, quarks, disability, illness) has led to a confused and mulled state of affairs with respect to what exactly is socially constructed about phenomena said to be social constructions.

In his aptly titled book *The Social Construction of What?* philosopher Ian Hacking asks the following types of questions: What does it mean to say that race, or a quark, or an illness is a social construct? Does it mean that we made these *things* and they would not exist as such if we had not made them, and/or we could have made them in a fundamentally different fashion? Or, does it mean that we made our *ideas* about these things, and we could have come up with very different ideas about these things? Does it mean that both the *things* and our *ideas* about the things are

socially constructed? Are all things and all ideas social constructions? Or, if all things and all ideas are not equally socially constructed, what makes some things and some ideas social constructions and not others?

Hacking and other analytic philosophers and philosophers of science raise important questions about social constructionism (Boghossian 2001; Hacking 1999; Searle 1995; Slezak 2000). Among the principal charges they raise are that social constructionism explicitly or implicitly denies the existence of the natural world (or at least denies the possibility that we can know about it with some degree of accuracy); and, relatedly, that the approach stumbles over questions concerning whether or not some ideas are better representations of the world than are others. Hacking also alleges that social constructionism inevitably reproduces a false binary between things that are *real* (and therefore have an entirely biophysical basis) and things that are *socially constructed* (and therefore have no biophysical basis whatsoever). As a result, Hacking contends, social constructionism fails to consider the possibility that something can be *both* real *and* socially constructed (Hacking 1999, 31). However, sociologists of medicine have often supported this view, insofar as they believe that the social forces constructing the definition and treatment of illness are themselves real phenomena that can be empirically studied (Brown 1995; Freidson 1971).

What many sociologists mean when they claim that an illness is socially constructed is that the experience of illness is shaped by social and cultural context. The earlier comments concerning the variability in the experience of illness across time (history) and space (culture) are illustrative. Many sociologists have pursued this line of reasoning and in so doing have given us powerful insights into the cultural fabric of illness. Without question, the experience of cancer, epilepsy, or anxiety differs greatly historically and cross-culturally. Insofar as all illness gains meaning within the context of human society, all illness is socially constructed. Yet, if all illnesses are social constructions, then there is no point in singling out any particular illness as being a social construct. In short, the social constructionist perspective loses its expository or investigatory power when followed to its logical conclusion. Even here, however, a core conceptual contribution of social constructionism to medical sociology remains intact: the distinction between the medical model, which emphasizes biological pathology, and the social model, which emphasizes the oft-neglected social causes and character of illness and impairment.

There still is the matter of the social construction of illnesses as things. A strict constructionist position would implicitly or explicitly hold that no illness—cancer, epilepsy, or anxiety—exists outside our socially and historically bound mental constructions. These things exist at all, or exist as they are, only because we created them. Although not about illness, this position, which effectively denies the existence of the ontological world or the reality of what Searle (1995) calls "brute facts" (i.e., facts about the physical and natural world), was famously mocked in 1996 when the physicist Alan Sokal published a hoax article in *Social Text*, a leading journal representing the postmodern critique of science's alleged objectivity in the so-called science wars. Despite the attention given the Sokal hoax and the vocal attacks against the relativism of social constructionism, it is difficult to find scholars who make these strict types of claims. Even Hacking (1999) admits that most social constructionists avoid this pitfall.

A line of inquiry pursued by medical sociologists that thoughtfully negotiates many of these logical problems emphasizes the social construction of medical knowledge. As described by Brown (1995, 37), the social construction of illness stresses the illness experience, whereas the social construction of medical knowledge "deals with the ways of knowing that are based on the dominant biomedical framework" and is chiefly concerned with professional beliefs and diagnoses. Of course, in our society it is impossible to fully disentangle these spheres given that people primarily make sense of and manage illness within the dominant biomedical framework (ibid.). In fact, it is difficult to overstate biomedicine's influence in shaping the prevailing ideas about illness in advanced capitalist societies. Among other things, biomedicine plays a dominant role in organizing our experiences and complaints into disease categories.

A disease does not exist, so to speak, until the social institution of medicine creates a representative diagnostic category (Brown 1995; Freidson 1971). For a disease to exist, in this limited sense, it must be identified. Disease begins with "social discovery" or the "the ways in which people, organizations, and institutions determine that there is a disease or condition" (Brown 1995, 38). This is not to suggest that there are no biological facts concerning disease, nor is the point merely one of semantics. As noted earlier, we can claim that a disease as defined in a diagnostic category is a social construction without implying that the suffering it represents has no biological basis. After all, social constructionists are primarily interested in the empirical adequacy of their own descriptions of the social forces behind medical ideas, be these forces at odds with or supplementary to the empirical adequacy of the corresponding biomedical ideas. Contrary to Hacking's allegations, medical sociologists and anthropologists clearly recognize the possibility that a condition can be both real and socially constructed (Brown 1995; Freidson 1971). For example, such a both/and stance vis-à-vis the real/social-construction dichotomy has been advanced in the case of post-traumatic stress disorder (Young 1995), mood disorders (Horwitz 2002), and anorexia nervosa (Brumberg 2009), to name but a few. Additionally, the social constructionist approach clearly addresses how diagnoses interact with the individuals who are diagnosed, again acknowledging social constructionism's both/and analytic potential (Brown 1995; Freidson 1971; Horwitz 2002).

But not all diseases, as captured in their diagnostic categories, are fundamentally or primarily social constructions. Sometimes the factors behind the creation of a new disease category and its application are straightforwardly biological. A particular type of human distress is linked to biological pathologies, and the new diagnosis represents progress in medical knowledge. In these instances it might be meaningful to talk about the social practices that resulted in the discovery of the disease and its application, but it would not be particularly meaningful to assert that the disease is a social construction simply because social activity led to its discovery. Here the deft historical accounts of the social processes leading up the discovery of tuberculosis (Tomes 1998), end-stage renal disease (Peitzman 1992), and HIV/AIDS (Epstein 1996) come to mind. Often, however, there is a level of arbitrariness concerning why a particular set of attributes comes to be organized and represented under a biomedical diagnosis. Cases characterized by apparent arbitrariness are of most interest to sociologists (Brown 1995). These cases are interesting not because they have no connection to biological facts, but because they demonstrate that "an entity that is regarded as an illness or disease is not ipso facto a medical problem; rather, it needs to become defined as one" (Conrad 2007, 5–6). Hence, the social construction of medical knowledge goes hand in hand with the process known as medicalization.

Biomedical Knowledge and Medicalization

Medicalization is the process by which an ever-wider range of human experiences comes to be defined, experienced, and treated as medical conditions.

One large sector includes the medicalization of deviance (Conrad and Schneider 1992). Calling a drunk an alcoholic or a gambler an addict are such examples. Social problems are also medicalized, as seen in the case of obesity and antisocial personality disorder (Lorber and Moore 2002). In some cases, "normal" human variation in such things as height, appearance, or temperament is defined as a medical problem and treated accordingly (Conrad 2007). In other instances, it is appropriate to speak of the medicalization of life itself. Medicine, Illich warned us, "can transform people into patients because they are unborn, newborn, menopausal, or at some other 'age of risk'" (Illich 1976, 78). The medicalization of life, therefore, includes natural physical changes ranging from the profound (e.g., senility) to the trivial (e.g., male-patterned baldness). Biotechnology promises to expand the frontier even further as genetic research medicalizes the state of being "at risk" (Skolbekken 2008). Through medicalization, natural human variation, normal experiences, routine complaints, and hypothetical scenarios become medical conditions.

Drawing on social constructionist tenets, feminist scholars have demonstrated how wom-

en's bodies and experiences have been particularly susceptible to medicalization. There are many complex reasons for this tendency, including medicine's conceptualization of male physiology as normative. Borrowing Simone de Beauvoir's (1989) central insight, men and men's bodies represent the biomedical standard and women and women's bodies are the biomedical other. It is but a short step to define normal aspects of women's embodiment as biologically aberrant. For example, women's natural reproductive functions are routinely medicalized (e.g., pregnancy, childbirth, menstruation, menopause) (Ehrenreich and English 1973; Lorber and Moore 2002, 2007; Martin 1987). That being said, women have themselves been proactive in processes of medicalization—perhaps because it represents one of a few avenues afforded them to pursue their needs and gain access to resources in a society characterized by gender inequality (Lorber and Moore 2002, 2007; Riessman 1983; Theriot 1993).

Medicalization is a complex process. Although the general historical trend has been toward ever-greater medicalization, it can be a bidirectional process, as the demedicalization of homosexuality and masturbation attest (Conrad 2007; Clarke et al. 2003). In the 1970s, at the height of the natural childbirth movement, childbirth became less medicalized (Lorber and Moore 2007). Although there is considerable evidence that this trend has reversed itself, the case of childbirth nevertheless illustrates the potential bidirectionality of medicalization. In a somewhat similar vein, there are individuals and groups who reject a medical classification of their behavior, as seen in the contemporary examples of pro-anorexia and self-injury (e.g., cutting, burning, etc.) groups (Adler and Adler 2007; Pascoe and Boero 2008). The actions of these groups have not led to demedicalization per se—the diagnoses these groups reject remain well established—but they do demonstrate pockets of resistance to the medicalization of deviant behaviors. Specifically, these groups actively produce counterconstructions of disordered eating and self-injury, affirm them as alternative lifestyles, and forge virtual subcultures, all far from the dictates of medical practitioners and the clinical gaze. Likewise, although parents and parent groups opposing childhood immunization don't undermine established medical protocol, they do show some individual and collective opposition to unlimited medicalization (Casiday 2007).

There can also be different levels or degrees of medicalization (Conrad 2007). A condition isn't necessarily medicalized or not medicalized. For instance, although a small number of individuals are treated medically for short stature (Conrad 2007), it would be an overstatement to suggest that the general public perceives shortness as an illness. Similarly, individuals who are dissatisfied with their bodily appearance can seek to have it medically altered, but so far being unattractive isn't considered an illness. In contrast to these cases of medical treatment in the absence of illness or disease, celiac disease is an illness without a medical treatment. In the case of celiac disease, the principal treatment is adherence to a gluten-free diet. Because celiac disease requires no medical intervention, it exists somewhere between a medicalized and nonmedicalized condition (Copeland and Valle 2009). Contested illnesses also illustrate different degrees of medicalization insofar as some of these conditions are further down the road toward accepted medical conditions than are others. Sociologists have referred to emergent or partial medicalization (Dumit 2006), or specified different medicalized classifications and categories (Brown 1995) to denote that certain human experiences hit a snag in the process of becoming institutionally accepted medical phenomena.

It is also clear that the principal forces behind medicalization in the present era differ from those that expanded medicine's jurisdiction up through the first three quarters of the twentieth century (Clarke et al. 2003; Conrad 2005). Dramatic changes in the organization of medicine toward the end of the twentieth century, most notably the rise of corporate managed care and the corresponding decline of physicians' professional power, underlie changing patterns of medicalization. One can briefly summarize the standard twentieth-century story of medicalization as follows: physicians carved out a professional niche for themselves by negating lay knowledge and practices and promoting the medical management of natural human experiences, social ills, and personal problems (Conrad and Schneider 1992; Freidson 1970; Illich 1976). The medicalization of childbirth and pregnancy are exemplars (Barker 1998; Wertz and Wertz 1979).

In contrast, when it comes to the forces promoting the expansion of medicine's jurisdiction in the current era, the role of physicians has declined in significance, while that of biotechnology (e.g., pharmaceuticals and genetics) and other corporate health industries (e.g., managed-care organizations), in tandem with the markets and consumers they create and serve, have increased in salience (Clarke et al. 2003; Conrad 2005). The popularity of elective cosmetic surgery and fertility treatments attests to consumer demands for medical solutions to personal problems and disappointments (Blum 2003; Conrad 2007). Direct-to-consumer pharmaceutical advertising encourages patients to ask their doctor about particular drugs to treat many previously normal or benign symptoms (e.g., toenail discoloration, heartburn) and to consider them specific medical conditions or diseases (e.g., dermatophytes, acid reflux disease) (Moynihan, Heath, and Henry 2002). The availability of a drug or other biotech treatment for a complaint significantly increases the likelihood that the compliant will be medicalized. This raises serious allegations that biotech corporations are engaging in "disease mongering" (Angell 2004; Conrad 2007; McCrea 1983).

There are important consequences of medicalization. By defining disease as a biological disruption residing with an individual human body, medicalization obscures the social forces that influence our health and well-being. Medicalization is depoliticizing: it calls for medical intervention (medication, surgery, etc.) when the best remedy for certain types of human suffering may be political, economic, or social change. Medicalization can also grant the institution of medicine undue authority over our bodies, minds, and lives, thereby limiting individual autonomy and functioning as a form of social control (Illich 1976; Zola 1972). Rarely, however, is medicalization exclusively the result of the medical profession's imperialistic claims. As patient consumers, we are increasingly active participants in the medicalization of our experiences as we earnestly seek to resolve and legitimate our suffering.

A social constructionist perspective that emphasizes the biological arbitrariness of certain diagnoses provides a powerful analytic framework for making sense of medicalization, or the process by which our complaints, disappointments, and experiences come to be defined and treated as medical conditions. In addition, such a perspective circumvents many of the critiques of social constructionism. A close examination of the social construction of contested illnesses further demonstrates these claims.

Contested Illnesses

Contested illnesses are conditions in which sufferers and their advocates struggle to have medically unexplainable symptoms recognized in orthodox biomedical terms, despite resistance from medical researchers, practitioners, and institutions (Barker 2008; Conrad and Stults 2008; Dumit 2006). In the last several decades there has been a notable increase in the number of contested illnesses and contested illness sufferers (Barsky and Borus 1999; Henningsen, Zipfel, and Herzog 2007; Manu 2004; Mayou and Farmer 2002). Tens of millions of Americans are diagnosed with one of several syndromes characterized by a cluster of common, diffuse, and disturbing symptoms, ranging from pain and fatigue to sleep and mood disorders. Some of these illnesses include chronic fatigue syndrome/myalgic encephalomyelitis (ME), fibromyalgia syndrome, irritable bowel syndrome, urologic chronic pelvic pain syndrome, temporomandibular dysfunction (TMJ), tension headache, multiple chemical sensitivity disorder, Gulf War syndrome, and sick building syndrome (Barsky and Borus 1999; Nimnuan et al. 2001; Wessley 2004) many sufferers and some clinician advocates suggest that these disorders—frequently called "functional somatic syndromes" in the medical literature—are unique disease entities with unique natural histories and specific characteristics. At this time, however, there is tremendous medical uncertainty concerning these conditions (Mayou and Farmer 2002).

At the very core of the uncertainty is a lack of medical consensus concerning the biological nature of these illnesses. Despite fierce claims to the contrary, none of these illnesses are associated with any specific organic abnormality. These conditions are not detectable in x-rays, blood tests, CAT scans, or any other high-tech diagnostic tool. Instead, they are diagnosed based on clinical observations and patients' subjective reports of symptoms. They are also diagnosed by exclusion, that is, after other possible explanations for the symptoms have been ruled out. Consequently, many physicians approach these "wastebasket" diagnoses, and those so diagnosed, with considerable skepticism. What is at issue is whether these syndromes are "real" (have organic biological origins) or not (are psychogenic, behavioral, or iatrogenic). With the exception of Gulf War syndrome, these disorders are highly feminized (Mayou and Farmer 2002). This unavoidable fact introduces ruminations that these diagnoses are modern-day labels for hysteria (Bohr 1995; Hadler 1997a, b; Showalter 1997).

The subjective experiences of these illnesses stand in sharp contrast to the medical uncertainty surrounding them. Individual sufferers provide persuasive accounts of their distress (Asbring and Narvanen 2003; Barker 2005; Hayden and Sacks 1998; Koziol et al. 1993; Kroll-Smith and Floyd 1997). They report significant reductions in functional abilities, health status, and quality of life, and little long-term improvement in well-being over time (Manu 2004; Nimnuan et al. 2001; Wessley, Nimnuan, and Sharpe 1999). Living with a contested illness, therefore, means managing a constellation of chronic and often debilitating symptoms, as well as coping with medical uncertainty, skepticism, and disparagement. Indeed these conditions are called "contested" illnesses precisely because of the clash between medical knowledge and patient experience (Conrad and Stults 2008; Dumit 2006; Moss and Teghtsoonian 2008).

A related line of investigation addresses contested environmental illnesses, or illnesses that involve "scientific disputes and extensive public debates over environmental causes" (Brown 2007, xiv). A growing body of research demonstrates that when individuals claim to have an illness caused by exposure to environmental hazards, they meet with considerable resistance (Brown et al. 2004; Zavestoski et al. 2004a, b).

Specifically, "corporate, government, and medical authorities" contest environmental illness claims in an effort to defend their organizational, professional, and economic interests (Cable, Mix, and Shriver 2008, 384). The principal contestation is over claims that a specific condition (e.g., breast cancer, asthma, lung cancer) is caused by exposure to a particular environmental hazard. In some cases, however, there are also disputes about the existence of the illness itself (e.g., Gulf War Syndrome, multiple chemical sensitivity disorder) said to be caused by environmental toxins (Kroll-Smith et al. 2000). These latter cases are examples of contested illness as defined in this chapter, but all contested environmental illnesses showcase conflicts between biomedical and lay ways of knowing, and hinge on the inability of medical experts to legitimate lay peoples' symptoms and suffering (ibid., 4).

According to Joseph Dumit (2006, 578), contested illnesses "are researched, discussed, and reported on, but no aspect of them is settled medically, legally, or popularly." Pamela Moss and Katherine Teghtsoonian (2008, 7) describe contested illnesses as "dismissed as illegitimate—framed as 'difficult,' psychosomatic, or even non-existent—by researchers, health practitioners, and policy makers operating within conventional paradigms of knowledge." More than a decade ago, Brown (1995) identified two types of conflictual or contested diagnoses: conditions that are generally accepted but to which a medical definition is not routinely applied (e.g., environmental diseases); and conditions that are not generally accepted but to which a medical definition is nevertheless often applied (e.g., chronic fatigue syndrome). In both cases, for different reasons, sufferers have to convince the institution of biomedicine that their condition is medical in character. Thus, the term "contested" denotes that these illnesses exist somewhere between entirely discredited and fully legitimate diseases.

The particulars concerning the knowledge and experience of individual contested illnesses differ. For example, each condition is coupled with a body of medical research and a case definition or diagnostic criteria (Dumit 2006; Wessley, Nimnuan, and Sharpe 1999). Having been the beneficiaries of more sympathy from mainstream medical professionals, some of these classifications are more widely applied (e.g., fibromyalgia syndrome, irritable bowel syndrome) than others (e.g., sick building syndrome, multiple chemical sensitivity disorder). These illnesses can also be differentiated on the basis of subjective features and accounts: the experience and meaning of living with fibromyalgia is distinct from that of multiple chemical sensitive disorder; and individuals and groups coalesce around specific diagnoses. Nevertheless, these illnesses share a number of key similarities that account for their contested status.

Given that sufferers and their advocates want medically unexplainable symptoms to be medically recognized and legitimated, contested illnesses are examples of conditions for which individual patients and patient groups demand medicalization.[2] That is, they are evidence of a shift in the engines of medicalization: the demands of patient-consumers, rather than the professional agendas of physicians, increasingly underlie medicine's jurisdictional expansion (Conrad 2005). In addition, contested illness and medicalization are tied together conceptually via social constructionism: "Both medicalization and contested illness highlight that illness categories (usually, but not always, diagnoses) are socially constructed and not automatically ascertained from scientific and/or medical discoveries" (Conrad and Stults 2008, 332). What follows is a descriptive account of the social construction of contested illnesses.

Of specific interest to us are the shared factors and influences in the social processes by which contested illnesses were created and propagated. These include public intolerance of or anxiety about medically unexplainable but highly common symptoms; the dynamics of doctor-patient encounters and the corresponding diagnostic imperative; lay knowledge production and the emergence of illness identities and communities; and bureaucratic and institutional demands and practices (Aronowitz 1997; Barsky and Borus 1995; Brown 1995; Freidson 1971; Showalter 1997). I address each in turn.

When delineating the factors contributing to the social construction of contested illnesses, ground zero, so to speak, is the ubiquity of the symptoms they represent. Contested-illness symptoms are widespread in the general public and are particularly common among women (Fillingim 2000; Lorber and Moore 2002; Mayou and Farmer 2002). For example, pain and fatigue are the most common physical aliments reported by the general public (Barsky and Borus 1999). Fatigue is so commonly reported that the acronym TATT (tired all the time) now appears regularly in medical and popular media. The additional symptoms that make up these disorders, including mood, sleep, and bowel disturbances, are also widely prevalent (Mayou and Farmer 2002). This is not to suggest that these disorders are much ado about nothing. Whether these symptoms are common or not, their cumulative effect can be overwhelming. Aggravating this tendency is our cultural impatience with discomfort (Barsky and Borus 1995; Kleinman 1988; Kleinman and Ware 1992).

Accordingly, individuals turn to the institution of medicine for an explanation and remedy. However, even with extensive and very expensive clinical workups, many common symptoms simply can't be explained in biomedical terms (Barsky and Borus 1995; Mayou and Farmer 2002). So it is that sufferers describe a protracted and troubling road into medical uncertainty. "Nothing is wrong," they are told by one doctor after another. And yet they feel very ill indeed. In turn, sufferers must reconcile a subjective certainty of their symptoms with a lack of objective medical evidence regarding the existence of their symptoms (Asbring and Narvanen 2001). Along the way, individuals experience real or perceived accusations that they are faking their symptoms, malingering, or "just plain crazy" (Dumit 2006, 578). Their credibility is called into question. Given the gulf between their distress and the growing mound of negative medical tests, even sufferers sometimes begin to doubt their own grip on reality (Asbring and Narvanen 2003; Banks and Prior 2001). Not surprisingly, many individuals doggedly continue their search for a biological explanation in an effort to prove to medical professionals, their families, and themselves that they really are ill (Dumit 2006). In her research on chronic fatigue syndrome, Pia Bülow (2008) aptly calls this arduous search the "pilgrimage."

The dynamics of countless medical encounters that make up many such pilgrimages stand behind the creation and application of these diagnoses. There are many reasons that doctor-patient encounters favor diagnosing. For the physician, a diagnosis represents codified knowledge about a patient's experience and indicates a treatment protocol. For the patient, a diagnosis gives meaning and legitimacy to worrying symptoms and provides a framework for what he or she is facing (Balint 1957). Thus, when a doctor encounters a patient with distressing symptoms, both parties benefit from a diagnosis: it effectively legitimizes both parties and the doctor-patient relationship itself. Before contested-illness diagnoses could serve this legitimating purpose, however, they had to be created.

The creation of these diagnoses, in terms of both the specific case definitions and the actors advancing those definitions, differ in their particulars (Barsky and Borus 1999; Wessley, Nimnuan, and Sharpe 1999), but two general points can be made. First, each of these diagnoses is a descriptive category or analytic abstraction that stands for otherwise medically unexplainable symptoms (Mayou and Farmer 2002). It has been argued that many medical specialties and subspecialties have at least one functional diagnosis at their disposal to manage a large population of patients whose symptoms lack an understood biological cause; hence the creation of several different, overlapping syndromes (e.g., rheumatology has fibromyalgia, neurologists have tension headache, gastroenterologists have irritable bowel syndrome, gynecologists have chronic pelvic pain) (Barsky and Borus 1999; Nimnuan et al. 2001). Second, although none of these diagnoses would have come about without the efforts of key players who pushed for their creation—"claims-makers," as Conrad and Schneider (1992) call them—those that were advanced primarily by specialists in the medical mainstream have moved further along in the medicalization process than have those that relied more heavily on lay advocacy or were associated with marginal medical professionals. Examples of the former include fibromyalgia and irritable bowel syndrome. Examples of the latter include multiple chemical sensitivity and chronic fatigue syndrome.[3]

Although some support from sympathetic medical professionals is a necessary part in disease discovery, medical professionals also resist discovery (Brown 1995). Again, this resistance is what defines contested illnesses. Reflecting the most contested end of the continuum, an article published in the prestigious *Annals of Internal Medicine* referred to multiple chemical sensitivity as a "cult" (quoted in Kroll-Smith and Floyd 1997, 29). But even the least contested of the contested illnesses, fibromyalgia, has been resolutely attacked. The essence of the charge, captured in the following quote from a leading rheumatology journal, points to the social construction of the diagnosis: "No one can have fibromyalgia. Fibromyalgia is just a word we use to represent the situation of someone complaining about widespread chronic pain, fatigue, and sleep disturbances. . . . It is not a disease, it's a description" (da Silva 2004, 828). The creation of contested illness diagnostic categories represents a decisive move toward the medicalization of common physical and mental distress, but none of these conditions is yet fully medicalized. In the absence of biomedical markers or efficacious treatments, medical professionals will continue to be skeptical of further medicalization.

Where diagnoses have been created—by whatever path and against whatever crystallized medical opposition—a number of factors have ensured their widespread application. First among these is a tendency within medicine to favor assigning illness over health. This is called the "decision rule" (Freidson 1971), but it might also be called the "diagnostic imperative." Concerned about their patients and trained to be proactive, physicians prefer to diagnose illness rather than health. Consequently, the existence of these diagnoses gives medical practitioners a new tool for managing the steady influx of patients with otherwise unexplainable symptoms. Under the weight of the decision rule, even physicians who are skeptical about contested illnesses are inclined to diagnose them.

The diagnosing behavior of physicians is only one side of the story. Once contested illnesses exist, again in the narrow sense of the creation of a diagnostic classification, individuals in distress encounter them. This makes possible perhaps the

most crucial moment in the patient's pilgrimage (Bülow 2008)—the moment when her suffering is at last given a name. A diagnosis brings a coherence and order to a collection of symptoms that have heretofore been incoherent and unruly. Perhaps even more important, the diagnosis validates the sufferer and her suffering after a protracted period of disparagement (Asbring and Narvanen 2003; Barker 2005; Dumit 2006). In practical terms, a diagnosis is required to receive health care, disability compensation, and other social reparations. For all these reasons, individuals often strongly identify with their diagnosis. These are also all key factors that motivate sufferers to demand greater medicalization of their condition.

The means by which individuals encounter their diagnosis is also of interest. In some instances, the patient learns about her diagnosis only when a sympathetic (or agnostic) medical provider diagnoses her. Increasingly, however, individuals discover their diagnosis without the aid of their health-care provider. Some happen upon their diagnosis by way of a family member or friend battling the same symptoms. Others come to their diagnosis after reading a magazine or newspaper article that describes a condition that fits their symptoms to a tee. As the Internet becomes a primary source of health-related information (Fox and Fallows 2003), an ever-greater number of individuals find their diagnosis by typing their symptoms into an online search engine. In turn they connect to an extensive network of commercial and nonprofit websites that describe their symptomatic experience as evidence of a diagnosable disease about which they were previously unaware (Barker 2008; and see Conrad and Stults, this volume). Now that the FDA has approved the first drug for the treatment of fibromyalgia, some individuals find out they have this disease courtesy of a direct-to-consumer pharmaceutical advertisement. Although commonplace, self-diagnosis is insufficient; individuals need medical corroboration. Sometimes doctors are amenable, especially given the inertia of the decision rule. But many clinicians are hesitant to diagnose patients with a contested illness. Some patients go from doctor to doctor in search of a willing diagnostician. For this reason, Dumit

(2006, 577) calls these "illnesses you have to fight to get." Again, issues surrounding self-validation and health/disability compensation make the fight for a diagnosis particularly salient.

Illness support communities also play an important role in the social construction of contested illnesses. Although patient advocacy, education, and mutual support are increasingly common in relation to many illnesses, contested-illness sufferers are particularly eager to affiliate with those who share their experiences. To use Bülow's (2008) metaphor again, these communities provide a welcomed shelter for the weary pilgrim. Through a variety of sources (e.g., best-selling self-help books, real and virtual support groups, and a host of advocacy organizational websites), individuals learn the biological facts—those denied by the uninformed in the medical mainstream—about their "real" disease. They also learn how to manage symptoms, deflect medical derision, and find a friendly provider who will diagnosis and treat their disease. Illness support communities produce and disseminate knowledge of sufferers' shared embodied experiences in an effort to support fellow sufferers, produce logical accounts of their distress, and challenge medical critics (Barker 2008; Dumit 2006; Kroll-Smith and Floyd 1997). At the level of experience, therefore, affiliation with a contested-illness community validates an individual's diagnosis and the diagnostic category. It would be difficult to overstate the degree to which the Internet has increased the reach and influence of these communities (Barker 2008; and see Conrad and Stults, this volume).

In this way, contested illnesses are examples of what Hacking (1999) calls "interactive kinds of things." Herein lies another important factor fueling the development of contested illnesses. In the case of interactive kinds of things, individuals react to being classified in particular ways. Unlike calling a quark a quark, which Hacking notes makes no difference to the quark, an individual reacts to being diagnosed with fibromyalgia or chronic fatigue syndrome or irritable bowel syndrome. Individuals come to see themselves as having a particular disease and reorient their symptoms and sense of self in relationship to that disease designation. This is starkly seen with re-

spect to the self-validation that being diagnosed represents. The diagnosis launches a particular illness career, contributes to the creation of an illness identity, and makes possible affiliation with an illness community. Additionally, the creation and application of these diagnoses result in their reification: although these diagnoses are conceptual abstractions, they have come to garner status as "things." Because contested illnesses include many common symptoms and provide no exclusionary criteria, sufferers can readily see the parallels between their own illness experience and the illness experience of fellow sufferers. Not only are contested illnesses interactive kinds of things in terms of how the designation interacts with the individual so designated, but their interactive quality also creates a cultural milieu wherein even more individuals, through their brief or extensive encounters with illness support communities, come to locate themselves within these designations.

Finally, organizational imperatives and dynamics also critically influence "the type and amount of conditions discovered" (Brown 1995, 45). Patients with unexplainable symptoms can be very costly. Although managed-care organizations erect barriers to limit health-care utilization, these barriers force patients to "express their 'disease' in more urgent and exaggerated terms in order to gain access to the physician" (Barsky and Borus 1995, 1931) Additionally, health-care providers use these diagnoses to help patients gain access to health-care resources within the constraints of managed care. Curiously, a case can also be made that these diagnoses might, in the end, work to the financial advantage of managed-care organizations. When patients with medically unexplainable symptoms are diagnosed with a contested illness in its early stages, health-care costs are reduced by limiting the number of expensive diagnostic tests, referrals to specialists, and surgical procedures that otherwise characterize the contested-illness experience. Because the standard treatment protocol is often relatively inexpensive (e.g., pain, sleep, and antidepressant medications, as well as behavioral and exercise therapies), managed-care organizations may use contested-illness diagnoses as part of their agenda for cost containment.

In sum, contested illnesses reveal the conceptual union between social constructionism and medicalization. Specifically, contested illnesses are social constructions that give biomedical meaning to a broad range of distress and suffering that characterize the lives of many individuals, especially women. The contested status of these diagnoses, however, signifies only partial medicalization. Whereas advocates for contested illnesses demand greater medicalization as a route to legitimate the sufferer and secure necessary health and welfare reparations, critics hope to stem the medicalization tide to which these diagnoses contribute (Conrad and Stults 2008). There are two obvious paths toward increasing the degree to which contested illnesses are medicalized. The first includes identifying biological markers upon which the "social legitimacy and intellectual plausibility of contemporary disease categorizations often hinge" (Shostak, Conrad, and Horwitz 2008, 310). For example, recent reports of potential genetic variations associated with restless leg syndrome bode well for this condition's further medicalization (Shostak, Conrad, and Horwitz 2008). The second path includes a specific treatment option. Based on my current research, for example, sufferers and their clinician-advocates have enthusiastically embraced the recent FDA approval of the first drug specifically for the treatment of fibromyalgia syndrome, more for the drug's disease-legitimating potential than for its therapeutic efficacy.

It is worth restating what it means to call contested illnesses socially constructed. As they currently exist, these diagnoses are best understood as intellectual categories whose social etiological is more clearly understood than is their biomedical etiology. The diagnostic criteria for these illnesses are descriptive, subjectively determined, and inexactly and inconsistently applied. The creation of these diagnostic categories has more to do with the social dictates of clinical encounters, the influence of illness communities, and institutional demands than with scientific or medical discoveries. Contested illnesses are very large conceptual tents under which many dissimilar types of symptoms and distress can be located. What is more, these types of symptoms and distress are widespread in general, and particularly common among women.

Calling these syndromes socially constructed, however, does not deny the reality of their symptoms. It is clear that the suffering of those so diagnosed is real: their quality of life is significantly eroded and they would do almost anything to be well (Asbring and Narvanen 2001; Bülow 2008; Kroll-Smith and Floyd 1997). Although the diagnostic labels are social constructions, they might, in fact, represent a number of things that have biomedical correlates that are currently unknown. The socially constructed meanings that mediate our experience of a disorder or condition can be overly simplistic, imperfect, or vague, but that does not mean that the symptoms that comprise the disorder have no biological basis or that they would cease to exist in the absence of a specific diagnosis. Instead, as Hacking has claimed, things can be *both* socially constructed *and* real; this may, in fact, prove to be the case with one or more contested illnesses.

Conclusion

All illnesses, not just those that are contested, are in some general sense socially constructed. Without exception, the meaning and experience of all illness is innately social. In this regard we can speak of the social construction of epilepsy. To be sure, the seizures are real. At the same time, however, the meaning of the seizures (possession vs. disease) and their experience (stigmatized vs. medicalized) is socially contingent. This chapter has emphasized the social construction of illness in a more limited or restricted sense, focusing on the social creation of new biomedical diagnostic categories for human experiences that do not lend themselves to such categorization, with contested illnesses as a case in point. A restricted definition of the social construction of illness gives medical sociologists a powerful expository tool for charting the concrete social forces that promote medicalization. Insofar as laypeople, not the medical profession, demand the medicalization of contested illnesses, the creation of contested-illness categories is paradigmatic of the shifting engines of medicalization (Conrad 2005).

It is important to put the social construction of contested illnesses into larger perspective.

Many widely accepted disorders are also characterized by uncertainties. Many uncontested conditions lack diagnostic precision or are difficult to diagnose (e.g., asthma, osteoarthritis, rheumatoid arthritis); the causal mechanisms of some illnesses are poorly understood or unknown (e.g., lupus, multiple sclerosis, scoliosis, allergies); and many conditions respond poorly or only marginally to medical therapeutics (e.g., Alzheimer's disease, pancreatic cancer). None of these disorders are discredited as biologically unreal on such grounds. Some of these conditions can hardly be in doubt, given that they dramatically and unambiguously manifest themselves in bodily disfigurement or death. But others are neither disfiguring nor deadly. In short, imperfect medical knowledge is ubiquitous to contemporary biomedicine.

One might argue that contested illnesses are but exaggerated or extreme cases of contemporary medicine's inevitable encounter with uncertainty. To a large degree, this can be attributed to the intrinsic difficulties many chronic conditions pose to conventional biomedicine, which proved far more effective in slaying our earlier infectious enemies. But biomedical uncertainty alone is an insufficient explanation. Biomedicine's lack of certitude about contemporary illnesses is also the result of its dealings with an ever-expanding range of complex human distresses. Uncertainty grows as patients and clinicians alike seek to frame multifaceted forms of human suffering within the confines of the conventional biomedical model. That is, uncertainty grows as we push for greater medicalization. Most of us live or will live with a number of long-term afflictions that are medically diffuse and elusive but that nevertheless, negatively and very tangibly, impact the quality of our lives. The creation of contested-illness diagnoses puts into sharp relief our sociocultural response to this larger dilemma, suggesting that we either come to acknowledge and address the normalization of suffering, or expect to see the creation of many new contested-illness diagnoses in the future.

Notes

Some of the material in this chapter appears in Barker 2002, 2005, and 2008.

1. Brown (1995, 34–35) suggests that there are three versions of social constructionism in medical sociology. The first emerges from social problems scholarship that addresses the contingent processes by which specific phenomena come to be identified as social problems. The second version draws on the Focauldian tradition and emphasizes how medical knowledge and discourse give meaning to illness. The third version, aligned with the interdisciplinary field of science studies, argues that the production of scientific facts emerges from everyday social actions and interactions in clinical settings.

2. Given the definition of contested illness, it is possible to consider post-traumatic stress disorder (PTSD) and attention deficit hyperactivity disorder (ADHD) under the rubric of contested illnesses. More generally, many mental illnesses are contested, since sufferers and advocates claim the existence of a biophysical basis for these conditions that is not currently acknowledged by medical experts. In this chapter, contested illnesses are limited to the overlapping conditions referred to as "functional" in the medical literature.

3. The campaign behind chronic fatigue syndrome originated with the claims of two physicians in Lake Tahoe concerning a link between mysterious symptoms and the Epstein-Barr virus. The subsequent path to medicalize CFS, however, was heavily lay forged (Aronowitz 1997; Showalter 1997). Along with other contested environmental illnesses, the emergence of multiple chemical sensitivity disorder also relied overwhelmingly on lay advocacy. The legitimacy of contested environmental illnesses has been further hindered (or at least not advanced) by their association with health professionals practicing in specialties that the American Medical Association does not recognize (e.g., clinical ecology and environmental medicine).

References

Adler, Patricia A., and Peter Adler. 2007. "The Demedicalization of Self-Injury: From Psychopathology to Sociological Deviance." *Journal of Contemporary Ethnography* 36:537–70.

Angell, Marcia. 2004. *The Truth about the Drug Companies*. New York: Random House.

Aronowitz, Robert. 1997. "From Myalgic Encephalitis to Yuppie Flu: A History of Chronic Fatigue Syndrome." In *Framing Disease*, ed. Charles Rosenberg and Janet Golden, 155–81. New Brunswick, N.J.: Rutgers University Press.

Asbring, Pia, and Anna-Liisa Narvanen. 2001. "Chronic Illness—A Disruption in Life: Identity-Transformation among Women with Chronic Fatigue Syndrome and Fibromyalgia." *Journal of Advanced Nursing* 34:312–19.

———. 2003. "Ideal versus Reality: Physicians' Perspectives on Patients with Chronic Fatigue Syndrome (CFS) and Fibromyalgia." *Social Science and Medicine* 57:711–20.

Balint, Michael. 1957. *The Doctor, His Patient and the Illness.* New York: International Universities Press.

Banks, Jonathan, and Lindsay Prior. 2001. "Doing Things with Illness: The Micro Politics of the CFS Clinic." *Social Science and Medicine* 52:11–23.

Barker, Kristin. 1998. "A Ship upon a Stormy Sea: The Medicalization of Pregnancy." *Social Science and Medicine* 47:1067–76.

———. 2002. "Self-Help Literature and the Making of an Illness Identity: The Case of Fibromyalgia Syndrome." *Social Problems* 49:279–300.

———. 2005. *The Fibromyalgia Story: Medical Authority and Women's Worlds of Pain.* Philadelphia: Temple University Press.

———. 2008. "Electronic Support Groups, Patient-Consumers, and Medicalization: The Case of Contested Illness." *Journal of Health and Social Behavior* 49:20–36.

Barsky, Arthur, and Jonathan Borus. 1995. "Somatization and Medicalization in the Era of Managed Care." *Journal of the American Medical Association* 274:1931–34.

———. 1999. "Functional Somatic Syndromes." *Annals of Internal Medicine* 130:910–21.

Berger, Peter, and Thomas Luckmann. 1967. *The Social Construction of Reality: A Treatise in the Sociology of Knowledge.* New York: Anchor.

Blum, Virginia. 2003. *Flesh Wounds: The Culture of Cosmetic Surgery.* Berkeley: University of California Press.

Boghossian, Paul. 2001. "What Is Social Construction?" *Times Literary Supplement,* February.

———. 2006. *Fear of Knowledge: Against Relativism and Constuctivism.* New York: Oxford University Press.

Bohr, T. W. 1995. "Fibromyalgia Syndrome and Myofascial Pain Syndrome: Do They Exist?" *Neurologic Clinics* 13:365–84.

Brown, Phil. 1995. "Naming and Framing: The Social Construction of Diagnosis and Illness." *Journal of Health and Social Behavior,* extra issue: 34–52.

———. 2007. *Toxic Exposures: Contested Illnesses and the Environmental Health Movement.* New York: Columbia University Press.

Brown, Phil, Stephen Zavestoski, Sabrina McCormick, Brian Mayer, Rachel Morello-Frosch, and Rebecca Gesior Altman. 2004. "Embodied Health Movements: New Approaches to Social Movements in Health." *Sociology of Health and Illness* 26:50–80.

Brumberg, Joan Jacobs. 2009. "Anorexia Nervosa in Context." In *The Sociology of Health and Illness:*

Critical Perspectives, 8th ed., ed. Peter Conrad, 107–20. New York: Worth.

Bülow, Pia H. 2008. "Tracing Contours of Contestation in Narratives about Chronic Fatigue Syndrome." In *Contesting Illness: Processes and Practices,* ed. Pamela Moss and Katherine Teghtsoonian, 123–41. Toronto: University of Toronto Press.

Cable, Sherry, Tamara L. Mix, and Thomas E. Shriver. 2008. "Risk Society and Contested Illness: The Case of Nuclear Weapons Workers." *American Sociological Review* 73:380–401.

Casiday, Rachel Elizabeth. 2007. "Children's Health and the Social Theory of Risk: Insights from the British Measles, Mumps and Rubella (MMR) Controversy." *Social Science and Medicine* 65:1059–70.

Clarke, Adele, Laura Mamo, Jennifer R. Fishman, Janet K. Shim, and Jennifer Ruth Fosket. 2003. "Biomedicalization: Technoscientific Transformations of Health, Illness, and U.S. Biomedicine." *American Sociological Review* 68:161–94.

Collins, Patricia Hill. 1991. *Black Feminist Thought: Knowledge, Consciousness, and the Politics of Empowerment.* New York: Routledge.

Copeland, D. A. and Valle, G. 2009. "You Don't Need a Prescription to Go Gluten-Free": The Scientific Self-Diagnosis of Celiac Disease. *Social Science and Medicine* 69:623–31.

Conrad, Peter. 2007. *The Medicalization of Society: On the Transformation of Human Conditions into Treatable Disorders.* Baltimore: Johns Hopkins University Press.

———. 2005. "The Shifting Engines of Medicalization." *Journal of Health and Social Behavior* 46:3–14.

Conrad, Peter, and Joseph W. Schneider. 1992. *Deviance and Medicalization: From Badness to Sickness.* Philadelphia: Temple University Press.

Conrad, Peter, and Cheryl Stults. 2008. "Contestation and Medicalization." In *Contesting Illness: Processes and Practices,* ed. Pamela Moss and Katherine Teghtsoonian, 323–35. Toronto: University of Toronto Press.

da Silva, Luiz Claudio. 2004. "Fibromyalgia: Reflections about Empirical Science and Faith." *Journal of Rheumatology* 31:827–28.

de Beauvoir, Simone. 1989 [1953]. *The Second Sex.* Translated by H. M. Parshley. New York: Knopf.

Dumit, Joseph. 2006. "Illnesses You Have to Fight to Get: Facts and Forces in Uncertain, Emergent Illnesses." *Social Science and Medicine* 62:577–90.

Ehrenreich, Barbara, and Deirdre English. 1973. *Complaints and Disorders: The Sexual Politics of Sickness.* New York: Feminist Press.

Epstein, Steven. 1996. *Impure Science: AIDS, Activism, and the Politics of Knowledge.* Berkeley: University of California Press.

Fillingim, Roger. 2000. *Sex, Gender, and Pain*. Seattle, Wash.: IASP Press.

Fox, Susannah, and Deborah Fallows. 2003. Internet Health Resources. Pew Internet and American Life Project. www.pewinternet.org. Accessed November 26, 2005.

Freidson, Eliot. 1970. *Profession of Medicine: A Study of the Sociology of Applied Knowledge*. New York: Harper and Row.

Hacking, Ian. 1998. *Mad Travelers: Reflections on the Reality of Transient Mental Illnesses*. Charlottesville: University of Virginia Press.

———. 1999. *The Social Construction of What?* Cambridge, Mass.: Harvard University Press.

Hadler, N. M. 1997a. "Fibromyalgia, Chronic Fatigue, and Other Iatrogenic Diagnostic Algorithms. Do Some Labels Escalate Illness in Vulnerable Patients?" *Postgraduate Medicine* 102:262–77.

———. 1997b. "La Maladie Est Morte, Vive le Malade." *Journal of Rheumatology* 24:1250–51.

Hayden, Lars-Christer, and Lisbeth Sacks. 1998. "Suffering, Hope and Diagnosis: On Negotiation of Chronic Fatigue Syndrome." *Health* 2:175–93.

Henningsen, P., S. Zipfel, and W. Herzog. 2007. "Management of Functional Somatic Syndromes." *Lancet* 369:946–55.

Horwitz, Allan V. 2002. *Creating Mental Illness*. Chicago: University of Chicago Press.

Illich, Ivan. 1976. *Medical Nemesis: The Expropriation of Health*. New York: Pantheon.

Kleinman, Arthur. 1988. *The Illness Narratives: Suffering, Healing and the Human Condition*. New York: Basic Books.

Kleinman, Arthur, and Norma C. Ware. 1992. "Culture and Somatic Experience: The Social Course of Illness in Neurasthenia and Chronic Fatigue Syndrome." *Psychosomatic Medicine* 54:546–60.

Knorr Cetina, Karin. 1997. "Sociality with Objects: Social Relations in Postsocial Knowledge Societies." *Theory, Culture and Society* 14:1–30.

Koziol, J. A., D. C. Clark, R. F. Gittes, and E. M. Tan. 1993. "The Natural History of Interstitial Cystitis: A Survey of 374 Patients." *Journal of Urology* 149(3): 465–69.

Kroll-Smith, Steve, Phil Brown, and Valerie J. Gunter. 2000. *Illness and the Environment: A Reader in Contested Medicine*. New York: New York University Press.

Kroll-Smith, Steve, and H. Hugh Floyd. 1997. *Bodies in Protest: Environmental Illness and the Struggle over Medical Knowledge*. New York: New York University Press.

Latour, Bruno. 1987. *Science in Action: How to Follow Scientists and Engineers through Society*. Cambridge, Mass.: Harvard University Press.

Lorber, Judith, and Lisa Jean Moore. 2002. *Gender and the Social Construction of Illness*. 2nd ed. Lanham, Md.: Rowman Altamira.

———. 2007. *Gendered Bodies: Feminist Perspectives*. Los Angeles: Roxbury Publishing.

Mannheim, Karl. 1936. *Ideology and Utopia*. New York: Harcourt, Brace.

Manu, Peter. 2004. *The Psychopathology of Functional Somatic Syndromes*. New York: Haworth Medical Press.

Martin, Emily. 1987. *The Woman in the Body: A Cultural Analysis of Reproduction*. Boston: Beacon Press.

Mayou, Richard, and Andrew Farmer. 2002. "Functional Somatic Symptoms and Syndromes." *British Medical Journal* 325:265–68.

McCrea, Frances. 1983. "The Politics of Menopause: The 'Discovery' of a Deficiency Disease." *Social Problems* 31:111–23.

Merton, Robert. 1973. *The Sociology of Science: Theory and Empirical Investigations*. Chicago: Chicago University Press.

Moss, Pamela, and Katherine Teghtsoonian. 2008. "Power and Illness: Authority, Bodies, and Context." In *Contesting Illness*, ed. Pamela Moss and Katherine Teghtsoonian, 3–27. Toronto: University of Toronto Press.

Moynihan, R., I. Heath, and D. Henry. 2002. "Selling Sickness: The Pharmaceutical Industry and Disease Mongering." *British Medical Journal* 324:886–91.

Nimnuan, Chaichana, Sophia Rabe-Hesketh, Simon Wessley, and Matthew Hotopf. 2001. "How Many Functional Somatic Syndromes." *Journal of Psychosomatic Research* 51:549–57.

Parsons, Talcott. 1951. *The Social System*. Glencoe, Ill.: Free Press.

Pascoe, C. J., and Natalie Boero. 2008. *No Wannarexics Allowed: An Analysis of Pro-Eating Disorder Online Communities*. Typescript.

Peitzman, Steven J. 1992. "From Bright's Disease to End-Stage Renal Disease." In *Framing Disease: Studies in Cultural History*, ed. Charles Rosenberg and Janet Golden, 3–19. New Brunswick, N.J.: Rutgers University Press.

Riessman, Catherine. 1983. "Women and Medicalization: A New Perspective." *Social Policy* 14:3–18.

Searle, John R. 1995. *The Construction of Social Reality*. New York: Free Press.

Shostak, Sara, Peter Conrad, and Allan Horwitz. 2008. "Sequencing and Its Consequences: Path Dependency and the Relationships between Genetics and Medicalization." *American Journal of Sociology* 114:287–316.

Showalter, Elaine. 1997. *Hystories: Hysterical Epidemics*

and Modern Media. New York: Columbia University Press.

Skolbekken, John-Arne. 2008. "Unlimited Medicalization? Risk and the Pathologization of Normality." In *Health Risk and Vulnerability*, ed. Ian Wilkinson, 16–29. New York: Routledge.

Slezak, Peter. 2000. "A Critique of Radical Social Constructionism." In *Constructivism in Education: Opinions and Second Opinions on Controversial Issues*, ed. D. C. Philips, 91–126. Chicago: University of Chicago Press.

Smith, Dorothy. 1987. *The Everyday World as Problematic: A Feminist Sociology*. Boston: Northeastern University Press.

Sokal, Alan. 1996. "Transgressing the Boundaries: Towards a Transformative Hermeneutics of Quantum Gravity." *Social Text* 46/47:217–52.

Starr, Paul. 1982. *The Social Transformation of American Medicine*. New York: Basic Books.

Tesh, Sylvia Noble. 1988. *Hidden Arguments: Political Ideology and Disease Prevention Policy*. New Brunswick, N.J.: Rutgers University Press.

Theriot, Nancy. 1993. "Women's Voices in Nineteenth-Century Medical Discourse: A Step toward Deconstructing Science." *Signs* 19:1–31.

Timmerman, Stefan. 2007. *Postmortem: How Medical Examiners Explain Suspicious Deaths (Fieldwork and Discoveries)*. Chicago: University of Chicago Press.

Tomes, Nancy. 1998. *The Gospel of Germs: Men, Women, and the Microbe in American Life*. Cambridge, Mass.: Harvard University Press.

Wertz, Richard, and Dorothy Wertz. 1979. *Lying-In: A History of Childbirth in America*. New York: Schocken.

Wessley, S. 2004. "There Is Only One Functional Somatic Syndrome: For." *British Journal of Psychiatry* 185:95–96.

Wessley, S., C. Nimnuan, and M. Sharpe. 1999. "Functional Somatic Syndromes: One or Many?" *Lancet* 354:936–39.

Young, Allan. 1995. *The Harmony of Illusions: Inventing Post-Traumatic Stress Disorder*. Princeton, N.J.: Princeton University Press.

Zavestoski, Stephen, Phil Brown, Sabrina McCormick, Brian Mayer, Maryhelen D'Ottavi, and Jamie C. Lucove. 2004a. "Embodied Health Movements and Challenges to the Dominant Epidemiological Paradigm." *Research in Social Movements, Conflicts and Change* 25:253–78.

———. 2004b. "Patient Activism and the Struggle for Diagnosis: Gulf War Illnesses and Other Medically Unexplained Physical Symptoms in the U.S." *Social Science and Medicine* 58:161–75.

Zola, Irving Kenneth. 1972. "Medicine as an Institution of Social Control." *Sociological Review* 20:487–504.

10

The Patient's Experience of Illness

David A. Rier, Bar-Ilan University

What happens when someone gets sick? What is it like to *be* sick? This review considers the patient's experience of illness, broadly defined. Rather than a comprehensive survey, it is a selective look at some of the main contributions of research on the illness experience over the years and, more briefly, certain newer research areas, some suggestions for future research, and an assessment of the field's contributions. Insofar as possible, it emphasizes topics less widely covered in earlier reviews or by other chapters in this volume.[1] Also, given the enormity of the literature, it deals mainly with qualitative research. The topic encompasses illness narratives, but this chapter deals more with content than with format and epistemology, which Bell's (2000) piece in the previous edition of this handbook addressed well.

One way to appreciate how medical sociology has changed in how it understands the experience of illness is to begin with Parsons's (1951) statement of the sick role, which will provide both framework and foil for parts of our discussion. This model involved a pair of duties and a pair of privileges. Specifically, the sick person must recognize that it's bad to be sick and must also seek competent help (i.e., consult a physician) and comply with treatment. The sick are excused from their normal obligations (to family, community, job, etc.), and are also excused from blame for becoming ill. This model helped set the terms of discussion for over a generation but has also sustained varied criticism from subsequent writers, fueling decades of debate (Parsons 1975; Levine and Kozloff 1978; Gallagher 1979; Gerhardt 1989;

Turner 1990; Williams 2005). Relevant to this chapter are criticisms of the model for ignoring self-management, for its paternalism, and for its simplistic conceptualization of time. Most relevant for our purposes is what now seems the glaring absence of the patient's perspective from the model.

This absence of patient perspectives also characterized the first edition of the *Handbook of Medical Sociology* (Freeman, Levine, and Reeder 1963), and subsequent generations of medical sociology textbooks and anthologies, which placed hospitals and physicians squarely at the center. There was little focus on patients beyond their interactions with the medical system, involving such issues as debates over Parsons's sick role, the sick "career," help-seeking behavior, and provider-patient relationships (Twaddle and Hessler 1977; Mechanic 1978; Jaco 1979; Wolinsky 1980; Maykovich 1980). Even in the fourth edition of this handbook (Freeman and Levine 1989), the section headings tell the story: after an introductory section composed of two pieces—"The Present State of Medical Sociology" and "Trends in Death and Disease and the Contribution of Medical Measures"—subsequent pieces were grouped under "Sociological Perspectives in Disease Causation," "The Organization of Health Services," "Use of Health Services," and "Health Care Providers."[2] All this reflects an era in which patients were not directly at the heart of medical sociology, and in which, even when their views were solicited, this was accomplished often through questionnaires designed around topics salient to researchers.

In medicine, too, the patient's perspective has not always received significant attention. Asymmetries in knowledge, status, and authority have traditionally helped doctors control communication with patients and compel patients to function according to the physician's definition of the situation (Anderson and Helm 1979). The physician's definition may differ substantially from that of the patient. According to Kleinman's (1988) distinction between disease and illness, disease is a physiological, clinical entity, which physicians are taught to approach in objective, empirical fashion. Illness, by contrast, is the subjective, lived experience of patients (and their families and perhaps social networks), within the context of their wider existence. It is comprised of elements such as fear, suffering, hope, stigma, support, and shame. Patients often frame their health problems as they subjectively experience them, as part of their lifeworlds. Yet Mishler's fine-grained analyses of patient-doctor communication demonstrated that, when seeing patients, doctors use various techniques, including interruptions, to guide patients into presenting their stories within the "disease" framework of biomedicine. This accords with biomedicine's goal of isolating and quantifying certain discrete, technical parameters for determining diagnosis and treatment. Mishler provides a powerful example of what this can mean in practice. In answer to a doctor's question about how long the patient had been drinking heavily, the patient answered, "Since I've been married." Rather than pursuing this comment as a clue to the patient's drinking problems, the doctor treated it as something of a non sequitur, asking, "How long is that?" (Mishler 1984, 114). As Anderson and Helm and Mishler suggest, doctor-patient communication partly represents a struggle between the voices of the lifeworld and biomedicine.

Mirroring in part a gradual recognition of the value of eliciting patients' perspectives in medicine (Armstrong 1984) and a wider interest in narrative among social scientists (Hydén 1997), contemporary medical sociology has helped reverse the inattention to patients and their perspectives by highlighting the voice and experience of the lifeworld (Rosenfeld 2006, 65). This reflects and contributes to a redirection of interest away from the medical profession to the patient as a focus of inquiry in medical sociology.

Some Highlights of Research on the Experience of Illness

Managing Chronic Illness

The overwhelming majority of research on the illness experience has involved chronic illness. Coping emerged early as a major concern. Strauss (1975), relying largely on sets of ethnographic studies, delineated key aspects of managing chronic illness. For example, he pointed out how coping with the daily regimens (of medication, exercise, therapy, etc.) necessary to preserve function and prevent further declines can take a major portion of one's time and energy and, in some cases, may even become the focal point of life. He described individuals' efforts to "normalize" their lives insofar as the disease allowed. Significantly, he also located problems of chronic illness in their wider policy context, such as when discussing the failure of U.S. communities to design facilities accessible to the chronically ill. Charmaz (1991), with greater use of direct interview data on the personal experience of illness, contributed additional insights. For example, she described trade-offs, compromises necessary in confronting the demands and limitations of the disease while preserving as much as possible of one's pre-illness life. A particularly valuable contribution has been her work on disclosure—the various calculations necessary to decide whether, when, how, and to whom one reveals one's physical condition (Strauss had discussed disclosure and concealment, but more briefly). Such maneuvering can leave the chronically ill maintaining complex webs of truth and lies. Crucially, Charmaz's analysis was also explicitly located within the dimension of time (to which we will return).

Definitions of Illness

Since Parsons (1951) published his original model of the sick role, numerous challenges have arisen. For example, determination of illness and assignment of the sick role are far from simple. Patients may struggle for years in their quest for the validation of an official diagnosis (Stewart and Sullivan 1982).

More recent work has highlighted other facets of the assignment of the sick role. First, there is the phenomenon of contested diseases and symptoms, in which providers and others reject patients' claims to be genuinely ill. Examples include chronic fatigue syndrome and myalgic encephalomyelitis, as well as unexplained constellations of symptoms (Cooper 1997; Nettleton et al. 2004; Sim and Madden 2008). Apart from the pain, loss of function, and other experiences common to various types of illnesses, in these cases patients' difficulty in securing a definitive diagnosis undermines their credibility with health providers and friends and family as well. Even patients themselves may question whether their ailments have psychological, rather than strictly somatic, origins. Back pain is among the most common forms of contested illness; absence of clinically observable signs means patients worry that others regard them as malingerers (Glenton 2005). Though Glenton regards Parsons's model of the sick role as inappropriate to the case of back pain, she observes that patients themselves *do* embrace its expectations, as they seek the legitimation and validation of a medical diagnosis (thus according the medical profession additional power). Indeed, she notes that, unlike most sufferers, for whom a medical diagnosis is generally unpleasant news, those living with back pain often welcome it as conferring a form of "absolution" (2249–50). But living with a contested disease may also politicize patients, causing them to resist (and lose faith in) their physicians. Discussing Gulf War syndrome, Brown and colleagues (2001) demonstrated how issues of contestation can play out against a wider social context of relations between laypersons, scientific expertise, and social activism. In this case, veterans pursued various strategies to legitimate their claims (disputed by government officials) to be suffering from service-related, somatic illnesses "worthy" of compensation. They met with only mixed success. Difficulties included incommensurable paradigms regarding disease criteria and standards of scientific evidence, bureaucratic inertia, and the fact that their claimed maladies

were not readily traceable to specific exposures. A special case of contested disease is the phenomenon of the "worried well," particularly as regards HIV/AIDS. This refers mainly to individuals who, despite not having been diagnosed as HIV+, are convinced that they have been infected with the virus (Lombardo 2004).

Contestation cuts both ways, however. Individuals may resist efforts of professionals and society to label them ill. By 1979, Lorde (1997) was already resisting social pressure to label her, following mastectomy, as disfigured and requiring concealment via prosthetics. Still, she certainly viewed breast cancer as an actual disease. Yet some deaf activists resist the view of deafness as disability, seeing it instead as membership in an alternative "linguistic minority" (Lane 2006). A striking example of resistance is the "pro-ana" movement (especially online), in which those living with anorexia attempt to dissuade others from pursuing recovery (Fox, Ward, and O'Rourke 2005b; Gavin, Rodham, and Poyer 2008).

Second, there is the rich body of work on medicalization (e.g., Conrad and Schneider 1992). Conditions such as hyperactivity, homosexuality, and alcoholism have undergone sociocultural shifts, leading them to be considered, at various times and places, as sins, crimes, diseases, normal, and alternative lifestyle choices. Indeed, medicalization is one segment of a spectrum that can include de- and remedicalization, with given conditions moving in and out of medical frameworks and jurisdictions at different times and places. More recently, Conrad (2007) and others have highlighted how enhancement and augmentation to correct or supplement "normal" attributes have become more popular. Here, too, contemporary research has taken us far beyond Parsons's original formulation, which did not treat the actual determination of disease or illness (hence, patient) status as especially problematic.

The Politics of Patienthood

Parsons defined the patient nearly completely in terms of his or her relationship with physicians. Yet it is now clear that this is far too narrow a model. First, at least for chronic illness, those dealing with illness spend only limited time in direct contact, *as patients*, with the medical system (particularly since hospitalizations have shortened over the past several decades.) Today, much of the illness experience takes place well beyond the doctor-patient relationship. In particular, the community—rather than the hospital or doctor's office—has become the locus of much management, with self-management an important element.

Second, patients themselves have demonstrated a far broader definition of their role. Not relying only on physicians, they rely on themselves, their families, and, via activist networks or online and offline support groups, on each other as well. Nowhere was this made more explicit than with the response to AIDS, where those living with HIV/AIDS engaged in informed critiques of the biomedical establishment's handling of research and policy; they even engaged in the production and dissemination of their own scientific data (Epstein 1996; Indyk and Rier 1993). One aspect of their activism was explicit resistance to the dominant model, which defined them, always, as patients. Consider AIDS activists' 1983 "Denver Principles" manifesto, which included the important statement: "we are only occasionally 'patients,' a term which implies passivity, helplessness, and dependence upon the care of others" (Advisory Committee of People with AIDS, quoted in Callen 1988, 294). By redefining patienthood and renegotiating definitions of expertise, AIDS activists have influenced activists for other diseases, from breast cancer to disability (Epstein 1996; Indyk and Rier 1993). As Prior (2003) shows, however, contemporary medical sociology may exaggerate such trends, sometimes conflating lay experiences with actual biomedical knowledge and expertise.

Internet

One realm in which individuals enact the post-Parsonian patient role, with its scope for much wider patient initiative and involvement, is on the Internet. The Internet arguably constitutes the single greatest change in the experience of illness over the last two decades. First, it is an extremely powerful tool for gaining information about symptoms, diagnosis, and treatment. There are now countless sites maintained by health authorities, universities, and various private and activist entities. There are also numerous sites operated by patients themselves. Often these take the form of support groups, in which those confronting various diseases post questions and comments and view the responses. Unlike traditional face-to-face support groups, participation is not limited to those who can fit in the same room at the same time; instead, membership can be truly global. To an extent Parsons could scarcely have envisioned in 1951, this helps individuals bypass their physicians and affords them wide access to those facing similar issues with whom to trade information and tips. Although it does not guarantee a revolution in doctor-patient relations (Broom 2005), such information empowers participants to question their doctor and form their own opinions about managing their illness (Hardey 1999; Ziebland 2004). Personal home pages become a means for private citizens to produce and disseminate their own information about illness (Hardey 2002).

Electronic groups also provide social and emotional support (Sharf 1997; Bar-Lev 2008). The anonymity they offer helps create an aura of a "safe space" where intimate issues can be discussed without fear of censure or stigma. Members may engage in intricate interactional practices to preserve this environment (Walstrom 2000). Online support groups may also serve as devices for communally debating, crystallizing, and attempting to enforce moral codes (Rier 2007a, b).

As suggested earlier, we may view the medical interview as partly a struggle between the voices of the lifeworld and of biomedicine. Online discussion and support groups, by contrast, are largely free of direct interference from professional and expert authorities (see Connery 1997). We might thus expect these channels to help liberate the traditionally subjugated voice of the lifeworld and create new, alternative types of illness discourses. However, such changes do not necessarily occur. Pitts (2004) has criticized the personal webpages of breast cancer patients for reproducing both biomedical linguistic framing and the wider societal discourse of personal responsibility. Fox, Ward, and O'Rourke (2005a) found, in their study of an online support group for users of a weight-loss drug, that the group helped develop informed patients, but that online discussions replicated biomedical and societal discourses regarding obesity and weight loss. A study of how online HIV/AIDS support groups discussed seropositivity disclosure found that most posts replicated traditional, offline views of moral responsibility (Rier 2007b). Studies of online HIV/AIDS (Bar-Lev 2008) and breast cancer (Sandaunet 2008) support groups found that, while these groups did offer alternative spaces for airing personal concerns and exchanging support, they did not encourage certain "negative," socially undesirable comments.

Apart from what it means for patients, the Internet can influence how researchers study the experience of illness. In her study of agency and empowerment, Pitts (2004) examined webpages of women who confronted breast cancer. The online DIPEx video archive (recently redesigned as healthtalkonline.org) affords researchers the opportunity to conduct secondary analysis of interviews with those (or actors playing them, speaking their words) living with a range of diseases (Ziebland and Herxheimer 2008). The transparency of many online support groups turns them into a fascinating opportunity for researchers to treat them as subject-initiated, floating focus groups in which crystallization of community norms—and their enforcement—can be tracked in real time (Rier 2007a, 244).

Time

Parsons's original model was based on a patient who is healthy, gets sick, seeks medical help, and then gets better. Yet much of the work on the experience of illness points to far more complicated temporal patterns. In fact, the dimension of time pervades research on the experience of illness.

TRAJECTORIES

At least since Roth's (1963) early work on the illness trajectory of hospital patients, and Davis's ([1963] 1991) study of the various stages through which families pass when a child contracts po-

lio, the time dimension has been a part of social science work on the illness experience. Strauss (1975, 47) noted, regarding chronic illness, that trajectories "may plunge straight down; move slowly but steadily downward; vacillate slowly, moving slightly up and down before diving downward radically; move slowly down at first, then hit a long plateau, then plunge abruptly, even to death." Charmaz (1991) devoted considerable attention to the dimension of time. She described how patients may subjectively experience illness: as interruption, intrusion, or immersion. Soon after onset, patients often viewed the illness as an interruption in the normal flow of their lives. They expect recovery and, as in Parsons's sick role, resumption of prior roles and identities. Often, however, patients came to experience their illness as a chronic, demanding intrusion requiring significant attention and trade-offs to manage their regimens, debilities, and other disruptions, while also trying to preserve as much day-to-day life as possible. More advanced, serious illness might lead to immersion, as the disease consumes more and more of one's daily life.

Yoshida (1993) contributed substantially to our grasp of the types of identity threat and reconstruction that can occur after disabling injury and how these unfold over time. Yoshida's mostly young respondents had experienced traumatic spinal cord injury. Though discussions of the illness trajectory had invariably portrayed it in linear fashion, Yoshida found that it described a pendular pattern. Specifically, these individuals oscillated between their "baseline" (preaccident) healthy, "whole" identity and the physically diminished, highly dependent self of their postaccident lives. Over time, the swings between these poles diminished, as the individuals settled into a middle ground in which they refashioned their identity to accommodate their disability without surrendering to it.

ILLNESS STATES

Questions of time also bear directly upon the definitions of illness states. For example, there is the increasing significance of the "preemptive" or "preliminary" sick role. For Parsons, the sick role effectively commenced with manifestation of physical restrictions on fulfilling normal roles.

Yet this is no longer true. By the 1980s, many confused testing seropositive for the HIV virus with being sick, triggering such risks as fear and stigma (Sontag 1990a, 120–21)—despite the fact that HIV+ individuals might not develop AIDS for years, if ever. The burdens of genetic testing provide another example. Cox and McKellin (1999) showed how healthy people known to be at risk for Huntington's disease apply a variety of subjective mental devices to decide whether to seek testing. Women with family risk of breast and ovarian cancer, even before the appearance of clinical signs of disease or definitive results of genetic testing, may regard themselves as bearing special responsibilities, particularly to their families. This can lead to phenomena such as high-risk women, with no evidence of actually having cancer, choosing elective, prophylactic mastectomy. Often, this choice involves complex feelings about their duties to their families, including questions of disclosure, such as to unmarried daughters (Hallowell 1999). The case of Machado-Joseph disease shows there may be feelings of guilt and responsibility among family members even when no genetic test exists (Boutte 1990). However, as genetic tests become increasingly available, these experiences will grow more common. Knowing one's genetic fate may be a mixed blessing, particularly in the absence of effective prevention or therapy (Kenen 1996). More recently, Arribas-Ayllon, Sarangi, and Clarke (2008) have detailed the dilemmas parents face regarding assuming or attributing responsibility for disclosing their children's genetic test results. A corollary category, resembling somewhat the experience of living with genetic risk, involves those receiving early detection of slow-moving cancers, such as prostate cancer (Oliffe et al. 2009). Such individuals confront not only existential uncertainty about their future, but also substantial clinical uncertainty about whether active management or "watchful waiting" is appropriate.

Time is also bound up with definitions of illness at the other end of the illness trajectory: the issue of resolution. Although in Parsons's model the patient simply seeks treatment, complies, and is cured, achieving such closure in practice is far from simple. With cancer, for example, even after passing the technical five-year survival milestone,

former patients still face the possibility that their apparent cure is merely a remission, subject to recurrence. Physicians often have great difficulty in answering such questions as, "What are my odds, Doc?" or "How much time have I got?" (Christakis 1999). Describing his status after treatment (including bone marrow transplantation) for his rare blood disorder, patient/physician Biro spoke for many: "My story is far from over. Questions remain. . . . Will my disease return . . . ? No answers. . . . Cure? Depends on what you mean, who you ask. In my book, no. I will always remain a patient" (Biro 2000, 286).

REMISSION, LIMINALITY, SURVIVAL

Indeed, Frank ([1991] 2002, 138–39) has written famously of a "remission society." Thanks to medical advances, it is inhabited by a growing number of people whose experiences of serious illness place them in a "chronically critical," indeterminate state between health and illness. Building partly on van Gennep's work on rites of passage, Miles Little and his colleagues (1998) formulated the concept of liminality as crucial for understanding this aspect of the illness experience. It highlights how disease removes individuals from their prior life but often, *contra* Parsons, the complete return to that life is far from seamless, or even impossible. Anthropologist Robert Murphy (1990, 131) claimed that the disabled spend their entire lives in the liminal stage. Experiencing chronic illness, or surviving a severe illness, places someone forever on a spectrum between, in Sontag's (1990b, 3) classic terms, the kingdom of the sick and the kingdom of the well. Following Bellaby (1995), we might regard the case of severe head trauma as involving double liminality: many such patients are young males who were already "liminal," located between adolescence and adulthood; then the accident removed them from their prior status while leaving uncertain their future status.

Beyond remission and liminality, there remains much to learn about what happens "after" illness. Thomas (2004, 13) observed that medical sociology has devoted scant attention to recovery and reengagement with pre-illness roles and identities. Since then, Ville (2005) has explored how those surviving severe spinal cord damage gradually confront the possibility of returning to work. Janet Parsons and her colleagues showed that, for young cancer patients, reentry to their normal social roles of completing their education and establishing their careers is complicated by the need to attend also to their disease and to the reconstruction and repair of their identities (Parsons et al. 2008).

HIV/AIDS disease in the current era of effective antiretroviral therapy is a particularly interesting site for examining reentry. By the late 1990s, the "Lazarus Syndrome" (Trainor and Ezer 2000) had been noted, in which those literally near the brink of death experienced seemingly miraculous recoveries. Their being, in Dickens's phrase, "recalled to life" challenged them to rebuild and reconstitute relationships, jobs, and other elements of their lives to which they had already bade farewell. Later, awareness of toxicity and other problems with the AIDS cocktails demonstrated that even patients who have entered what is sometimes considered a type of remission might face severe medical problems. As one informant remarked about the difficulties others had in grasping his fluid health status: "They wouldn't dream that I have AIDS and that I'm attached to an IV pole once a week . . . and yet it's true, and both realities are true: The Thursday afternoons at the gym is true, and the Wednesday afternoons at the clinic is true" (ibid., 652). Significantly, each of the seven respondents in Trainor and Ezer's study reported that adjusting to their new situation was more difficult than when they had been dying; in the latter instance, they at least had a clearly defined social role to play.

Frank (1995) has examined survival as project, in explicitly moral terms, such as the obligation to bear witness. He has likened survival to craft work, documenting two very different socially constructed templates through which survivors might define what their illness experience implies for their subsequent lives (Frank 2003). According to the narrative of extensive responsibility, survivors see their experience as imposing some duty, essentially a calling, on them. This might involve engaging in activism, providing support, or simply bearing witness. By contrast, the narrative of limited liability regards the illness as an obstacle to be surmounted and then left behind.

Looking at cancer survivors, Kaiser (2008) used interviews with women who had completed breast cancer treatment to show how the "breast cancer culture" influenced cultural scripts and expectations, and how women sometimes resisted these expectations and even the survivor identity itself. Some defined themselves as survivors not because they thought they actually had beaten cancer, which they believed could always recur, but because they had fought the disease as best they could. Also, even Kaiser's "relatively homogenous" sample of women interviewed at similar stages of breast cancer survival varied substantially among themselves in how they understood survival (86).

This work suggests that the post-illness phase merits closer attention. Future studies could compare what survival and recovery mean across disease, age, sex, ethnic, class, and cultural categories, and how these definitions change over time. Reminding us that some patients actually do get better, just as Parsons's model assumed, Thomas (2004) has proposed a sociology of recovery which, on the microsociological level, would explore such areas as physical and psychological restoration and exiting the patient role.

SOME METHODOLOGICAL IMPLICATIONS

Another significant point about time is methodological. Pierret (2001, 2007) and Trainor and Ezer (2000) have demonstrated the value of returning to the field at various time intervals. Such long-range perspectives are particularly important for understanding the experiences of illnesses that are rapidly moving targets, such as HIV/AIDS. Indeed, Baumgartner (2007) has recently shown how identity shifted across three time points over a period of almost five years. Though this range was not particularly large, it coincided with the introduction of antiretroviral treatment that helped redefine AIDS from terminal to chronic illness. However, there has not been enough of such work, presumably because of logistic difficulties such as deadline pressure and limited budgets.

Not only is it valuable to collect data at different points over a patient's illness experience, it can be most fruitful to *analyze* data at different points in a researcher's career. Riessman (1990) detailed the rhetorical strategies of impression management employed by a man suffering from multiple sclerosis to present himself either as successful or as mostly blameless for a life that was (by most objective measures) in profound disarray. Over a decade later, Riessman (2003) published a follow-up piece in which she returned to this man's story, pointing out several ways in which her initial "reading" had evolved since she had originally analyzed it, several years before publishing the first article. In this newer reading, she located his story within the wider context of contemporary disability politics and a critique of market capitalism. These perspectives helped her understand his social isolation as an unemployed disabled man. Surely, many studies would yield new insights if investigators returned to their data at various points in their intellectual development, political awareness, and ideological orientations. This point mirrors an insight about patients' narrative recounting over time encapsulated in Gareth Williams's (1984, 179) citation of R. G. Collingwood's observation that "every present has a past of its own."

Newer Topics of Interest

The previous section presented highlights of research on the patient's experience of illness. This section focuses specifically on two types of diseases to which this literature has only recently begun to attend.

Alzheimer's

The perspectives of Alzheimer's patients were long ignored in the literature (MacRae 2008, 397; Beard and Fox 2008, 1510). Traditionally, senile dementia has been regarded as a form of social death, as Sweeting and Gilhooly's (1997) research on family caretakers of such individuals illustrated. Yet the Alzheimer's patients Snyder (1999) interviewed were often able to articulate the accretion of losses—of memory, of independence, of identity, of social ties—that their condition brought in its wake. One declared, "I want to cry and whine and kick!" (71). In describing her situation, an-

other offered one of the most arresting remarks in the entire literature on the illness experience: "You aren't you anymore" (62). As Charmaz had noted about the chronically ill, persons living with Alzheimer's often must fight to preserve as much of their original routines as possible. For—though the popular image is dominated by latter stages of the disease, in which people may not recognize even close family—Snyder's informants remind us that declines can be gradual. Such Alzheimer's patients occupy a liminal stage in which they remain aware enough to recognize and describe what is happening, and integrated enough into their pre-disease roles, networks, and identities to be able to mourn their losses.

Subsequent work has confirmed the ability of Alzheimer's patients movingly to describe their inner and social worlds (Clare 2003), even when already confined to institutions (Clare et al. 2008). MacRae (2008) demonstrated how such early-stage Alzheimer's patients—much like the disabled discussed in Lutz and Bowers (2005)—resist stereotypical constructions of their situation as devastated victims, and employ numerous coping mechanisms to preserve their identities and manage others' perceptions of them. These include such techniques as positive thinking, humor, cultivating hope, preemptive disclosure, and normalization (in which patients attempt to integrate their disease into their daily lives). Beard and Fox (2008) showed how, beyond resisting dominant constructions, Alzheimer's patients can manipulate their diagnosis, using it as a resource for managing their condition. Beard and Fox also examined how support groups shape the illness experience, in this case by discussing how these groups influenced constructions of illness identities. Medical advances in earlier detection present the possibility of additional research into the subjective experience of dementia, since the illness trajectory has effectively been extended backward in time to a period in which those affected remain articulate and reflective.

Mental Illness

Another example of interesting new work in previously neglected areas is research into the experience of mental illness (Kangas 2001). Karp (1996, 11) has observed that when he first began writing on depression, the existing literature contained the voices of countless experts but never those of the depressed themselves. Based on interviews with a diverse sample of individuals with depression, Karp's sociologically grounded analysis explored topics such as the threat to one's identity, the web of family and friends who may attempt to lend emotional support and instrumental assistance, and the range of coping strategies employed to negotiate daily life. Karp attempted to link the growing prevalence of depression in the United States to wider structural and sociocultural trends. These included: a "therapeutic," self-help culture, postmodern social alienation, postindustrial economic dislocation and loss of valued identities, and consumerism that converts happiness (and other emotions) into marketable commodities.

Kangas (2001) examined lay sense making and attribution among the depressed. Emslie and her colleagues (2006) discussed how depressed men attempted to preserve or reconstruct their masculine identities as part of recovery. Pollock (2007) detailed how, during doctor visits, her sample of depressed individuals engaged in face-saving strategies that could undermine their treatment by leading them to deny the extent of their illness, including in response to their doctors' queries. Often, patients feared to drop their "masks" of normalcy and admit to their illness. Sometimes, however, they were attempting to protect the doctor from the time and bother of confronting a difficult problem, and so concealed it. More generally, according to Pollock, these patients attempted to make the visit proceed smoothly, as a social encounter; they felt that admitting the extent of their depression would spoil this interaction. Such practices, Pollock concluded, impeded treatment.

Despite the existence of research on depression, the sociological literature includes less material on other forms of mental illness. Among the limited body of work not specifically dealing with depression, Crossley and Crossley (2001) cleverly documented changes over time in how persons diagnosed as mentally ill constructed their identity. They compared narratives published in two

anthologies, *The Plea for the Silent* (published in 1957) and *Speaking Our Minds* (published in 1996). These titles alone eloquently attest to significant changes. Similarly, Cresswell (2005) has described how those suffering from "self-harm" came to define themselves as "survivors"—not of mental illness, but of psychiatric *treatment*— and began to practice a form of self-advocacy that asserted their right to voice their views. They resisted or rejected certain professional and societal labels, and offered alternative "truth-claims" grounded in their personal experiences, which Cresswell defined as "testimony." Lester and Tritter (2005) conducted focus groups with those experiencing schizophrenia, depression, and other significant mental problems. Participants described such difficulties as service access, unemployment, medication side effects, and social isolation. Many wished to volunteer to help others navigate services. Most recently, Moses (2009) used a mixed-method approach, including semi-structured interviews, to explore how adolescents receiving mental health services related to mental illness labels. Most were either unsure whether, or denied that, they were mentally ill; some moved in and out of accepting this identity. Only one-fifth clearly accepted this label.

Despite such studies, we still know comparatively little about the experience even of such common conditions as schizophrenia and phobia. Additional research is needed to examine more fully such questions as: How does society label and stigmatize the mentally ill? How do they manage their disease across its particular trajectory? Do they attempt to resist their diagnosis and its attendant stigma? If so, how successfully? How do these patterns vary by gender, class, and ethnicity?

Uncharted Territory: Critical Illness

The existing sociological literature on the illness experience has focused on chronic (Bell 2000) rather than on acute (Faircloth et al. 2004; Rosenfeld 2006) and critical (Rier 2000) illness. Sociological (Zussman 1992) and anthropological (Cassell 2005; Kaufman 2005) ethnographies have explored the intensive care unit (ICU). But

Zussman and Cassel related to patients only as passive objects, while Kaufman emphasized end-of-life decisions rather than patients' experiences.

First-person, nonacademic accounts (Simpson 1982; Baier and Schomaker [1986] 1995; Bauby 1997) have shed some light on patients' experiences of critical illness. The latter two works deserve special mention for opening up new worlds in our understanding. The authors were both paralyzed and ventilator dependent; they communicated and dictated their thoughts by blinking their eyes. Perhaps their single greatest contribution lies in their having revealed what even many ICU staff may not recognize: that such patients, despite their dire physical condition, retained awareness, hopes, dreams—in short, an inner life. Simpson wrote wisely about the cultivation of hope, and how this might require lying to critically ill patients (32, 108, 116).

Yet, with such limited exceptions as first-hand accounts (Robillard 1994; Richman 2000; Rier 2000), the sociology literature says little about the experiences of the critically ill (Rier 2000, 2008). Therefore, debates over such questions as autonomy, paternalism, empowerment, and disclosure of information to patients take place with little input from patients themselves (Rier 2000, 2008). In particular, critical illness still awaits its Strauss (1975) and Charmaz (1991), who bequeathed to students of chronic illness a magnificent set of conceptual tools for their work. One major difference between most chronic illness and critical illness is that, whereas the former typically involves the struggle to integrate illness into the routines of one's daily life, critical illness is likelier to *replace* one's existing life (Rier 2000, 72) in a more advanced form of the "immersion" (Charmaz 1991) described earlier.

A major reason for the lack of focus on the ICU patient experience is the significant methodological difficulty in studying these patients. ICUs have high mortality rates, many survivors are too weak to be interviewed, and many remember very little of their experiences, particularly given the heavy sedation they often received. One attempt to address such limitations comes from the nursing/critical care literatures, where researchers have interviewed ICU patients about their experiences (e.g., Granberg, Engberg, and Lundberg 1998; Johnson 2004; Magarey and McCutcheon 2005; Karlsson and Forsberg 2008). This work has yielded important insights into elements of the experience, such as dreams, fears, and feelings of helplessness. However, such studies have typically been based on small samples.

Some studies (e.g., Bergbom et al. 1999; Bäckman and Walther 2001; Combe 2005; Egerod and Christensen 2009; Egerod et al. 2007; Roulin, Hurst, and Spirig 2007) have used ICU "diaries," summaries of daily events in the ICU written by nurses and family on behalf of and for the patient, not by the patient. Such texts clearly help former patients make sense of their time in the ICU. Yet, authored by others, these top-down diaries cannot necessarily help patients recapture their inner world or restore their voice; neither can they really help us understand what such patients experience. Therefore, Rier (2000) has proposed a method of offering nonvocal patients the chance to write as a means of communication while in the ICU, then using this writing as a memory aid for postdischarge interviews.[3]

That so few studies of the ICU patient experience engage with the rich medical sociology literature leaves much work for sociologists. For example, the contemporary, post-Parsonian discourse of patient empowerment may not be relevant to the high dependency of the ICU (Rier 2000). Among other areas for research are gender (which existing studies of the critical illness experience rarely address) and the timing and extent of disclosure of information to ICU patients. Another area arises from the fact that, partly as a means of controlling infection, newer ICUs often have individual patient rooms. Little is known about how such ecological changes in the ICU affect patients.

Conclusion

Over the past generation or so, the patient has emerged as a focus of medical sociology research, joining providers, hospitals, and health systems. Studying patients' experiences has taught us much about how body, self, and society interact. This includes such specific topics as: identity; support; how patients integrate their illness into daily routines and family, community, and work lives; how patients resist or negotiate professional authority, societal labels, and sociocultural expectations; moral dilemmas; and how the illness experience develops over time. It is interesting to speculate, How might Parsons's sick-role model have looked, had his generation already produced a substantial body of research on patient experiences?

Research on patient experiences also allows physicians to transcend blood gases and x-rays, teaching them about pain, loneliness, dread— but also hope, dreams, courage. It underscores the humanity and agency of disabled, demented, and mentally, critically, and terminally ill persons. Clinicians are learning to apply illness narratives to improve how they communicate with, support, and treat their patients (Charon 2006; Overcash 2003). Such research is also a tool for medical education (Childress 2002) and bioethics (Charon and Montello 2002). Without understanding the meanings patients give to central elements of their experiences such as pain, fear of death, guilt, and quality of life, clinicians and bioethicists may be reduced to guessing patients' needs. Clinicians are currently developing illness narratives as a form of evidence-based medicine (Charon and Wyer 2008), treating them as one source of data, alongside more traditional sources such as randomized clinical trials, for improving clinical decision making.

Yet so much remains undone. Recovery (i.e., actually getting better) has received insufficient attention. Immense work remains in understanding different forms of mental illness. Sociological research on the patient's critical illness experience has barely begun. Also, if physicians must look beyond their biomedical measures to the wider psychosocial context, social scientists must look beyond the psychosocial context to attend to the body and its pathology as direct influences on the illness experience (Timmermans and Haas 2008). Research on illness trajectories does typically correlate experience with disease stage. Yet sociological writing too often brackets off the actual physical disease, ignoring the proverbial elephant in the room in an attempt to highlight purely social aspects of illness. Taking the body seriously, for example, would provide a useful counterweight to radical critiques of disability as a purely social construct (Bury 2000). Methodologically,

moreover, it is sloppy to interview, say, dozens of cancer patients without careful attention to, not just age or sex, but also disease stage, symptoms, and side effects. Despite various obstacles to gaining access to clinical charts, correlating biomedical status with lifeworld experience can yield rich benefits. In fact, perhaps the disease/illness distinction has by now been overstated.

Still, research on the illness experience is flourishing. It is a large, lively, diverse field. Thus, there is ample reason to expect that it will continue to illuminate new areas of the illness experience, generating insights for social science, health practice and policy, and beyond.

Notes

The author gratefully acknowledges his conversations with Miles Little and Hilary Thomas, and the editorial advice of Stefan Timmermans.

1. There exist numerous social science reviews of the large body of literature on the illness experience. Bury (1991) and Charmaz (2000) focused on chronic illness. Frank (1995), Hydén (1997), and Bell (2000) reviewed the narrative recounting of such experiences. Anthropologists Kleinman and Seeman (2000) located the illness experience within a socially and politically critical framework. Lawton (2003) and Pierret (2003) focused specifically on material published in the first quarter-century of the journal *Sociology of Health and Illness*.

2. However, the fifth edition of this handbook (Bird, Conrad, and Fremont 2000) included Bell's chapter on illness narratives plus Bury's theoretical chapter on chronic illness and disability. Also, the third edition of Graham Scambler's (1991) medical sociology text already included Locker's chapter on living with chronic illness.

3. Development of this technique parallels use of a set of techniques described in recent studies employing photography as a means through which the sick can capture and reconstruct their experiences and narrate their own stories (Bell 2002; Radley and Taylor 2003a, b; Oliffe and Bottorff 2007; Frith and Harcourt 2007).

References

Anderson, W. Timothy, and David T. Helm. 1979. "The Physician-Patient Encounter: A Process of Reality Negotiation." In *Patients, Physicians, and Illness*, 3rd ed., ed. E. Gartly Jaco, 259–71. New York: Free Press.

Armstrong, David. 1984. "The Patient's View." *Social Science and Medicine* 18(9): 737–44.

Arribas-Ayllon, Michael, Srikant Sarangi, and Angus Clarke. 2008. "Managing Self-Responsibility through Other-Oriented Blame: Family Accounts of Genetic Testing." *Social Science and Medicine* 66(7): 1521–32.

Bäckman, C. G., and S. M. Walther. 2001. "Use of a Personal Diary Written on the ICU during Critical Illness." *Intensive Care Medicine* 27(2): 426–29.

Baier, Sue, and Mary Z. Schomaker. [1986] 1995. *Bed Number Ten*. Reprint. Boca Raton, Fla.: CRC Press.

Bar-Lev, Shirly. 2008. "'We Are Here to Give You Emotional Support': Performing Emotions in an Online HIV/AIDS Support Group." *Qualitative Health Research* 18(4): 509–21.

Bauby, Jean-Dominique. 1997. *The Diving-Bell and the Butterfly*. Translated by Jeremy Leggatt. New York: Vintage.

Baumgartner, Lisa M. 2007. "The Incorporation of the HIV/AIDS Identity into the Self over Time." *Qualitative Health Research* 17(7): 919–31.

Beard, Renee L., and Patrick J. Fox. 2008. "Resisting Social Disenfranchisement: Negotiating Collective Identities and Everyday Life with Memory Loss." *Social Science and Medicine* 66(7): 1509–20.

Bell, Susan, 2000. "Experiencing Illness in/and Narrative." In *Handbook of Medical Sociology*, 5th ed., ed. Chloe E. Bird, Peter Conrad, and Allen M. Fremont, 184–99. Upper Saddle River, N.J.: Prentice Hall.

———. 2002. "Photo Images: Jo Spence's Narratives of Living with Illness." *Health* 6(1): 5–30.

Bellaby, Paul. 1995. "The World of Illness of the Closed Head Injured." In *Worlds of Illness: Biographical and Cultural Perspectives on Health and Disease*, ed. Alan Radley, 161–78. London: Routledge.

Bergbom, Ingegerd, Carina Svensson, Elisabeth Berggren, and Marie Kamsula. 1999. "Patients' and Relatives' Opinions and Feelings about Diaries Kept by Nurses in an Intensive Care Unit: Pilot Study." *Intensive and Critical Care Nursing* 15(4): 185–91.

Bird, Chloe E., Peter Conrad, and Allen M. Fremont, eds. 2000. *Handbook of Medical Sociology*. 5th ed. Upper Saddle River, N.J.: Prentice Hall.

Biro, David. 2000. *One Hundred Days: My Unexpected Journey from Doctor to Patient*. New York: Pantheon.

Boutte, Marie I. 1990. "Waiting for the Family Legacy: The Experience of Being at Risk for Machado-Joseph Disease." *Social Science and Medicine* 30(8): 839–47.

Broom, Alex. 2005. "Virtually He@lthy: Impact of Internet Use on Disease Experience and the Doctor-Patient Experience." *Qualitative Health Research* 15(3): 324–45.

Brown, Phil, Stephen Zavetoski, Sabrina McCormick,

Meadow Linder, Joshua Mandelbaum, and Theo Luebke. 2001. "A Gulf of Difference: Disputes over Gulf War–Related Illnesses." *Journal of Health and Social Behavior* 42(3): 235–257.

Bury, Mike. 1991. "The Sociology of Chronic Illness: A Review of Research and Prospects." *Sociology of Health and Illness* 13(4): 451–68.

———. 2000. "On Chronic Illness and Disability." In *Handbook of Medical Sociology*, 5th ed., ed. Chloe E. Bird, Peter Conrad, and Allen M. Fremont, 173–83. Upper Saddle River, N.J.: Prentice Hall.

Callen, Michael, ed. 1988. *Collected Wisdom*. Vol. 2 of *Surviving and Thriving with AIDS*. New York: People with AIDS Coalition.

Cassell, Joan. 2005. *Life and Death in Intensive Care*. Philadelphia: Temple University Press.

Charmaz, Kathy. 1991. *Good Days, Bad Days: The Self in Chronic Illness and Time*. New Brunswick, N.J.: Rutgers University Press.

———. 2000. "Experiencing Chronic Illness." In *The Handbook of Social Studies in Health and Medicine*, ed. Gary L. Albrecht, Roy Fitzpatrick, and Susan C. Scrimshaw, 277–92. London: Sage.

Charon, Rita. 2006. *Narrative Medicine: Honoring the Stories of Illness*. Oxford: Oxford University Press.

Charon, Rita, and Martha Montello, eds. 2002. *Stories Matter: The Role of Narrative in Medical Ethics*. London: Routledge.

Charon, Rita, and Peter Wyer [for the NEBM Working Group]. 2008. "Narrative Evidence Based Medicine." *Lancet* 371(9609): 296–97.

Childress, Marcia D. 2002. "Of Symbols and Silence: Using Narrative and Its Interpretation to Foster Physician Understanding." In *Stories Matter: The Role of Narrative in Medical Ethics*, ed. Rita Charon and Martha Montello, 119–25. London: Routledge.

Christakis, Nicholas A. 1999. *Death Foretold: Prophecy and Prognosis in Medical Care*. Chicago: University of Chicago Press.

Clare, Linda. 2003. "Managing Threats to Self: Awareness in Early-Stage Alzheimer's Disease." *Social Science and Medicine* 57(6): 1017–29.

Clare, Linda, Julia Rowlands, Errollyn Bruce, Claire Surr, and Murna Downs. 2008. "'I Don't Do Like I Used to Do': A Grounded Theory Approach to Conceptualising Awareness in People with Moderate to Severe Dementia Living in Long-Term Care." *Social Science and Medicine* 66(11): 2366–77.

Combe, Denise. 2005. "The Use of Patient Diaries in an Intensive Care Unit." *Nursing in Critical Care* 10(1): 31–34.

Connery, Brian A. 1997. "IMHO: Authority and Egalitarian Rhetoric in the Virtual Coffeehouse." In *Internet Culture*, ed. David Porter, 161–79. New York: Routledge.

Conrad, Peter. 2007. *The Medicalization of Society: On the Transformation of Human Conditions into Treatable Disorders*. Baltimore: Johns Hopkins University Press.

Conrad, Peter, and Joseph W. Schneider. 1992. *Deviance and Medicalization: From Badness to Sickness*. 2nd ed. Philadelphia: Temple University Press.

Cooper, Lesley. 1997. "Myalgic Encephalomyelitis and the Medical Encounter." *Sociology of Health and Illness* 19(2): 186–207.

Cox, Susan M., and William McKellin. 1999. "'There's This Thing in Our Family': Predictive Testing and the Construction of Risk for Huntington Disease." *Sociology of Health and Illness* 21(5): 622–46.

Cresswell, Mark. 2005. "Psychiatric 'Survivors' and Testimonies of Self-Harm." *Social Science and Medicine* 61(8): 1668–77.

Crossley, Michelle L., and Nick Crossley. 2001. "'Patient' Voices, Social Movements and the Habitus: How Psychiatric Survivors 'Speak Out.'" *Social Science and Medicine* 52(2): 1477–89.

Davis, Fred. [1963] 1991. *Passage through Crisis: Polio Victims and their Families*. Reprint. New Brunswick, N.J.: Transaction.

Egerod, Ingrid, and Doris Christensen. 2009. "Analysis of Patient Diaries in Danish ICUs: A Narrative Approach." *Intensive and Critical Care Nursing* 25(5): 268–77.

Egerod, Ingrid, Kathrine H. Schwartz-Nielsen, Glennie M. Hansen, and Eva Laerkner. 2007. "The Extent and Application of Patient Diaries in Danish ICUs in 2006." *Nursing in Critical Care* 12(3): 159–67.

Emslie, Carol, Damien Ridge, Sue Ziebland, and Kate Hunt. 2006. "Men's Accounts of Depression: Reconstructing or Resisting Hegemonic Masculinity?" *Social Science and Medicine* 62(9): 2246–57.

Epstein, Steven. 1996. *Impure Science: AIDS, Activism, and the Politics of Knowledge*. Berkeley: University of California Press.

Faircloth, Chris A., Craig Boylstein, Maude Rittman, Mary E. Young, and Jaber Gubrium. 2004. "Sudden Illness and Biographical Flow in Narratives of Stroke Recovery." *Sociology of Health and Illness* 26(2): 242–61.

Fox, Nick, Katie Ward, and Alan O'Rourke. 2005a. "The 'Expert Patient': Empowerment or Medical Dominance? The Case of Weight Loss, Pharmaceutical Drugs and the Internet." *Social Science and Medicine* 60(6): 1299–1309.

———. 2005b. "Pro-anorexia, Weight-Loss Drugs and the Internet: An 'Anti-Recovery' Explanatory Model of Anorexia." *Sociology of Health and Illness* 27(7): 944–71.

Frank, Arthur W. 1995. *The Wounded Storyteller: Body, Illness, and Ethics*. Chicago: University of Chicago Press.

———. [1991] 2002. *At the Will of the Body: Reflections on Illness*. Reprint. Boston: Houghton Mifflin.

———. 2003. "Survivorship as Craft and Conviction: Reflections on Research in Progress." *Qualitative Health Research* 13(2): 247–55.

Freeman, Howard E., and Sol Levine. 1989. *Handbook of Medical Sociology*. 4th ed. Englewood Cliffs, N.J.: Prentice Hall.

Freeman, Howard E., Sol Levine, and Leo G. Reeder. 1963. *Handbook of Medical Sociology*. Englewood Cliffs, N.J.: Prentice Hall.

Frith, Hannah, and Diana Harcourt. 2007. "Using Photographs to Capture Women's Experiences of Chemotherapy: Reflecting on the Method." *Qualitative Health Research* 17(10): 1340–50.

Gallagher, Eugene B. 1979. "Lines of Reconstruction and Extension in the Parsonian Sociology of Illness." In *Patients, Physicians, and Illness*, 3rd ed., ed. E. Gartly Jaco, 162–83. New York: Free Press.

Gavin, Jeff, Karen Rodham, and Helen Poyer. 2008. "The Presentation of 'Pro-Anorexia' in Online Group Interactions." *Qualitative Health Research* 18(3): 325–33.

Gerhardt, Uta. 1989. *Ideas about Illness: An Intellectual and Political History of Medical Sociology*. New York: New York University Press.

Glenton, Claire. 2005. "Chronic Back Pain Sufferers: Striving for the Sick Role." *Social Science and Medicine* 57(11): 2243–52.

Granberg, Anetth, Ingegerd Bergbom Engberg, and Dag Lundberg. 1998. "Patients' Experience of Being Critically Ill or Severely Injured and Cared for in an Intensive Care Unit in Relation to the ICU Syndrome. Part 1." *Intensive and Critical Care Nursing* 14(6): 294–307.

Hallowell, Nina. 1999. "Doing the Right Thing: Genetic Risk and Responsibility." *Sociology of Health and Illness* 21(5): 597–621.

Hardey, Michael. 1999. "Doctor in the House: The Internet as a Source of Lay Health Knowledge and the Challenge to Expertise." *Sociology of Health and Illness* 21(6): 820–35.

———. 2002. "'The Story of My Illness': Personal Accounts of Illness on the Internet." *Health* 6(1): 31–46.

Hydén, Lars-Christer. 1997. "Illness and Narrative." *Sociology of Health and Illness* 19(1): 48–69.

Indyk, Debbie, and David A. Rier. 1993. "Grassroots AIDS Knowledge: Implications for the Boundaries of Science and Collective Action." *Knowledge: Creation, Diffusion, Utilization* 15(1): 3–43.

Jaco, E. Gartly, ed. 1979. *Patients, Physicians, and Illness*. 3rd ed. New York: Free Press.

Johnson, Patricia. 2004. "Reclaiming the Everyday World: How Long-Term Ventilated Patients in Critical Care Seek to Gain Aspects of Power and Control over Their Environment." *Intensive and Critical Care Nursing* 20(4): 190–99.

Kaiser, Karen. 2008. "The Meaning of the Survivor Identity for Women with Breast Cancer." *Social Science and Medicine* 67(1): 79–87.

Kangas, Ilka. 2001. "Making Sense of Depression: Perceptions of Melancholia in Lay Narratives." *Health* 5(1): 76–92.

Karlsson, Veronika, and Anna Forsberg. 2008. "Health Is Yearning: Experiences of Being Conscious during Ventilator Treatment in a Critical Care Unit." *Intensive and Critical Care Nursing* 24(1): 41–50.

Karp, David A. 1996. *Speaking of Sadness*. Oxford: Oxford University Press.

Kaufman, Sharon R. 2005. . . . *And a Time to Die: How Hospitals Shape the End of Life*. Chicago: University of Chicago Press.

Kenen, Regina H. 1996. "The At-Risk Health Status and Technology: A Diagnostic Invitation and the 'Gift' of Knowing." *Social Science and Medicine* 42(11): 1545–53.

Kleinman, Arthur. 1988. *The Illness Narratives*. New York: Basic Books.

Kleinman, Arthur, and Don Seeman. 2000. "Personal Experience of Illness." In *The Handbook of Social Studies in Health and Medicine*, ed. Gary Albrecht, Roy Fitzpatrick, and Susan C. Scrimshaw, 230–42. London: Sage.

Lane, Harlan. 2006. "Construction of Deafness." In *The Disability Studies Reader*, 2nd ed., ed. Lennard Davis, 79–92. New York: Routledge.

Lawton, Julia. 2003. "Lay Experiences of Health and Illness: Past Research and Future Agendas." *Sociology of Health and Illness* 25(3): 23–40.

Lester, Helen, and Jonathan Q. Tritter. 2005. "'Listen to My Madness': Understanding the Experiences of People with Serious Mental Illness." *Sociology of Health and Illness* 27(5): 649–69.

Levine, Sol, and Martin A. Kozloff. 1978. "The Sick Role: Assessment and Overview." *Annual Review of Sociology* 4:317–43.

Little, Miles, Christopher F. C. Jordens, Kim Paul, Kathleen Montgomery, and Bertil Philipson. 1998. "Liminality: A Major Category of the Experience of Cancer Illness." *Social Science and Medicine* 47(10): 1485–94.

Locker, David. 1991. "Living with Chronic Illness." In *Sociology as Applied to Medicine*, ed. Graham Scambler, 81–92. London: Bailliere Tindall.

Lombardo, Anthony P. 2004. "Anatomy of Fear: Mead's Theory of the Past and the Experience of the HIV/ AIDS 'Worried Well.'" *Symbolic Interaction* 27(4): 531–48.

Lorde, Audre. 1997. *The Cancer Journals*. Special ed. San Francisco: Aunt Lute.

Lutz, Barbara J., and Barbara J. Bowers. 2005. "Disability in Everyday Life." *Qualitative Health Research* 15(8): 1037–54.

MacRae, Hazel. 2008. "'Making the Best You Can of It': Living with Early-Stage Alzheimer's Disease." *Sociology of Health and Illness* 30(3): 396–412.

Magarey, Judith M., and Helen H. McCutcheon. 2005. "'Fishing with the Dead': Recall of Memories from the ICU." *Intensive and Critical Care Nursing* 21(6): 344–54.

Maykovich, Minako K. 1980. *Medical Sociology*. Sherman Oaks, Calif.: Alfred Publishing.

Mechanic, David. 1978. *Medical Sociology*. 2nd ed. New York: Free Press.

Mishler, Elliot G. 1984. *The Discourse of Medicine: Dialectics of Medical Interviews*. Norwood, N.J.: Ablex.

Moses, Tally. 2009. "Self-Labeling and Its Effects among Adolescents Diagnosed with Mental Disorders." *Social Science and Medicine* 68(3): 570–78.

Murphy, Robert F. 1990. *The Body Silent*. New York: W. W. Norton.

Nettleton, Sarah, Lisa O'Malley, Ian Watt, and Philip Duffey. 2004. "Enigmatic Illness: Narratives of Patients Who Live with Medically Unexplained Symptoms." *Social Theory and Health* 2(1): 47–66.

Oliffe, John L., and Joan L. Bottorff. 2007. "Further Than the Eye Can See? Photo Elicitation and Research with Men." *Qualitative Health Research* 17(6): 850–58.

Oliffe, John L., B. Joyce Davison, Tom Pickles, and Lawrence Mróz. 2009. "The Self-Management of Uncertainty among Men Undertaking Active Surveillance for Low-Risk Prostate Cancer." *Qualitative Health Research* 19(4): 432–43.

Overcash, Janine A. 2003. "Narrative Research: A Review of Methodology and Relevance to Clinical Practice." *Critical Reviews in Oncology/Hematology* 48(2): 179–84.

Parsons, Janet A., Joan M. Eakin, Robert S. Bell, Renée-Louise Franche, and Aileen M. Davis. 2008. "'So, Are You Back to Work Yet?' Re-conceptualizing 'Work' and 'Return to Work' in the Context of Primary Bone Cancer." *Social Science and Medicine* 67(11): 1826–36.

Parsons, Talcott. 1951. *The Social System*. Glencoe, Ill.: Free Press.

———. 1975. "The Sick Role and Role of the Physician Reconsidered." *Milbank Memorial Fund Quarterly* 53(3): 257–78.

Pierret, Janine. 2001. "Interviews and Biographical Time: The Case of Long-Term HIV Nonprogressors." *Sociology of Health and Illness* 23(2): 159–79.

———. 2003. "The Illness Experience: State of Knowledge and Perspectives for Research." 25(3): 4–22.

———. 2007. "An Analysis over Time (1990–2000) of the Experiences of Living with HIV." *Social Science and Medicine* 65(8): 1595–1605.

Pitts, Victoria. 2004. "Illness and Internet Empowerment: Writing and Reading Breast Cancer in Cyberspace." *Health* 8(1): 33–59.

Pollock, Kristian. 2007. "Maintaining Face in the Presentation of Depression: Constraining the Therapeutic Potential of the Consultation." *Health* 11(2): 163–80.

Prior, Lindsay. 2003. "Belief, Knowledge and Expertise: The Emergence of the Lay Expert in Medical Sociology." *Sociology of Health and Illness* 25(3): 41–57.

Radley, Alan, and Diane Taylor. 2003a. "Images of Recovery: A Photo-Elicitation Study on the Hospital Ward." *Qualitative Health Research* 13(1): 77–99.

———. 2003b. "Remembering One's Stay in Hospital: A Study in Photography, Recovery and Forgetting." *Health* 7(2): 129–59.

Richman, Joel. 2000. "Coming out of Intensive Care Crazy: Dreams of Affliction." *Qualitative Health Research* 10(1): 84–102.

Rier, David A. 2000. "The Missing Voice of the Critically Ill: A Medical Sociologist's First-Person Account." *Sociology of Health and Illness* 22(1): 68–93.

———. 2007a. "The Impact of Moral Suasion on Internet HIV/AIDS Support Groups: Evidence from a Discussion of Seropositivity Disclosure Ethics." *Health Sociology Review* 16(3–4): 237–47.

———. 2007b. "Internet Support Groups as Moral Agents: The Ethical Dynamics of HIV+ Status Disclosure." *Sociology of Health and Illness* 29(7): 1043–58.

———. 2008. "'The Missing Voice of Critical Illness,' Ten Years Later: In Sociology, Still Missing." Presented to the American Sociological Association 103rd Annual Meeting, Boston, August 1–4.

Riessman, Catherine K. 1990. "Strategic Uses of Narrative in the Presentation of Self and Illness: A Research Note." *Social Science and Medicine* 30(11): 1195–1200.

———. 2003. "Performing Identities in Illness Narrative: Masculinity and Multiple Sclerosis." *Qualitative Research* 3(1): 5–33.

Robillard, Albert B. 1994. "Communication Problems in the Intensive Care Unit." *Qualitative Sociology* 17(4): 383–95.

Rosenfeld, Dana. 2006. "Similarities and Differences between Acute Illness and Injury Narratives and Their Implications for Medical Sociology." *Social Theory and Health* 4(1): 64–84.

Roth, Julius. 1963. *Timetables: Structuring the Passage of Time in Hospital Treatment and Other Careers*. Indianapolis: Bobbs-Merrill.

Roulin, Marie-José, Samia Hurst, and Rebecca Spirig. 2007. "Diaries Written for ICU Patients." *Qualitative Health Research* 17(7): 893–901.

Sandaunet, Anne-Grete. 2008. "A Space for Suffering? Communicating Breast Cancer in an Online Self-Help Context." *Qualitative Health Research* 18(12): 1631–41.

Scambler, Graham, ed. 1991. *Sociology as Applied to Medicine*. London: Bailliere Tindall.

Sharf, Barbara F. 1997. "Communicating Breast Cancer On Line: Support and Empowerment on the Internet." *Women and Health* 26(1): 65–84.

Sim, Julius, and Sue Madden. 2008. "Illness Experience in Fibromyalgia Syndrome: A Metasynthesis of Qualitative Studies." *Social Science and Medicine* 67(1): 57–67.

Simpson, Elizabeth L. 1982. *Notes on an Emergency: A Journal of Recovery*. London: W. W. Norton.

Snyder, Lisa. 1999. *Speaking Our Minds: Personal Reflections from Individuals with Alzheimer's*. New York: W. H. Freeman.

Sontag, Susan. 1990a. "AIDS and Its Metaphors." In *Illness as Metaphor and AIDS and Its Metaphors*, 93–183. New York: Anchor Books/Doubleday.

———. 1990b. "Illness as Metaphor." In *Illness as Metaphor and AIDS and Its Metaphors*, 3–87. New York: Anchor Books/Doubleday.

Stewart, David C., and Thomas J. Sullivan. 1982. "Illness Behaviors and the Sick Role in Chronic Disease: The Case of Multiple Sclerosis." *Social Science and Medicine* 16(15): 1397–404.

Strauss, Anselm L. 1975. *Chronic Illness and the Quality of Life*. St. Louis: C. V. Mosby.

Sweeting, Helen, and Mary Gilhooly. 1997. "Dementia and the Phenomenon of Social Death." *Sociology of Health and Illness* 19(1): 93–117.

Thomas, Hilary. 2004. "From Patient to Person: Identifying a Sociology of Recovery." Paper presented at the American Sociological Association 99th Annual Meeting, San Francisco, August 14–17.

Timmermans, Stefan, and Steven Haas. 2008. "Towards a Sociology of Disease." *Sociology of Health and Illness* 30(5): 659–76.

Trainor, Andrea, and Hélène Ezer. 2000. "Rebuilding Life: The Experience of Living with AIDS after Facing Imminent Death." *Qualitative Health Research* 10(5): 646–60.

Turner, Bryan S. 1990. *Medical Power and Social Knowledge*. London: Sage.

Twaddle, Andrew C., and Richard M. Hessler. 1977. *A Sociology of Health*. St. Louis: C. V. Mosby.

Ville, Isabelle. 2005. "Biographical Work and Returning to Employment Following a Spinal Cord Injury." *Sociology of Health and Illness* 27(3): 324–50.

Walstrom, Mary K. 2000. "'You Know, Who's the Thinnest?': Combating Surveillance and Creating Safety in Coping with Eating Disorders Online." *CyberPsychology and Behavior* 3(5): 761–83.

Williams, Gareth. 1984. "The Genesis of Chronic Illness: Narrative Re-construction." *Sociology of Health and Illness* 6(2): 175–200.

Williams, Simon J. 2005. "Parsons Revisited: From the Sick Role to . . . ?" *Health* 9(2): 123–44.

Wolinsky, Frederick D. 1980. *The Sociology of Health: Principles, Professions, and Issues*. Boston: Little, Brown.

Yoshida, Karen K. 1993. "Reshaping of Self: A Pendular Reconstruction of Self and Identity among Adults with Traumatic Spinal Cord Injury." *Sociology of Health and Illness* 15(2): 217–43.

Ziebland, Sue. 2004. "The Importance of Being Expert: The Quest for Cancer Information on the Internet." *Social Science and Medicine* 59(9): 1783–93.

Ziebland, Sue, and Andrew Herxheimer. 2008. "How Patients' Experiences Contribute to Decision Making: Illustrations from DIPEx (Personal Experiences of Health and Illness)." *Journal of Nursing Management* 16(4): 433–39.

Zussman, Robert. 1992. *Intensive Care: Medical Ethics and the Medical Profession*. Chicago: University of Chicago.

11

The Internet and the Experience of Illness

Peter Conrad, Brandeis University

Cheryl Stults, Brandeis University

Sociologists have studied the experience of illness for at least the past four decades (Conrad 1987). The earliest studies focused on how patients managed the sick role (Parsons 1951) or how they maneuvered through the stages of an illness career (Suchman 1965). Beginning with the work of Anselm Strauss and his colleagues (Glaser and Strauss 1965; Strauss and Glaser 1975), sociological researchers started investigating the experience of illness by examining the illness experience from the patient's viewpoint. This has led to several lines of work that focused on how people live with and in spite of their illness, the subjective experience of illness, and strategies sufferers develop to manage their illnesses and lives (e.g., Charmaz 1999; Bury 1982; Bell 2000). Researchers have typically used qualitative research methods, especially interviews, to examine the experience of illness (Conrad 1987; Charmaz 1999) and have studied stigmatized illnesses like epilepsy (Schneider and Conrad 1983) and HIV/AIDS (Weitz 1991; Klitzman and Bayer 2003), contested illnesses like fibromyalgia (Barker 2005), psychiatric disorders like major depression (Karp 1997), and medical conditions such as infertility (Greil 1991) and genetic disorders (Cox and McKellin 1999). Numerous studies have focused on how sufferers manage their identity (Charmaz 1991), stigma (Weitz 1991), biographical disruption (Bury 1982), or narrative reconstruction (Williams 1984).

Two consistent findings from experience-of-illness studies through roughly the year 2000 are that with few exceptions there were no illness subcultures and that illness was a profoundly privatizing experience. In an early statement, Parsons and Fox (1952, 137) observed that "illness usually prevents the individual from attaching himself to a solidary subculture of similarly oriented deviants." Sociologists who studied the experience of illness studied individuals through interviews and, in contrast to a field like deviance, could not render ethnographies of illness subcultures, for they essentially did not exist. There were a few cases where sociologists could study patient subcultures in hospitals, the most famous of which are the classic studies of TB hospitals (Roth 1963) and mental institutions (Goffman 1961), but these were studies of the experience of patienthood more than of the experience of illness. Other than hospitals, there were few settings where people with the same illness interacted with one another. There have been a few studies of self-help groups for people with illness, especially post-illness, but studies of these were more about self-help than about the experience of illness (Borkman 1999). In a few rare instances, such as the early days of end-stage renal disease (ESRD), there was sufficient interaction to begin to create some kind of illness subculture (e.g., Kutner 1987), but for the most part patients were treated separately and rarely interacted in meaningful ways with others who had the same illness. One can say with reasonable certainty that there were very few illness subcultures (had there been more, sociologists and others would certainly have studied them.)

Until recently, illness in general was a privatizing experience discussed only with one's doctor, family, and perhaps a few good friends. It was not unusual for individual sufferers of an illness never to have spoken to another person with the same illness or to have known someone who shared the same illness. In a 1983 study of the experience of epilepsy, when Schneider and Conrad interviewed eighty people with epilepsy, no more than five had ever spoken to another person with epilepsy about their illness experience. It may be in part the stigma that discouraged revealing one's illness and communication, but for the overwhelming majority of those interviewed illness remained a private experience. With specific illnesses such as HIV/AIDS, where a large and active gay subculture organized around the illness, there was surely more interaction among those with the illness. But this was an unusual situation; typically illnesses were privatized, and most sufferers had little or no communication with people suffering the same disorder.

In the past two decades the Internet has changed all that. There are now hundreds, probably thousands, of illness subcultures on the Internet, and illness is now a public as well as a private experience. In short, for many people, the Internet has changed the experience of illness.

Coming of the Internet

What we now term "the Internet" began in 1969 when four computers in the United States were linked together to pass military information to one another. Until the late 1980s, most communication over the Internet was text-based e-mails (Hardey 1999). The initial Web browser, the World Wide Web (WWW), was created to allow users to search for information rather than rely on authors to distribute it. The WWW "through a browser enables users to point and click their way across the Internet," placing information at only a mouse click away (Hardey 1999, 825). The first browser for the masses, Mosaic, appeared in 1993; Google as an Internet search engine appeared in 1998. This access to online information

and interconnectivity has impacted many aspects of communication, including business and commerce, government, education, news, personal communication, and information acquisition.

The Internet has grown enormously in the past fifteen years, as has the number of users, with roughly 360 million users in 2000 and an estimated 1.5 billion in 2007 (Internet World Stats 2008). The greatest penetration of usage is of course in the developed world, but China has pulled ahead of the United States with the largest number of Internet users (Barboza 2008); according to recent statistics, North America has roughly 250 million Internet users. It has become increasingly easier to access the Internet with computers in all schools, most businesses, public libraries, Internet cafés, and millions of homes. And the Internet is available 24/7; it never shuts down. Sophisticated search engines like Google make accessing relevant information quick and simple. It is not an exaggeration to observe that despite the existence of a real but shrinking Internet divide (Marriott 2006), there has been a digital revolution in the past two decades. Virtually everything about the Internet is growing or increasing. The Internet revolution has affected health information and communication as well.

Estimates of Internet use vary and change by the month. In the United States, nearly 100 million people regularly access the Internet for health information, and most (66 percent) are searching for information about specific diseases (Fox 2005; Blumenthal 2002). Other sources suggest that 80 percent (113 million) of adults who use the Internet have searched for health information online, a 250 percent increase since 1998 (Miah and Rich 2008; Ayers and Kronenfeld 2007). Health-related websites and discussion lists are some of the most popular resources on the Web (Miah and Rich 2008). On any given day more people in the United States go online for health information than consult a health professional (Ayers and Kronenfeld 2007; Nettleton, Burrows, and O'Malley 2005). However, while on some level the Internet is the great equalizer, allowing individuals the same access to information as the experts, a digital divide has emerged. People with lower incomes access or utilize the Internet less often for health information than do people with higher incomes (Ayers and

Kronenfeld 2007). Somewhat more whites than African Americans utilize the Internet for health information (Fox and Fallows 2003, 5; cf. Lieberman et al. 2005). Women utilize the Internet more for health information than men do (54 percent to 46 percent) and report significantly more interest in information about specific diseases (69 percent to 58 percent) and certain treatments than do men (54 percent to 47 percent) (Fox 2006). In addition to women, individuals with more education, health insurance, and younger persons are those more likely to use the Internet to search for health information (Ayers and Kronenfeld 2007). The digital gap among minority groups is decreasing, with 43 percent of African Americans and 59 percent of Hispanics reporting access to the Internet (Lieberman et al. 2005).

Individuals who access the Internet are able to locate vast amounts of information about any health condition from sites sponsored by governments, hospitals, national organizations, medical information collections, and even individuals. Beyond these institutional sites (including megasites like WebMD.com), one finds personal webpages, weblogs (blogs), online chat rooms, bulletin boards, and discussion sites where individuals can participate and share their knowledge and experience. Many sites allow participation or interaction by posting, or individuals can choose to be "lurkers," who read the messages but do not post or add to the conversations. The number of lurkers on a site can greatly exceed the number of active members—one study found twenty lurkers for each participant (Loader et al. 2002). Thus Internet participation can occur in both interactional and observational ways. The net accumulation is a tremendous amount of health information available on the Internet, some scientific, some personal or experiential, and some commercial. While virtually any illness now has its own site or numerous electronic support groups (ESGs) or informational sites, the actual information must be evaluated with a careful eye. The quality of information may be improving, however; in a recent study analyzing 343 websites about breast cancer, the authors found that only 5.2 percent of the sites contained inaccurate information (Bernstam et al. 2008).

While the Internet has helped patients become more active consumers by providing them a means for finding information and occasionally purchasing treatments, it has also transformed individuals into producers of knowledge. In this Web 2.0 (more interactive) era, individuals can construct their own websites or home pages or develop blogs about their health issues, transforming them from "consumers of health information and care to producers of health information and care" (Hardey 2002, 31). In his study, Hardey (2002) chose 132 webpages through search engines (Yahoo, Alta Vista, Dogpile), newsgroups, and ICQ ("I seek you") chat rooms; 74 webpage constructors returned an e-mail questionnaire that investigated information not included on the websites. Based on these two sources (home pages and questionnaires), Hardey generated four categories of motives for constructing these pages: (1) explain illness; (2) give "expert advice" to others: (3) promote an approach to the illness; and (4) indirect or direct selling of products. "Explaining myself" was one of the main reasons indicated by 43 percent of respondents for placing information on their webpage. Many, in the midst of their narrative, included a hypertext link to a particular aspect of their account (e.g., treatment regimen). Hardey found that while many were skeptical about the efficacy of traditional medicine, they were just as skeptical about alternative treatments. These webpage producers presented information as if they were the "experts" because they had experienced the illness. At times, they felt that this experience was more valid than medical training. Finally, in several cases, the websites not only provided experience-based advice but also a "sales pitch" for a particular treatment.

Internet sources such as personal websites, bulletin boards, and electronic support groups produce a significant amount of lay knowledge based on embodied expertise that can be shared and that sometimes is used to challenge physician or dominant medical perspectives (Barker 2008). While experiential knowledge was embedded in sources like the feminist book *Our Bodies, Ourselves*, published in 1970, the Internet, due to its vast nature and accessibility, amplifies such knowledge and in its sheer ubiquity helps legitimize it as well. This blurs some distinctions between patient and expert, developing what Collins and Evans (2002, 238) call "experience-based experts," who have "special technical expertise by virtue of experience that is not recognized by degrees or other certificates."

The Internet can also empower patients with knowledge and options by offering information previously limited to medical experts (or available only through extensive library research) and the potential to increase control over their health. Pitts (2004) examined fifty personal webpages of women with breast cancer to see if their information and stories portrayed evidence of empowerment. She found the women often referred to the Internet as a "virtual library" where they could "arm themselves" with information that they could take to medical appointments to challenge or question doctors about the care and treatments they felt they should be receiving. The process of writing out their experiences helped them better understand medical language. Several women portrayed the Internet as a "beacon of hope," since it can potentially provide life-saving information. However, this may become a double-edged sword if women blame themselves if the treatment or course of illness goes awry, despite the illness trajectory being beyond their control. As Pitts notes: "The idea that breast cancer kills only the unaware is blatantly wrong—it also kills the aware, the 'tested'—and implies that women who do get sick or die could have prevented this fate" (48). Thus, women feel a responsibility to save themselves in what Pitts calls the "individual responsibility ethic." Pitts shows that while the Internet can be empowering and creates something of a cyberspace breast cancer community, it also reinforces dominant cultural norms like femininity, consumerism, and individualism. It enables women to feel that they "were not alone" and that it was their "ethical imperative" and responsibility to share their experience so that it might benefit others. This empowerment provides a venue for activism in order to possibly "ameliorate the alienating aspects of medicine" (ibid.) and, perhaps unwittingly, transform breast cancer from a personal to a public issue.

Support Groups

In-person self-help groups have a long and winding history with health and illness but are actu-ally quite limited in their population penetration (Borkman 1999). In a way, the Internet is just an extension of the self-help tradition, but it also revolutionizes it. The Internet has most directly and dramatically altered the experience of illness through online electronic support groups (ESGs). For most people, as noted earlier, illness was a private affair before the advent of the Internet, often isolating individuals; most people didn't communicate with others who suffered from the same illness. Through interconnectivity on the Internet, we have seen the emergence of illness subcultures and, for many people, illness is now a more shared and public experience. As Barker (2008, 21) notes: "The process of understanding one's embodied distress has been transformed from an essentially private affair between doctor and patient to an increasingly public accomplishment among sufferers in cyberspace." Increasingly, individuals are also communicating with others who have the same illness, thereby creating thousands of virtual self-help groups incorporating nearly all illnesses, many with a range of groups from different sources and angles. Many "connectors" have been around for years, as the first newsgroups appeared on the Internet in 1981 (Richardson 2005). What began with illness-oriented newsgroups and bulletin boards has expanded to a large variety of interactive virtual realms, facilitated by expanding Web access and the speed of broadband cable Internet.

An estimated 9 percent of Internet users have visited online support groups (Lieberman et al. 2005). Tens of thousands of ESGs are "accessed as bulletin boards, newsgroups, listserves, and chat rooms" in postings of individuals (Barker 2008, 20). In another vein, computer-mediated social support (CMSS) occurs when medical consultations, prescriptions, and advice from health-care providers can be accessed by the patient, that is, the patient can receive information about diagnosis and treatment. But beyond accessing knowledge, patients can connect with other individuals who are having similar experiences. As just one example, in 2002 Usenet was estimated to have 15,000+ newsgroups and 20,000 people posting 300,000 messages daily (Loader et al. 2002). No doubt with today's greater variety of venues, these numbers are much larger.

The disorders represented on the Internet differ from traditional self-help groups. Davison Pennebaker, and Dickerson (2000) investigated community-based (in-person) and Internet-based self-help groups (5,440 Internet posts to news-groups and bulletin boards over a two-week period) for twenty illnesses in four metropolitan areas. The most common community-based self-help group was Alcoholics Anonymous (AA), while chronic fatigue syndrome in-person self-help groups were uncommon. In contrast, chronic fatigue syndrome had the most self-help groups on the Internet, while AA was not among the top three. This suggests that Internet-based self-help groups may be especially attractive to individuals who experience chronic illnesses or illnesses that have contested viewpoints. As the authors note: "The on-line domain may be particularly useful in bringing together those who suffer from rare and debilitating conditions, in which getting together physically would present a number of practical barriers" (8). In addition, Internet technology may allow individuals who experience contested illnesses like fibromyalgia and chronic fatigue syndrome or socially stigmatizing illnesses such as epilepsy and sexually transmitted diseases (STDs) to communicate with others who have the same condition in relative privacy and without fear of discrimination. The anonymity of the Internet, buffered by the ability to create screen names and extended by the possibility of simply lurking to view others' experience, creates a relatively safe and private environment for communication and observing others' illness experience.

The "compensation model of Internet use" posits that those who are the most socially awkward will utilize and derive more "benefit" from the Internet (Guo, Bricout, and Huang 2005). The experience of those suffering from stigmatized illnesses, physical disabilities, and multiple chronic illnesses could potentially be the most affected by Internet interaction. In a national survey, Berger, Wagner, and Baker (2005) studied how U.S. adults utilize the Internet for health conditions. Comparing nonstigmatized and stigmatized illnesses, they found that those with stigmatized illness were statistically significantly more likely to use the Internet to obtain health information, communicate with health-care prac-

titioners about their condition, and apply the information they had found to increase their utilization of health care. However, no statistically significant relationship occurred between length of time spent online, frequency of Internet usage, satisfaction with discovered health information, and discussing findings with health care providers. They then separated the group "stigmatized illnesses" into four specific conditions: anxiety, depression, herpes, and urinary incontinence. Upon comparison, the psychiatric stigmatized illnesses (anxiety and depression) were more likely to go online to find health information and to converse with a health provider. These results suggest that overall, individuals with stigmatized illnesses utilize the Internet more than do those with nonstigmatized conditions; however, differences emerge among types of stigmatized illnesses, with higher use by those with psychiatric illnesses (Berger, Wagner, and Baker 2005). Internet communication is particularly attractive to people suffering from physical disabilities and mobility impairments. Individuals with disabilities can access information from their homes.

Guo, Bricout, and Huang (2005) surveyed Internet users in China with a disability about their online interactions. One benefit of online communication was that it allowed disabled individuals to choose whether or not to disclose their disability to other users. Fifty-four percent of respondents felt that the Internet reduced the amount of social discrimination they experience, while 77 percent expressed that online use provided them increased social integration and reduced isolation. Only 32 percent responded that online interactions increased societal concern for disabilities. While their individual isolation was lessened, the Internet appears to have a limited impact on real-world change. Thus, "the Internet cannot by itself remedy the social exclusion faced by persons with disabilities, but must instead be part of a larger programme fueled by social development" (65).

Uncertainty about illness seems to be a factor driving Internet usage. According to a recent study, individuals with multiple chronic illnesses utilized the Internet more than did other respondents (regardless of conditions) due to an increased amount of uncertainty with their situations (Ayers and Kronenfeld 2007). These users seek information to attempt to decrease both social and medical uncertainty. But not all users envisage Internet use in the same way. One study that compared prostate and breast cancer online message boards found different emphases for men and women. Consistent with other studies, both men and women could mention topics that they might not feel comfortable discussing in person. Women allowed more direct emotional expressions of support and criticized the health information found on Internet; men were more likely to search for information about treatments/diseases (Seale, Ziebland, and Charteris-Black 2006).

We know little about what differentiates individuals who do not participate in ESGs from those who do. One study of Norwegian breast cancer patients provides us a little insight. Breast cancer patients are among the illness groups that have the highest participation in both online and offline support groups, according to Sandaunet (2008), who examined why individuals do not join ESGs or become members and then leave them. She found that among her sample, those who did not participate (or left) online breast cancer support groups did so because they did not like to hear stories about death, given their own mortal situations. Other nonparticipators felt that they were not "ill enough" or that they did not have anything to contribute to the discussion. Some women felt that if they participated in the online group, their posts would contain "too much complaining." Sandaunet's results align with previous findings that Western illness narratives are often mediated by a moral imperative to be "successfully ill" and to "rise to the occasion" when sick (Miah and Rich 2008, 62).

Moral or value issues are common among ESGs. Rier researched HIV message boards and found that besides giving emotional support, moral dilemmas about living with HIV were debated online, bringing out sharp moral judgments. This research demonstrates that this new medium, the Internet, does not necessarily mean a new message is being conveyed: "If these boards are seldom generators of genuinely new moral discourse, they do seem clearinghouses for and *transmitters* of existing alternative discourses. De-bates over disclosure ethics were witnessed not only by active posters, but also those merely lurking on the boards" (Rier 2007, 1054).

The emergence and popularity of ESGs for virtually any illness may be the most unique and consequential effect of the Internet on illness experience. Not only are these active illness subcultures, but also they move the illness experience from the private to the public sphere and in some cases, allow a kind of collective activism in the name of whatever illness the group represents.

Internet Illness Social Movements

Another manifestation of illness on the Internet has been the rise of what might be termed "online social movements." In general these are not extensions of extant social movements but phenomena spawned on the Internet and largely a function of Internet interaction. In this instance, groups move beyond experiential exchange and support to advocate for an alternative interpretation of an illness or the recognition of a previously unknown condition as an illness.

The most developed examples of such social movements are the so-called pro-anorexia (pro-ana) websites. The pro-ana sites have their origin as support groups but have become online communities for people with eating disorders that challenge the dominant medical treatment model of anorexia (see Miah and Rich 2008, 91–106). Pro-ana groups present a very different viewpoint: they attempt to help members and visitors become "better" anorexics, with information as to how to eat fewer calories and survive, hide their anorexia from friends and family, share "anorexic tricks," and avoid medical treatment. They extol the joys and benefits of extreme thinness and develop a counternarrative to the medical view, such as "anorexia is a lifestyle, not an illness." They often consider themselves an "Anorexic Nation." Part of many pro-ana sites is "thinspiration," photos ranging from ultrathin models to skin-and-bones anorexic women who look to most people emaciated and sickly. Beyond message boards, thinspiration videos have begun to emerge on the Internet. Most videos have no dialogue but show faceless, still photos of ultrathin bodies (Heffernan 2008). One video placed a line of text underneath the photos: "Time spent wasting is not wasted time" (ibid.).

Among the few studies of pro-ana websites is a study of an online support group, Anagrl, in which Fox, Ward, and O'Rourke (2005b) found that the participants viewed the site as a "refuge" for anorexics. Many of the participants did not want the site to become a place to "teach" individuals about how to become an anorexic; rather, the goal of this pro-ana site is to "sustain life in the healthiest way possible for an anorexic" and not force individuals into treatment and eradicate their lifestyle choice (959). The authors termed this view the "anti-recovery stance," meaning that "the movement is there to support its members through life problems, helping them manage anorexia safely, without removing the crutch that it provides them" (963). The response of one Anagrl member described the difference of this site as being "proanorectics," not "proanorexia" (ibid.).

One of the main arguments supporting the pro-anorexia "community" is that the Internet creates "the first truly equal communications platform" by providing a medium where people are not judged upon their appearance—race/ethnicity, gender, or social class—but where all are "neutral and unmarked" (Ferreday 2003, 279). But Ferreday argues that bodies still matter, since they are what house the virtual subject. She suggests there is a powerful resistance to the pro-ana sites because they are uniting individuals based upon how their body looks. These sites post images on their thinspiration pages of anorexic torsos and links to potentially anorexic models to entice others to investigate this whole process. This imagery demonstrates "the hypocrisy of a society that positions anorexics as sick, while continually celebrating and displaying extremely thin bodies" (286).

Pro-ana groups have become very controversial. Nonanorexic viewers often comment that anorexics don't know how "disgusting their bodies are" (Ferreday 2003, 288), although many lurkers visit the sites. Critics have accused the pro-ana sites of recruiting young women to extreme dieting and thinness, teaching them how to become anorexics, or at least glorifying what can be a deadly disorder. Many Internet service providers have removed or blocked their sites in the name of public health, but the sites keep reappearing. In April 2008, the lower house of France's parliament proposed banning any "online incitement" to anorexia, which includes thinspiration videos and more than four hundred websites (Heffernan 2008).

The Internet has also become a forum for conditions or desires once considered anomalies or oddities to develop a collective voice. There have probably always been rare individuals who admired amputees, for example, and a few who desired to become one. These individuals, if they expressed or acted out on their desires, were likely considered disturbed or even mentally ill. The idea of a perfectly healthy individual who has an intense desire to have an amputation of one (or multiple) limbs, or someone who has actually performed a self-amputation of an extremity, is a rare condition (First 2004). The technical term for the attraction to becoming an amputee is "apotemnophilia," coined in 1977 by Johns Hopkins psychologist John Money (Elliott 2000). On the Internet there are now websites created by and catering to "wannabes," which is how these individuals refer to themselves (for "wannabe" an amputee). They write about how this leg shouldn't be there, it's not meant to be their leg, and they need to have it removed to become their ideal self. They have found support and solace in the hundreds of other wannabes worldwide who post on the sites and exchange information about seeking (with little success) surgeons to remove their "unnecessary" limb or other ways that individuals could reach an amputee state. While the medical world in general opposes the amputation of healthy limbs, wannabes are working to get their disorder legitimated in the next edition of the DSM, perhaps as "amputee identity disorder" or "body integrity identity disorder" (BIID), with the hope that this would enable them to find physicians to "treat" their disorder with surgery (Elliott 2000). The wannabes use a claim similar to that of transsexuals—they are "trapped in the wrong body," and medical treatment could fix this.

In another frame, these two examples illustrate that the Internet can be a conduit for issues around medicalization (Conrad 2007). Pro-ana groups are a movement seeking the demedicalization of anorexia, while the wannabes are seeking medicalization as BIID in their quest to become amputees. Both are using the Internet to legitimize their views of what others might well see as illnesses. Recently there has been an upsurge of interest in a new contested illness called Morgellons syndrome, an alleged skin disorder with protruding florescent fibers that is eschewed by dermatologists but that the Centers for Disease Control has actually begun to investigate (Fair 2010). The Internet can operate as an organizing vehicle for or against medicalization of a particular problem and as a medium for the wider dissemination of medicalized claims and counterclaims.

Other illness-oriented groups that have used the Internet as a basis for social movements include mental illness web activists who are trying to reclaim "mad" as a positive term, similar to the way gay activists reclaimed the term "queer." One site has expanded offline to face-to-face support groups in some areas. From its five thousand unique monthly visitors, a New York–based online support group, the Icarus Project, has formed local chapters in Oregon, Missouri, and Virginia (Glaser 2008). HIV-AIDS activism is also visible on the Internet. Gillet (2003) found numerous activist orientations on AIDS websites, going far beyond the interests of AIDS ESGs. These websites both reflect and reinforce other media activism, but what makes them different is they are explicitly located in the illness experience of individuals. It seems clear that many illness experiences can lead to some kind of activism and social movement activity; the pro-ana and wannabe cases are unique in that they would not exist without the Internet. As Epstein (2008, 514) notes: "In a globally wired world, location doesn't *always* matter—at least not always to the same degree—and the birth and development of the Internet is . . . why patient and health movements have taken particular forms in recent years."

Challenging Physician Authority?

If the Internet provides patients with independent health information, and if ESGs provide external support and empowerment, is the Internet a medium for challenging physician authority? Blumenthal suggests patients' online interactions will lead to diminished physician authority since the medical information available on the Internet reduces the patients' dependence upon the physician as the "expert" but may also lead to a new role for physicians as consultants. Such a consultant plays two roles: "decision analyst" and "health care informatician." A decision analyst is able to make rational decisions in the presence of uncertainty that also incorporate the patient's preferences. A health-care informatician is an expert in all information technologies, having a vast knowledge of what is available. The acquisition of these skills is a double-edged sword: if the doctor consults a computer in front of some patients, it may undermine the patient's confidence in the physician; but if doctors are unacquainted with technologically advanced sources, many patient-consumers may lose confidence in them as well. Overall, Blumenthal (2002) concludes that while information technologies will cause a decline in physician authority, they will change but not remove the importance and functions of an expert physician. Some have suggested that the Internet and the wide access to medical information give the appearance of informational empowerment for patients but "may be *extending* the reach and power of medicine by creating a kind of 'indirect management of the population'" (Pitts 2004, 53).

The new information available on the Internet is not just replacing previous knowledge but is merging with a mix of sources. All this knowledge has escaped from the sole control of medical experts, potentially reducing their authority. One important area that needs to be studied is how medical professionals are regulating, using, and responding to this knowledge that is widely available to the public. This "e-scaped medicine" is a shift away from the expert provider toward the individuals who are learning and gathering information about their health concerns (Nettleton and Burrows 2003). Overall, it is likely that Internet-based medical information will become an additional resource for patients to manage their experience of illness. Some researchers have shown that the Internet is not used in place of physicians but rather as a supplement. According to one study, 61 percent of Internet health searchers sought health information online in conjunction with their physician visit, to supplement and "get more" from their visit (Ayers and Kronenfeld 2007).

Based on interviews with physicians in Australia, Broom found that doctors responded to the Internet-informed patient in a strategic way to avoid a breakdown of their authority. Several Australian practitioners encouraged their patients to seek information on the Internet, believing that an informed patient could improve the doctor-patient relationship by taking an active role with aspects of their health: "What emerged from these interviews was a view of the 'active' patient or 'informed' patient as safer than the so-called 'obedient' or 'passive' patient" (Broom 2005, 326). However, not all physicians' views of informed patients were so positive and cooperative. Many doctors liked having informed patients because they were more "compliant" with the treatment options prescribed to them (ibid.). These examples suggest that the Internet may alter ways in which physicians interact with their patients but has not eliminated the need for them. Some might argue that with so much information out there, patients are in greater need of physicians to clarify it.

In sum, our understanding of the impact of the Internet on physician authority is limited. There is considerable evidence that physician authority is decreasing (Mechanic 1996; McKinlay and Marceau 2002), so it would not be surprising if the Internet reinforced this decline. Our best guess now is that the Internet empowers patients, supplements and sometimes challenges physicians' expertise, and provides broader perspectives on illness experience. This probably does erode physician authority to some degree, but to what extent and with what consequences are not yet understood.

Evaluation of Information on the Internet

Sociological research on the Internet and health has focused upon the interaction of patients and consumers with the vast amount of information found on the Internet. Some articles frame their research in terms of a "reliability discourse" about the quality of health information on the Web and the ability of patients to evaluate it. Vari-

ous organizations including "the Federal Trade Commission and the U.S. science panel on interactive health communication have warned that much of the information available online may be misleading and potentially harmful" (Miah and Rich 2008, 44). Some critics suggest a paradox, when "such highly rational productions result in the incredible irrationality of information overloads, misinformation, disinformation, and out-of-control information. At stake is a disinformed society. . . . Thus, while we may appear to be 'smarting up,' the sheer proliferation of decontextualized information means that we are, in fact, experiencing a 'dumbing down'" (Nettleton and Burrows 2003, 174). While this is clearly an overstatement, there is some truth to the contention that there is much bad, wrong, and misleading information on the Internet and that consumers need to be able to evaluate online sources. In a study of the accuracy of information, Loader and colleagues (2002) asked four consultant diabetologists to evaluate sixty-one threads on an Internet newsgroup to determine if there was a gap between lay information and a more traditional medical view. Of the sixty-one, forty were graded B ("less good, some details") or C ("poor, little detail"), with 137 of 242 replies being personal opinion/anecdote. Only 5 of the 242 replies were "possibly dangerous," such as recommending more insulin for exercise.

One common criticism is that Internet information may be "problematic or even harmful" due to its potential to sway individuals away from biomedical treatments with inaccurate information or "unproven" complementary or alternative medical (CAM) treatments. To test this allegation, Broom and Tovey (2008) interviewed cancer patients from around the United Kingdom. Patients who used the Internet for CAM sought validation of the presented claims of others like family members, friends, or physicians. Several patients were skeptical not only of CAM but also of biomedicine information on the Internet and trusted only a few institutional sites. Overall, the Internet reenforced medical views: "Particularly for cancer patients who are CAM users, the Internet can be a form of virtual re-biomedicalization, imposing the biomedical diagnosis and prognostic knowledge in a context where they are attempting to pursue alternative models of healing" (150). So Internet information, even about CAM, did not necessarily undermine strong biomedical perspectives.

Finally, a word about ESGs, because of their interconnectivity and because they are perhaps the most unique aspect of the Internet. It seems clear that participants in Internet online illness groups are self-selected. While many individuals may access ESGs, only a small proportion seems to actually participate or post messages (Barker 2008; Stults 2007). There may be some evidence that individuals who have more difficulties with their illness, its treatment, or their medical care are more likely to post or seek information or affirmation (Ayers and Kronenfeld 2007). This could possibly self-select for the more severe forms of the illness, or individuals who are more apt to be dissatisfied or frustrated with their experience. Our assumption is that individuals with few problems with their illness might be less likely to participate or post in online groups. One outcome of this might be that ESGs can present an unbalanced picture of the experience of illness.

Emerging Directions of Illness on the Internet

While online electronic support groups have been one of the most transformational aspects of the experience of illness, other forms of interactive sites are starting to emerge. A major Internet development of the 2000s has been the emergence of social networking sites such as Facebook or My Space. These sites allow Internet users to join groups connected with their university, hometown, occupation, or hobby. Illness groups too have formed on Facebook, creating new links among people around the world. These connections are similar to Internet support groups, creating online links and community, yet they differ in that the individuals are linked to individual profile pages. These social network groups seem to be replacing the older bulletin board or chat room groups; illness becomes just another way of having some interest in common with other people.

A different kind of online networking illness site has emerged that may be a harbinger of fu-

ture sites. An exemplar is Patients Like Me, an innovative and expanding site where individuals not only connect and report their symptoms, pains, experiences, or treatment regimens, but also quantify these aspects of their illness: "They note what hurts, where and for how long. They list their drugs and dosages and score how well they alleviate their symptoms. All this gets compiled over time, aggregated and crunched into tidy bar graphs and progress curves by the software behind the site" (Goetz 2008). All this information is available for other group members to examine and evaluate against their own graphs. With so much information available, "the members of PatientsLikeMe are creating a rich database of disease treatment and patient experience" (Goetz 2008). The site began in 2004 with a group of individuals with amyotrophic lateral sclerosis (ALS), or Lou Gehrig's disease. As of July 2008, Patients Like Me had organized communities for anxiety, bipolar, depression, HIV/AIDS, multiple sclerosis, obsessive-compulsive disorder, Parkinson's disease, progressive muscular atrophy, primary lateral sclerosis, and post-traumatic stress disorder. The website creators note that they began this site to help empower patients: "We're here to give patients the power to control their disease and to share what they learn with others." The funding for the site comes from health-care providers, pharmaceutical and medical device companies, research institutions, and nonprofit organizations, who pay to utilize the anonymous data from the members to "drive treatment research and improve medical care" (PatientsLikeMe 2008). Pharmaceutical companies and other research groups conducting clinical trials can advertise on the site for member participation. While such sites provide illness sufferers with comparative information they never had before, there is of course a real danger of this experiential information being appropriated by corporate interests for commercial purposes.

There is always the risk that the Internet may be creating "cyberchondria," a condition in which individuals read too much into the information they unearth about diagnoses and think they are suffering from six or seven "problems" (Gray et al. 2005, 1473). Beyond the problem of excessive self-diagnosis, the Internet allows easy and accessible purchasing of many "prescription" drugs without a prescription. Some sites supply prescription drugs according to an online questionnaire the consumer completes (Fox et al. 2005a). Other suppliers in foreign countries like Canada or Mexico do not require prescriptions for most of their pharmaceuticals; patients may have these medications—some of which have not been officially approved by the U.S. Food and Drug Administration—shipped to them in the United States. Clearly this goes beyond the experience of illness, but such increased access to pharmaceuticals can affect how individuals manage their symptoms and illness. One of the most recent proposals has been to place patients' complete medical records online through providers like Google and Microsoft. These consumer-driven online electronic health records in theory should be able to link up with the records from doctors and hospitals, which could greatly ease the communication among physicians and providers to better coordinate care and reduce medical errors and records available in potentially lifesaving situations. The issues of privacy and confidentiality of these records remain an issue, with concern about the potential of inappropriate disclosure of patient information to unauthorized providers (Lohr 2008). But it seems likely that the Internet will become more of a repository of medical and experiential information about one's illness, and at least some of that will be available to others.

The extant sociological knowledge about the impact of the Internet on illness is still preliminary. At the moment we have growing evidence of the impact of the Internet on illness experience. But as yet, we have no publicly available data that have measured whether utilizing the Internet for illness has any effect on the morbidity or trajectory of the condition itself. A different kind of research will be necessary to ascertain whether Internet usage has any impact on health outcomes, and if it does, the type, extent, and context of such use. But it is clear that it can have a transformative effect on subjective aspects of illness.

In conclusion, the Internet has revolutionized aspects of illness experience in less than two decades. We now see established online illness subcultures, growing venues of social support for specific illnesses, important sources of informa-

tion and information exchange, and increased accessibility to and perhaps value of experiential illness information. Advancing technology, innovative communication media, and increased global accessibility suggest that we may be only beginning to recognize the impacts of the Internet on the experience of illness.

Note

Our thanks to Kristin Barker and Stefan Timmermans for comments on an earlier draft of this chapter.

References

Ayers, Stephanie L., and Jennie Jacobs Kronenfeld. 2007. "Chronic Illness and Health Seeking Information on the Internet." *Health: An Interdisciplinary Journal for the Social Study of Health, Illness and Medicine* 11(3): 327–47.

Barboza, David. 2008. "China Passes U.S. in Number of Internet Users." *New York Times*, July 26.

Barker, Kristin K. 2005. *The Fibromyalgia Story.* Philadelphia: Temple University Press.

———. 2008. "Electronic Support Groups, Patient-Consumers, and Medicalization: The Case of Contested Illness." *Journal of Health and Social Behavior* 49:20–36.

Bell, Susan. 2000. "Narratives." In *Handbook of Medical Sociology*, 5th ed., ed. Chloe Bird, Peter Conrad, and Allen Fremont, 184–99. New York: Prentice Hall.

Berger, Magdalena, Todd H. Wagner, and Lawrence C. Baker. 2005. "Internet Use and Stigmatized Illness." *Social Science and Medicine* 61:1821–27.

Bernstam, Elmer V., Muhammed F. Walji, Smitha Sagaram, Deepak Sagaram, Craig W. Johnson, and Funda Meric-Bernstam. 2008. "Commonly Cited Website Quality Criteria Are Not Effective at Identifying Inaccurate Online Information about Breast Cancer." *Cancer* 112(6): 1206–13.

Blumenthal, David. 2002. "Doctors in a Wired World: Can Professionalism Survive Connectivity?" *Milbank Quarterly* 80(3): 525–46.

Borkman, Thomasina. 1999. *Understanding Self-Help/ Mutual Aid: Experiential Learning in the Commons.* New Brunswick, N.J.: Rutgers University Press.

Broom, Alex. 2005. "Medical Specialists' Accounts of the Impact of the Internet on the Doctor/Patient Relationship." *Health: An Interdisciplinary Journal for the Social Study of Health, Illness and Medicine* 9(3): 319–38.

Broom, Alex, and Philip Tovey. 2008. "The Role of the Internet in Cancer Patients' Engagement with Complementary and Alternative Treatments."

Health: An Interdisciplinary Journal for the Social Study of Health, Illness and Medicine 12(2): 139–55.

Bury, Michael. 1982. "Chronic Illness as Biographical Disruption." *Sociology of Health and Illness* 4:167–82.

Charmaz, Kathy. 1991. *Good Days, Bad Days.* New Brunswick, N.J.: Rutgers University Press.

———. 1999. "Experiencing Chronic Illness." In *Handbook of Social Studies in Health and Medicine*, ed. Gary L. Albrecht, Ray Fitzpatrick, and Susan Scrimshaw, 277–92. Thousand Oaks, Calif.: Sage.

Collins, H. M., and Robert Evans. 2002. "The Third Wave of Science Studies: Studies of Expertise and Experience." *Social Studies of Science* 32(2): 235–96.

Conrad, Peter. 1987. "The Experience of Illness: Recent and New Directions." In *The Experience and Management of Chronic Illness*, ed. Peter Conrad and Julius A. Roth, 1–32. Vol. 6 of *Research in the Sociology of Health Care*. Greenwich, Conn.: JAI Press.

———. 2007. *The Medicalization of Society: On the Transformation of Human Conditions into Treatable Disorders.* Baltimore: Johns Hopkins University Press.

Cox, Susan, and William McKellin. 1999. "'There's This Thing in our Family': Predictive Testing and the Construction of Risk for Huntington Disease." In *Sociology Perspectives in the New Genetics*, ed. Peter Conrad and Jonathan Gabe, 121–47. Oxford: Blackwell.

Davison, Kathryn P., James W. Pennebaker, and Sally S. Dickerson. 2000. "Who Talks? The Social Psychology of Illness Support Groups." *American Psychologist* 55:205–17.

Elliott, Carl. 2000. "A New Way to Be Mad." *Atlantic Monthly* 286:72–84.

Epstein, Steven. 2008. "Patient Groups and Health Movements." In *The Handbook of Science and Technology Studies*, 3rd ed., ed. Edward J. Hackett, Olga Amsterdamska, Michael Lynch, and Judy Wacjman, 499–539. Cambridge, Mass.: MIT Press.

Fair, Brian. 2010. "Morgellons: Contested Illness, Diagnostic Compromise, and Medicalisation." *Sociology of Health and Illness* 32(4):597–612.

Ferreday, Debra. 2003. "Unspeakable Bodies: Erasure, Embodiment and the Pro-Ana Community." *International Journal of Cultural Studies* 6(3): 277–95.

First, Michael B. 2004. "Desire for Amputation of a Limb: Paraphilia, Psychosis, or New Type of Identity Disorder." *Psychological Medicine* 34:1–10.

Fox, N. J., K. J. Ward, and A. J. O'Rourke. 2005a. "The 'Expert Patient': Empowerment or Medical Dominance? The Case of Weight Loss, Pharmaceutical Drugs, and the Internet." *Social Science and Medicine* 60:1299–1309.

———. 2005b. "Pro-anorexia, Weight-Loss Drugs, and the Internet: An 'Anti-Recovery' Explanatory Model of Anorexia." *Sociology of Health and Illness* 60:944–71.

Fox, Susannah. 2005. "Health Information Online." Pew Internet and American Life Project. pewinternet. org/~/media//Files/Reports/2005/PIP_Healthtopics_May05.pdf.pdf.

———. 2006. "Online Health Search 2006." Pew Internet and American Life Project. pewinternet. org/~/media//Files/Reports/2006/PIP_Online_Health_2006.pdf.pdf.

———. 2008. "The Engaged E-patient Population." Pew Internet and American Life Project. pewinternet.org/~/media//Files/Reports/2008/PIP_Health_Aug08.pdf.pdf.

Fox, Susannah, and Deborah Fallows. 2003. "Internet Health Resources." Pew Internet and American Life Project. pewinternet.org/~/media//Files/Reports/2003/PIP_Health_Report_July_2003.pdf.pdf.

Gillet, James. 2003. "Media Activism and Internet Use by People with HIV/AIDS." *Sociology of Health and Illness* 25(6): 608–42.

Glaser, Barney G., and Anselm L. Strauss. 1965. *Awareness of Dying.* Chicago: Aldine.

Glaser, Gabrielle. 2008. "'Mad Pride' Fights a Stigma." *New York Times*, May 11.

Goetz, Thomas. 2008. "Practicing Patients." *New York Times Magazine*, March 23.

Goffman, Erving. 1961. *Asylums.* New York: Doubleday.

Gray, Nicola J., Jonathan D. Klein, Peter R. Noyce, Tracy S. Sesselberg, and Judith A. Cantrill. 2005. "Health-Information Seeking Behavior in Adolescents: The Place of the Internet." *Social Science and Medicine* 60:1467–78.

Greil, Arthur L. 1991. *Not Yet Pregnant: Infertile Couples in Contemporary America.* Philadelphia: Temple University Press.

Guo, Baorong, John C. Bricout, and Jin Huang. 2005. "A Common Open Space or a Digital Divide? A Social Mobility Perspective on the Online Disability Community in China." *Disability and Society* 20(1): 49–66.

Hardey, Michael. 1999. "Doctor in the House: The Internet as a Source of Lay Health Knowledge and the Challenge to Expertise." *Sociology of Health and Illness* 21(6): 820–35.

———. 2002. "'The Story of My Illness': Personal Accounts of Illness on the Internet." *Health: An Interdisciplinary Journal for the Social Study of Health, Illness, and Medicine* 6(1): 31–46.

Heffernan, Virginia. 2008. "The Medium: Narrow Minded." *New York Times*, May 25.

Internet World Stats. 2008. "Usage and Population Statistics." internetworldstats.com/stats.htm.

Karp, David. 1997. *Speaking of Sadness.* Oxford: Oxford University Press.

Klitzman, Robert, and Ronald Bayer. 2003. *Mortal Secrets: Truth and Lies in the Age of AIDS.* Baltimore: Johns Hopkins University Press.

Kutner, Nancy. 1987. "Social Worlds and Identity in End Stage Renal Disease." In *The Experience and Management of Chronic Illness,* ed. Peter Conrad and Julius A. Roth, 33–72. Vol. 6 in *Research in the Sociology of Health Care.* Greenwich, Conn.: JAI Press.

Lieberman, Morton A., Andre Winzelberg, Mitch Golant, Mari Wakihiro, Mariann DiMinno, Michael Aminoff, and Chadwick Christine. 2005. "Online Support Groups for Parkinson's Patients: A Pilot Study of Effectiveness." *Social Work in Health Care* 42(2): 23–38.

Loader, Brian D., Steve Muncer, Roger Burrows, Nicholas Pleace, and Sara Nettleton. 2002. "Medicine on the Line? Computer-Mediated Social Support and Advice for People with Diabetes." *International Journal of Social Welfare* 11:53–65.

Lohr, Steve. 2008. "Most Doctors Aren't Using Electronic Health Records." *New York Times,* June 19.

Marriott, Michel. 2006. "Digital Divide Closing as Blacks Turn to Internet." *New York Times,* March 31.

McKinlay, John B., and Lisa D. Marceau. 2002. "The End of the Golden Age of Doctoring." *International Journal of Health Services* 32:379–416.

Mechanic, David. 1996. "Changing Medical Organization and Erosion of Trust." *Milbank Quarterly* 74:171–89.

Miah, Andy, and Emma Rich. 2008. *The Medicalization of Cyberspace.* New York: Routledge.

Nettleton, Sarah, and Roger Burrows. 2003. "E-scaped medicine? Information, Reflexivity, and Health." *Critical Social Policy* 23(2): 165–85.

Nettleton, Sarah, Roger Burrows, and Lisa O'Malley. 2005. "The Mundane Realities of the Everyday Lay Use of the Internet for Health, and Their Consequences for Media Convergence." *Sociology of Health and Illness* 27(7): 972–92.

Parsons, Talcott. 1951. *The Social System.* New York: Free Press.

Parsons, Talcott, and Renée Fox. 1952. "Illness, Therapy and the Modern American Family." *Journal of Social Issues* 8:31–44.

PatientsLikeMe. 2008. patientslikeme.com/.

Pitts, Victoria. 2004. "Illness and Internet Empowerment: Writing and Reading Breast Cancer in Cyberspace." *Health: An Interdisciplinary Journal for the Social Study of Health, Illness, and Medicine* 8(1): 33–59.

Richardson, Jane C. 2005. "Establishing the (Extra)ordinary in Chronic Widespread Pain." *Health: An Interdisciplinary Journal for the Social Study of Health, Illness, and Medicine* 9(1): 31–48.

Rier, David. 2007. "Internet Social Support Groups as Moral Agents: The Ethical Dynamics of HIV+ Status Disclosure." *Sociology of Health and Illness* 29(7): 1043–58.

Roth, Julius A. 1963. *Timetables.* Indianapolis: Bobbs-Merrill.

Sandaunet, Anne-Grete. 2008. "The Challenge of Fitting In: Non-Participation and Withdrawal from an Online Self-Help Group for Breast Cancer Patients." *Sociology of Health and Illness* 30(1): 131–44.

Seale, Clive, Sue Ziebland, and Jonathan Charteris-Black. 2006. "Gender, Cancer Experience, and Internet Use: A Comparative Keyword Analysis of Interviews and Online Cancer Support Groups." *Social Science and Medicine* 62:2577–90.

Schneider, Joseph W., and Peter Conrad. 1983. *Having Epilepsy: The Experience and Control of Illness.* Philadelphia: Temple University Press.

Strauss, Anselm, and Barney G. Glaser. 1975. *Chronic Illness and the Quality of Life.* St. Louis: Mosby.

Stults, Cheryl. 2007. "Chronic Pain on the Internet: The Case of Arthritis and Fibromyalgia." Presented at the annual meeting of the Society for the Study of Social Problems, New York, August.

Suchman, Edward A. 1965. "Social Patterns of Illness and Medical Care." *Journal of Health and Human Behavior* 6:114–28.

Weitz, Rose. 1991. *Life with AIDS.* New Brunswick, N.J.: Rutgers University Press.

Williams, Gareth. 1984. "The Genesis of Chronic Illness: Narrative Reconstruction." *Sociology of Health and Illness* 6:175–200.

12

The Sociology of Disability
Historical Foundations and Future Directions

Gary L. Albrecht, University of Illinois at Chicago, University of Leuven, and Belgian Academy of Science and Arts

Disability is a high-profile issue situated at the intersection of the social sciences, health, and medicine. The definition of disability as a medical and social problem and proposed responses to it are central to discussions of health care and social welfare policies across the world today. The salience of disability issues is underscored by the recent high-level attention they are receiving from distinguished national and international organizations. Based on a coordinated analysis of more than a hundred recent national data surveys, the World Health Organization and the World Bank estimate in the 2010 "World Report on Disability and Rehabilitation" that 17 percent of the world's population (more than one billion people) currently experience disability.

Recognizing the enormity of the problem, the United Nations Convention on the Rights of Persons with Disabilities (2008) and the European Union Disability Strategy embodying the Charter of Fundamental Rights (2000) were passed to affirm that disabled people have the right to acquire and change nationalities, to retain their ability to exercise liberty, to have freedom of movement, to leave any country including their own, and to enter their own country and have access to the welfare and benefits afforded to any citizen of their country. These efforts elaborate and emphasize disability rights legislation like the American with Disabilities Act of 1990 and its amendments, the UK Disability Discrimination Act of 1995, the Disabled Person's Fundamental Law of Japan revised in 1993, and anti-discrimination laws passed in Russia in 1995 and South Africa in 1996. In the United States, disability has received heightened attention in two recent Institute of Medicine reports, *The Future of Disability in America* (2007) and *Improving the Presumptive Disability Decision-Making Process for Veterans* (2008).

Sociologists have long contributed to research and social policy discussions on disability and are counted among the leaders in the disability movement. As this chapter reflects, the sociology of disability has become a vibrant subspecialty in medical sociology and has attracted the attention of researchers in other sociological specialty areas like mental health and population demography. Here I highlight the key contributions that sociologists have made to the study of disability, show how sociologists are building on previous work and using cross-disciplinary perspectives to recast the critical issues facing disability researchers, and evaluate the strengths and weaknesses of the sociological approaches to disability.

How Sociologists Have Looked at Disability

The Concept and Problem of Disability

A persistent problem of conceptualizing disability has been understanding the relationships among disease, diagnosis, chronic illness, and disability, partly because instruments designed for description and diagnosis were often not appropriately operationalized for use in research. As a result, there was a historical disjunction between health-care practitioners, who required diagnostic categories to classify illnesses and conditions for the practice of medicine and for reimbursement under insurance schemes, and health-service researchers, demographers, and public health epidemiologists, who sought to understand the connections among diseases, illnesses, and disability. Beginning in the eighteenth century, numerous schemas were developed to classify diseases. By 1893 the Bertillon index of diseases was adopted by the International Statistics Institute at a meeting in Chicago to codify diseases. Since that time, the World Health Organization (WHO) has led efforts to untangle myriad measurement and classification problems by developing and standardizing an International Classification of Diseases (ICD) model, now in its tenth revision (ICD-10), to classify diseases and health conditions in the world.

These efforts also raised the problem of measuring and classifying disabilities. Key sociologists were central to these undertakings. In a 1965 publication, Nagi developed a disability model relating pathology, impairment, functional limitation, and disability that remains influential. According to Nagi, pathology represents an interruption in normal body processes as the body attempts to restore itself to its normal state. Impairment was defined in terms of anatomical or physiological abnormalities such as an amputated limb or multiple sclerosis. Functional limitations were conceived in terms of the restrictions that impairments placed on an individual's ability to perform activities and usual roles. Nagi saw disability as a "pattern of behavior that evolves in situations of long term or continued impairments that are associated with functional limitations"

(1965, 103). In this tradition, Phillip Wood in collaboration with Mike Bury developed the WHO *International Classification of Functioning, Disability and Health* (ICIDH), published in 1980, which was widely adopted to classify health-related domains that are associated with health conditions, some of which may result in restrictions in activity and role performance. The ICIDH-2 was organized into two parts, functioning and disability, and contextual factors.

While some sociologists participated in the first steps to define and understand disability, other sociologists (Oliver 1990; Higgins 1992) and disability activists (Pfeiffer 1998; Corker 1998; Shakespeare 2006) were critical of these initial efforts because they tended to medicalize disability, concentrated on deficits rather than differences in individuals, encouraged labeling, reinforced the passivity of disabled people, ignored or deemphasized the place of the physical and social environment in producing disability, did not adequately recognize the power of stigma and discrimination, diminished the responsibilities of the state in addressing disability issues, and failed to emphasize the fundamental rights of all human beings. The WHO responded to these concerns by developing a new, carefully vetted and field tested International Classification of Diseases and Functioning and Disability (ICF), which was approved at the World Health Assembly in 2001.

Sociologists and disability activists were also actively involved in the development of the ICF. There were key distinctions between U.S., Swedish, and British conceptions of disability that shaped early discussions on the ICF. U.S. conceptual models and research in the 1960s through the beginning of the 1990s emphasized the distinction between the able bodied and the disabled, focused on individuals, and stressed therapeutical interventions aimed at improving functional levels and enhancing role performance. This approach was focused on the individual and was strongly affected by the medical model. By contrast, Swedish researchers and policy makers in the 1970s conceived of disability as a difference among humans, a result of the interaction between individuals and their environments, and placed emphasis on adapting the environment to individuals and "normalizing" their lives (Söder 2006). This approach fit the concept of the Swedish welfare tradition, distinct from the U.S. concept of rugged individualism.

The British social model of disability was developed in the 1970s by the Union of the Physically Impaired against Segregation (UPIAS) who, inspired by Marxist politics, asserted that disability should be defined as the relationship between people with impairments and the society that excludes them (Shakespeare 2006). Oliver (1990) advocated for this approach in *The Politics of Disablement*, arguing that disability is a form of social oppression and should be addressed accordingly. The British sociologists Shakespeare (2006) and Barnes (1991) further elaborated the concept of disability in terms of the interaction between impaired individuals and their physical, social, and political environments. In Canada, Fougelrollas and Beauregard (2001) produced a similar model.

In the United States, Hahn (1988) developed a minority-group model of disability similar to those proposed in the race, gender, and ethnicity social movements of the 1960s and 1970s; his model served as a basis for the arguments in the Americans with Disabilities Act of 1990. Among sociologists, Zola set the tone in the United States for the disabled scholar-activist. In 1982, he recounted in *Missing Pieces: A Chronicle of Living with a Disability* his transformative experience of living for a short time in Het Dorp, an accessible residential facility in the Netherlands. While there, he decided that he would more publicly announce and celebrate his disability, encourage young disabled scholars in academic careers, and help develop an interdisciplinary disability studies specialty grounded in sociology. In the same year he along with four other sociologists—Daryl Evans, Steve Hey, Gary Kiger, and John Seidel—founded the Section for the Study of Chronic Illness, Impairment and Disability (SSCIID) of the Western Social Science Association, which became the Society for Disability Studies in 1986. In 1982 Zola also began editing the *Disability and Chronic Disease Newsletter* from Brandeis University, which in 1986 became the *Disability Studies Quarterly*. With these moves, Zola abandoned the

value neutrality of Max Weber and embraced the sociological activism of C. Wright Mills. He provided an example of applying sound theory and research to public sociology.

Based on the social model and minority-group models of disability, Pfeiffer (1998), in a critique of the medical model, proposed that the WHO ICIDH required major revision to be credible and useful.

It was these sociologists and kindred social scientists who led the charge for refining disability concepts and models, put pressure on the WHO to revise its definitions and measurement of disability, and demonstrated how sociological theory and research can be combined with personal experience to make important contributions to public sociology.

Issues Defined and Theories and Perspectives Employed

The critical issues addressed by sociologists interested in disability reflected the brief history of the development of disability definitions, the models just reviewed, and the larger issues within the sociology of the time. Certainly, early work in the sociology of disability was influenced by sociology inside and outside medicine (Bloom 2002). The first people in the area either were studying chronic illness and rehabilitation from a medical perspective and based in schools of medicine or were interested in deviance, identity, social class, professions, organizations, family, and labeling as applied to disability and situated in departments of sociology. Three early works—*Sociology and Rehabilitation* (1965), edited by Sussman and published by the American Sociological Association, and *The Sociology of Physical Disability and Rehabilitation* (1976) and *Cross National Rehabilitation Policies* (1981), edited by Albrecht—are indicative of the discussions of the time. In these volumes, Nagi raised issues of definition and models; Gove and Becker, of societal reaction theory and labeling; Alexander and Featherman, of social class; Sussman, of disabled people, their families, and the rehabilitation system; Stone and Krause, of political economic perspectives; Davis, Roth, and Zola, of the personal experience of disability; Anselm Strauss, of chronic illness and disability across the life course; Albrecht and Levy, of the social construction of disability as a social problem; Shanas and Haug, of disability and aging; and Freidson and Krause, of medical professions and rehabilitation work.

The theory development and research of the 1960s through the 1980s reflected divisions in how scholars defined and parsed disability. In demographic and epidemiological studies undertaken by the U.S. Census Bureau, its counterparts around the world, and the WHO, World Bank, and Centers for Disease Control (CDC), disability is considered a causative factor in restricting physical function, social activity, and participation. Yet sociologists and other social scientists who were not epidemiologists or demographers worked within rather tightly constricted areas such as types of physical disability; mental illness; and developmental, intellectual, cognitive, and sensory disabilities. Each of these research areas produced classic work that not only highlighted different types of disability but also developed an armamentarium of concepts and theories (Bury 2000). Examples include Roth's (1963) *Timetables: Structuring the Passage of Time in Tuberculosis Treatment and Other Careers*, which explored the notions of time and patient careers in rehabilitating from chronic illnesses and disabilities. His subsequent work with Eddy, *Rehabilitation for the Unwanted* (1967), drew early attention to the institutionalization of people who seemed deviant so that they could be resocialized before they were admitted back into society. Scott (1968) showed how blind men were "made" through socialization processes inside and outside institutions. Strauss and colleagues (1975) built on such work by introducing a life-span perspective into the study of chronic illness and disability and asking how it affected quality of life. Bury (1982) added to this line of work by conceiving of chronic illness and disabilities as "biographical disruptions," events and experiences that altered one's identity, plans, and expectations. Charmaz (1991) introduced the idea of an ebb and flow of feelings, function, and identity through the course of the chronic illness and disability experience. These seminal works developed concepts, theories, and metaphors that were later used to expand analyses

of disability across the life span, of the power of socialization and resocialization in shaping disability identity and expectations, and of the place of emotions and function in determining self-worth in the disability experience.

Goffman's (1963) work on stigma continues to be one of the major contributions to the study of disability in terms of concepts and content. His distinctions among stigmas due to abominations of the body, blemishes of individual character, and tribal stigmas of race, nation, and religion generated a body of work that flourishes to this day. This research drew attention to distinctions between visible and invisible disabilities and the differential moral evaluations that society and cultures associated with different types of disabling conditions, from spinal cord injury to HIV/AIDS. Labeling theory, also referred to as societal reaction theory, which developed out of sociological theories of deviance, focused on majority representations of "different" people as being deviant, subsequently "labeled," treated stereotypically, and often discriminated against (Becker 1963). In a study of intellectual disability, Mercer (1973) used this framework to analyze how clinicians and schools classify students as "mentally retarded" and what the consequences were of the labeling. Working in this tradition as well, Higgins (1980) used a deviance and labeling perspective to examine how deaf people were perceived as deviant by the general public, and how, within the deaf community, people who sold pencils or begged in public places were seen as deviant.

During the 1960s through the 1980s, the development of sociological research on mental illness as a disability ran a parallel but somewhat separate course from that of physical, intellectual, cognitive, and sensory disabilities. The reasons lie in historical events, some differences in method and theoretical frameworks, and funding sources. Whereas sociologists working on the types of disability just discussed generally relied on case and community-based studies and qualitative research methods, early sociological research on mental illness was more epidemiological in nature—focused on neighborhoods and mental health catchment areas—was quantitative in methodology, and was often funded by the National Institutes of Mental

Health (NIMH). As a consequence, much of this work is survey based or observational, or consists of evaluations of institutional and community interventions. Hollingshead and Redlich's 1958 study of the epidemiology of mental illness in New Haven and Srole's 1962 Midtown Manhattan Study were two of the first sociologically oriented studies funded by NIMH. While all the members of the National Advisory Mental Health Council at the time initially were physicians, sociologists found a research home in the early days of NIMH. Clausen, Brim, Srole, Kohn, and Pearlin were among the sociologists whose early work on mental illness was supported by NIMH. In fact, many of them worked at NIMH at this point in their careers. Because of the nature of the funding institution, much of the work reflected the interests of the then-current social psychiatry. The initial work on psychosocial epidemiology continues today, with a fundamental interest in the social class determinants of health (Kessler and Wang 2008; Adler and Rehkopf 2008). Clausen and Brim's interests in socialization and life-span approaches to mental illness and aging were expressed in streams of research. Kohn and Pearlin did foundational work on cross-cultural differences in health and illness and on the family's role in health. At NIMH, Pearlin developed models of stress, coping, buffers to the effects of mental illness, and caregiving that were undergirded with years of survey research.

Further work on mental illness produced concepts and perspectives that were fruitfully applied to studies of both mentally and physically disabled people. During this period, Mechanic began his work on the illness experience, the organization and financing of care for the severely mentally ill, and the criminalization of mental illness. Goffman's concepts of stigma and total institutions and labeling theory also stimulated a plenitude of research in mental illness. Scheff's *Being Mentally Ill* (1966) sparked a debate between labeling theorists and Gove (1978). In general terms, Scheff argued that society views certain behaviors as deviant and frequently labels people mentally ill because they exhibit these behaviors. The process becomes mutually reinforcing because people who are labeled mentally ill increasingly live up to those expectations. Society, then, according to this position, makes people mentally ill by its need to categorize and explain deviant behavior. Gove countered that the public's perception of behaviors that suggest mental illness is indeed based on observable behavior and not just on socially produced labels. Link and colleagues (1989), Thoits (1999), and other researchers have conducted numerous studies which suggest that labeling does affect the classification, expectations, and treatment of the mentally ill but that these processes are affected by the history of the behavior, the situation, the environment, and more recently, biological factors (Major and O'Brien 2005).

Research on the medicalization of deviant behavior (Zola 1972; Conrad and Schneider 1992; Conrad 2007) built upon the arguments of labeling theory, social construction, and analyses of the professional dominance of medicine (Freidson 1970) to show how common conditions like hyperactivity, erectile dysfunction, and "feeling down or blue" were defined as deviant and made into health problems worthy of medical attention. As such deviant conditions were medicalized, they also became conceptualized as impairments and viewed behaviorally as disabilities. Within the medical arena of disability and rehabilitation, medicalizaton also occurred when, to enhance the body, athletic performance, and subjective perceptions of well-being, health-care professionals expanded the use of procedures and drugs developed for serious and unusual conditions. For example, techniques developed to repair serious facial injuries incurred in automobile accidents or in war were later employed to do cosmetic surgery. Similarly, corticosteroids were injected near the point of injury of individuals suspected of suffering a spinal cord injury to reduce inflammation and pressure on the spinal cord and subsequent paralysis. But these and anabolic steroids used to treat anemia were later employed singly or in combination by athletes to improve performance and by the general public to enhance their looks. Likewise, serotonin reuptake inhibitors (SRIs) developed to control severe depression were later prescribed and used by a wide public to enhance general feelings of well-being. Such analyses of medicalization drew renewed attention to the questions, What is normal and what is not? What are impairments and disabilities?

The disability rights movement originating in the United States and the UK presented a further critique of the medicalization of disability. Much of this movement was grassroots in origin and involved sociologists or those with sociological training (Zola 1982; Scotch 1984; 1988; Oliver 1990; Barnes 1991; Charlton 1998; Shakespeare 2006). In 1972, three spinal cord–injured people with connections to the University of California, Berkeley, led by Ed Roberts, formally incorporated the first Center for Independent Living (CIL) in the United States This revolutionary movement redefined the power dynamics between the medical establishment, the state, and disabled people because CILs are run and controlled by disabled people and are located in the community, not in institutions. Disabled people became active participants in their own lives, care, and destinies. They campaigned for inclusion in society, embracing the slogan, "Nothing about us without us." Such grassroots efforts directly confronted the forces of medicalization and successfully resulted in the Rehabilitation Act of 1973, Section 504, which asserts that people with disabilities have equal rights that prevent discrimination based on the disability in programs or activities that receive federal funding. Further activism and lobbying produced the Americans with Disabilities Act of 1990 (ADA) which expanded previous legislation by prohibiting discrimination in employment, housing, public accommodations, education, and public services.

Concurrent with this movement in the United States, the Union of the Physically Impaired against Segregation (UPIAS) in the UK published a paper in 1975 that reconceptualized the concept of disability from a deficit within the individual in need of medical and social intervention to a condition produced by a discriminatory physical, social, political, and economic environment. The resulting "social model" of disability was at once a stirring critique of the medical model of disability and a conceptual basis for the international disability rights movement as it spread around the world, culminating in a series of UN declarations condemning discrimination and recognizing the human rights of disabled people.

The U.S. civil rights movement, the global women's movement, and the disability rights movement called attention to the issue of being multiply discriminated against on the basis of race, gender, and disability. These multiple stigmas created serious health disparities and resulted in constrained life chances for disabled women, particularly if they were minorities. They are poorer than disabled men, are more likely to be heads of households, are often viewed as "asexual," are at greater risk for sexual abuse than are nondisabled women, receive less education than do nondisabled women or disabled men, and have less access to services than do men with disabilities (Bowe 1984; G. Frank 2000; Lorber 2000; Peters and Opacich 2006). The condition and rights of disabled women have become critical arenas for studying the cumulative effects of bearing multiple stigmas, effects of health and welfare disparities, and discrimination among the most vulnerable.

Early seminal work on disability and the family focused attention on how disabled family members produced stigma and stress, altered social structures and roles within the family, changed family relationships within the community, evoked the need for a caregiving system, and developed as a coping unit. For example, Farber's study (1962) of families with a severely developmentally disabled (DD) child suggested that placement of a young, male DD child outside the home had beneficial effects on the parents and female siblings who were relieved from child-care duties. This early work focused attention on caretaker burden and coping mechanisms to deal with a disabled family member. Likewise, Sussman's (1987) work over thirty years drew attention to how a disabled family member modified family structure, rearranged social roles, and altered the family as an economic unit. Later research summarized by Ferguson (2001) suggested that disability did affect family life but that responses to a disabled family member were highly variable within families and that responses to disability depended on family resources, on the type and severity of the disability, and on coping mechanisms. Taken in concert, these theories, concepts, and studies provide a flavor of the contributions that sociologists have made historically to the field of disability.

Sociologists have made critically important conceptual and theoretical contributions to the study of disability through their work on disability definitions, models of the disabling process, socialization into disability roles, disability identity and experience, deviant behavior and normalization, life stages, stigma and discrimination, stress and coping, institutionalization, social class, stratification and deprivation, culture, and quality of life as applied to disabled people and their worlds. Their empirical work was influenced by history and the social movements of the times. For example, much work was done on disabled veterans after World War II, the Korean conflict, and the Vietnam War. Studies on the creation of disability were related to social and behavioral issues like hyperkinesis in children, attention deficit disorder, and cognitive changes in the behavior of the elderly that were defined as deviant behaviors and social problems and were medicalized. Research and social activism based on the social movements surrounding race and gender informed studies of the formation and development of the disability movement (Scotch and Schriner 1997).

Much of the best work in the sociology of disability was affected by sociologists' personal experiences. Prominent sociologists of these times had served in the military and deeply appreciated the effects of combat and stress on disability. Other sociologists tackled problems related to their own disabilities and family or work experiences. Roth spent time in a tuberculosis hospital, Zola lived with the effects of polio, Higgins had deaf parents, and Charmaz built on her experiences as a therapist.

Sociological research on disability was also shaped by the settings in which sociologists worked, who their colleagues were, and who supported their research. Goffman was a classic ethnographer who labored alone, spending considerable time in a mental hospital observing daily behavior, routines, and decision making, and analyzing the organization and operations of the institution. Hollingshead and Redlich were funded by the nascent NIMH to do a large-scale mental health epidemiological study in the community of New Haven. Clausen, Kohn, and Pearlin conducted their early research as employees of NIMH, where the leaders were physicians and psychiatrists who were open to sociological research. Research in this environment by the very nature of the setting and colleagues focused on mental illness generally as seen from a medical perspective. By contrast, Scheff and Becker, working in traditional sociology departments and not receiving major funding for their work, developed labeling and societal reaction theory based on theories of deviant behavior.

As sociologists began to work outside sociology departments, they began to do more interdisciplinary research. The resulting studies profited from being informed by sociological concepts and theories but were grounded in the situation. The growth of government funding agencies like the U.S. Census Bureau, the Department of Health and Human Services (DHHS), the Social Security Administration (SSA), the National Institutes of Health (NIH), the NIMH and Rehabilitation Services Administration (RSA), the Centers for Disease Control (CDC), and private foundations enabled sociologists to conduct large multidisciplinary surveys, community studies, and evaluation research on disability. In these environments, sociologists worked in teams with demographers, epidemiologists, physicians, therapists, economists, and psychologists. The resulting research produced a broader and more nuanced view of disability and more methodologically sophisticated studies.

Sociologists moved from the development of concepts and theory to designing and undertaking a broad range of qualitative, case, community-based, survey, and evaluation studies that accumulated evidence to test and refine their perspectives and hypotheses about disability. Arguments were increasingly supported by accumulating evidence that forced the modification and elaboration of previous positions. More attention was given to what data one had to support an argument and how to design and execute the next studies to test revised hypotheses. The resulting evidence was then used to inform government social policy, indicate unmet public health and welfare needs, and suggest intervention programs.

Historically, sociological work in disability was segregated into different camps and spheres of influence based on physical, mental, intellectual, cognitive, and sensory disabilities. This was in part due to traditional divisions in the specialties in medicine that dealt with various impairments. Internal medicine, neurology, surgery, psychiatry, and physical medicine and rehabilitation concentrate on different problems. Sociologists studying a particular impairment or disability were forced by the nature of these divisions to follow preestablished medical road maps. Another reason for the balkanization of disabilities is the power of special interest groups and foundations to focus attention and resources on their disabilities of choice. For instance, the Kennedy family advocated for the study and treatment of intellectual disabilities; the Hogg Foundation, for depression and mental illness; Christopher Reeves, for spinal cord injury; and the Robert Wood Johnson Foundation, for childhood obesity, in an effort to prevent impairments and disabilities later in life.

During the last forty years, numerous professional organizations have recognized the study of disability. There are now sections of the American Sociological Association (ASA) devoted to disability and mental illness, and others like medical sociology, aging and the life course, and population that represent strong disability interests. The American Psychological Association (APA) has had a long-standing rehabilitation division, the American Public Health Association has a disability special interest group, and there is a Society for Disability Studies. Sociologists within the HIV/AIDS arena have also come to the realization that with improved treatment regimens, AIDS is a chronic condition with many disabling consequences. The sociologists have also been instrumental in producing the *Handbook of Disability Studies* (Albrecht, Seelman, and Bury 2001) and the *Encyclopedia of Disability* (Albrecht 2006).

How Sociologists Are Moving the Study of Disability Forward

Social Networks

While appreciative of previous contributions, current thinking on disability is moving beyond the influence of functionalism, deviance, labeling,

minority-group, and social movement models to consider disability as the result of the interrelationship among individuals, the social groups to which they belong, and their physical and social environments. From this perspective, social networks are important to understanding people's activities and participation in society. A social network is a social structure comprised of nodes, which are usually persons or organizations, tied together by communication and some type of interdependency such as kinship, friendship, trade, financial exchange, political persuasion, and values. Social networks bind people and organizations together, allowing them to work in concert to accomplish individual and group goals. Social network analysis shows graphically which actors in a network have the most social capital—the ability to influence the behavior of others in the network. This type of analysis also demonstrates how membership and position influence behavior patterns and changes in the network.

The contributions of Latour (2005) to actor-network theory and Pescosolido's (2001; Pescosolido and Wright 2004) use of social network models to understand physical and mental disabilities in terms of social relationships and social structure point the way for future disability research. Laumann's (Cornwell, Laumann, and Schumm 2008) examination of the social glue that holds groups together provides insights into the role of social connectedness in facilitating participation in society and mitigating the effects of aging and disability. Christakis's (Christakis and Fowler 2007; Smith and Christakis 2008) emerging body of work examines how one's membership and place in social networks affect health. Specifically, he and his colleagues have shown that health conditions such as obesity and behaviors such as smoking which lead to disability are spread through social ties in networks. Researchers could be well advised to use similar approaches to investigate the epidemiology of disability, the influence of social class on social networks, social ties to knowledge and care, support networks, and quality of life for disabled people. Barker (2008), for instance, suggests that electronic support groups clustered around specific illnesses generate an increased level of lay knowledge that empowers members and gives them knowledge to be informed consumers. By extension, the quality of disability diagnosis, treatment, and prognosis would benefit from network analysis of groups connected electronically around certain types of impairments like autism, depression, and Parkinson's disease. Social network models and analysis point the way to better conceptualizing the interactive nature of disability and the epidemiology of conditions and suggests public health interventions and policies that could positively alter the lives of disabled people. From a methodological viewpoint, it is also important to examine whether or not the descriptive patterns and relationships that are being uncovered through network analysis are merely correlations or indicate causal forces at work.

Sociology of the Body

Another fruitful approach to understanding disability is captured in the concept of the sociology of the body. From this perspective, disability is a way of being physically and socially embedded in the world. Much of this work has been done in Europe and Australia or by social scientists in other disciplines in the United States but offers considerable promise for researchers in the sociology of disability. Bryan Turner broke new ground with *The Body and Society* (1984), where he explored two versions of the sociology of the body in contemporary social thought. The first approach, stimulated by Foucault (1965, 1973), analyzed how the human body is socially produced, governed, and regulated. This view leads to an exploration of how disability is socially constructed and how rehabilitation is way of "normalizing" aberrations of the body. According to this perspective, medicine and government combine to exercise normative control over the self. The second approach has intellectual origins in Merleau-Ponty's (1961) analysis of the phenomenology of the body, in which he recognized the complex interaction between the objectified body of medical discourse, the subjective body of personal experience, and the body image that "embodies" the space between identity, experience, and social relationships. This approach suggests research on how disabled people recognize and deal with con-

flicting information and expectations obtained from health-care professionals, their own experience, and the expectations of others encountered in their social networks.

Bryan Turner (2001a) summarized his long-stated position that the theory and concepts developed around the sociology of the body could be fruitfully applied to research on disability. Using this framework, Seymour (1989, 1998) examined how medicalization of patients and the enforcement of the medical model had negative consequences for disabled patients in the Australian health-care system. In the United States, Zola (1991) echoed these sentiments in his ASA awards presentation on "bringing ourselves and our bodies back in." There he called for medical sociologists to refocus their work on the subjective experience, meaning, and consequences of disability. He pointed out that with the aging of populations the distinction between being "able-bodied" and "disabled" was becoming blurred, and that disability policy ought to be universalized to include all types of disability and extend to those who someday may share the disability experience (Zola 1989). In a later study, Brown and his colleagues (2004) show how the body perspective can aptly be applied to the study of health movements. They argue that embodied health movements are unique in focusing on the personal experience of disabled people, challenging existing medical knowledge and practice and involving disability activists along with health professionals in research and practice enterprises. Schilling (2007) more recently reviewed the current of research in the sociology of the body, calling for more sociologists to reconsider the importance of the body in their studies.

Disability Inequalities

While an enormous amount of research has been conducted over the years on health disparities (House et al. 1988; Siegrist and Marmot 2006; Braveman 2006; Agency for Healthcare Research and Quality 2008; Gehlert et al. 2008; Adler and Rehkopf 2008), less attention has been given to applying these concepts to disability. Therefore, examination of disability disparities is an area ripe for research. We know from the health disparities literature that being poor, being an immigrant, belonging to a racial or ethnic minority, living in a poor neighborhood, having limited access to care, and being exposed to other environmental barriers cumulatively cause a downward spiral in terms of illness and disease for both individuals and populations. This is also true of disability. Disabled people tend to be poor, disenfranchised, or both. Either they are poor and disabled to start with, or the experience of disability leads them on a trail to poverty. For instance, in the United States, about half the severely disabled people who cannot work because of their condition are totally dependent on government programs for health care and income support. Most often these benefits, insufficient to meet their needs, place them at or below the official designated poverty level (Batavia and Beaulaurier 2001). Those with less serious disabilities often have inadequate health insurance or none at all. This forces them to consume all their own resources before they reach levels of need where they are eligible for additional government benefits. The interrelationship between poverty and disability is so acute that the World Bank sees this as an enormous threat to development and has responded by launching a global program to reduce poverty and hence disability (Disability and Development Team 2004; Miller and Ziegler 2006).

It is also interesting to note that although the majority of disability activists are well educated and privileged, few speak for poor, uneducated, and generally unseen disabled people. As a result, research findings from studies on the most visible groups are often assumed to be generalizable to the less privileged and less noticeable groups, with erroneous conclusions. For instance, seriously disabled people do not necessarily have a poorer quality of life than have less disabled people or the larger population (Albrecht and Devlieger 1999) and poor blacks do not have as highly developed a disability culture as working and middle-class whites have (Devlieger, Albrecht, and Hertz 2007). And for all the attention given to immigrants, disability is not seen as an important issue for them. Yet recent research indicates that disability is a major understudied issue in the study of immigration (Albrecht, Devlieger, and

Van Hove 2008). Thus, the multilayered issues of disability disparities require further attention.

Citizenship and Human Rights

Citizenship and human rights perspectives on disability have also opened up productive lines of research. Traditionally, citizenship has been defined as membership in a political or geographic community where citizens are accorded basic rights and are expected to have corresponding duties and responsibilities. There are two components of citizenship: juridical status, which conveys civil rights and political liberties on members of a nation-state, and social membership in the nation-state, which permits citizens to benefit from the social and economic rewards of being a member. Both juridical and social membership are key to the well-being of disabled citizens, for without being recognized they would have difficulty accessing health care and social welfare benefits and being integrated into social support networks.

In general, there is increased interest among sociologists about what it means to be a citizen of the world or an immigrant, to be multicultural, or to live an international life, and what challenges such individuals present to the nation-state (B. Turner 2001b; Bloemraad, Korteweg, and Yurdakul 2008). This research is pertinent to the study of disability because many people are migrating today from conflict zones and areas of civil unrest and drought with disabilities incurred or exacerbated by their environment. As they move, they put enormous stress on the recipient country or international aid organizations. Derose, Escarce, and Lurie (2007) indicate that these are very vulnerable people. In light of these facts, sociologists could contribute by studying the experiences of disabled immigrants, the consequences for the communities where they land, and the state welfare systems of the recipient countries.

At the same time, there is increased emphasis on the human rights of disabled people, exemplified by the UN Convention on the Rights of Persons with Disabilities (2008). Half the countries of the world have recently signed this accord. The recognition of fundamental human rights for disabled people has been facilitated by an increasing public appreciation of global interdependency and by media attention to wars, failed states, natural disasters, and famine. Some examples include the movie *Hotel Rwanda* and video reports from war zones that show how armed conflicts produce disabled people. The Special Olympics for disabled athletes now runs along with the world Olympics, is broadcast worldwide, and demonstrates what disabled people can do. Mainstreaming disabled students in classrooms puts all students, teachers, and parents in contact with disabled youngsters. Curb cuts, motorized wheelchairs, and prosthetics have enabled disabled people to venture out frequently in public. As a consequence, people seem to be more aware of the plight of vulnerable people and more receptive to doing something about it. Human rights activities are based on values and moral beliefs, respect for others, and acknowledgement of mutual responsibility in a global world. In terms of disability research, this would stimulate studies of changing values, perceived vulnerability, reassessment of responsibilities, and respect for the other as related to disabled people.

Physical and Social Environments

An additional area of interest and opportunity for sociologists is the study of the physical and social environments of disabled people. The WHO's ICF and emerging models of disability emphasize the role of the environment in producing and maintaining barriers for disabled people. In fact, breaking down barriers is a key social policy approach to integrating disabled people into the community and increasing their levels of independence, activity, and participation. In the UK, Imrie (2000) and Edwards and Imrie (2008) have illustrated how the geography of access dramatically influences activity levels and perceived quality of life among disabled people. At the University of Leuven in Belgium, Devlieger and colleagues (2006) worked with blind and visually impaired people to ascertain what changes could be made in private and public spaces to transform the city into a welcoming space for people with a broad range of physical and sensory disabilities.

The theoretical consideration of observing how individuals observe and interact with their environments resulted in pragmatic changes such as curb cuts, ramps, accessible restrooms, auditory signals at crosswalks, and signage changes in the train station and elevators throughout the university that made the urban space friendlier to a wide variety of people. In the United States, architects and engineers engendered the universal design model to build spaces that were hospitable to people across the life span and at different levels and types of disability. Such planning has also been built into information technologies like computer designs, hardware, software, and smart houses that will interact with the inhabitants. MIT has been a leader in designing Internet courses and materials that are accessible to people with sensory disabilities. This represents a movement toward modifying our virtual environments to make them more user friendly.

The sociological study of the real and virtual environment should be a natural area for development in disability research that builds on the tradition of the Chicago school of sociology, where attention was directed on how urban areas, neighborhoods, and public spaces interacted with peoples' behavior, social structures, organizations, and community. Sampson and colleagues (1997, 2002, 2008) hint at how this work might be undertaken in their studies of neighborhood effects on crime, perceptions of vulnerability, and reproduction of racial inequality. This work also employs multilevel modeling so that individual, structural, and neighborhood effects can be disentangled. Similar approaches to the study of disability in the community would help us understand better how individuals interact with their environments. For example, it would be useful to know what effects resource-rich environments would have on the activity, performance, and quality of life of disabled people and, obversely, how poor neighborhoods with high crime rates isolate and alienate them.

Political Economy

Stone (1984) and Albrecht (1992) have suggested that more research on disability be informed by a political economic perspective to understand the interplay of the major structural forces that influence how disability is defined as a social problem and responded to. In these analyses, Stone used the analogy of the disabled state to examine how the government defines disability, and what programs are developed and resources allocated by the government to address the problem. Albrecht employed the metaphor of the disability business to show how the definition of disability as a social problem and the rehabilitation response in health care and social services in the United States were based on an American form of capitalism and the state that emphasized health care as a commodity that can be marketed and sold for a profit. Light (2001) lays out a strong argument for the importance of studying health-care—and, by inference, disability—markets from a sociological perspective. This work indicates that important research remains to be done to understand the structure, organization, rationing, and outcomes of the disability marketplace.

Disability and Biology

After some years of hesitation, compared to their colleagues in public health and psychology, sociologists are now actively engaged in sociological research that combines social, health, and biological marker variables in one study. Among early sociological leaders in this field was Udry, who worked with sociologists, physicians, and geneticists since the late 1960s on large studies that combined demographic and social variables with measures of hormone levels and other biological measures in survey, clinical, and cohort studies to understand sexual behavior, violence and delinquent behavior, and school and marriage behavior (Udry and Morris 1970; Udry 1988). More recently, the Institute of Medicine (2001) has encouraged the development of interdisciplinary research that studies the interplay of biological, behavioral, and social variables on health outcomes, and the NIH and foundations are funding this work. As this research became more mainstream among sociologists, young researchers are being cross-trained in sociology, biology, and genetics. Freese, Li, and Wade (2003) suggested that the incorporation of biology and

genetics into sociological work and vice versa will increase the power and range of our explanations. This work concentrates on nature-nurture kinds of issues such as gene-environment interactions related to health behaviors, the effects of hormone levels on social behavior, the combined effect of exposure to a risky environment (Agent Orange in Vietnam, combat in Iraq and Afghanistan; high HIV prevalence; poor neighborhoods), and traditional sociological variables.

Future research will examine how social, structural, and biological variables interact to explain behavior and how social conditions affect biological mechanisms. Two recent examples of this work are Boardman and colleagues (2008), who have studied how school settings may moderate the genetic effects of smoking, and Seltzer and colleagues (2009), who showed that, compared with other parents, parents of disabled children had elevated levels of stress, negative affect, and physical symptoms. Furthermore, their diurnal rhythm of cortisol expression differed significantly from the comparison group, suggesting that having a disabled child in the family has simultaneously social, biological, and health consequences.

Clearly this type of research is pertinent to understanding better the origins, dynamics, and consequences of disability. While sociologists have turned their lenses on medicalization, ethics, and the social context of the new genetics (Shakespeare 2006), few have joined with geneticists, biologists, and physicians to explore how disability is understood on the social and biological levels considered conjointly. Some examples of this kind of research are examining how modifying environments, social expectations, and schools can change the lives of those with Down's syndrome, and studying the effects of targeted gene and hormone therapies on levels of activity and participation among disabled people.

Evidence, Methods, and Measurement

Social, medical, and management sciences are placing increased attention on evidence and outcomes. This movement has strong sociological roots in a Durkheimian emphasis on facts and particularly on "social facts." Current research is also characterized by the rapidity with which research is conducted and reported around the world, thanks to electronic publishing, the global nature of the research enterprise, and recognition that interdisciplinary research is becoming a standard for understanding complex issues. Within this context there are a number of trends that will improve the type and quality of disability research.

The first is looking at disability across classification boundaries. R. Jay Turner (2006) has been a leader in this regard by investigating the relationship between physical disability, mental health, and substance disorders. His work on stress underscores the importance of considering the mental health effects of dealing with a physical disability (Reynolds and Turner 2008). It is also not a surprise that individuals with physical and mental disabilities often have problems with substance abuse, since many are using multiple medications and dealing with pain and psychological distress. In the disability arena, it is imperative to recognize that most disabled individuals are dealing with multiple disabilities and comorbidities at the same time. Sociologists can further contribute to the study of disability by taking the whole person as the unit of analysis, perhaps within a sociology of the body perspective, to examine how multiple types of disability coalesce around the same person to create complicated problems that can best be appreciated in context. Yet, even though physical and mental disabilities are beginning to be addressed together sociologically, little comparable work has been done on the conjunction of intellectual, cognitive, and sensory disabilities with other physical and mental disabilities. This should be on the future agenda.

The second methodological trend is using multilevel modeling techniques to jointly analyze the effects of variables at different levels of analysis on a selected outcome. This permits the simultaneous analysis of data collected from biological, social, and environmental variables to observe their relative effects on the production of disability and on disabled peoples' activity and participation. A third methodological contribution is grounded in building longitudinal data sets using cohort designs to sort out causation; temporal sequence is integrated into the design. Such designs also allow disability researchers to concentrate on transition state analyses. Most studies of disability are based on surveys, cross-sectional designs, and point estimates (Altman and Barnartt 2000; Mont 2007). Yet we know from qualitative methods and case studies that disability is a condition that can come and go in a person's life. Transition state analyses borrowed from demographic studies of migration and research on economic cycles would permit investigators to ask what factors explain the onset of disability and movement in and out of the disabled state. Such research is critical for understanding health, illness, and disability across the life course and for designing effective interventions to assist disabled people and their families.

A fourth major contribution to disability studies is the increasing use of mixed methods research to construct a more holistic view of the disability process and of disabled people. While surveys and cohort studies are essential in the study of disability, qualitative, case study, and focus group methods are necessary to reach difficult-to-find people like immigrants and many types of disabled people (A. Frank 1995). By analyzing the content of major sociological journals, Seale (2008) noted clear differences in the types of research being done in medical sociology in the UK and the United States in terms of theory, method, and content. U.S. journals are more quantitative in orientation, publish more on race and social divisions in American society, and draw less on social constructionism and a range of social theories than do their British counterparts. Seale implies that work on both sides of the Atlantic could be improved by using multiple methods, engaging issues that concern nonsociologists, and being more outward looking and international in scope. This is certainly true in disability research (Winance, Ville, and Ravaud 2007).

A final methodological advance of note is engaging more in participatory action research in which disabled people and the people from the communities being studied are treated as equal partners in designing the research and in collecting and interpreting the data (Cargo and Mercer 2008). Zola (1991) was a proponent of this approach, which embodies the disability activist mantra, "Nothing about us without us" (Charlton 1998). This approach addresses numerous threats to validity in disability research and involves disabled people in ways that may have policy implications for their lives (Iezzoni and O'Day 2006).

These five methodological advances are important because they permit disability to be studied in context rather than piecemeal, variable by variable. One of the interesting and frustrating aspects of studying disability is that it is terribly complex. These new methodological approaches permit researchers to study disability in its complexity and to disentangle directions of effect and the interaction of variables at multiple levels of analysis, and to "embody" investigations informed by the knowledge and experience of disabled people. Such an approach is more likely to paint an accurate picture of disability and to address multiple threats to validity.

Strengths and Weaknesses of Sociological Approaches to Disability

This chapter concludes by drawing attention to the strengths and weaknesses of the sociological approaches to disability and suggesting how this work can be advanced. In sum, on the one hand, sociology provides useful theory in terms of stigma, stress, medicalization, labeling, social networks, health disparities, and neighborhood contexts in addressing disability. Sociological research findings have contributed much to what we know about the social and behavioral aspects of disability. Sociologists have been key figures in designing and undertaking large national studies and now multinational studies on disability with focuses on general disability, activity and participation, stigma, HIV/AIDS, mental illness, and work. Sociologists have been major participants in helping develop the field of disability studies. They have been part of the grassroots movement to put sociology into practice. Sociologists have been key contributors in fielding studies where the people to be studied are included on the research team to help focus the issues, design the study, and develop the methods of participatory action research.

On the other hand, much of the work in the sociology of disability is American and generally very Western oriented and may not apply well to the rest of the world. This raises questions of ex-

ternal validity. The world population today is 6.7 billion people and rising. Most of the research on medical sociology and disability is conducted by researchers in the United States, Canada, the twenty-seven-member European Community, Australia, and New Zealand. These nations comprise 12.8 percent of the world's population. We have to ask, What do we know about the other 87.2 percent of the rest of the world, where there are many forms of government, race, culture, and religion?

Considerable attention also needs to be given to the way in which physical and mental disabilities are often experienced simultaneously by disabled people but studied separately. Furthermore, sociologists have generally not worked closely with geneticists, neurobiologists, and epidemiologists using biomarkers to investigate how behavior is shaped by the interaction of social, biological, and environmental variables that are crucial to understanding disability. In addition, sociologists have not given full attention to the physical, social, political, and cultural environments of disabled people as they affect levels of activity and participation or developed sound measures of these environments. Finally, cohort studies are necessary to examine the transitions of people moving in and out of disabled states and the cumulative effect of social networks and environments on disabled people. The sociology of disability can move ahead by building on the historical strengths of the discipline but also by attending to some apparent limitations. The scope and importance of this work will be determined by whether this is good sociology, is interesting to scientists outside the field, provides the foundations for sound social policy, and makes a difference in the lives of disabled people.

Note

This research was supported in part through a fellowship to the author from the Royal Flemish Academy in Belgium for Science and the Arts, Brussels, 2006–2008.

References

Adler, Nancy E., and David H. Rehkopf. 2008. "U.S. Disparities in Health: Descriptions, Causes, and Mechanisms." *Annual Review of Public Health* 29:235–52.

Agency for Healthcare Research and Quality. 2008. *A*

National Healthcare Disparities Report. ahrq.gov/qual/nhdro6/nhdror.htm. Accessed November 2, 2008.

Albrecht, Gary L., ed. 1976. *The Sociology of Physical Disability and Rehabilitation.* Pittsburgh: University of Pittsburgh Press.

———, ed. 1981. *Cross National Rehabilitation Policies: A Sociological Perspective.* Beverly Hills: Sage.

———. 1992. *The Disability Business: Rehabilitation in America.* Thousand Oaks, Calif.: Sage.

———, ed. 2006. *Encyclopedia of Disability.* 5 vols. Thousand Oaks, Calif.: Sage.

Albrecht, Gary L., and Patrick J. Devlieger. 1999. "The Disability Paradox: High Quality of Life against All Odds." *Social Science and Medicine* 48:977–88.

Albrecht, Gary L., Patrick J. Devlieger, and Geert Van Hove. 2008. "The Experience of Disability in Plural Societies." *ALTER: European Journal of Disability Research* 2:1–13.

———. 2009. "Living on the Margin: Disabled Iranian Immigrants in Belgium." *Disability and Society* 24:259–71.

Albrecht, Gary L., Katherine D. Seelman, and Michael Bury, eds. 2001. *Handbook of Disability Studies.* Thousand Oaks, Calif.: Sage.

Altman, Barbara M., and Sharon N. Barnartt, eds. 2000. *Expanding the Scope of Social Science Research in Disability.* Stamford, Conn.: JAI Press.

Barker, Kristin K. 2008. "Electronic Support Groups, Patient-Consumers, and Medicalization: The Case of Contested Illness." *Journal of Health and Social Behavior* 49:20–36.

Barnes, Colin. 1991. *Disabled People in Britain and Discrimination.* London: Hurst.

Batavia, Andrew I., and Richard L. Beaulaurier. 2001. "The Financial Vulnerability of People with Disabilities: Assessing Poverty Risks." *Journal of Sociology and Social Welfare* 28:139–62.

Becker, Howard S. 1963. *Outsiders.* New York: Free Press.

Bloemraad, Irene, Anne Korteweg, and Gökçe Yurdakul. 2008. "Citizenship and Immigration: Multiculturalism, Assimilation, and Challenges to the Nation State." *Annual Review of Sociology* 34:8.1–8.27.

Bloom, Samuel W. 2002. *The Word as Scalpel: A History of Medical Sociology.* Oxford: Oxford University Press.

Boardman, Jason D., Jarron M. Saint-Onge, Brett C. Haberstick, David S. Timberlake, and John K. Hewitt. 2008. "Do Schools Moderate the Genetic Determinants of Smoking?" *Behavior Genetics* 38:366–81.

Bowe, Frank. 1984. *Disabled Women in America: A Statistical Report Drawn from Census Data.*

Washington, D.C.: President's Committee on Employment of the Handicapped.

Braveman, Paula. 2006. "Health Disparities and Health Equity: Concepts and Measurement." *Annual Review of Public Health* 27:167–94.

Brown, Phil, Stephen Zavestoski, Sabrina McCormick, Brian Mayer, Rachel Morello-Frosch, and Rebecca Gasior Altman. 2004. "Embodied Health Movements: New Approaches to Social Movements in Health." *Sociology of Health and Illness* 26:50–80.

Bury, Michael. 1982. "Chronic Illness as a Biographical Disruption." *Sociology of Health and Illness* 4:167–82.

———. 2000. "On Chronic Illness and Disability." In *Handbook of Medical Sociology,* ed. Chloe E. Bird, Peter Conrad, and Allen Fremont, 173–82. Englewood Cliffs, N.J.: Prentice Hall.

Cargo, Margaret, and Shawna L. Mercer. 2008. "The Value and Challenges of Participatory Research: Strengthening Its Practice." *Annual Review of Public Health* 29:325–50.

Charlton, James I. 1998. *Nothing about Us without Us: Disability, Oppression and Empowerment.* Berkeley: University of California Press.

Charmaz, Kathy. 1991. *Good Days, Bad Days: The Self in Chronic Illness and Time.* New Brunswick, N.J.: Rutgers University Press.

Chatterji, Somnath, Paul Kowal, Colin Mathers, Nirmala Naidoo, Emese Verdes, James P. Smith, and Richard Suzman. 2008. "The Health of Aging Populations in China and India." *Health Affairs* 27:1052–63.

Christakis, Nicholas A., and James H. Fowler. 2007. "The Spread of Obesity in a Large Social Network over 32 Years." *New England Journal of Medicine* 357:370–79.

Conrad, Peter. 2007. *The Medicalization of Society.* Baltimore: Johns Hopkins University Press.

Conrad, Peter, and Joseph W. Schneider. 1992. *Deviance and Medicalization: From Badness to Sickness.* Expanded ed. Philadelphia: Temple University Press.

Convention on the Rights of Persons with Disabilities. 2008. New York: United Nations. un.org/disabilities/convention.

Corker, Mairian. 1998. *Deaf and Disabled, or Deafness Disabled?* Buckingham, UK: Open University Press.

Cornwell, Benjamin, Edward O. Laumann, and L. Philip Schumm. 2008. "The Social Connectedness of Older Adults: A National Profile." *American Sociological Review* 73:185–203.

Derose, K. P., J. J. Escarce, and N. Lurie. 2007. "Immigrants and Health Care: Sources of Vulnerability." *Health Affairs* 26:1258–69.

Devlieger, Patrick, Gary L. Albrecht, and Miriam Hertz. 2007. "The Production of Disability Culture among

Young African American Men." *Social Science and Medicine* 64:1948–59.

Devlieger, Patrick, Frank Renders, Hubert Froyen, and Kristel Wildiers, eds. 2006. *Blindness and the Multi-Sensorial City.* Antwerp, Neth.: Garant.

Disability and Development Team. 2004. *Poverty Reduction Strategies: Their Importance for Disability.* Washington, D.C.: World Bank.

Edwards, C., and Rob Imrie. 2008. "Disability and the Implications of the Well-Being Agenda." *Journal of Social Policy* 37:337–55.

European Disability Forum. 2003. *Disability and Social Exclusion in the European Union: Time for Change, Tools for Change.* Athens: Greek National Confederation of Disabled People.

European Union Charter of Fundamental Rights. 2000. European Parliament. europarl.europa.eu/charter.

Farber, Bernard. 1962. "Effects of a Severely Mentally Retarded Child on the Family." In *Readings on the Exceptional Child: Research and Theory*, ed. E. P. Trapp and P. Himelstein, 227–46. New York: Appleton-Century-Crofts.

Ferguson, Philip M. 2001. "Mapping the Family: Disability Studies and the Exploration of Parental Response to Disability." In *Handbook of Disability Studies*, ed. Gary L. Albrecht, Katherine D. Seelman, and Michael Bury, 373–95. Thousand Oaks, Calif.: Sage.

Foucault, Michel. 1965. *Madness and Civilization: A History of Insanity in the Age of Reason.* London: Tavistock.

———. 1973. *The Birth of the Clinic: An Archeology of Medical Perception.* New York: Pantheon.

Fougelrollas, Patrick, and Line Beauregard. 2001. "An Interactive Person-Environment Social Creation." In *Handbook of Disability Studies*, ed. Gary L. Albrecht, Katherine D. Seelman, and Michael Bury, 171–94. Thousand Oaks, Calif.: Sage.

Frank, Arthur W. 1995. *The Wounded Storyteller.* Chicago: University of Chicago Press.

Frank, Gelya. 2000. *Venus on Wheels.* Berkeley: University of California Press.

Freese, Jeremy, Jui-Chung Allen Li, and Lisa Wade. 2003. "The Potential Relevance of Biology to Social Inquiry." *Annual Review of Sociology* 29:233–56.

Freidson, Eliot. 1970. *Profession of Medicine.* New York: Dodd, Mead.

Gehlert, Sarah, Dana Shimer, Tina W. Sacks, Charles Mininger, Martha McClintock, and Olufunmilayo Olopade. 2008. "Targeting Health Disparities: A Model Linking Upstream Determinants to Downstream Interventions." *Health Affairs* 27:339–49.

Goffman, Erving. 1963. *Stigma: Notes on the Management of Spoiled Identity.* Englewood Cliffs, N.J.: Prentice Hall.

Gove, Walter. 1978. "Sex Differences in Mental Illness among Adult Men and Women: An Examination of Four Questions Regarding Whether or Not Women Actually Have Higher Rates." *Social Science and Medicine* 12:187–98.

Hahn, Harlan. 1988. "The Politics of Physical Differences: Disability and Discrimination." *Journal of Social Issues* 4:39–44.

Higgins, Paul C. 1980. *Outsiders in a Hearing World: A Sociology of Deafness.* Beverly Hills, Calif.: Sage.

———. 1992. *Making Disability: Exploring the Social Transformation of Human Variation.* Springfield, Ill.: Charles C. Thomas.

Hollingshead, August B., and Frederick C. Redlich. 1958. *Social Class and Mental Illness.* New York: Wiley.

House, James S., K. R. Landis, and Debra Umberson. 1988. "Social Relationships and Health." *Science* 241:540–45.

Iezzoni, Lisa I., and Bonnie L. O'Day. 2006. *More Than Ramps.* Oxford: Oxford University Press.

Imrie, Rob. 2000. "Disabling Environments and the Geography of Access: Policies and Practices." *Disability and Society* 15:5–24.

Institute of Medicine. 2001. *Health and Behavior: The Interplay of Biological, Behavioral and Societal Influences.* Washington, D.C.: National Academies Press.

———. 2007. *The Future of Disability in America.* Washington, D.C.: National Academies Press.

Kessler, Ronald C., and Philip S. Wang. 2008. "The Descriptive Epidemiology of Commonly Occurring Mental Disorders in the United States." *Annual Review of Public Health* 29:115–29.

Latour, Bruno. 2005. *Reassembling the Social: An Introduction to Actor-Network Theory.* Oxford: Oxford University Press.

Light, Donald. 2001. "The Sociological Character of Health-Care Markets." In *The Handbook of Social Studies in Health and Medicine*, ed. Gary L. Albrecht, Ray Fitzpatrick, and Susan C. Scrimshaw, 394–409. London: Sage.

Link, Bruce G., Francis T. Cullen, Elmer Struening, Patrick E. Shrout, and Bruce P. Dohrenwent. 1989. "A Modified Labeling Theory Approach to Mental Disorders: An Empirical Assessment." *American Sociological Review* 54:400–423.

Lorber, Judith. 2000. "Gender Contradictions and Status Dilemmas in Disability." In *Expanding the Scope of Social Science Research on Disability*, ed. Barbara M. Altman and Sharon N. Barnartt, 85–103. Greenwich, CT: JAI Press.

Major, B., and L. O'Brien. 2005. "The Social Psychology of Stigma." *Annual Review of Psychology* 56:393–421.

Mercer, Jane. 1973. *Labeling the Mentally Retarded: Clinical and Social System Perspectives on Mental Retardation.* Berkeley: University of California Press.

Merleau-Ponty, Maurice. 1961. *Phenomenology of Perception.* London: Routledge Kegan Paul.

Miller, Ursula, and Stephanie Ziegler. 2006. *Making Poverty Reduction Strategy (PRSP) Inclusive.* Munich: Handicap International and Christoffel-Blindenmission.

Mont, D. 2007. "Measuring Disability Prevalence." World Bank Working Paper. Washington, D.C.: World Bank.

Nagi, Saad Z. 1965. "Some Conceptual Issues in Disability and Rehabilitation." In *Sociology and Rehabilitation*, ed. Marvin B. Sussman, 100–113. Washington, D.C.: American Sociological Association.

———. 1991. "Disability Concepts Revisited: Implications for Prevention." In *Disability in America: Toward a National Agenda for Prevention*, ed. Andrew M. Pope and Alvin R. Tarlov, 309–27. Washington, D.C.: National Academy Press.

Oliver, Michael. 1990: *The Politics of Disablement.* New York: St. Martin's Press.

Pescosolido, Bernice A. 2001. "The Role of Social Networks in the Lives of Persons with Disabilities." In *Handbook of Disability Studies*, ed. Gary L. Albrecht, Katherine D. Seelman, and Michael Bury, 468–89. Thousand Oaks, Calif.: Sage.

Pescosolido, Bernice A., and Eric R. Wright. 2004. "The View from Two Worlds: The Convergence of Social Network Reports between Mental Health Clients and Their Ties." *Social Science and Medicine* 58:1795–1806.

Peters, Karen E., and Karin Opacich. 2006. "Gender." In *Encyclopedia of Disability*, ed. Gary L. Albrecht, 2:760–64. Thousand Oaks, Calif.: Sage.

Pfeiffer, David. 1998. "The ICIDH and the Need for Its Revision." *Disability and Society* 13:503–23.

Reynolds, John R., and R. Jay Turner. 2008. "Major Life Events: Their Personal Meaning, Resolution, and Mental Health Significance." *Journal of Health and Social Behavior* 49:223–37.

Roth, Julius. 1963. *Timetables: Structuring the Passage of Time in Tuberculosis Treatment and Other Careers.* Chicago: University of Chicago Press.

Roth, Julius A., and Elizabeth M. Eddy. 1967. *Rehabilitation for the Unwanted.* New York: Atherton Press.

Samet, Jonathan M., and Catherine C. Bodurow, eds. 2008. *Improving the Presumptive Disability Decision-Making Process for Veterans.* Washington, D.C.: National Academies Press.

Sampson, Robert J., Jeffrey D. Morenoff, and Thomas Gannon-Rowley. 2002. "Assessing Neighborhood Effects: Social Process and New Directions in Research." *Annual Review of Sociology* 28:443–78.

Sampson, Robert J., Stephen W. Raudenbush, and Felton Earls. 1997. "Neighborhoods and Violent Crime: A Multilevel Study of Collective Efficacy." *Science* 277:918–24.

Sampson, Robert J., and Patrick Sharkey. 2008. "Neighborhood Selection and the Social Reproduction of Concentrated Racial Inequality." *Demography* 45:1–29.

Scheff, Tomas. 1966. *Being Mentally Ill: A Sociological Theory.* Chicago: Aldine.

Schilling, Chris. 2007. "Sociology and the Body: Classical Traditions and New Agendas." *Sociological Review* 55:1–18.

Scotch, Richard K. 1984. *From Good Will to Civil Rights: Transforming Federal Disability Policy.* Philadelphia: Temple University Press.

———. 1988. "Disability as the Basis for a Social Movement: Advocacy and the Politics of Definition." *Journal of Social Issues* 44:159–72.

Scotch, Richard K., and Kay Schriner. 1997. "Disability as Human Variation: Implications for Policy." *Annals of the American Academy of Political and Social Science* 549:148–59.

Scott, Robert. 1968. *The Making of Blind Men: A Study in Adult Socialization.* New Brunswick, N.J.: Transaction.

Seale, Clive. 2008. "Mapping the Field of Medical Sociology: A Comparative Analysis of Journals." *Sociology of Health and Illness* 30:677–95.

Seltzer, Marsha M., David M. Almeida, Jan S. Greenberg, Jyoti Savla, Robert S. Stawski, Jinkuk Hoong, and Julie Lounds Taylor. 2009. "Psychological and Biological Markers of Daily Lives of Midlife Parents of Children with Disabilities." *Journal of Health and Social Behavior* 50:1–15.

Seymour, Wendy. 1989. *Body Alterations: An Introduction to a Sociology of the Body for Health Workers.* Sydney: Allen and Unwin.

———. 1998. *Remaking the Body: Rehabilitation and Change.* St. Leonards, UK: Allen and Unwin.

Shakespeare, Tom. 2006. *Disability Rights and Wrongs.* London: Routledge.

Siegrist, Johannes, and Michael Marmot, eds. 2006. *Social Inequalities in Health.* Oxford: Oxford University Press.

Smith, Kirsten P., and Nicholas A. Christakis. 2008. "Social Networks and Health." *Annual Review of Sociology* 34:405–29.

Söder, Martin. 2006. "Social Model: Sweden." In *Encyclopedia of Disability*, ed. Gary L. Albrecht, 4:1465–67. Thousand Oaks, Calif.: Sage.

Srole, Leo. 1962. *Mental Health in the Metropolis.* New York: McGraw-Hill.

Stiker, Henri-Jacques. 1999. *A History of Disability.* Ann Arbor: University of Michigan Press.

Stone, Deborah A. 1984. *The Disabled State.* Philadelphia: Temple University Press.

Strauss, Anselm, ed. 1975. *Chronic Illness and the Quality of Life.* St. Louis: Mosby.

Sussman, Marvin B., ed. 1965. *Sociology and Rehabilitation.* Washington, D.C.: American Sociological Association.

———. 1987. *Childhood Disability and Family Systems.* Binghamton, N.Y.: Haworth Press.

Thoits, Peggy A. 1999. "Sociological Approaches to Mental Illness." In *A Handbook for the Study of Mental Health*, ed. Allan V. Horwitz and Teresa L. Scheid, 121–38. Cambridge: Cambridge University Press.

Turner, Bryan S. 1984. *The Body and Society.* London: Blackwell.

———. 2001a. "Disability and the Sociology of the Body." In *Handbook of Disability Studies*, ed. Gary L. Albrecht, Katherine D. Seelman, and Michael Bury, 252–66. Thousand Oaks, Calif.: Sage.

———. 2001b. "The Erosion of Citizenship." *British Journal of Sociology* 52:189–210.

Turner, R. Jay, Donald A. Lloyd, and John Taylor. 2006. "Physical Disability and Mental Health: An Epidemiology of Psychiatric and Substance Disorders." *Rehabilitation Psychology* 51:214–23.

Udry, J. Richard. 1988. "Biological Predispositions and Social Control in Adolescent Sexual Behavior." *American Sociological Review* 53:709–22.

Udry, J. Richard, and Naomi M. Morris. 1970. "The Effect of Contraceptive Pills on the Distribution of Sexual Activity in the Menstrual Cycle." *Nature* 227:502–3.

Winance, Myrian, Isabelle Ville, and Jean-Francois Ravaud. 2007. "Disability Policies in France: Changes and Tensions between the Category-Based, Universalist and Personalized Approaches." *Scandinavian Journal of Disability Research* 9:160–81.

WHO [World Health Organization]. 2001. *International Classification of Functioning, Disability and Health.* Geneva: WHO.

———. In press. *World Report on Disability and Rehabilitation.* Geneva and Washington, D.C.: WHO and World Bank.

Zola, Irving Kenneth. 1972. "Medicine as an Institution of Social Control." *Sociological Review* 20:487–504.

———. 1982. *Missing Pieces: A Chronicle of Living with a Disability.* Philadelphia: Temple University Press.

———. 1989. "Toward the Necessary Universalizing of a Disability Policy." *Milbank Quarterly* 67:401–27.

———. 1991. "Bringing Our Bodies and Ourselves Back In: Reflections on the Past, Present and Future of Medical Sociology." *Journal of Health and Social Behavior* 32:1–16.

13

Death, Dying, and the Right to Die

Clive Seale, Queen Mary, University of London

Death in late-modern mass societies has a particular character which sociological analysis, informed by historical, anthropological, and demographic studies, is well suited to bring out. Such analysis exposes the underlying dynamics of common ethical dilemmas in end-of-life care, showing that subjective experiences otherwise thought to be purely psychological in origin—dying, grief, care provision—are shaped by historical and social forces. This chapter reviews some important features of modern societies that influence and explain our experience of death, focusing on the desire of many modern individuals—manifest in the growth of right-to-die social movements—to benefit from an open awareness of dying and to control the manner in which death is experienced.

There is considerable cross-cultural variation in the degree to which personal control of the dying process is seen to be desirable, partly influenced by level of affluence, education, and religiosity, as well as cultural patterns associated with race or ethnicity. For example, the right-to-die movement largely prospers in wealthier societies and appeals most to educated sections of the population that have good access to health care. The desire to benefit psychologically from awareness of dying has particular appeal in cultural groups where freedom of choice is embraced as a duty of citizenship, and self-identity is taken to be a personal, worked-upon project. Much of the detailed empirical work reviewed in this chapter describes such variation.

Death in Modern Societies

The modern experience of dying is highly influenced by a transformation in life expectancy and in the pattern of disease in modern societies. In 2006 the average life expectancy at birth worldwide was sixty-seven years, having risen from just forty-eight years in 1955 (WHO 1988, 2008). Historical data for England going back to 1541 (Wrigley and Schofield 1981) show life expectancy fluctuating below forty years until the 1830s, after which it began a steady rise to the 2006 averages of seventy-seven for men and eighty-one for women (WHO 2008). The drop in the infant and child mortality rates and decline of deaths in middle-aged groups that has accompanied raised life expectancy means that in the wealthier countries of the world, death is typically experienced at the end of a long life. Thus the experience of dying is increasingly linked to the more general experience of being old (Seale 2000).

Again in wealthier countries in particular, changing patterns of disease also influence the experience of dying. Broadly speaking, death from infectious disease, epidemics, and malnutrition has largely been replaced by death from cancer, heart disease, and stroke. A rising incidence of dementia in later life adds to the social care needs of people approaching death. The position of elderly women in terms of access to informal care and financial resources is more difficult than that of elderly men (Arber and Ginn 1991). Kellehear (2007) argues that, increasingly, people are living longer than they want to, so the social exclusion of elderly people and their placement in care homes where many experience a "shameful" death is an unwelcome feature of contemporary societies. He relates a relatively high rate of suicide among elderly people to the desire to avoid such circumstances.

Additionally, the management of death has become increasingly subject to professional management and sequestration in institutions, reflected most obviously in the rising proportion of deaths that occur within hospitals and the decline in home deaths in wealthier countries. This has led to a common perception, often aired in mass media discourse, that modern society is "death denying," by which is usually meant that modern individuals rarely encounter dying people and are relatively unskilled in managing the realities of death, both in terms of responding to the emotions of dying and bereavement and in dealing with the physical aspects of dying and dead bodies. This denial-of-death thesis has attracted careful critical examination by sociologists, including Talcott Parsons (1978; Parsons and Lidz 1967), who argues that in an important sense modern societies are remarkably death affirming, being effectively organized to control death as part of a primary cultural pattern of activism. This involves the use of health care to resist premature death and alleviate the physical suffering of dying, and the control of deliberately imposed death by state management of warfare, violence, and capital punishment. Premature death has thus come to be regarded as an unnatural violation of a normal lifespan.

The concept of "death brokering" (Timmermans 2005) has been helpful in understanding the contemporary medical role in the management of dying and the construction of meaning around death. Timmermans argues that medical authorities, through clinical and forensic activities, are dominant in providing acceptable explanations for death, thus rendering it "culturally manageable and understandable" (2005, 1005). Forensic medical investigation, by ensuring that the cause of each death is securely located within an explanatory system for bodily events, renders even

the most mysterious type of death understandable. Clinical activities involve an active approach to the management of the physiological aspects of dying, as well as the expectations of patients and relatives. Thus they enable the pursuit of an ideal death (for example, one that is explainable as the result of a physical disease process, free of uncontrolled physical suffering, predictable so that it is preceded by the right amount of time spent "dying," and accompanied by an appropriate degree of emotion). Sometimes, of course, efforts to provide for such a death fail, but, argues Timmermans, these serve only to mark out a realm for further activity by medical authorities, maintaining the continuing cultural authority of medicine over the meaning of modern dying.

More broadly, as Blauner (1966) pointed out, the retirement and replacement of older people ensures the continuity of modern institutions. Specialized professions and institutions—health-care staff, hospitals and other places of care —complete the sequestration of dying people from mainstream social life, ensuring the minimum of disruption to the smooth functioning of social institutions. All this might be regarded, as in Parsons, as part of facing up to the reality of death rather than denying it. Nevertheless, such sequestration means that many people lack personal familiarity with death when compared with individual experience in smaller, premodern social groups, where the end of a life is generally witnessed and, in many cases, experienced as very disruptive to the continuity of group social life. Funerals in such groups are then rituals to revive community spirit as well as to address personal grief (Hertz 1960). There is a greater focus on mourning rather than on the emotions of dying in such pre-modern societies because of the unpredictability of death, which means "dying" people cannot readily be labeled as such (Kellehear 2007).

The growth in popularity of life insurance, overcoming religious objections, is an indicator of the acknowledgment of the reality of death that is typical of modern mass societies. Zelizer (1978), who studied its introduction in the nineteenth-century United States, demonstrates that the ministry initially opposed life insurance, viewing it as a gamble on the outcome of the divine will. But families living in urban conditions without the safety net of a supportive local community increasingly experienced destitution on the death of a breadwinner. Taking out life insurance was gradually reinterpreted as the moral duty of responsible fatherhood, eventually becoming an aspect of the risk planning that characterizes a modern approach to life (Beck 1992; Giddens 1990, 1991). By this means modern individuals take charge of their destinies and attempt to control the effects of adverse life events.

But the insurance industry is just one example of a broad range of social institutions that contribute to this sense of control. The chief institution is, of course, medicine and the health care system, including public health and associated state sponsorship of health-promoting (and therefore death-avoiding) lifestyles. The works of Arney and Bergen (1984), Armstrong (1987), and Prior (1989), examples of sociological work informed by Foucauldian theory, bring out this particular character of modern societies. These authors show that the most basic contribution of the medical perspective is to locate death in the body as the natural outcome of disease, so that medical endeavors in combating disease then become part of the "sheltering canopy" (Berger and Luckmann 1971) constructed by human activity as a shield against death. As the technical efficacy of medical science has improved, this contribution has largely substituted for religious defenses against death, or adds to them for individuals able to hold on to both scientific and religious understandings of life. There is a sense, then, in which health promotion is a religion, and the zeal with which some people devote themselves to health and fitness regimes is considerable (Glassner 1989).

Death certification is an important social instrument for locating death in the body. Bloor's (1991) study shows that doctors in Scotland, whose training in the practice is minimal, experience it as a minor routine. This means that certification is done in sometimes idiosyncratic ways by doctors whose main concern may be to fulfill the legal requirement of ruling out such "unnatural" causes as murder or accident (Bloor 1994). Yet, in spite of its limitations as an accurate descrip-

tion of bodily processes, certification follows certain principles. Prior (1989) observes that we no longer find "intemperate living," "want," or "cold and whiskey" written on certificates, or "poverty," "bad luck," or "the will of God." Instead, a causally linked chain of bodily processes resulting in death is required. Certification rules out understandings of death, social causes, and human agency and is a pure assertion of the bodily containment of death, a ritualized identification of the workings of natural disease within the body. As medicine holds out the possibility of successful intervention into the course of natural disease, so the death certificate is an indirect promise to the living that death can be controlled.

Interactions between medical staff and relatives at the time of death continue to describe death as the outcome of bodily events, as medical sociologists studying observations of death announcements by hospital staff (Sudnow 1967) and coroners' officials (Charmaz 1976) show. Charmaz notes that key tasks which must be achieved by coroners' deputies in notifying relatives of a sudden unexpected death (apart from preserving composure and ensuring acceptance of burial costs by relatives) are to make the death credible, accountable, and "acceptable" to relatives. A common strategy is to delay announcing a death until details of an accident or collapse have been given as "cues," which ideally prompt the relative to jump to the conclusion that a death has occurred. For example: "I tell them that he collapsed today while at work. They asked if he is all right now. I say slowly, 'Well, no, but they took him to the hospital.' They ask if he is there now. I say, 'They did all they could do—the doctors tried very hard.' They say, 'He is dead at the hospital?' Then I tell them he's at the coroner's office" (Charmaz 1976, 78).

To the question that then follows—What must I do?—the deputy points the shocked recipient toward activity to deal with the death. Sudnow (1967) notes that in every such hospital announcement scene he witnessed, a "historical reference" was made to a medically relevant antecedent "cause of death" such as a heart attack. Talk then proceeds to further elaboration on this cause, to a discussion of whether the person had "suffered," and to assurances that all that could have been done was done. On this last matter, Sudnow records occasions where this impression was made easier to sustain by artificially delaying the appearance of the medical announcer to suggest that heroic but futile rescue attempts were made. On the matter of suffering, Sudnow notes that "doctors . . . routinely lie in their characterizations of death as painless" (1967, 146), an impression that relatives are often equally keen to sustain. In these various ways people learn about deaths and participate in the confirmation of death as the outcome of bodily processes.

Practices such as these can be understood as similar in their function to the mortuary rites described by anthropologists studying tribal or traditional societies (Bloch and Parry 1982). The task of the living is to enclose and explain death, reduce its polluting effects, and symbolically place individual deaths in a context that helps survivors turn away from death and toward continuing life. In other words, medicine writes a cultural script that enables participants to engage in a resurrective practice (Seale 1998).

Palliative Care

On the whole, the demographic transition means that dying trajectories for those in wealthier countries tend to be longer and, particularly in the case of cancer, more predictably threatening to life. A form of terminal care has emerged that is largely predicated on the existence of cancer, finding its expression in the hospice and palliative care movement. In many respects this movement has promoted a model for what dying should be like: something that involves emotional accompaniment, awareness of oncoming death, and psychological and relationship development during the final phase of last farewells, coupled with expert medical and nursing care devoted to the alleviation of suffering (Kubler-Ross 1969; Saunders and Baines 1983). As Kellehear (2007) argues, this continues conceptions of the "good death" that were developed when societies changed from hunter-gatherer to pastoral modes of life.

Walter (1994) has described the ideas promoted by the hospice and palliative care movement as "revivalist," incorporating a critique of the "modern" way of death that had developed in Western societies up until the mid-twentieth century, which influential commentators such as Gorer (1965) perceived as involving a taboo. The revivalist alternative that developed and gathered strength through the 1960s and continues to the present day resists the consequences of sequestration, or the hiding away of dying and bereavement, so that these are subject to greater public attention as well as psychological and medical expertise. Revivalism enables people encountering bereavement and death to engage in institutionalized practices (such as hospice care or grief counseling) that include their experience in a publicly available discourse or cultural script, providing a sense of community membership that combats the isolation and abandonment otherwise experienced by dying and bereaved people. Drawing on this perspective, Arnarson (2007) argues that bereavement counseling serves to regenerate the sense of autonomy that drives a modern image of self-identity.

The microinteractions involved in providing a sense of membership have been studied by a number of sociologists, including Hunt (1991a, b) whose ethnomethodological account of home palliative care nurses "being friendly and informal" describes processes reminiscent of Hochschild's (1983) account of the emotional labor of flight attendants. Hunt (1991b) describes nurses performing their tasks informally, wearing nonuniform clothing, and beginning a home visit with small talk that continues, interspersed with clinical questioning, as the visit proceeds. Professional friendliness is distinguished from friendship by the degree to which self-disclosure is reciprocal, and Hunt shows that nurses only rarely make such disclosures, though families often do. At the same time, such nurses are carrying out important tasks such as identifying who in the family might be expected to provide care and indeed who might be constituted as "family" (Hunt 1991a). Perakyla (1991), in similar vein, has brought an ethnomethodological perspective to bear on the "hope work" done in care settings for the terminally ill.

The hospice and palliative care social movement that began in the 1960s and rapidly spread through the UK, North America, and other

Anglophone countries in the 1970s, subsequently influencing terminal care worldwide, is subject to certain tensions which sociologists have documented. Early work by Abel (1986) and Paradis and Cummings (1986) argued that U.S. hospice care, initially the product of grassroots activism to rehumanize dying, had rapidly moved toward organizational homogeneity through a process of institutionalization. In part this was due to the narrow vision of health-insurance agencies, which could not incorporate a service with diffuse aims, intangible psychosocial interventions, and unquantifiable gains in their reimbursement systems. Abel echoes the concern of Dooley (1982, 37), who observed the danger that care then came increasingly to look like "traditional health care service with hospice overtones." Paradis and Cummings identify the "normative" influence exercised by the influx of staff from orthodox care settings who were not fully acculturated into hospice ways. The professionalization of hospice nursing was also a sign of encroachment and corruption of the ideal.

In the United Kingdom, James and Field (1992) put forth a similar argument, drawing some of their empirical data from James's experiences as a participant observer in a palliative care unit within the NHS (James 1986), where James identified a dilution of hospice ideals that led to an emphasis on physical rather than psychosocial care. James and Field (1992) draw on Weberian ideas to describe the routinization of hospice care, the reestablishment of interprofessional hierarchies that the early hospice movement had challenged, and a resurgence in rule-bound behavior, rationalization, and the commodification of humanitarian values through processes of audit, measurement, and marketing.

There is no doubt that palliative care as a nursing and medical specialty is now securely established within the health-care systems of many developed countries and is beginning to be taken up in different forms in developing regions where terminal care has become more relevant with the changing patterns of disease that accompany growing wealth and better health (Wright et al. 2008). With institutional success comes an input of resources, so the decline in the initial idealism of the movement may be no bad thing. Addition-

ally, as Giddens (1990) has observed about the assumption that bureaucratization is restrictive, "rather than tending inevitably towards rigidity, [such] organisations [can] produce areas of autonomy and spontaneity which are actually often less easy to achieve in smaller groups" (1990, 138). The extent to which this is true of modern palliative care requires further empirical sociological work.

Hospice and palliative care services largely provide for people with cancer; for many in Western societies, this provides a model of what it is like to die. However, cancer causes a minority of deaths, albeit a fairly large minority, in the societies where hospice and palliative care services have developed, with heart disease, strokes, old age, and other conditions eventually carrying off the majority of the population. These conditions have somewhat different trajectories from cancer and different degrees of predictability that they will end in death (Kellehear 2007; Seale 1991, 2000). Indeed, Logue (1994) points out the limitations of hospice-style care for elderly people with dementia or for those experiencing social care needs rather than terminal illness, who are not seen to be appropriate clients of palliative care services. This author has noted elsewhere that the demographic profile of the elderly population, coupled with the disadvantages experienced by elderly women, means that the quality of care provision for very elderly women is a "women's issue" (Logue 1991, 97). Indeed, as we will see, gender is also an important consideration in relation to the right-to-die social movement, which represents an alternative method to that of hospice care in influencing the timing and manner of death.

Awareness of Dying

No account of the sociology of dying can avoid the conclusion that the work of Glaser and Strauss (Glaser and Strauss, 1965, 1968; Strauss and Glaser 1977) for the project that also saw the launch of grounded theory (Glaser and Strauss 1967) represents a foundational moment. Their account of "awareness contexts" in *Awareness of Dying* (Glaser and Strauss 1965) deserves particular attention in this review, because it permits a reevaluation and reinterpretation of that work from the perspective of contemporary sociological thinking. Broadly speaking, this involves looking back from a sociological viewpoint that is somewhat influenced by poststructuralism and postscientism to see that this seminal work which presents itself as an objective and scientific account is in fact very much a product of its time and culture—a "story" about dying, in fact. This perspective is consistent with a view that sees research reporting in the human sciences as an artful practice whose texts may be deconstructed in that light (Clifford and Marcus 1986; Atkinson 1990). I will contrast *Awareness of Dying* with later work in institutional ethnography by Lawton (1998, 2000) that reflects a more contemporary but nevertheless realist perspective that draws on the sociology of the body.

The main purpose of *Awareness of Dying* is to describe four "awareness contexts"—closed, suspicion, pretense, and open—in which dying can occur. In the first of these, the dying person is unaware that they are dying but relatives and caregivers are aware; in the last of these all openly acknowledge the person's terminal disease. The other two contexts represent stages between these points. The typology is based on observations across a range of institutional settings in which people die. Much of the book explores the conditions under which movement from one context to another occurs, as well as the consequences of each context for interaction between the parties involved. Glaser and Strauss are critical of the sociologist who develops a theory "that embodies, without his realization, the sociologist's ideals, the values of his occupation and social class, as well as popular views and myths" (260). The contrast to this is the systematic induction of theory grounded in data, which ensures both objectivity and practical relevance to a broad variety of situations.

Yet, read as a literary production, *Awareness of Dying* reveals itself as a dramatic parable of revivalism (Walter 1994), in which dying people are portrayed as romantic heroes struggling with diminishing resources against an iron cage of modernist bureaucracy. Doctors, as chief system representatives, call the shots, and in a subdrama to the main plot, nurses stressfully vacillate between the roles of patient advocate and the instrument of doctors' will. As a "side interest," relatives hover in the background, occupying a role whose tensions resemble those of nurses.

The main plot concerns the dying patient versus the impersonal forces of the hospital, a "single individual . . . who is pitted against" staff (Glaser and Strauss 1965, 12). Suspicion awareness is a "contest" or a "fencing match" (47) or a matter of "tactics" (53), in which "the patient's actual resources are exceedingly slim" (51). Unlike wives who suspect a cheating husband, say the authors, patients do not have intimate knowledge of their opponent, are physically somewhat immobile, and cannot pay private detectives. Unlike spies, the patient has no team but "faces an organized team" (52) that is unlikely to contain any allies.

Doctors in *Awareness of Dying* behave like tricksters or con men when a patient is in closed awareness. Possessing the advantage of membership on an experienced team they will, for example, "make meaningless trips" (186) to the bedside to maintain an illusion of a commitment to cure. More worrying, they may add to this a layer of inhumanity, discounting dying patients' requests to withdraw from clinical trials and restricting levels of analgesic medications in case they become confounded with the effects of the experimental treatment. Doctors may keep patients alive "for the rest of the semester" if they present "interesting" teaching material, forcing a patient to "have to ask for his own death" (186). Little evidence is provided for these claims in the text; we do not know how the authors determined whether particular visits to the bedside were "meaningless" in medical terms, or how many (and why) terminal patients were or were not allowed to withdraw from trials, or how they came to the view that particular patients were kept alive for teaching purposes. In Baruch's (1981) terms, these are "atrocity stories" which align the reader with the authors' judgments through an appeal to emotion. Additionally, the depiction of doctors is striking for what it omits. We are not told how things seem from their point of view (unlike nurses, whose position is explored in more sympathetic terms). The effect is to present doctors as impersonal system representatives, without humanity.

Glaser and Strauss promote in this book a particular model for desirable dying. First, there is the rhetorical strategy of inciting talk about death by claiming the existence of a widespread culture of death denial: "typical Americans . . . are unlikely to initiate . . . a conversation [about a patient's impending death]" (1965, 67), and "Americans are characteristically unwilling to talk openly about the process of dying" (3). As the Foucauldian sociologist Armstrong (1987) has pointed out, such silence about death has been constituted as a "lie," and therefore to be condemned, only since the late 1950s. Up until that point, "to keep death a secret was justifiable because patients inevitably feared death and relied on the hope which the secret gave them" (1987, 653). After this point, a new regime of truth emerged, which meant that the announcement by Glaser and Strauss of a prohibition against talking about death was an invitation to break the taboo. The new system prioritized the subjective experience of the dying person, so that in Armstrong's words, "the chief mourners become the dying themselves" (654).

Glaser and Strauss's open awareness context provides for this self-mourning role. The authors point out that "there is much to recommend giving the patient an opportunity actively to manage his own dying" (1965, 135), including the chance for all concerned to prepare themselves, say goodbyes and "close their lives with proper rituals" (43). These psychological benefits are "of course not available to unaware patients in the closed awareness situation" (43). Such patients fail to prioritize important things, make unrealistic plans, and may even hasten their deaths by not realizing why they should cooperate with treatment (43–44). Thus these sociologists are fully aligned with the ideals of the nascent hospice movement of the time, itself informed by a philosophy expressed by the humanist physician Kübler-Ross, whose account of the psychological and spiritual benefits of acceptance of death in *On Death and Dying* (1969) became an international best seller. The emerging psychosocial discipline of thanatology was informed by such ideals, prompting the observation from one enthusiast: "We begin to live the moment we begin to die" (Kalish 1980, 7).

We can see now, with the benefit of more than forty years' hindsight, that *Awareness of Dying* presents a particularly culture-bound portrayal of dying. That it does this under the cloak of a supposedly objective, scientific methodology should prompt reflection on broader issues of method in sociological research. Evidence from cultures where personal projects of self identity are less intense and care of the self is more readily given over to others contribute to the view that open awareness of dying is evaluated in more widely varying ways than Glaser and Strauss acknowledged. What in Anglophone culture may be seen as a conspiracy of silence that abandons the patient may in other societies be regarded as an appropriate way of protecting dying persons by allowing others to shoulder the responsibility of decision making on their behalf (see studies reviewed in Seale 1998, 110–12).

Sociology of the Body

All sociological writing relies on rhetorical devices that construct realities reflecting the times in which the writer lives. This does not necessarily entail dismissal of the insights contained in such work. The work of Glaser and Strauss continues to be highly influential, prompting further modifications to the theory of awareness contexts. Mamo (1999), for example, is critical of the emphasis placed on information and cognition in the work of Glaser and Strauss, proposing that the role of emotional work done by both care providers and patients should be recognized as a part of the maintenance and negotiation of awareness contexts. Lawton's (1998, 2000) ethnography of care of dying people in a hospice setting is of particular note in its explicit contrast with the work of Glaser and Strauss; Lawton places the deteriorating body, and its consequences for social interaction and selfhood, at the center of the analysis. In so doing, she provides an implied critique of the impetus toward death awareness to which the work of Glaser and Strauss contributes.

Lawton draws on the historical work of Elias (1978, 1982) concerning the civilizing process, whereby the physical and animal aspects of human life—bodily functions, illness, death—have become increasingly regulated and controlled. In modern European societies, Elias argues, the growth of "manners" means that we no longer blow our noses on our sleeves, eat from communal bowls with our fingers, or urinate in full view of others. Hygiene as a rationale for the decline of these practices masks their relation to social practices that developed in courtly European society in response to the political needs of a central royal authority, and thereafter spread through the bourgeoisie as markers of social distinction. Lawton interprets the sequestration of the dying in hospice care as a part of the "civilized" hiding away of bodily decay that has become increasingly disturbing to modern sensibilities and is now regarded as unmanageable in family settings. She presents particularly harrowing case studies of bodily deterioration and "unboundedness" that involve the leakage of bodily fluids and associated smells to demonstrate her thesis that the experience of dying from advanced cancer often included a loss of personhood, a state in which benefiting from awareness and acceptance of dying appears impossible.

A number of patients observed by Lawton withdrew socially before their deaths in response to the experience of their deteriorating bodies. They also sometimes asked for euthanasia, as in the case of "Dolly":

> Dolly . . . had cancer of the colon and was admitted after becoming chronically incontinent at home. Her husband informed me that every time she had a severe bout of diarrhoea she begged him to help her take her own life. Dolly's requests for euthanasia continued during the first week of her stay in hospice. The staff were unable to get her diarrhoea under control. In addition, she went into obstruction. The tumour mass expanded and blocked her colon and, as a consequence, digested food would reach her lower gut and then come back up as faecal vomit. Around the time Dolly went into total obstruction staff observed a notable change in her behaviour. Dolly stopped requesting euthanasia; in fact she stopped talking altogether. When the nurses came to turn her in bed or to attend to her care she would close her eyes and totally ignore them. As one nurse observed: "it's as if she's shut the outside world out and herself off in the process." (Lawton 1998, 129–30)

Through such case studies Lawton's work demonstrates the body's central role in enabling a performance of self through social interaction,

reflecting the growing interest of sociologists in embodiment that has occurred since Glaser and Strauss (Malacrida and Low 2008). Reading Lawton, it becomes difficult to regard with equanimity statements like Kalish's, just quoted, about dying being an opportunity for new life: these are people who are experiencing "social death" (Sudnow 1967) before they die, as their bodies cease to provide them with possibilities for meaningful existence.

The Right-to-Die Movement

The desire to control the timing and manner of death before the experience of such assaults on self-identity is a particular aim of the right-to-die movement, represented by such organizations as the Hemlock Society (United States until 2003), Compassion and Choices (United States), Dignity in Dying (UK), and the World Federation of Right to Die Societies. This new social movement has the particular political agenda of overturning legal prohibitions against assisted dying (euthanasia and physician-assisted suicide), and an educational agenda in arguing for the need to exercise a right to die; more controversially in some jurisdictions, it disseminates information on practical methods for ending life (McInerney 2000; Fox, Kamakahi, and Capek 1999).

The movement is particularly developed in North America, several European countries including the UK, and Australia and New Zealand, consistent with the view that it is a phenomenon of wealthier countries with extensive health-care coverage. Additionally, the members of right-to-die movements tend to be more affluent and educated than the general population (Fox, Kamakahi, and Capek 1999). Studies of euthanasia movements in the UK (Kemp 2002) and the United States (Emanuel 1994) show that in their early history (the late Victorian period and first half of the twentieth century), eugenicist ideas about improving population health and aspirations to conserve scarce societal resources provided an impetus—termed "social Darwinism" by Emanuel (1994). Though somewhat controversial even before the Second World War, these arguments were later downplayed in the light of the horrors of the Nazi euthanasia program. Members of the right-to-die movement now stress the humanitarian goal of relieving suffering that is intractable by other means. Sociologically it is clear, then, that the claim for a right to die in such countries is an expression of the individualism that pervades Western nations, representing resistance to using readily available medical technology to preserve life at the expense of its quality. By contrast, opposition to the right to die stems at least in part from a religious and communitarian conception of human existence, which downplays individual needs in favor of a divine will or the needs of the community at large.

A familiar communitarian argument against the legalization of euthanasia is that of the "slippery slope," which claims pressure will be brought to bear on vulnerable people who will interpret the "right to die" as a "duty to die" (Saunders 1992). In particular, elderly people without resources, who feel themselves to be a burden on others, are likely to feel an obligation to opt for assisted dying. As Logue (1991) points out, elderly women are likely to feel this because of their multiple disadvantages in later life. Some empirical support for this view has been provided in a survey of relatives of people who die, where elderly women with no family members with an emotional investment in the continuation of their lives were shown to be more likely than others to feel that they were better off dead (Seale and Addington-Hall 1995).

The slippery-slope argument, though, also alerts us to a particular feature of the assisted dying debate: it arises in wealthier countries with relatively good health-care coverage and, as we shall see, is supported by people in countries with particularly good access to health care who fear excessive provision of life-sustaining care at a time when it will damage quality of life. Where people are poor and have inadequate access to health care, there is far less concern about the dangers of excessive medical care being provided. King and Wolf (1997–1998) document the long history of discrimination and disadvantage experienced by African Americans whose autonomy of decision making is compromised because of their race. Noting that U.S. opinion polls show greater support among the white than among the

black population for legalizing euthanasia, they suggest that African Americans see legalization of physician-assisted suicide not as the opening up of an opportunity, but merely as permission for another way of ending black lives. They quote the account of an elderly black woman from Dula's (1994) report: "Look like every time I turn on the TV, somebody's talking about euthanasia, and doctors helping kill off old and sick folks. Well, I ain't seen them ask nary a elderly black on none of them TV shows and news programs what they thought about euthanasia. I believe the Lord will take me away when it's time to go" (King and Wolf 1997–1998, 1022).

Sleeboom-Faulkner's account of death and health care in China provides a further twist. She notes that surveys show a majority of the Chinese population to be in favor of allowing euthanasia, but not for the same reasons as in the individualistic West, where the specter of Nazi eugenics rules out any appeal to societal betterment through disposing of people who are a drain on scarce resources. It is clear that Chinese support for euthanasia involves a communitarian justification of self-sacrifice in the interests of society. Thus party secretary comrade Deng Yingchao was reported in 1989 to have stated: "A Communist Party member before death faces a revolution once more. When I am about to pass away, by all means do not try to save me by applying medication. It would be a waste of effort and resources. Please organize criteria for legalising euthanasia" (Sleebohm-Faulkner 2006, 207). Other statements on euthanasia in China, occurring for example in the medical textbooks surveyed by Sleebohm-Faulkner, involve the view that relatives should have the right to ask for euthanasia for a patient and the idea that people with Alzheimer's are suitable candidates. She points out that this situation contrasts markedly with that in the Netherlands and warns against any assumption that the Dutch example can be easily transferred to a country with such a different history and culture.

Opinion polls in Western countries where the right-to-die movement is strong show widespread public support for the legalization of assisted dying. This support has grown since the mid-twentieth century (Emanuel 2002; Seale 2009b) as consumerism in health care and more general societal stress on a way of life that requires people "to understand and enact their lives in terms of choice" (Rose 1999, 87) has gained ground. The mass media of these countries are in general sympathetic to cases of "mercy killing" because these provide opportunities to tell human-interest stories of individuals battling for the right to die against tragic circumstances and apparently unsympathetic legislators or medical authorities (Clarke 2005–2006; Hausmann 2004; McInerney 2006, 2007; Pollock and Yulis 2004). It is perhaps more difficult to construct attractive human-interest stories that oppose euthanasia, as there are no evident "victims" of a pro-euthanasia policy that has not yet been implemented. Emanuel (1994) also relates rising support for assisted dying in these countries to increasing willingness to question the cultural authority of doctors: "The interest in euthanasia may be the culmination of the 20-year effort to curtail physician authority over end-of-life decisions" (1994, 800).

Perhaps understandably, doctors are on the whole less likely than the public to endorse the idea that medically assisted dying should be sanctioned by law (Seale 2009b). Where there are exceptions to this rule, the law can change as a result. The passage of legislation permitting physician-assisted suicide in Oregon in the United States was made easier when the Oregon Medical Association adopted a formal position of neutrality on the bill, in spite of pressure from the American Medical Association to oppose it (Fox, Kamakahi, and Capek 1999). In the Netherlands too, a country with a long history of a permissive approach to euthanasia, the support of the Royal Dutch Medical Association has been crucial in implementing the practice and eventually in passing a permissive law. In the UK, changing the briefly held neutral policy of the British Medical Association to restore its formal opposition to euthanasia became a focus for campaigners in a failed 2004 attempt to pass permissive legislation (Sommerville 2005).

Assisted dying presents a dilemma for doctors, whose professional ethics commit them to providing patients with comfort yet enshrine the historical role of medicine as a defense against death. The majority of deaths do not require doctors to confront the possibility of actively assisting in dying, and withdrawing or withholding treatment or providing medications that may shorten life as a secondary effect have increasingly become normal parts of end-of-life care (Seale 2006, 2009a). Yet some deaths cannot be managed by these means and continue to present doctors with the dilemma of how to help. Individual doctors solve this in a variety of ways in jurisdictions where euthanasia and physician-assisted dying is illegal, and studies have demonstrated that medical assistance is responsible for a small proportion of deaths in many countries where these actions are against the law (van der Heide et al. 2003; Kuhse et al. 1997; Emanuel 2002; Seale 2006). Research also shows that some doctors, as well as other health-care providers, became involved in covert acts of assisting dying in deaths from AIDS for a brief period in the 1980s and 1990s, providing fertile ground for sociologists exploring covert euthanasia.

AIDS and the Euthanasia Underground

In the 1980s and 1990s the high AIDS mortality in wealthier countries such as Australia, Canada, and the United States included younger people who would not otherwise have expected to confront death until later in life. Additionally, AIDS mortality disproportionately included people who by virtue of their social identity as urban-dwelling gay men tended to be marginalized, somewhat critical of mainstream social norms, and particularly used to formulating their own meanings for life events. They faced the prospect of a distressing death, often already witnessed in others, which could involve a variety of wasting syndromes, cancers, infections of the central nervous system, AIDS-related dementia, and the like. All these assaulted the capacity of individuals to maintain control over both body and self-identity, leading many HIV-infected individuals to consider the prospects for influencing the manner and timing of their death in a way that was consistent with their hard-won image of who they were and how they wanted to appear to others. Now that HAART (highly active antiretroviral [anti-HIV]) therapy has transformed the picture for mortality from AIDS for those with good access to it (Bhaskaran et al. 2008), it can be assumed that this demand for control over dying will have declined. This was therefore a time-limited social and medical phenomenon that provides revealing insights into the sociological basis of the desire for assisted dying.

Lavery and colleagues interviewed thirty-two people with HIV in Toronto, Canada, showing that the desire for an assisted death arose from an anticipation of personal disintegration and loss of community, resulting in a loss of self. One person who had also acted as a caregiver expressed personal disintegration:

> You turn them over, they're in pain. They're going to shit themselves, they're going to piss themselves, they're going to lie there and have someone do all their bodily functions and just, there's going to be no happiness, they're going to go down to 60–70 pounds, they're just going to, their whole last weeks of life is just going to be pain and agony and people coming in, people being upset, them being upset. (Lavery et al. 2001, 363–64)

Such indignities could be accompanied by dependency on others that the dying person experienced as intolerable. Loss of community, for these authors, described a progressive diminishment in the capacity to maintain social relationships. This could arise from stigmatization by others who rejected the person with AIDS, as well as from a declining inner desire to maintain contacts with others, associated with lowered levels of energy or loss of function. The resultant loss of self led to the perception that euthanasia could both limit the experience of decline and restore a sense of mastery over events, as in the following account:

> If I'm going to be rolling around in my own faeces because I have no control, then forget it. . . . It's the dignity and wholeness of my body, as well as spirit. And, it is, it's cruel too for others to have to do this when there's no end in sight, other than death. To just, to clean me up. I just don't want that . . . Dignity is that I have control over my body, when, when, not, not a virus that is going to take my life. I'm the one who is going to decide when my life will end, not a virus, and not with great pain. Not anything else other than in, in my control. It is my control, my choice to do. (365)

Magnusson's (2002) study of the "euthanasia underground" in San Francisco, Sydney, and Melbourne makes a persuasive case for understanding opposing views in the euthanasia debate as a clash of worldviews. On the one hand, those opposed to legalization are likely to draw on religious justifications about the sanctity of life, or to uphold communitarian values through arguments such as the "slippery slope." Those in favor of legislation, on the other hand, tend to espouse liberal rather than conservative values, emphasize individual needs, and reject religion as a basis for moral choices.

Magnusson explores the fine detail of individual cases with considerable sensitivity, exposing dilemmas that are experienced when particular circumstances cannot easily be fitted to the pre-existing categories made available by the conflicting cultural scripts for thinking about assisted dying. For example, interviewees told him that some individuals experience "shifting goalposts" whereby they enter states of being which previously they had thought would be intolerable, yet seem to manage: "it's sort of snuck up on them," one interviewee said, "and it's not as bad as they thought it was going to be" (2002, 82). Another interviewee recalled a man who had earlier asked friends to "take him home and kill him" (83) but later experienced ambivalence, finding it difficult to confess that he now wanted to live. Yet sometimes the request for euthanasia is persistent and the goalposts do not shift. It appears that many in the euthanasia underground are then ready to help out.

A diversity of attitudes by members of the euthanasia underground—many of whom were doctors and other health-care workers—toward assisting in a death was evident in this study, ranging from outright opposition through ambivalence to radical pro-euthanasia activism. The ambivalent were people who were willing to help individuals to die but felt uncomfortable with breaking the law. The radicals were often themselves gay men who felt alienated from the values of the mainstream medical establishment. Some radicals resisted the proposal that euthanasia be legalized because they felt this would result in unwelcome regulation of their activities. Magnusson describes a number of disturbing features of the illegal practice of euthanasia, some of which are reminiscent of the scenarios painted by those warning of slippery-slope consequences of legalization. These include sometimes ill-considered decisions to go ahead with euthanasia after the most superficial of explorations of the desire for an assisted death, occasional cases of a lack of professional distance that led to considerable distress and dubious ethical decision making, and an arbitrarily variable level of access to skilled assistance, meaning that there were botched attempts at both assisted suicide and euthanasia. These led Magnusson to argue that legalization might result in "harm reduction" by exposing these practices to quality control.

The Slippery Slope? Euthanasia in Practice

Another case that has been intensively observed by researchers is the Netherlands, where euthanasia has been permitted since the early 1990s. Study of assisted dying in this country has been supplemented by studies of Switzerland and Oregon, in both of which jurisdictions forms of assisted dying are permitted. They provide a good opportunity to explore the view that legalization of assisted dying results in a slide down the slippery slope, whereby vulnerable people come under pressure to end their lives, or whether Magnusson's "harm reduction" argument has some force.

Statistical reports from the Netherlands (van der Heide et al. 2007) show that the proportion of Dutch deaths from euthanasia has varied between 1.7 percent and 2.6 percent between 1991 and 2005. A much smaller percentage of deaths are physician-assisted suicides, and from 0.4 percent to 0.8 percent involve people whose lives are ended without an explicit request, usually because they were unable to communicate but had requested this in the past and were hours from death, which was judged clinically beneficial because of signs of unrelieved distress. In addition, much higher proportions of deaths were cases where a person's death may have been hastened by a decision to withhold or withdraw treatment, or involved giving medication such as morphine in doses that doctors estimated might have contrib-

uted to the end of life. A particular phenomenon of the Dutch situation is a growing recognition that continuous deep sedation until death occurs in a high proportion of deaths—8.2 percent in 2005—meaning that doctors can often avoid becoming involved in actions deliberately designed to end life.

If evidence for the slippery slope were to be derived from such studies, one might expect to see disproportionately higher rates of assisted dying, or perhaps of continuous deep sedation, among very elderly people, women, or noncancer deaths, but data presented by van der Heide et al. (2007) do not show this, instead demonstrating that these acts are more common in younger dying people, men, and cancer deaths.

Ganzini (2004) reports the characteristics of people who carried out physician-assisted suicide under the Oregon Death with Dignity Act over a period of six years (1998–2003), showing that these did not include any African Americans, were almost all covered by health insurance, were largely affected by cancer, were either enrolled in hospice programs or had declined enrollment, were slightly more likely to be men, and had a higher than average level of education. Although the interpretation of the Oregon figures is not uncontroversial (Foley and Hendin 2002), these do not on the surface appear to provide evidence of a slippery slope.

Bosshard, Ulrich, and Bar (2003) report on 748 cases of suicide assisted by the main Swiss right-to-die association during a ten-year period (1990–2000) and reveal a picture that is somewhat more disturbing for those concerned with the slippery-slope argument. Unlike the Netherlands or Oregon, such deaths were more likely to involve women, particularly where older groups were involved, and 21 percent of the dying suffered from nonfatal conditions such as rheumatoid arthritis, osteoporosis, chronic pain syndrome, or blindness. In this last group, 76 percent were women and tended to be of higher mean age. In a few cases the wish to die was related to depression or another mental illness, with no concomitant disease. Over the study period the number of such deaths per year rose threefold. On the surface, then, it appears that the Swiss situation may have slid down the slippery slope for those who believe assisted dying ought to be confined to clear cases of terminal illness.

Swiss regulations concerning assisted dying are more open than those of Oregon and the Netherlands, where medical second opinions are required. In Oregon a terminal illness must be present and in the Netherlands, where the medical profession has been intimately involved in drawing up guidelines for euthanasia practice, doctors must be convinced that the patient is facing unremitting and unbearable suffering. Exit, the Swiss organization responsible for assisting the 748 deaths reported by Bosshard, Ulrich, and Bar (2003), by contrast has a history of conflict with the Swiss medical association (Bosshard, Fischer, and Bar 2002) and is a citizen organization with some involvement of sympathetic doctors.

The evidence of these statistical studies in Switzerland, the Netherlands, and Oregon and the earlier evidence about underground euthanasia suggests that an approach which permits but firmly regulates the practice of medically assisted dying is more likely to protect the socially disadvantaged and is a strategy described by Magnusson (2002) as a "harm reduction" approach, drawing on a vocabulary developed for dealing with illegal drug usage. Clearly the evidence base for such policies remains somewhat thin and there remain many opportunities for policy-oriented sociologists and social researchers to explore and illuminate this important issue.

Conclusion

The research highlighted in this chapter provides evidence supporting the view that the experience of dying is determined by social, historical, and cultural conditions, as well as by physical events in the body. Historically and cross-culturally informed medical sociology is well placed to bring this evidence out. At various points medical sociology diverges from psychologically informed ideas about dying, most obviously in relation to views about the "denial of death," which many psychologists as well as cultural commentators in the mass media perceive to be a widespread feature of modern life. As this chapter has shown, Parsons's view that modern society is a particu-larly death-affirming one is supported by sociological investigation and appropriate theoretical reflection.

This chapter has reported that in a great variety of ways, members of modern societies are organized to manage the problem of dying people, with medical endeavors and health-care institutions providing for their specialist treatment, as well as being part of the larger medical system for the avoidance of illness and death. Because of the demographic transition undergone by developed countries, dying is largely confined to the elderly in modern societies, and the pattern of disease results in different dying trajectories, notably a rise in the incidence of cancer as a terminal illness. Specialized services to manage the dying process for people with cancer have been associated with the promotion of the benefits of "death awareness," a phenomenon documented by sociologists, whose culture-bound character has also been made clear through study of dying in several cultures.

More recent medical sociology has brought the life (and death) of the body to center stage, demonstrating through the study of dying how central the body is for adequate social interaction. Much care of the dying can be interpreted as managing the boundary between social and bodily existence. It is clear, too, that the activist orientation of many people in developed countries expresses itself in movements that argue for the right to die. This chapter has reported that such movements draw support from more affluent sectors of the population whose access to health care is such that they fear an excessive application of life-sustaining technology. Such fears are less likely to be shared by the more disadvantaged. Additionally, like the "death awareness" movement, which similarly seeks to influence the manner of dying, the right to die is conceived of as an individual matter. Studies have been reviewed which show that in societies that place individual needs second to the good of the community, the call for euthanasia has a complexion that many Western supporters would find unacceptable.

Sociologists have much to contribute in future research to the important field of end-of-life decision making. For example, continuous deep sedation is increasingly common in the care of dying people and in some respects may have become an alternative to euthanasia. The circumstances that lead to the decision to use this medication and the communication and ethical issues that this procedure involves are topics that deserve further investigation. Additionally, there is a widespread belief that people prefer, where possible, to die at home rather than in institutions. To some extent this belief may be fueled by the negative imagery of institutional dying associated with the "denial of death" thesis. Empirical investigation of preferences and factors associated with place of death, particularly for people dying with nonmalignant diseases such as heart failure, stroke, or respiratory conditions, offers many opportunities for sociologists to make original contributions. In general, the investigation of care of the dying allows for the empirical investigation of ethical dilemmas, and nowhere is this more evident than in the debate over the legalization of euthanasia. The tension here between the rights of individuals and the concerns of the community is classic sociological territory, and we may look forward to studies that illuminate and inform ethical and policy debates in this important area.

References

Abel, Emily K. 1986. "The Hospice Movement: Institutionalising Innovation." *International Journal of Health Services* 16:71–85.

Arber, Sara, and Jay Ginn. 1991. *Gender and Later Life: A Sociological Analysis of Resources and Constraints.* London: Sage.

Armstrong, David. 1987. "Silence and Truth in Death and Dying." *Social Science and Medicine* 24(8): 651–57.

Arnarson, Arnar. 2007. "'Fall Apart and Put Yourself Together Again': The Anthropology of Death and Bereavement Counselling in Britain." *Mortality* 12:48–65.

Arney, William R., and Bernard J. Bergen. 1984. *Medicine and the Management of Living: Taming the Last Great Beast.* Chicago: University of Chicago Press.

Atkinson, Paul. 1990. *The Ethnographic Imagination: Textual Constructions of Reality.* London: Routledge.

Baruch, Geoffrey. 1981. "Moral Tales: Parents' Stories of Encounters with the Health Profession." *Sociology of Health and Illness* 3(3): 275–96.

Beck, Ulrich. 1992. *Risk Society: Towards a New Modernity.* London: Sage.

Berger, Peter L., and Thomas Luckmann. 1971. *The Social Construction of Reality.* Harmondsworth, Eng.: Penguin.

Bhaskaran, Krishnan, Osamah Hamouda, Mette Sannes, Faroudy Boufassa, Anne M. Johnson, Paul C. Lambert, and Kholoud Porter. 2008. "Changes in the Risk of Death after HIV Seroconversion Compared with Mortality in the General Population." *Journal of the American Medical Association* 300(1): 51–59.

Blauner, Robert. 1966. "Death and Social Structure." *Psychiatry* 29:378–94.

Bloch, Maurice, and Jonathan Parry, eds. 1982. *Death and the Regeneration of Life.* Cambridge: Cambridge University Press.

Bloor, Michael. 1991. "A Minor Office: The Variable and Socially Constructed Character of Death Certification in a Scottish City." *Journal of Health and Social Behavior* 32:273–87.

———. 1994. "On the Conceptualisation of Routine Medical Decision-Making: Death Certification as an Habitual Activity." In *Qualitative Studies in Health and Medicine*, ed. Michael Bloor and Patricia Taraborelli, 96–109. Aldershot, Eng.: Avebury,

Bosshard, Georg, Stephen Fischer, and Walter Bar. 2002. "Open Regulation and Practice in Assisted Dying: How Switzerland Compares with the Netherlands and Oregon." *Swiss Medical Weekly* 132:527–34.

Bosshard, Georg, Esther Ulrich, and Walter Bar. 2003. "748 Cases of Suicide Assisted by a Swiss Right-to-Die Organisation." *Swiss Medical Weekly* 133:310–17.

Charmaz, Kathy C. 1976. "The Coroner's Strategies for Announcing Death." In *Toward a Sociology of Death and Dying*, ed. Lyn Lofland, 61–81. Beverly Hills: Sage.

Clarke, Juanne N. 2005–2006. "Death under Control: The Portrayal of Death in Mass Print English Language Magazines in Canada." *Omega: Journal of Death and Dying* 52(2): 153–67.

Clifford, James, and George E. Marcus, eds. 1986. *Writing Culture: The Poetics and Politics of Ethnography.* Berkeley: University of California Press.

Dooley, J. 1982. "The Corruption of Hospice." *Public Welfare*, spring, 35–39.

Dula, Annette. 1994. "The Life and Death of Miss Mildred . . . The Life Story of an Elderly Black Woman in the Rural South." *Clinics in Geriatric Medicine* 10(3): 419–30.

Elias, Norbert. 1978. *The History of Manners.* Vol. 1 of *The Civilizing Process.* Oxford: Blackwell.

———. 1982. *State Formation and Civilization.* Vol. 2 of *The Civilizing Process.* Oxford: Blackwell.

Emanuel, Ezekiel J. 1994. "The History of Euthanasia

Debates in the United States and Britain." *Annals of Internal Medicine* 121:793–802.

———. 2002. "Euthanasia and Physician-Assisted Suicide: A Review of the Empirical Data from the United States." *Archives of Internal Medicine* 162:142–52.

Foley, Kathleen, and Herbert Hendin. 2002. "The Oregon Experiment." In *The Case against Assisted Suicide: For the Right to End-of-Life Care*, ed. Kathleen Foley and Herbert Hendin, 144–74. Baltimore: Johns Hopkins University Press.

Fox, Elaine, Jeffrey J. Kamakahi, and Stella M. Capek. 1999. *Come Lovely and Soothing Death: The Right-to-Die Movement in the United States*. New York: Twayne.

Ganzini, Linda. 2004. "The Oregon Experience." In *Physician-Assisted Dying: The Case for Palliative Care and Patient Choice*, ed. Timothy E. Quill and Margaret P. Battin, 165–83. Baltimore: Johns Hopkins University Press.

Giddens, Anthony. 1990. *The Consequences of Modernity*. Cambridge: Polity Press.

———. 1991. *Modernity and Self-Identity: Self and Society in the Late Modern Age*. Cambridge: Polity Press.

Glaser, Barney G., and Anselm L. Strauss. 1965. *Awareness of Dying*. Chicago: Aldine.

———. 1967. *The Discovery of Grounded Theory: Strategies for Qualitative Research*. Chicago: Aldine.

———. 1968. *Time for Dying*. Chicago: Aldine.

Glassner, Barry. 1989. "Fitness and the Postmodern Self." *Journal of Health and Social Behavior* 30(2): 180–91.

Gorer, Geoffrey. 1965. *Death, Grief and Mourning*. London: Cresset.

Hausmann, Elke. 2004. "How Press Discourse Justifies Euthanasia." *Mortality* 9(3): 206–22.

Hertz, Robert. 1960. *Death and the Right Hand: A Contribution to the Study of the Collective Representation of Death*. Translated by Rodney Needham and Claudia Needham. First published 1907. Glencoe, Ill.: Free Press

Hochschild, Arlie R. 1983. *The Managed Heart: Commercialisation of Human Feeling*. Berkeley: University of California Press.

Hunt, Maura W. 1991a. "Being Friendly and Informal: Reflected in Nurses', Terminally Ill Patients', and Relatives' Conversations at Home." *Journal of Advanced Nursing* 16:929–38.

———. 1991b. "The Identification and Provision of Care for the Terminally Ill at Home by 'Family' Members." *Sociology of Health and Illness* 13(3): 375–95.

James, Veronica. 1986 "Care and Work in Nursing the Dying: A Participant Study of a Continuing Care Unit." PhD thesis, University of Aberdeen.

———. 1989. "Emotional Labour: Skill and Work in the Social Regulation of Feelings." *Sociological Review* 37:15–42.

James, Veronica, and David Field. 1992. "The Routinization of Hospice: Charisma and Bureaucratization." *Social Science and Medicine* 34(12): 1363–75.

Kalish, Robert A., ed. 1980. *Caring Relationships: The Dying and the Bereaved*. Farmingdale, N.Y.: Baywood.

Kellehear, Alan. 2007. *A Social History of Dying*. New York: Cambridge University Press.

Kemp, Nick D. A. 2002. *Merciful Release: The History of the British Euthanasia Movement*. Manchester, Eng.: Manchester University Press.

King, Patricia A., and Leslie E. Wolf. 1997–1998. "Empowering and Protecting Patients: Lessons for Physician-Assisted Suicide from the African-American Experience." *Minnesota Law Review* 82:1015–43.

Kubler-Ross, Elisabeth. 1969. *On Death and Dying*. New York: Macmillan.

Kuhse, Helga, Peter Singer, Peter Baume, Malcolm Clark, and Maurice Rickard. 1997. "End-of-Life Decisions in Australian Medical Practice." *Medical Journal of Australia* 166:191–96.

Lavery, James V., Joseph Boyle, Bernard D. Dickens, Heather Maclean, and Peter A. Singer. 2001. "Origins of the Desire for Euthanasia and Assisted Suicide in People with HIV-1 or AIDS: A Qualitative Study." *Lancet* 358:362–67.

Lawton, Julia. 1998. "Contemporary Hospice Care: The Sequestration of the Unbounded Body and 'Dirty Dying.'" *Sociology of Health and Illness* 20:121–43.

———. 2000. *The Dying Process*. London: Routledge.

Logue, Barbara. J. 1991. "Taking Charge: Death Control as an Emergent Women's Issue." *Women and Health* 17(4): 97–121.

———. 1994. "When Hospice Fails: The Limits of Palliative Care." *Omega—Journal of Death and Dying* 29(4): 291–301.

Magnusson, Roger S. 2002. *Angels of Death: Exploring the Euthanasia Underground*. New Haven, Conn.: Yale University Press.

Malacrida, Claudia, and Jacqueline Low. 2008. *Sociology of the Body: A Reader*. Oxford: Oxford University Press.

Mamo, Laura. 1999. "Death and Dying: Confluences of Emotion and Awareness." *Sociology of Health and Illness* 21(1): 13–36.

McInerney, Fran. 2000. "'Requested Death': A New Social Movement." *Social Science and Medicine* 50:137–54.

———. 2006. "Heroic Frames: Discursive Constructions around the Requested Death

Movement in Australia in the Late 1990s." *Social Science and Medicine* 62:654–67.

———. 2007. "Death and the Body Beautiful: Aesthetics and Embodiment in Press Portrayals of Requested Death in Australia on the Edge of the 21st Century." *Health Sociology Review* 16(5): 384–96.

Paradis, Leonora Finn, and Scott B. Cummings. 1986. "The Evolution of Hospice in America toward Organizational Homogeneity." *Journal of Health and Social Behavior* 27:370–86.

Parsons, Talcott. 1978. "Death in the Western World." *Action Theory and the Human Condition*, 331–51. New York: Free Press.

Parsons, Talcott, and Victor Lidz. 1967. "Death in American Society." In *Essays in Self Destruction*, ed. Edwin S. Shneidman, 133–70. New York: Science House.

Perakyla, Anssi. 1991. "Hope Work in the Care of Seriously Ill Patients." *Qualitative Health Research* 1(4): 407–33.

Pollock, John C., and Spiro G. Yulis. 2004. "Nationwide Newspaper Coverage of Physician-Assisted Suicide: A Community Structure Approach." *Journal of Health Communication* 9(4): 281–307.

Prior, Lindsay. 1989. *The Social Organization of Death*. Basingstoke and London: Macmillan.

Rose, Nikolas. 1999. *Powers of Freedom: Reframing Political Thought*. Cambridge: Cambridge University Press.

Saunders, Cicely. 1992. "Voluntary Euthanasia." *Palliative Medicine* 6:1–5.

Saunders, Cicely, and Mary Baines. 1983. *Living with Dying: The Management of Terminal Disease*. Oxford: Oxford University Press.

Seale, Clive. 1991. "Death from Cancer and Death from Other Causes: The Relevance of the Hospice Approach." *Palliative Medicine* 5:12–19.

———. 1998. *Constructing Death: The Sociology of Dying and Bereavement*. Cambridge: Cambridge University Press.

———. 2000. "Changing Patterns of Death and Dying." *Social Science and Medicine* 51:917–30.

———. 2006. "National Survey of End-of-Life Decisions Made by UK Medical Practitioners." *Palliative Medicine* 20(1): 3–10.

———. 2009a. "End-of-Life Decisions in the UK Involving Medical Practitioners." *Palliative Medicine* 23(3): 198–204.

———. 2009b. "Legalisation of Euthanasia or Physician-Assisted Suicide: Survey of Doctors' Attitudes." *Palliative Medicine* 23(3): 205–12.

Seale, Clive, and Julia Addington-Hall. 1995. "Dying at the Best Time." *Social Science and Medicine* 40(5): 589–95.

Sleeboom-Faulkner, Margaret. 2006. "Chinese Concepts of Euthanasia and Health Care." *Bioethics* 20(4): 203–12.

Sommerville, Ann. 2005. "Changes in BMA Policy on Assisted Dying." *British Medical Journal* 331:686–88.

Strauss, Anselm L., and Barney G. Glaser. 1977. *Anguish: A Case Study of a Dying Trajectory*. London: Martin Robertson.

Sudnow, David. 1967. *Passing On: The Social Organization of Dying*. Englewood Cliffs, N.J.: Prentice Hall.

Timmermans, Stefan. 2005. "Death Brokering: Constructing Culturally Appropriate Deaths." *Sociology of Health and Illness* 27(7): 993–1013.

van der Heide, Agnes, Luc Deliens, Karin Faisst, Tore Nilstun, Michael Norup, Eugenio Paci, Gerrit van der Wal, and Paul J. van der Maas. 2003. "End-of-Life Decision-Making in Six European Countries: Descriptive Study." *Lancet* 362:345–50.

van der Heide, Agnes, Bregie D. Onwuteaka-Philipsen, Mette L. Rurup, Hilde M. Buiting, Johannes J. M. van Delden, Hanssen-Johanna E. de Wolf, Anke G. J. M. Janssen, Roeline W. Pasman, Judith A. C. Rietjens, Cornelis J. M. Prins, Ingeborg M. Deerenberg, Joseph K. M. Gevers, Paul J. van der Maas, and Gerrit van der Wal. 2007. "End-of-Life Practices in the Netherlands under the Euthanasia Act." *New England Journal of Medicine* 356(19): 1957–65.

Walter, Tony. 1994. *The Revival of Death*. London: Routledge.

WHO [World Health Organisation]. 1988. *World Health Statistics*. Geneva: WHO.

———. 2008. *World Health Statistics*. Geneva: WHO. who.int/whosis/whostat/2008/en/index.html.

Wright, Michael, Justin Wood, Tom Lynch, and David Clark. 2008. "Mapping Levels of Palliative Care Development: A Global View." *Journal of Pain and Symptom Management* 35(5): 469–85.

Wrigley, Edward A., and Roger S. Schofield. 1981. *The Population History of England, 1541–1871: A Reconstruction*. London: Edward Arnold.

Zelizer, Viviana A. 1978. "Human Values and the Market: The Case of Life Insurance and Death in 19th Century America." *American Journal of Sociology* 84(3): 591–610.

PART III

Health-Care Organization, Delivery, and Impact

14

Gender and Health Care

Renee R. Anspach, University of Michigan

The health-care system is a deeply gendered social institution, often affecting men and women in dramatically different ways. In the United States and many European countries, health-care occupations are sex segregated: men constitute a majority of physicians, while women are concentrated in occupations that are less prestigious and poorly paid. Because women are more likely than men to seek medical treatment, they are the principal consumers of health care. However, more than three decades of research has demonstrated differences in the kind of health care men and women receive—differences that often place women at a disadvantage. Gender is a significant dimension of social stratification that affects men and women as both providers and recipients of health care. Together with inequalities of race, socioeconomic status, and age, gender shapes both the health-care delivery system and the quality of health care men and women receive. This chapter reviews work on gender and health care, focusing primarily on theory and research in sociology.

Origins of Interest in Gender and Health Care

Interest in gender and health care developed from the engagement of the social sciences with the second wave of feminism, which flourished in the United States and Western Europe in the 1970s. Feminists made medicine the centerpiece of their analysis, arguing that no institution so clearly epitomized women's subjugation. In a series of widely read books, feminist writers developed a far-reaching critique of the health-care system, attacking the medical profession for excluding women from medicine; overusing and misusing drugs, surgery, and technology; withholding important information from women patients; and trivializing women patients' concerns (Arms 1975; Corea 1977). Like members of other new social movements that challenged and demystified medicine's "cultural authority" (Starr 1982), feminists asserted the right to be full and equal participants in medical decisions.

The women's health movement was particularly influential in the social sciences as historians, anthropologists, and sociologists tested and extended feminist ideas. In medical sociology, researchers challenged the prevailing view that professionals are recruited according to strict meritocratic criteria and treat all patients equally (Parsons 1951). Theory and research on gender and health care have also challenged fundamental assumptions of the medical model (Mishler 1981). Researchers have challenged the assumption that definitions of health and illness are unaffected by the social context by showing them to be culturally variable and historically contingent: what is designated an illness varies according to time, place, or social context. Studies revealing gender bias in medical texts have challenged the assumption that medicine is scientifically neutral. The highly sex-segregated nature of the professional division of labor demonstrates that recruitment into medicine continues to have ascriptive elements. At the level of social interaction, medicine's scientific neutrality and its universalism have been challenged by studies showing that men and women patients presenting the same symptoms receive different diagnoses and treatments. These challenges have resulted in a body of theory and research demonstrating that the very acts of defining and treating illness are consummately social and cultural processes. Researchers in gender and health care, then, were at the forefront of the movement to create a sociological perspective on health and medicine.

Gender and the Medical Division of Labor: The Persistence of Ascription

Gender and Healing: A Brief Historical Overview

Both men and women have been healers, although their roles have varied historically. Most historical accounts focus on medieval Europe and the nineteenth-century United States. The Middle Ages laid the foundations for a structure that was to continue in many European countries until the nineteenth century: a largely male stratum, consisting of guilds and dominated by university-trained physicians; and midwives and folk healers, usually women, who served the rest of the population (Ehrenreich and English 1978).

In nineteenth-century America, multiple healing paradigms existed in competition. The predominately male "regulars" served a wealthy clientele in Eastern cities. Regulars were known—and sometimes dreaded—for their harsh treatments, such as bleeding and purging. Women were often rejected by regular medical schools and forced to attend women's colleges, proprietary colleges, or the schools of the sects that proliferated during the period. In contrast to regulars, sectarians avoided harsh remedies, and most served a rural or working-class clientele (Ehrenreich and English 1978).

At the beginning of the twentieth century, the leadership of the regular physicians, influenced by progressivism, began a campaign to make medical education more "scientific," culminating in the Flexner Report of 1910, a study of medical education commissioned by the Carnegie Foundation. As a result of both licensing and the Flex-

ner Report, medical education became university based and grounded in instruction in laboratory science (Starr 1982; Burrow and Burgess 2001). There were, however, additional consequences. Lacking the resources to build laboratories, many proprietary and sectarian colleges saw their enrollments dwindle. As these colleges closed their doors, most women (as well as African Americans) could no longer obtain a medical education. In the aftermath of the Flexner Report, medicine became a profession of a white, male elite. The process continued as many states outlawed midwives (Burrow and Burgess 2001; Starr 1982; Achterberg 1990).

Excluded from medicine, many women chose the fledgling profession of nursing. In England and the United States, the first professional nursing programs were established in the nineteenth century after Florence Nightingale successfully commanded a contingent of nurses during the Crimean War. Some of Nightingale's views were to become a mixed blessing in the twentieth century, such as her ruling that no nurse could act without explicit orders from a doctor. Throughout the twentieth century, nursing has struggled to regain the autonomy from medicine that Nightingale forfeited (Freidson 1970).

The Contemporary Medical Division of Labor

For most of the twentieth century, the gender composition of U.S. health-care occupations has followed a single principle: the higher the prestige, power, and pay of the occupation, the smaller the proportion of women. Table 14.1 presents the gender composition of the health-care occupations and the 2005 median salaries of each occupation. Figure 14.1 represents the median incomes and percent women in selected medical specializations. Both clearly show an inverse correlation between occupational salaries and the percentage of women in each occupation.

The occupational division of labor can be loosely divided into three strata (Table 14.1): At the top of the salary hierarchy are the predominately white and male health professions. At the middle level—allied health practitioners such as nurses, dieticians, and therapists—the majority is

Table 14.1. Percentage of women employees and annual income in selected occupations, 2005

Occupation	Number employed	Percent women	Median annual income AMGA[a]	MGMA[b]
Health-care practitioners				
Physicians	902,053	27.1		
Pediatrics	72,288	53.1	$184,900	$167,570
Obstetrics/gynecology	42,600	42.5	$275,800	$272,369
Psychiatry	41,598	33.5	$183,900	$190,965
Family Practice	81,701	33.5	$177,900	$165,135
General internal medicine	154,002	31.2	$180,800	$175,935
Anesthesiology	40,494	22.2	$322,900	$338,722
Emergency medicine	29,144	22.1	$232,400	$226,768
Radiology	8,813	15.2	$385,400	$411,131
General surgery	37,857	14.4	$320,200	$306,490
Orthopedic surgery	24,140	0.05	$373,656	$314,056
Chiropractors	82,000	21.8	$82,060	$67,200
Dentists	164,000	22.5	$133,680	$125,300
Veterinarians	61,000	38.7	$77,710	$68,910
Midlevel providers				
Pharmacists	248,000	48.3	$89,820	
Respiratory therapists	94,000	58.8	$45,140	
Physicians' assistants	74,000	62.1	$72,030	
Physical therapists	177,000	68.9	$63,080	
Speech-language pathologists	98,000	92.0	$54,880	
Registered nurses	2,426,000	92.3	$54,670	
Occupational therapists	85,000	92.9	$56,860	
Dieticians	68,000	95.3	$44,940	
Emergency medical technicians and paramedics	155,000	31.3	$26,080	
Clinical laboratory technologists and technicians	334,000	74.2	$39,705	
Medical records and health information technicians	121,000	86.6	$26,690	
Dental hygienists	132,000	97.1	$60,890	
Licensed practical and licensed vocational nurses	510,000	93.4	$35,230	
Health-care service occupations				
Dental assistants	259,000	96.1	$29,520	
Nursing, psychiatric, and home-health aides	1,900,000	88.7	$21,053	

Sources: Smart 2007; U.S. Department of Labor 2006, 2007; MGMA 2006. Statistics in preceding two sources are also reported in *Modern Healthcare* 2006.

Note: Only the ten largest medical specialties and subspecialties are included in this table. To be listed in this table, an occupation must appear in both the Current Population Survey and the Occupational Employment Survey, which use different job-classification systems.

a. American Medical Group Association

b. Medical Group Management Association

male. Finally, at the lowest level—health service workers, many of whom are women of color—women represent about 90 percent (Olesen 1997).

Medicine

Medicine, the most lucrative and prestigious occupation in the United States, remains a predomi-nately male profession. Although the number of women physicians has increased dramatically since 1970, in 2008 less than one-third of all physicians were women. Moreover, only 6.2 per-cent of all physicians, and fewer than 2 percent of all *women* physicians, are African American (U.S. Department of Labor 2009).

Since 1970, the number of women physicians has increased tenfold (AMA 2009). However,

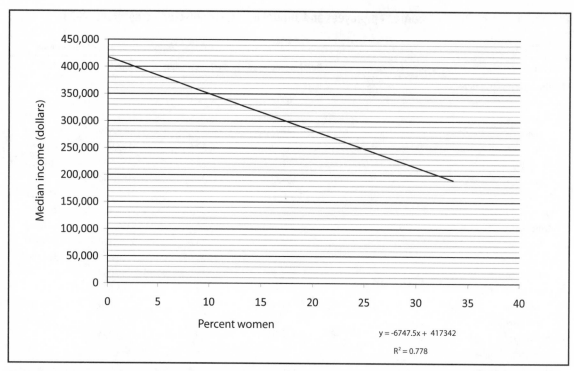

Figure 14.1. Median annual income and gender composition of selected specialties and subspecialties, 2005. Specialties and subspecialties include pediatrics, OB/GYN, psychiatry, family practice, general internal medicine, anesthesiology, emergency medicine, radiology, general surgery, and orthopedic surgery.

despite this major change, medicine remains internally stratified by gender (see Table 14.1 and Figure 14.1). Women are generally concentrated in the medical specialties having the lowest incomes, such as pediatrics, psychiatry, and family practice, which involve considerable direct patient contact. Conversely, the lowest proportions of women are found in the most lucrative surgical specialties, which involve medical procedures and require less patient contact. The single exception to this pattern is OB-GYN, a relatively remunerative occupation, in which 40 percent of practitioners are women (U.S. Department of Labor 2006, 2009a, b; Smart 2007; AMA 2009a, b).

In addition, the medical subspecialties are themselves internally stratified by gender. Very few women enter the most lucrative surgical subspecialties, such as orthopedic surgery. Within internal medicine, the proportion of women is lowest in cardiology and gastroenterology, subspecialties similar to surgery in their use of

procedures and their salary structures (U.S. Department of Labor 2006, 2009a, b; Smart 2007).

The practice patterns of men and women physicians also place women at a disadvantage: women are more likely than men to work in the least lucrative practice arrangements—that is, to be salaried employees rather than partners in a medical practice (Boulis and Jacobs 2008; AMA 2009a, b). Since 1970, the absolute number of women in administration and teaching more than doubled (AMA 2009b). However, as Boulis and Jacobs note, the number of women physicians in leadership positions has not kept pace with the entry of women into the profession. Moreover, women administrators remain in the "less prestigious, less well reimbursed" areas of medicine (Boulis and Jacobs 2008, 202). In 2005, the same authors report, women represented almost half of all medical students, but only 10 percent of department chairs were women.

Discrimination against women physicians

extends to medicine's informal structure: women physicians report instances of discrimination and sexual harassment (Boulis and Jacobs 2008) and experience what Lorber (2000) calls "covert discrimination"; they are often excluded from sponsorship networks that channel medical students into prestigious specialties and enable younger physicians to establish practices.

The entry of increasing numbers of women into medicine during the last three decades of the twentieth century—a trend likely to continue—raises the question of whether women physicians provide care that differs qualitatively from the care provided by male physicians. Although this question makes the essentialist, binary assumption of categorical differences between men and women (Olesen 1997; West 1993; Bird and Rieker 2008; see also Rieker, Bird, and Lang, this volume), it merits an answer. The many studies that have examined whether male and female physicians differ in attitudes and values, choice of medical treatment, or interactive styles present a mixed picture. On the one hand, male and female family practitioners do not differ in their evaluations of common medical problems. On the other hand, women physicians are more likely to perform preventive screening exams, to use a more collaborative mode of interaction, to engage in discussion of psychosocial issues, to deal with emotions, and to create opportunities for their patients to participate in the medical exchange (Flocke and Gilchrist 2005; Roter and Hall 2006). In a 1993 study, West found male physicians more likely to use the imperative, whereas women make requests rather than issue commands, thereby creating more symmetry in the doctor-patient relationship. In most cases, then, the physician's gender is more likely to affect the *style* of communication than the *content* of medical decisions (for a discussion, see Roter and Hall 2006; Roter, Hall, and Aoki 2002).

More recently, researchers have focused on the effects of gender concordance on the medical encounter. Concordance research moves away from an exclusive emphasis on gender differences to focus on the social situation in which patient and doctor find themselves. Like the studies just reviewed, however, concordance research presents a mixed picture: On the one hand, concordance

increases patient trust (Bonds et al. 2004), and physicians are likely to spend more time with patients of the same sex (Franks and Bertakis 2003). Because male (or female) physicians have more experience treating gender-specific problems, physicians are more likely to perform gender-specific screening (e.g., breast exams) on patients of the same sex (Roter and Hall 2006; Franks and Bertakis 2003). On the other hand, doctor-patient gender concordance has not been shown to increase rates of gender-neutral diagnostic screening (Flocke and Gilchrist 2005) or to increase rates of detection of mental health problems (Chan et al. 2006).

Some observers have cautioned that increasing the number of women physicians may not in itself transform U.S. health care. First, sex role socialization is only one of many forces that shape physicians' attitudes and behavior. Its effects diminish as men and women undergo similar training and encounter pressures arising from similar work environments (Olesen 1997). This consideration suggests that increasing the number of women in medicine is a necessary but ultimately insufficient condition for creating a humane health-care system responsive to the diverse needs of both men and women. It is necessary because of what women contribute to the medical encounter. It is insufficient, however, because of the absence of women of color and because more women physicians remain underrepresented in the highest reaches of the profession (Boulis and Jacobs 2008). What is needed are more women who occupy positions of leadership within medicine and are able to reshape the medical curriculum (Lorber 2000), revise the textbooks, and influence funding priorities.

Second, as Boulis and Jacobs (2008) note, both male and female physicians face unprecedented structural challenges to their ability to deliver quality health care. Cost-containment concerns, shrinking reimbursements, and pressures on productivity have forced many primary-care providers to see more patients per day and spend significantly less time with any one of them. In the face of these constraints, the number of men and women entering primary care is shrinking. With this flight from primary care, midlevel health-care providers—physician assistants and advanced-practice nurses—are increasingly filling the niche many physicians have vacated. Thus, the doctor-patient relationship may one day not involve a doctor at all.

Midlevel Providers

Contrasting with the profession of medicine is a middle level consisting of the allied health professions—registered nurses, pharmacists, dieticians, and therapists—as well as licensed medical technicians. Women predominate in most of these occupations (see Table 14.1). These professions are also stratified according to race, with the largest percent of women of color found in the occupations with the lowest salaries (Olesen 1997).

Women allied health professionals and technicians usually advance more slowly than men in those occupations. For example, the small number of men who have entered nursing have been promoted very quickly to administrative positions (C. Williams 1992). Women earn less than men who do the same work, and they also earn less than men in predominately male occupations who do different but comparable work. Pharmacy, a predominately male allied health profession, is also the most lucrative. Pharmacists earn more than nurse supervisors, even though researchers found the latter job to be more demanding (Achterberg 1990).

Of the allied health professions, nursing has fought hardest to improve its status and attain autonomy from medicine. The decline of three-year diplomate nursing programs and the growth in baccalaureate programs have contributed to nursing's independent professional identity (Chambliss 1996). One sign of nursing's success is the growth of advanced-practice nursing, such as certified nurse midwives and nurse practitioners. Despite some opposition from medicine to their growing independence, advanced-practice nurses have thrived in a climate of cost containment. At the same time, however, pressures for cost containment have worked to the detriment of the majority of nurses who have worked in hospitals, as administrators attempt to replace them with less-trained aides and assistants.

Part of nursing's warrant for autonomy rests on its claim, often articulated by educators, that nursing offers a philosophy of healing that differs fundamentally from that of medicine—one premised on caring rather than curing. For this reason, some observers have asked whether this philosophical difference translates into differences in the kind of care nurses provide. Again, the empirical evidence presents a mixed picture. On the one hand, researchers have suggested that caring for the socioemotional needs of patients and families is an integral facet of nurses' work (Chambliss 1996); that nurses are more likely than physicians to adopt a more egalitarian communication style (Fisher 1995); and that they are more likely to conclude that care should be withdrawn from terminally ill patients (Anspach 1993; Zussman 1992). On the other hand, researchers have noted that caring is not the only or even the most important part of nursing work. Nurses are, for example, as likely as physicians to attend to the technical aspects of care and to treat the patient as an object when the situation requires it (Anspach 1993; Chambliss 1996). Both technical and socioemotional labor, then, are parts of nursing. Which side prevails is likely to depend in part on the social contexts in which health care is delivered.

Health Service Occupations: Paid and Unpaid

At the bottom of the occupational hierarchy are the health service occupations, consisting primarily of aides, orderlies, and attendants. Women represent nearly 90 percent of this group, which also has the greatest proportion of African American workers. Although hospitals could not function without health service work, it is typically characterized by low pay, low prestige, and limited prospects for advancement. As care of the chronically ill has moved out of the hospital and into the home, the number of home-health aides has increased. These jobs, typically performed by women of color and immigrants, lack the fringe benefits that come with hospital work and are compensated at levels at or below the poverty line (Olesen 1997; U.S. Department of Labor 2006, 2009b).

Most research on health-care occupations focuses on the occupations with higher status. We know more about medicine than about nursing, more about nurses than about technicians, and we know the least of all about health aides, janitors, and cafeteria employees. This gap exists despite the fact that these occupations are an integral part of a hospital's infrastructure. Until these occupations are studied, knowledge of the hospital's social organization will be incomplete.

Women also perform most of the unpaid, informal caregiving for sick relatives in the home—a phenomenon that has also increased with "dehospitalization" (Glazer 1990). Caregiving entails a number of strains, including: loss of social relationships outside the family, interference with work roles, and the strain of performing multiple caregiving roles simultaneously (Olesen 1997). At the same time, McLaughlin (2009) shows that caregiving is a complex, multifaceted phenomenon that has its rewards. For some women, for example, advocating for children fueled their political consciousness. Perhaps the greatest strain arises from the assumption, often unquestioned, that responsibility for providing care rests exclusively with women.

Particularism in the Medical Encounter: Are Men and Women Patients Treated Differently?

Although women's reentry into medicine in the twentieth century has been one of the most important developments in the history of the profession, as I have noted, women remain underrepresented in leadership positions, a trend which may have limited their influence on medical practice. Moreover, the typical medical encounter with a *specialist* is still likely to involve a male physician and a female patient. These patterns invite the question of whether physicians treat their male and female patients differently, that is, whether physicians are universalistic (Parsons 1951) or particularistic (Freidson 1970) in their treatment of patients.

Differential treatment can assume two forms. First, physicians can interact differently with female than with male patients by adopting a more controlling communication style or by giving women less information. Second, physicians may give a different diagnosis or recommend a different treatment to male and female patients with similar medical problems.

Gender and Communication

Some of the first studies to identify the structure of the medical interview were conducted in obstetrical and gynecological clinics. These studies found that physicians persuaded patients to use or forego specific treatments by presenting information selectively; made recommendations that reflected cultural assumptions about gender (e.g., only married women should have children); and gave poor women fewer choices than they gave educated, middle-class patients (Fisher 1986; Todd 1989).

These studies show that assumptions about gender affect the content of the medical encounter but do not demonstrate that male and female patients are treated differently. Studies comparing physicians' communication with male and female patients present contradictory findings. On the one hand, physicians spend more time with female patients and give more explanations, possibly because women present more symptoms and ask more questions (Elderkin-Thompson and Waitzkin 1999). On the other hand, communication between male doctors and female patients is likely to be viewed as problematic: physicians report preferring male patients, and women are more likely to report that male physicians talked down to them and trivialized their concerns (Elderkin-Thompson and Waitzkin 1999). As observers have noted, the medical encounter is highly asymmetrical: physicians interrupt patients and deflect their concerns within the first moments of the interview (Beckman and Frankel 1984). However, physicians heighten this asymmetry when they "do gender" by interrupting women patients (West 1984).

Gender and Medical Decision Making

The second question regarding differential treatment—whether gender influences medical decision making—has been studied extensively.

Research undertaken in the 1970s and 1980s tested the hypothesis that primary care physicians share the commonsense stereotype of women as more emotional than men and are more likely to interpret women's physical complaints as psychogenic—a pattern that may cause doctors to overlook a physical disease or incorrectly diagnose a psychological disorder. Studies of routine decisions of internists and family practitioners provide strong support for the hypothesis that physicians stereotype female patients as more emotional and weaker than men, more equivocal support for the hypothesis that stereotypes result in unequal treatment (see Weiss and Lonnquist 2005). What are needed are studies that determine whether these patterns obtain today.

Beginning in the 1980s and 1990s, research on gender bias focused on specialists' decisions, particularly those involving "high technology medicine." Several studies have suggested that women are less likely to be treated aggressively than are male patients with similar conditions. For example, women are less likely than men to receive organ transplants (Elderkin-Thomson and Waitzkin 1999; Schaubel et al. 2000) and less likely to receive intensive antiretroviral therapies for AIDS (Anderson and Mitchell 2000), invasive cardiac diagnostic studies, or coronary bypass treatment (see Schelfer, Escarce, and Schulman 2000).

With increased understanding that heart disease is also a woman's disease (see Bird and Rieker et al. 2008), the focus shifted to the diagnosis and treatment of cardiovascular disease (CVD). By 2010, there were more than a thousand studies comparing the treatment of male and female patients showing signs of CVD. These include studies with retrospective and prospective research designs; studies using clinical samples and population-based samples; studies that use information from case records; and studies that ask physicians to respond to hypothetical vignettes. Virtually every point in the decision-making process has been examined.

Even after adjusting for confounding variables, many studies have found male and female patients with heart disease to be treated differently at one or more of the following decision points: women are less likely than men to be included in clinical trials of anticholesterol drugs (Bandyopadhyay, Bayer, and O'Mahony 2001; Abuful, Gidron, and Henkin 2005); to undergo noninvasive diagnostic studies such as treadmill tests and imaging (Williams, Bennett, and Feely 2003; Peterson, Masoudi, and Rumsfeld 2005); and to receive invasive diagnostic procedures such as catheterization (Daly et al. 2006; Schelfer, Escarce, and Schulman 2000; Gopalakrishnan, Ragland, and Tak 2009). Once a heart attack has been diagnosed, women are less likely than men to be treated with thrombolytics ("clot busters") and less likely to receive a cardiology consult (Peterson, Masoudi, and Rumsfeld 2005). Women, particularly African American women, are less likely than men to undergo angioplasty or coronary bypass surgery (Wenger 2003; Smedley et al. 2003). When they do receive angioplasty or surgery, they are referred later in the course of their disease than men are—a pattern that may contribute to women's higher surgical mortality (see Beery 1995). Most of these studies involve patients presenting in emergency rooms or hospitals with possible symptoms of a heart attack, but gender disparities also occur in ambulatory care. Bird and her colleagues (2007) found that among individuals with insurance and a diagnosis of diabetes or coronary heart disease, women are less likely than men to be screened for cardiovascular risk factors or to receive treatment such as beta-blockers or ACE inhibitors, a difference that persists in intermediate outcomes (see also Chou et al. 2007).[1]

These findings should be interpreted cautiously for two reasons. First, a substantial number of studies have failed to find evidence of gender differences in one or more of the treatments of heart disease that have been mentioned (see Ghali et al. 2002; Blum et al. 2003). Second, because these studies use information extracted from written documents, they do not reveal the actual decision-making process culminating in differential treatment. Several plausible explanations of these findings have been proposed (Beery 1995):

(1) *Perceived risk of procedures.* Physicians may be reluctant to perform angioplasty and cardiac bypass surgery on female patients because they view these procedures as more risky for women.

In fact, women who undergo bypass surgery are older, have higher comorbidity, and are at a later stage in their disease. However, this pattern may also reflect physicians' reluctance to diagnose and treat women with heart disease at earlier stages (Beery 1995).

(2) *Beliefs about heart disease.* The misconception that heart disease is a man's disease may prevent physicians from recognizing the symptoms of heart disease in their women patients. In fact, in a content analysis of 919 cardiovascular advertisements in general medicine and cardiology, Ahmed et al. (2004) found that only 20 percent of the advertisements depicted women patients—a pattern that may contribute to the view of CVD as a man's disease. This misconception also exists outside of medicine: in a survey by the American Heart Association, 54 percent of women respondents were unaware that heart disease was a major cause of death among women (Mazzaferri and Limacher 2005). This belief may also account for women's greater tendency to delay seeking treatment—a pattern that further complicates their clinical course and prognosis.

(3) *Different symptoms.* Women are more likely to present atypical symptoms. For both men and women, chest pain is the most frequently reported symptom of a heart attack (Gopalakrishnan, Ragland, and Tak 2009). However, women are more likely to report epigastric pain, fatigue, nausea, shortness of breath, or lower back pain—more subtle and diffuse symptoms that overlap with other possible diagnoses (Arslanian Engoren 2000; Gopalakrishnan Ragland, and Tak 2009). A recent study of patients in an emergency department, however, found that gender bias in cardiovascular testing persisted even after adjusting for patients' presenting symptoms (Chang et al. 2007).

(4) *Cultural assumptions about gender.* In addition to the factors just mentioned, cultural assumptions about gender may lead physicians to miss a diagnosis of heart disease. This explanation receives some empirical support from a study of chest pain evaluation in an emergency room, which found men more likely to receive emergency cardiology consults, nitroglycerin, aspirin, and thrombolytic agents and women more likely to receive antianxiety drugs (Lehmann et al.

1996). This finding suggests that physicians may fail to diagnose heart disease in female patients partly because of a belief that their symptoms are psychosomatic.

(5) *Presentation style.* Some writers suggest that women's greater tendency to introduce contextual information into the medical interview may cause their complaints to be discounted or interpreted as psychosomatic (Elderkin-Thompson and Waitzkin 1999).

To summarize: there is considerable evidence that women are less likely than men to be treated aggressively for heart disease. Because disparities in quality of care contribute to morbidity and mortality from CVD, it is imperative that health-care organizations assess and report variation in the quality of health care by gender (Fremont, Correa-de-Araujo, and Hayes 2007). At the same time, despite evidence that gender bias exists, how and why this bias occurs remains poorly understood. To understand the causal pathways leading to gender bias, we need to understand the cognitive schemas and micropolitical processes that culminate in a biased decision. In addition to the research designs that have been widely used, we need research examining decision making directly (for an example, see Lutfey and McKinlay 2009). These patterned differences in the treatment of men and women may contribute to women's greater mortality from heart attacks that occur later in life. They also raise questions about medicine's scientific neutrality and universalism and suggest that diagnosis and treatment decisions contain particularistic assumptions. In this case, research on gender and health care provides a powerful demonstration of a key discovery of medical sociologists: that medical decision making is a social process.

Gender and the Social Construction of Illness

In the last section, I argued that research on gender and health care has challenged the medical model at the level of social interaction. In this section, I turn to the level of culture and suggest that research has challenged the view of health and illness as generic or invariant (Mishler 1981).

Drawing on Freidson's (1970) conception of illness as socially constructed, writers have shown that conceptions of illness are historically contingent, culture bound, and ineluctably tied to the social contexts out of which they arise. Both discourse and practice are important, for changing ideas about medical problems have profoundly affected how patients have been treated (for a discussion of the social construction of illness, see Barker, this volume).

Cultural Constructions of the Body

Since the 1980s, historians have examined how the human body has been viewed and represented. According to historical accounts, the very idea of fundamental anatomical differences between the male and female body did not emerge until the eighteenth and nineteenth centuries. Before the Enlightenment, anatomists from Galen to Vesalius depicted the female body as a similar, though less developed, version of male anatomy. Around 1750, these ideas gave way to the conception of fundamental differences between the male and female body. The key to these incommensurable differences between the sexes was the female reproductive system, now viewed as differing dramatically from that of the male (Laqueur 1990). Nineteenth-century anatomical drawings depict the female skeleton as much smaller than that of the male, with a larger pelvis and smaller brain, reflecting the woman's ostensibly greater suitability for bearing children and lesser aptitude for intellectual and economic pursuits (Schiebinger 1987).

According to nineteenth-century conceptions of the body, the female reproductive system was the foundation of womanhood that enabled women to fulfill their most important role—bearing children (Laqueur 1990). These ideas about female sexuality shaped the ways nineteenth-century physicians treated the affluent women who sought treatment for a variety of complaints diagnosed as "hysteria" or "neurasthenia." This epidemic of "female invalidism" was a form of symbolic resistance to the enforced idleness that pervaded affluent women's lives. Rather than recognizing the social source of women's

complaints, physicians located their cause in the female reproductive system. Female complaints, physicians argued, resulted from adverse effects on the uterus and ovaries brought about by deviation from prescribed gender roles. The treatments ranged from "rest cures" that forced women into idleness, to sexual surgery to remove the uterus or ovaries (Ehrenreich and English 1978). The medical response to female complaints illustrates how ostensibly scientific ideas about the body can be used ideologically to justify prescriptive claims about gender and women's place.

Gender, Medicalization, and Health Care

Although these ideas no longer hold sway, in the twentieth century, as in the nineteenth, the body continues to serve as a metaphor for cultural assumptions about the body politic. A notable example in the United States and Europe is the extension of the medical model to an increasing number of deviant behaviors and natural processes. Women, particularly middle-class women, have been deeply affected by the medicalization of natural processes or the tendency to treat the reproductive phases in the female life course—childbirth, menstruation, and menopause—as illnesses (Riessman 1983; see also Barker, this volume).[2]

Throughout the last two centuries, childbirth, particularly in the United States, has been gradually transformed from a natural event, taking place at home and assisted by midwives, into a medical event managed by obstetricians (Wertz and Wertz 1977). By the middle of the twentieth century childbirth in the United States had been medicalized to an extent unparalleled in the world. Women have been subjected to myriad medical procedures, including epidural anesthesia, forceps, and fetal monitors—technologies with questionable therapeutic value. Despite U.S. medicine's use of medical technology, infant mortality rates in the United States continue to lag behind those of other European countries in which medicalization has been less extensive (Riessman 1983).

Of these interventions, it is electronic fetal monitoring that has evoked the most criticism.

As early as 1979, questions were raised about its cost effectiveness (Banta and Thacker 1979). In a 1996 meta-analysis of twenty years of clinical trials, the U.S. Preventive Services Task Force found electronic fetal monitoring (EFM), particularly in high-risk pregnancies, to be of limited use in reducing perinatal morbidity and mortality. It was during this period, in the face of mounting evidence against its effectiveness, that the use of electronic fetal monitoring increased to about three-fourths of all live births (USPSTF 1996). Why do U.S. hospitals continue to use an intervention that has not been cost effective? A frequently cited factor in the use of EFM is the desire to avoid litigation. In addition, even if an intervention has limited medical value, it nevertheless may have *ritual* value, initiating the woman into a technological conception of childbirth (Davis-Floyd 2004).

Medicalization is also behind the controversial definition of premenstrual syndrome (PMS) as a psychiatric disorder. Despite the lack of consensus as to how the condition should be defined and despite the lack of evidence that women's moods vary according to their menstrual cycles, Premenstrual Dysphoric Disorder (PMDD) remains listed in the American Psychiatric Association's *Diagnostic and Statistical Manual*, has been treated with hormones and antidepressants, and has even been proposed as a criminal defense (see Tavris 1992; Figert 1996; Offman and Kleinplatz 2004). Between 2000 and 2003, the Food and Drug Administration approved four drugs (Prozac, Paxil, Lexapro, and Zoloft) for the treatment of PMDD—a move that has proven controversial (see Daw 2002). In 2003 the European Union's Committee for Proprietary Medicinal Products removed PMDD from the list of approved indications for Prozac (Moynihan 2004) but now seems likely to reverse this position (European Medicines Agency 2009). The medicalization of PMS can be a double-edged sword. On the one hand, women may be relieved to learn that they suffer from a "real" illness. On the other hand, the medicalization of PMS in the courts may revive the nineteenth-century view that the reproductive system controls women's mental lives.

In Europe and the United States, menopause, once viewed as a natural process, has been defined as a disease requiring medical treatment. Inequalities of age and gender combine to create a highly negative view of menopause in medical texts, which depict menopause as "hormonal failure" having far-reaching consequences for the heart, the skin, and the skeleton and, until 2002, requiring treatment with hormone replacement therapy. Underlying the discourse on menopause are assumptions that menopause is a hormone deficiency disease; that the menopausal body is unproductive; that the female body is designed primarily for reproduction; and that the youthful body is the gold standard of health against which the menopausal woman should be judged and found wanting (Lock 1993; S. Bell 1995).

Anthropologists have shown that these views of both PMS and menopause are deeply culture bound. Since 1931, descriptions of PMS have varied widely. Only during periods in which women were expected to leave the labor market were the symptoms of PMS depicted as debilitating. Further, whether or not women experience PMS also varies by social class: although middle-class women interviewed in one study viewed themselves as suffering from PMS, working-class women did not believe in its existence (E. Martin 1987).

Menopause shows similar cultural variation. In Japan, menopause has not been medicalized, although aging women are nevertheless stigmatized as unemployed caretakers. Since Japanese women are viewed as natural caretakers, government officials have suggested that women should become full-time caregivers of both aging parents and aging in-laws. It is these issues, rather than their hormones, that concern Japanese women (Lock 1993). The medicalization of childbirth, PMS, and menopause, then, demonstrate the power of culture to shape the experience of "natural" processes.

Gender and Medical Technology

Medicalization is often accompanied by the growth of medical technologies. In fact, medicalization is fueled by the pharmaceutical companies, who have a stake in promulgating the idea that pregnancy, PMS, and menopause are diseases requiring treatment. Medicalization is that point where cultural beliefs about gender converge with a health-care system organized for profit.

Feminists were among the first critics of the iatrogenic consequences and rapid diffusion of reproductive technologies. Early studies of estrogen replacement therapy, of the synthetic estrogen drug diethylstilbestrol (DES), and of the Dalkon shield, a contraceptive intrauterine device, focused on their diffusion into medical practice before their consequences had been fully assessed and on the drug companies' delay in recalling these technologies even after their risks had become apparent (e.g., Kaufert and McKinlay 1985)—a pattern that has been observed in other medical technologies unrelated to women's health.

Cultural beliefs about gender and the life course have been implicated in the growth and diffusion of some medical technologies. In her analysis of the language and logic of an expert panel queried by the Food and Drug Administration in 1941 about prescribing DES to menopausal women, Susan Bell (1995) suggests that a need to regulate and restore order to the menopausal body led experts to misattribute the drug's side effects to physician or patient error, leading to widespread use of the drug and dangerous health consequences for women.

This rapid diffusion has only accelerated in the last two decades as the pharmaceutical and biotechnology industries have promoted new drugs directly to consumers, or sought approval for new indications of existing products. Some observers have suggested that the pharmaceutical and biotechnical industry has supplanted professionals as a new "engine" of medicalization (Conrad 2005). The result has been the manufacture of new drugs (e.g., synthetic human growth hormone) and new indications for old drugs (Zoloft for PMDD), as what had once been considered mere variation is transformed into *deviation*.[3] These technologies may have gendered consequences. For example, short stature is believed to be a more serious problem for men, who are supposed to be the "taller" sex, than for women (Conrad and Potter 2004), but short women experience pervasive infantilization (Rott 2009). Human growth hormone is thus used to treat

boys for violating heteronormative masculinity, but used to treat girls for exaggerated conformity to stereotypical femininity. Technologies to treat short stature are used for both boys and girls, but gender is the lens through which the meaning of short stature is refracted.

Gender may also propel the diffusion of some medical technologies. In fact, in their quest for new markets, pharmaceutical companies may try to extend a profitable concept from one gender to the other. Thus pharmaceutical executives have lured researchers to develop a "male pill" (Oudshoorn 2003) or "female Viagra" (Hartley 2009). Thus diffusion across gender lines is one path medicalization can follow.

Commentators have examined not only the diffusion and health consequences but also the social consequences of reproductive technologies such as genetic screening, in vitro fertilization, and fetal surgery. Support for these reproductive technologies is grounded in the Enlightenment's promise that science and technology can empower. Critics suggest, however, that some reproductive technologies have not made good on the promise to enhance women's control over reproduction. Instead, they have diminished women's control in decision making, while augmenting the power of professionals, social movements, or the state. For example, the use of implantable contraceptives by the poor or by women in developing nations raises the specter of a powerful group or society controlling the fertility of the less powerful (Pies 1997). New diagnostic technologies diminish the importance of women's experience of their bodies and cause them to depend on experts to interpret the new technologies (Reiser 1978). With the development of ultrasound, for example, women became less reliant on their own experience of fetal movement and more reliant upon experts to help them "see" the fetus in an otherwise obscure sonogram (Duden 1993).

Moreover, commentators fear the potential of some new medical technologies to devalue the mother while increasing the social value of the fetus (Rothman 1989). For example, the new specialty of fetal surgery results in the creation of an unborn patient—the fetus—while the mother becomes peripheral to the treatment process (Casper 1998). The culmination of this devaluation of the mother and valorization of the fetus is the fetal rights movement, in which (poor, African American) mothers have been prosecuted for allegedly endangering fetal health (Roberts 1998). In these cases, women lose control of reproduction, which has been taken over by the state.

Most critics of new medical technologies do not assume that all medical technologies are intrinsically harmful to women (or men). Rather, most take the more nuanced view that the consequences of any technology depend largely on the social context in which it is deployed. Some technologies, such as birth control, can benefit some groups to the detriment of others—an issue I revisit in the last section.

Medicalization, Demedicalization, and Resistance

Some early feminist accounts portrayed treated women as passive victims of drug companies and physicians who convinced them that natural processes were serious conditions requiring medical treatment (see K. Martin 2003). In fact, many women have embraced medicalization through myriad technologies of the body, from dieting and exercise to weight-loss surgery to the vast array of chemicals that promise to keep aging at bay. Through these technologies of the self, along with efforts to be nice patients, women discipline themselves from within, often embracing medicalization in the process (K. Martin 2003). Moreover, organized consumers, many of them women, have been a potent force for medicalization as they have fought to define contested illnesses as legitimate medical diseases (see Barker, this volume).

But it is the feminist movements that have attempted to demedicalize childbirth that have left an enduring institutional legacy. In the 1960s and 1970s, some middle-class parents sought alternatives that provided a more radical challenge to the medical model, even to the extent of bypassing the hospital altogether and turning to lay midwives. At the same time, the women's health movement challenged professional dominance, sometimes usurping what had been considered professional prerogatives (Ruzek 1978). It is in

this context that feminist health centers, lay midwifery, and the home-birth movement emerged.

As a result of these social movements, three alternatives to traditional labor and delivery have developed: home births using lay midwives, home births using nurse-midwives, and delivery by nurse-midwives in freestanding birth centers (Sullivan and Weitz 1988; Rothman 1983; Riessman 1997). Each alternative offers a demedicalized childbirth that encourages mothers and families to become actively involved in the birth process, avoids technological interventions, and relies on hospitals only when complications arise. All three settings define providers as equals who share specific knowledge and skill rather than as professional experts.

While organized medicine has fought home births and attempted to regulate freestanding birth centers, hospitals have accommodated the demands of many parents for a less medicalized childbirth by creating alternative birth centers in hospitals and by offering Lamaze classes—changes that do not fundamentally challenge a technological and interventionist model of childbirth (Sullivan and Weitz 1988).

Despite opposition, home births and freestanding birth centers have continued through the beginning of the twenty-first century. However, these social movements have foundered because they have appealed exclusively to a small, educated, middle-class clientele—a limitation I discuss in the next section.

Intersecting Inequalities

In the past two decades, research on gender and health care has moved away from an exclusive focus on gender toward an understanding of the intersection of gender with race, class, and other forms of inequality. The impetus for this focus on differences among women came from developments both inside and outside academia. Influenced by postmodernism, academic feminists have criticized earlier feminist work for its essentialism, a binary view of inequality (see Rieker, Bird, and Lang, this volume) that treats gender as a unitary category having fixed and stable attributes, thereby ignoring the social relations and historical contexts within which categories take on meaning. Such essentialism, it is argued, elides important differences among women.

Outside the academy, women's health activists struggled to understand why their programs and political agenda appealed primarily to white middle-class women and failed to attract older women, working-class women, and women of color. Ultimately, it became apparent that some women had perspectives and interests that differed from those of white middle-class women. Both academics and activists have come to understand that it is misleading to extrapolate from their own experiences and project them onto women as a whole. Bearing these realizations in mind, researchers have focused on the intersection of gender with other forms of inequality in the context of health care. This focus on differences among women has opened several avenues of inquiry, and I explore two of them.

Inequalities as Policy

One line of inquiry has examined the role of race, class, and gender in shaping reproductive policies. In a classic study, Gordon (1982) examined ideological shifts in the birth control movement. At the turn of the century, Margaret Sanger viewed birth control as a way of enhancing the reproductive freedom of all women through "voluntary motherhood"—the right of all women to have (or not to have) children. As control of the movement shifted to physicians and eugenicists, its focus shifted to population control and was directed toward controlling the fertility of those deemed "unfit": poor women, immigrant women, and women with disabilities. In Margaret Sanger's words, the slogan of the movement shifted from "voluntary motherhood" to "more children from the fit, less children from the unfit" (Gordon 1982, 167).

At various points in the twentieth century, reproductive policies have enhanced middle-class women's control over reproduction but have attempted to control the reproduction of poor women or women of color. Policy discourse has depicted the infertility of middle-class women as a public problem while condemning the fertility

of the poor (A. Bell 2009, forthcoming). In the 1970s, for example, middle-class women struggled to retain the reproductive freedom they had won in *Roe v. Wade*. During that same period, the discourse on Zero Population Growth converged with the politics of class, as social workers were required to counsel women with "too many" children or children that were "inadequately spaced" about "family planning."[4] At the same time, in Los Angeles County General Hospital, several Latina immigrant women underwent sterilization without their informed consent, culminating in the 1978 lawsuit *Madrigal v. Quilligan* (Gutierrez 2008).

This concern with the fertility of poor women—sometimes depicted as "bad mothers"—was a leitmotif running through the doctrine of "fetal rights" (A. Bell 2009, forthcoming; Roberts 1998). In a series of "fetal abuse" cases, African American women accused of using crack cocaine were prosecuted, forced to relinquish their babies to the state, and occasionally jailed or forced to undergo caesarian sections. These mothers were not punished for drug abuse but rather for the decision to become pregnant and carry their infants to term while addicted (Roberts 1998). At a more mundane level, this concern with poor women's fertility is reflected in Medicaid policies that finance contraception but refuse to pay for infertility treatment (A. Bell 2009, forthcoming). How policies benefit some groups to the detriment of others, opening options for some but constraining choices for others, deserves further study (see Bird and Rieker 2008).

Inequalities as Prism

These events, etched in the collective memory of diverse groups, help explain why women differ systematically and dramatically in their attitudes toward health-policy issues. Many white middle-class women, whose access to medical care is unproblematic, question the quality of health care they receive. For these women, the problem is the medicalization of pregnancy and childbirth or, in other words, too much technology. By contrast, nonwhite women and women of low socioeconomic status, lacking access to high-technology medicine (Smedley, Stith, and Nelson 2003) and basic health care, and sometimes the targets of cost containment, seek access to the high-technology medicine they view as the best medicine has to offer. White middle-class women view access to contraception and abortion as fundamental reproductive freedoms. By contrast, a history of forced sterilization leads women of color to recognize the potential of these technologies to undermine their reproductive freedom (Ruzek, Clarke, and Olesen 1997). Middle-class women, concerned with the prospect of raising a child with serious disabilities, view access to prenatal screening and abortion on demand as reproductive rights. Disability rights activists, however, while not opposed to abortion on demand, oppose prenatal testing and the selective abortion of "defective" fetuses—policies that, in their view, symbolically devalue persons with disabilities and carry the implication that their lives are not worth living (Gill 1997; Ruzek, Clarke, and Olesen 1997). Middle-class working mothers who also care for aging parents or children with serious disabilities can complain about "caregiver burden." From a disability-rights perspective, however, the discourse on caregiver burden is concerned exclusively with the interests of the caregiver while reducing the person under her care to a "burden" (McLaughlin 2009). In all these cases, intersecting inequalities, symbolism, and collective memory are prisms through which perspectives on policy are refracted. At the very least, these prisms are topics for future research.

The mandate to study differences among women has yielded a richer, more complex picture of diverse women whose interests sometimes collide and at other times coincide. Once these differences have been identified, it may be possible to draw more meaningful generalizations about the kind of health care that serves diverse women.

Concluding Comments

This review tells three stories. The first is a story of the interplay between a social movement and academic inquiry. The women's movement not only was a source of research questions but, in addition, led scholars to reexamine critically their presuppositions about the needs and interests of diverse women. The second is the story of how the field of gender and health care developed, a story of growing depth, complexity, and sophistication. The dominant issues moved away from the exclusion of women from medicine toward awareness that including them was a necessary but insufficient condition for fundamental change in the content of medical knowledge. Having identified the harmful physical and social consequences of medicalization and the proliferation of medical technology, many commentators concluded that these technologies could benefit some women and harm others. Finally, scholars subjected their own fundamental analytic concept—gender—to critical scrutiny. The third narrative is about how the field of gender and health care contributed to medical sociology. Research on gender and health care challenged the idea that achievement and universalism were the defining attributes of a profession by demonstrating how the behavior of physicians departed from these ideals. This research also challenged the medical model by showing, for example, how ideas about the body, the life course, and illness are socially constructed and by demonstrating that diagnosis and treatment decisions are based on social as well as medical considerations. Research on gender and health, then, played a critical part in the move to create a post-Parsonian, critical sociology of health and medicine, a perspective that has influenced three generations of sociologists and remains influential today.

Notes

I am very grateful to James S. House for comments on a much earlier, related paper and to Chloe Bird for commenting on several drafts of this paper.

1. Bird et al. (2007) found that women with diabetes were 19 percent less likely than men to have their low-density lipoprotein level controlled. However, as the authors acknowledge, this difference in intermediate outcomes may not be due to differential treatment of male and female patients. If future studies find that gender differences in outcomes persist despite equivalent treatment, these disparities may be due to differences in the disease process or in health behavior.

2. Although medicalization affects both men and women, as Casper and Moore (2009) suggest, until

recently issues concerning men's health, particularly men's genitalia, have not been discussed. For this reason, this part of the review focuses on women.

3. The last two decades have seen dramatic developments in biology, medicine, and health care (for the most comprehensive discussion, see Clarke et al. 2003). So striking are these transformations, Clarke and her associates argue, that they signify a shift from an "age of medicalization" to one of "biomedicalization," a move that coincides with the transition from late modernity to postmodernity. According to the authors, the term "biomedicalization" encompasses a wide range of developments, such as increasing privatization of medicine, research, and health care; expanding the techniques of health surveillance and identifying an increasing number of persons as being "at risk" for medical disorders; rationalizing health care through computerized data banks, practice guidelines, and evidence-based medicine; disseminating biomedical knowledge through the Internet to the general public with efforts by pharmaceuticals to capture this new consumer market; and a shift from controlling bodies to transforming them and creating new identities (Clarke et al. 2003). The boundaries of the biomedicalization concept are not clear. Some of the developments described as "biomedicalization" have long histories. For example, identity-transforming surgery, such as sex-change operations, has existed since the 1970s. Efforts to rationalize health care through data banks and practice guidelines may actually represent new forms of bureaucratization, a quintessentially modern, rather than a postmodern, phenomenon. In other cases, the boundaries between medicalization and biomedicalization are blurred. It is clear that medicalization has assumed new forms, but it is not clear whether trends described as "biomedicalization" differ *qualitatively* from medicalization (Conrad 2005). For example, in direct marketing to consumers on the Internet, pharmaceutical companies use traditional medicalization rhetoric when they assert that "premenstrual dysphoric disorder . . . [is] a real medical condition [that] causes real suffering" (Pfizer Inc. 2002). Finally, it is not clear whether the disparate developments discussed under the rubric of "biomedicalization" constitute a single phenomenon. How these issues are resolved—whether we find evidence of a new age or a continuation of the old, a single trend or many—depends in part on our reading of the historical record.

4. I was one of those social workers.

References

Abuful, Akram, Yehuda Gidron, and Ya'akov Henkin. 2005. "Physicians' Attitudes toward Preventive Therapy for Coronary Artery Disease: Is There a Gender Bias?" *Clinical Cardiology* 28:389–93.

Achterberg, Jeanne. 1990. *Woman as Healer*. Boston: Shambhala Publications.

Ahmed, Sofia B., Sherry L. Grace, Henry Thomas Stelfox, George Tomlinson, and Angela Cheung. 2004. "Gender Bias in Cardiovascular Advertisements." *Journal of Evaluation in Clinical Practice* 10(4): 531–38.

Aiken, Linda H. 2002. "Allied Health Professionals." In *International Encyclopedia of the Social and Behavioral Sciences*, ed. Neil Smelser and Paul Baltes, 6591–98. London: Elsevier.

AMA [American Medical Association]. 2008. *Health Care Careers Directory: 2008–2009*. Chicago: American Medical Association.

———. 2009a. "Careers in Health Care." ama-assn .org/ama/pub/education-careers/careers-health-care/ health-care-income.html. Retrieved August 21, 2009.

———. Women Physicians Congress. 2009b. "Statistics and History." ama-assn.org/ama/pub/about-ama/ our-people/member-groups-sections/women -physicians-congress/statistics-history.html. Retrieved August 21, 2009.

AMGA [American Medical Group Association]. 2005. "2005 Medical Group Compensation and Financial Survey." Excerpted in *Unique Opportunities: The Physician's Resource*. udworks.com. Retrieved August 27, 2009.

———. 2009. "Physician Compensation Data." Excerpted from *2008 Physician Compensation Survey*. Cejka Search. cejskasearch.com. Data also available at ama-assn.org/go/hpsalary. Retrieved August 22, 2009.

Anderson, Katherine H., and Jean M. Mitchell. 2000. "Differential Access in the Receipt of Antiretroviral Drugs for the Treatment of AIDS and Its Implications for Survival." *Archives of Internal Medicine* 160(20): 3114–20.

Anspach, Renee R. 1993. *Deciding Who Lives: Fateful Choices in the Intensive-Care Nursery*. Berkeley: University of California Press.

Arms, Suzanne. 1975. *Immaculate Deception: A New Look at Women and Childbirth in America*. Boston: Houghton Mifflin.

Arslanian-Engoren, Cynthia. 2000. "Gender and Age Bias in Triage Decisions." *Journal of Emergency Nursing* 26(2): 117–24.

Bandyopadhyay, Syamasis, A. J. Bayer, and M. Sinead

O'Mahony. 2001. "Age and Gender Bias in Statin Trials." *Quarterly Journal of Medicine* 94(3): 127–32.

Banta, H. David, and Stephen B. Thacker. 1979. "Policies toward Medical Technology: The Case of Electronic Fetal Monitoring." *American Journal of Public Health* 69(9): 931–34.

Beckman, Howard B., and Richard M. Frankel. 1984. "Effect of Patient Behavior on Collection of Data." *Annals of Internal Medicine* 102:520–28.

Beery, Theresa A. 1995. "Gender Bias in the Diagnosis and Treatment of Coronary Artery Disease." *Heart and Lung Journal of Critical Care* 24:427–35.

Bell, Ann V. 2009. "'It's Way Out of My League': Low-Income Women's Experiences of Medicalized Infertility." *Gender and Society* 23(5): 688–709.

———. Forthcoming. "Beyond (Financial) Accessibility: Inequalities within the Medicalisation of Infertility." *Sociology of Health and Illness.*

Bell, Susan E. 1995. "Gendered Medical Science: Producing a Drug for Women." *Feminist Studies* 21(3): 469–500.

Bird, Chloe E., Allen Fremont, Arlene Bierman, Steve Wickstrom, Mona Shah, Thomas Rector, Thomas Horstman, and José J. Escarce. 2007. "Does Quality of Care for Cardiovascular Disease and Diabetes Differ by Gender for Enrollees in Managed Care Plans?" *Women's Health Issues* 17(3): 131–38.

Bird, Chloe E., and Patricia P. Rieker. 2008. *Gender and Health: The Effects of Constrained Choices and Social Policies.* Cambridge: Cambridge University Press.

Blum, Michael, Martin Slade, Donna Boden, Henry Cabin, and Teresa Caulin-Glaser. 2003. "Examination of Gender Bias in the Evaluation and Treatment of Angina Pectoris by Cardiologists." *American Journal of Cardiology* 93(6): 1724–27.

Bonds, Denise E., Kristie Foley, Elizabeth Dugan, Mark A. Hall, and Pam Extrom. 2004. "An Exploration of Patients' Trust in Physicians in Training." *Journal of Health Care for the Poor and Underserved* 15(2): 294–306.

Boulis, Ann K., and Jerry A. Jacobs. 2008. *The Changing Face of Medicine: Women Doctors and the Evolution of Health Care in America.* Ithaca, N.Y.: Cornell University Press.

Burrow Gerard N., and Nora L. Burgess. 2001. "The Evolution of Women as Physicians and Surgeons." *Annals of Thoracic Surgery* 71(2), suppl.: S27–29.

Casper, Monica J. 1998. *The Making of the Unborn Patient: A Social Anatomy of Fetal Surgery.* New Brunswick, N.J.: Rutgers University Press.

Casper, Monica J., and Lisa Jean Moore. 2009. *Missing Bodies: The Politics of Visibility.* New York: New York University Press.

Chambliss, Daniel F. 1996. *Beyond Caring: Hospitals, Nurses, and the Social Organization of Ethics.* Chicago: University of Chicago Press.

Chan, Kitty S., Chloe E. Bird, Robert Weiss, Naihua Duan, Lisa S. Meredith, and Cathy D. Sherbourne. 2006. "Does Patient-Provider Gender Concordance Affect Mental Health Care Received by Primary Care Patients with Major Depression?" *Women's Health Issues* 16:122–32.

Chang, Anna Marie, Mumma Byrne, Keara L. Sease, Jennifer L. Robey, Frances S. Shofer, and Judd E. Hollander. 2007. "Gender Bias in Cardiovascular Testing Persists after Adjusting for Presenting Characteristics and Cardiac Risk." *Academic Emergency Medicine* 14:599–606.

Chou, Ann F., Sarah Hudson Scholle, Carol S. Weisman, Arlene S. Bierman, Rosaly Correa-de-Araujo, and Lori Mosca. 2007. "Gender Disparities in the Quality of Cardiovascular Disease Care in Private Managed Care." *Women's Health Issues* 17(3): 120–30.

Clarke, Adele E., Laura Mamo, Jennifer M. Fishman, Janet K. Shim, and Jennifer Ruth Fosket. 2003. "Biomedicalization: Technoscientific Transformations of Health, Illness and U.S. Biomedicine." *American Sociological Review* 68(2): 161–94.

Conrad, Peter. 2005. "The Shifting Engines of Medicalization." *Journal of Health and Social Behavior* 46 (March): 3–14.

Conrad, Peter, and Deborah Potter. 2004. "Human Growth Hormone and the Temptations of Biomedical Enhancement." *Sociology of Health and Illness* 26(2): 184–215.

Corea, Gena. 1977. *The Hidden Malpractice: How American Medicine Treats Women as Patients and Professionals.* New York: Morrow.

Daly, Caroline, Felicity Clemens, Jose L. Lopez Sendon, Luigi Tavazzi, Eric Boersma, Nicholas Danchin, Francois Delahaye, Anselm Gitt, Desmond Julian, David Mulcahy, Witold Ruzyllo, Kristian Thygesen, Freek Verheugt, and Kim M. Fox. 2006. "Gender Differences in the Management and Clinical Outcome of Stable Angina." *Circulation* 113:490–98.

Davis-Floyd, Robbie E. 2004. *Birth as an American Rite of Passage.* 2nd ed. Berkeley: University of California Press.

Daw, Jennifer. 2002. "Is PMDD Real?" APA Online: Monitor on Psychology (October 2002). apa.org/monitor/oct02/pmdd.html. Retrieved September 12, 2009.

Duden, Barbara. 1993. *Disembodying Women: Perspectives on Pregnancy and the Unborn.* Cambridge, Mass.: Harvard University Press.

Ehrenreich, Barbara, and Deidre English. 1978. *For Her*

Own Good: 150 Years of the Experts' Advice to Women. Garden City, N.Y.: Anchor Press.

Elderkin-Thompson, Virginia, and Howard Waitzkin. 1999. "Differences in Clinical Communication by Gender." *Journal of General Internal Medicine* 14:112–21.

European Medicines Agency, Committee for Medicinal Product for Human Use. 2009. "Concept Paper on the Need for a Guideline on the Treatment of Premenstrual Dysphoric Disorder (PMDD)." emea.europa.eu/pdfs/human/ewp/1187709en.pdf. Retrieved September 12, 2009.

Figert, Ann. 1996. *Women and the Ownership of PMS: The Structuring of a Psychiatric Disorder.* Chicago: Walter De Gruyter.

Fisher, Sue. 1986. *In the Patient's Best Interest.* New Brunswick, N.J.: Rutgers University Press.

———. 1995. *Nursing Wounds: Nurse Practitioners, Doctors, Women Patients and the Negotiation of Meaning.* New Brunswick, N.J.: Rutgers University Press.

Flocke, Susan A., and Valerie Gilchrist. 2005. "Physician and Patient Gender Concordance and the Delivery of Comprehensive Clinical Preventive Services." *Medical Care* 43:486–92.

Franks, Peter, and Klea D. Bertakis. 2003. "Physician Gender, Patient Gender, and Primary Care." *Journal of Women's Health* 12:73–80.

Fremont, Allen M., Rosaly Correa-de-Araujo, and Sharonne N. Hayes. 2007. "Gender Disparities in Managed Care: It's Time for Action." *Women's Health Issues* 17:116–19.

Freidson, Elliot. 1970. *Profession of Medicine: A Study in the Sociology of Applied Knowledge.* New York: Dodd, Mead.

Ghali, William A., Peter D. Faris, Diane Galbraith, Colleen M. Norris, Michael J. Curtis, L. Duncan Saunders, Vladimir Dzavik, Brent Mitchell, and Merril K. Knudtson. 2002. "Sex Differences in Access to Coronary Revascularization after Cardiac Catheterization: Importance of Detailed Clinical Data." *Annals of Internal Medicine* 136(10): 723–32.

Gill, Carol J. 1997. "The Last Sisters: Health Issues of Women with Disabilities." In *Women's Health: Complexities and Differences,* ed. Sheryl B. Ruzek, Virginia L. Olesen, and Adele E. Clarke, 96–112. Columbus: Ohio State University Press.

Glazer, Nona Y. 1990. "The Home as Workshop: Women as Amateur Nurses and Medical Care Providers." *Gender and Society* 4:479–99.

Gopalakrishnan, Prabhakaran, Moluk Mirrasouli Ragland, and Tahir Tak. 2009. "Gender Differences in Coronary Artery Disease: Review of Diagnostic Challenges and Current Treatment." *Postgraduate Medicine* 121(2): 60–67.

Gordon, Linda. 1982. "The Politics of Birth Control, 1920–1940: The Impact of Professionals." In *Women and Health: The Politics of Sex in Medicine,* ed. Elizabeth Fee, 151–75. Farmingdale, N.Y.: Baywood.

Gutierrez, Elena. 2008. *Fertile Matters: The Politics of Mexican Origin and Women's Reproduction.* Austin: University of Texas Press.

Hartley, Heather. 2009. "Efforts to Create and Repackage Sex Drugs." In *The Sociology of Health and Illness,* 8th ed., ed. Peter Conrad, 287–95. New York: Worth.

Kaufert, Patricia, and Sonia McKinlay. 1985. "Estrogen Replacement Therapy: The Production of Medical Knowledge and the Emergence of Policy." In *Women, Health and Healing,* ed. Ellen Lewin and Virginia Olesen, 113–38. London: Tavistock.

Kee, Frank. 1995. "Gender Bias in Treatment for Coronary Heart Disease: Fact or Fallacy?" *Quarterly Journal of Medicine* 8:587–96.

Laqueur, Thomas. 1990. *Making Sex: Body and Gender from the Greeks to Freud.* Cambridge, Mass.: Harvard University Press.

Lehmann, Joan B., Wehner P. Christopher, U. Lehmann, and Linda M. Savory. 1996. "Gender Bias in the Evaluation of Chest Pain in the Emergency Department." *American Journal of Cardiology* 77:641–44.

Lock, Margaret. 1993. "The Politics of Mid-Life and Menopause: Ideologies for the Second Sex in North America and Japan." In *Knowledge, Power, and Practice: The Anthropology of Medicine and Everyday Life,* ed. Shirley Lindenbaum and Margaret Lock, 330–63. Berkeley: University of California Press.

Lorber, Judith. 2000. "What Impact Have Women Physicians Had on Women's Health?" *Journal of the American Medical Women's Association* 55(1): 13–15.

Lorber, Judith, and Lisa Jean Moore. 2002. *Gender and the Social Construction of Illness.* 2nd ed. Walnut Creek, Calif.: Alta Mira Press.

Lutfey, Karen E., and John B. McKinlay. 2009. "What Happens along the Diagnostic Pathways to CHD Treatment? Qualitative Results Concerning Cognitive Processes." *Sociology of Health and Illness* 31(7): 1077–92.

Malat, Jennifer. 2000. "Racial Differences in Norplant Use in the United States." *Social Science and Medicine* 50(9): 1297–1308.

Martin, Emily. 1987. *The Woman in the Body: A Cultural Analysis of Reproduction.* Boston: Beacon Press.

Martin, Karin A. 2003. "Giving Birth Like a Girl." *Gender and Society* 17(1): 54–72.

Mazzaferri, Ernest, Jr., and M. C. Limacher. 2005. "Changing Patterns of CAD Therapy and Hormone Usage for Women." *Cardiology Review* 22(3): 32–37.

McLaughlin, Janice. 2009. "How Do Citizenship and

Care Intersect in the Lives of Mothers of Disabled Children?" Presented at the annual meeting of the American Sociological Association, August 11, San Francisco.

MGMA [Medical Group Management Association]. 2006. *2005 Physician Compensation Survey.* reeves-associates.com/2005survey.htm. Retrieved August 22, 2009.

Mishler, Elliot G. 1981. "Viewpoint: Critical Perspectives on the Biomedical Model." In *Social Contexts of Health, Illness, and Patient Care*, ed. Elliot G. Mishler, Lorna R. Amarasingham, Stuart T. Hauser, Nancy E. Waxler, and Ramsay Liem, 1–22. Prospect Heights, Ill.: Waveland Press.

Modern Healthcare. 2006. *2005–2006 Physician Compensation Review: A Compendium of Physician Compensation Studies Annually Profiled in Modern Healthcare.* merritthawkins.com/pdf/2005_Modern_Healthcare_Physician_Compensation_Review.pdf. Retrieved August 22, 2009.

Moynihan, Ray. 2004. "Controversial Disease Dropped from Prozac Product Information." *British Medical Journal* 328:7436.

Offman, Alla, and Peggy J. Kleinplatz. 2004. "Does PMDD Belong in the DSM? Challenging the Medicalization of Women's Bodies." *Canadian Journal of Human Sexuality* 13. findarticles.com/p/articles/mi_go1966/is_1_13/ai_n7459081/. Retrieved August 22, 2009.

Olesen, Virginia L. 1997. "Who Cares? Women as Informal and Formal Caregivers." In *Women's Health: Complexities and Differences*, ed. Sheryl Burt Ruzek, Virginia L. Olesen, and Adele E. Clarke, 397–424. Columbus: Ohio State University Press.

Oudshoorn, Nelly. 2003. *The Male Pill: A Biography of a Technology in the Making.* Chapel Hill, N.C.: Duke University Press.

Parsons, Talcott. 1951. *The Social System.* Glencoe, Ill.: Free Press.

Peterson, Pamela L., Frederick A. Masoudi, and John S. Rumsfeld. 2005. "Gender Differences in the Epidemiology and Treatment of Heart Failure." *Cardiology Review* 22(3): 24–29.

Pfizer Inc. 2002. "Learn about PMDD." zoloftforpmdd.com/. Retrieved August 29, 2009.

Pies, Cheri A. 1997. "The Ongoing Politics of Contraception: Norplant and Other Emerging Technologies." In *Women's Health: Complexities and Differences*, ed. Sheryl Ruzek, Virginia L. Olesen, Adele E. Clarke, 397–424. Columbus: Ohio State University Press.

Reiser, Stanley Joel. 1978. *Medicine and the Reign of Technology.* Cambridge: Cambridge University Press.

Riessman, Catherine Kohler. 1983. "Women and Medicalization: A New Perspective." *Social Policy* 14:3–18.

———. 1997. "Improving the Health Experiences of Low-Income Patients." In *The Sociology of Health and Illness: Critical Perspectives*, ed. Peter Conrad, 436–39. New York: St. Martin's Press.

Roberts, Dorothy E. 1998. "Punishing Drug Addicts Who Have Babies: Women of Color, Equality, and the Right to Privacy." In *Abortion Wars: A Half Century of Struggle, 1950–2000*, ed. Rickie Solinger, 124–56. Berkeley: University of California Press.

Roger, Véronique L., Michael E. Farkouh, Susan A. Weston, Guy S. Reeder, Steven J. Jacobsen, Alan R. Zinsmeister, Barbara P. Yawn, Stephen L. Kopecky, and Sherine E. Gabriel. 2000. "Sex Differences in Evaluation and Outcome of Unstable Angina." *Journal of the American Medical Association* 283(5): 646–52.

Roter, Debra L., and Deirdre Hall. 2006. *Doctors Talking with Patients/Patients Talking with Doctors.* 2nd ed. Westport, Conn.: Praeger.

Roter, Debra L., Judith A. Hall, and Yuko Aoki. 2002. "Physician Gender Effects in Medical Interview: A Meta-Analytic Review." *Journal of the American Medical Association* 288(6): 756–64.

Rothman, Barbara Katz. 1983. "Midwives in Transition: The Structure of a Clinical Revolution." *Social Problems* 30:262–71.

———. 1989. *Recreating Motherhood: Ideology and Technology in a Patriarchal Society.* New York: W. W. Norton.

Rott, Leslie R. 2009. "The Dual Role of Normalisation and Stigmatisation in the Experience of Growth Hormone Treatment." Presented at the annual meeting of the American Sociological Association, August 11, San Francisco.

Ruzek, Sheryl Burt. 1978. *The Women's Health Movement: Feminist Alternatives to Medical Control.* New York: Praeger.

Ruzek, Sheryl Burt, Adele E. Clarke, and Virginia L. Olesen. 1997. "What Are the Dynamics of Difference?" In *Women's Health: Complexities and Differences*, ed. Sheryl Burt Ruzek, Virginia L. Olesen, and Adele E. Clarke, 51–95. Columbus: Ohio State University Press.

Schaubel, Douglas E., Donna E. Stewart, Howard I. Morrison, Deborah L. Zimmerman, Jill I. Cameron, John J. Jeffery, and Stanley S. A. Fenton. 2000. "Sex Inequality in Transplantation Rates." *Archives of Internal Medicine* 160(15): 2349–54.

Schelfer, Stuart E., Jose J. Escarce, and Kevin A. Schulman. 2000. "Race and Sex Differences in the Management of Coronary Artery Disease." *American Heart Journal* 139(5): 848–57.

Schiebinger, Londa. 1987. "Skeletons in the Closet:

The First Illustrations of the Female Skeleton in Eighteenth-Century Anatomy." In *The Making of the Modern Body: Sexuality and Society in the Nineteenth Century*, ed. Catherine Gallagher and Thomas Laqueur, 42–82. Berkeley: University of California Press.

Smart, Derek R. 2007. *Physician Characteristics and Distribution in the U.S., 2007 Edition*. Chicago: American Medical Association.

Smedley Brian D., Adrienne Y. Stith, and Alan R. Nelson, eds. 2003. *Unequal Treatment: Confronting Racial and Ethnic Disparities in Health Care*. Washington, D.C.: National Academies Press.

Starr, Paul. 1982. *The Social Transformation of American Medicine*. New York: Basic Books.

Sullivan, David A., and Rose Weitz. 1988. *Labor Pains: Modern Midwives and Home Birth*. New Haven, Conn.: Yale University Press.

Tavris, Carol. 1992. *The Mismeasure of Women*. New York: Simon and Schuster.

Todd, Alexandra Dundas. 1989. *Intimate Adversaries: Cultural Conflict between Doctors and Women Patients*. Philadelphia: University of Pennsylvania Press.

U.S. Department of Labor. Bureau of Labor Statistics. 2006. "Women in the Labor Force: A Databook." Current Population Survey Report 996 (September 2006). bls.gov/cps/wlf-databook.pdf. Retrieved August 24, 2009

———. 2007. "Occupational Employment and Wages, May 2005." Bureau of Labor Statistics Bulletin 2585. Revised May 2007. bls.gov/oes/oes_pub_2005.htm. Retrieved August 20, 2009.

———. 2009a. "Annual Tables: Employment by Detailed Occupation and Sex." Labor Force Statistics from the Current Population Survey. bls.gov/cps/cpsaat11.pdf. Retrieved August 2, 2009.

———. 2009b. "Occupational Employment and Wages, 2008." Revised and released, May 29, 2009. bls.gov/oes/ocwage08.oes.pdf. Retrieved August 20, 2009.

USPSTF [U.S. Preventive Services Task Force]. 1996. *Guide to Clinical Preventive Services*. 2nd ed. Baltimore: Williams and Wilkins.

Weiss, Gregory L., and Lynne E. Lonnquist. 2005. *The Sociology of Health, Healing, and Illness*. 5th ed. Upper Saddle River, N.J.: Prentice Hall.

Wenger, N. K. 2003. "Coronary Heart Disease: The Female Heart Is Vulnerable." *Progress in Cardiovascular Disease* 46(3): 199–229.

Wertz, Richard W., and Dorothy C. Wertz. 1977. *Lying-In: A History of Childbirth in America*. New York: Free Press.

West, Candace. 1984. *Routine Complications: Troubles with Talk between Doctors and Patients*. Bloomington: Indiana University Press.

———. 1993. "Reconceptualizing Gender in Physician-Patient Relationships." *Social Science and Medicine* 36:57–66.

Williams, Christine L. 1992. "The Glass Escalator: Hidden Advantages for Men in the 'Female' Professions." *Social Problems* 39:253–67.

Williams, David, Kathleen Bennett, and John Feely. 2003. "Evidence for an Age and Gender Bias in the Secondary Prevention of Ischaemic Heart Disease in Primary Care." *British Journal of Clinical Pharmacology* 55:604–8.

Zussman, Robert. 1992. *Intensive Care: Medical Ethics and the Medical Profession*. Chicago: University of Chicago Press.

15

Institutional Change and the Organization of Health Care

The Dynamics of "Muddling Through"

Peter Mendel, RAND Corporation

W. Richard Scott, Stanford University

Many observers of the health-care system in the United States, including medical and organizational sociologists, have noted the profound changes that have occurred over the last four decades, particularly since the advent of the managed care "revolution" in the 1980s. From a highly stable sector that for decades was dominated by medical professionals and had long exhibited "dynamics without change" (Alford 1972), the sector experienced an influx of new types of organizations, models of service delivery and financing, and approaches to regulation inspired by corporate and managerial ideologies previously marginalized within mainstream health care (Alexander and D'Aunno 1990; Burns 1990; Mechanic 1994; Mick and Wyttenbach 2003).

Here we build on a study of these changes and their precursors from the 1940s through the 1990s (Scott et al. 2000), and the framework it developed for analyzing organizational fields, to understand more recent changes over the past decade in U.S. health care. Inspired by institutional theory from sociology and organization studies, this framework defines an organizational field as "those organizations that, in the aggregate, constitute a recognized area of institutional life" (DiMaggio and Powell 1983). An organizational field is similar to standard notions of an industry—that is, organizations providing similar services or products—but incorporates both competing and cooperating organizations, such as major suppliers and consumers, as well as the regulatory agencies, funding bodies, and interest groups, often at distant locations, that affect their operation. Thus the concept of field exploits the insight that "local social orders" constitute the building blocks of contemporary societies and represent an important level of social structure between society at large and particular types of organizations or groups of stakeholders (Scott 2008a, forthcoming).

Key components of organization fields under this framework include field actors, institutional logics, and governance mechanisms. *Field actors* include the basic types of actors, both individual roles and organizational models, that inhabit a field, as well as their relative numbers and how they relate among each other. Within any given field, there are usually a delimited number of roles for participating and models for organizing, for example, individual roles such as doctor, health administrator, and health economist, and organizational models such as community acute-care hospitals, academic medical centers, medical groups, and private health-insurance companies. *Institutional logics* are the cultural frames and belief systems that define and justify the roles of certain actors, help actors within the field to interpret events, and provide routines and rationales defining appropriate ways to carry on work. *Governance mechanisms* are arrangements that support the regularized control, whether by mutual agreement, legitimate authority, or coercive power, of some subset of actors by others. These mechanisms in the United States usually include mixes of public, professional, and private (both for-profit and nonprofit) players. The changing distributions of types of actors, logics, and governance mechanisms constitute some of the distinguishing and most recognizable features of the health-care field over time, such as the role and authority of professionals and changing emphases on quality, access, and cost containment.

As DiMaggio and Powell (1983; DiMaggio 1991) have pointed out, organization fields vary in the nature and degree of their "structuration"— the extent to which a small number of recognizable organization archetypes exists, the density of relations among them, the nature of their governance structures, and the degree of consensus on and coherence of institutional logics utilized and prevalent within the field at any given time.

From this perspective, the era of managed care in the 1980s and 1990s heralded an influx of new actors, logics, and governance mechanisms which tended to add to and compete with, rather than entirely supplant, the incumbents (Scott, Mendel, and Pollack 1996; Caronna 2004). As a result, these changes, although rooted in precursors from earlier eras, represented a process of rapid destructuration along a number of field-level dimensions within the health-care sector, such as increased fragmentation of funding and governance, dissensus on logics, and blurring of organizational and field boundaries (Scott et al. 2000).

Similar institutional frameworks have been used to compare the key structural composition and dynamics across organizational fields such as accounting, architecture, and higher-education publishing (Thornton, Jones, and Kury 2005). This approach has also been used to analyze how structuration of fields varies across levels, as well as across sectors and over time. Scott et al. (2000), for instance, documented differences in the composition of health-care actors, logics, and gover-

nance systems at the national, state (California), and local (San Francisco Bay Area) levels during the latter half of the twentieth century, and differing responses of various kinds of organizations to these changes in the Bay Area. Understanding how changes play out with varying impact between broad societal levels, more intermediate field-level structures, and local communities and markets—as well as how changes and influences travel upward—has been a focus shared by other institutional and organizational researchers (e.g., Ferlie and Shortell 2001; Alexander and D'Aunno 2003; Schneiberg and Soule 2005).

Thus, a strength of the institutional approach is its emphasis on studying and conceptualizing the context—social, political, and cultural, as well as economic and resource aspects—within which the delivery of health care takes place. This emphasis includes attention to the unique features of the health-care field, as well as to the multiple levels of social structure that guide, enable, and constrain behavior (see also Rieker, Bird, and Lang, this volume). It likewise attends to the process of change—who the stakeholders and decision makers are and how their preferences, interests, and organizational actions evolve and interact within these contexts over time (Wells and Banaszak-Holl 2000; Flood and Fennell 1995). As a result, the approach developed here offers a historical perspective that helps contrast how recent developments differ from earlier ones, in order to highlight the defining character of current changes and more accurately gauge the dynamics and direction of present trends. Knowing where we're coming from can help our understanding of where we are and where we seem to be going.

Using this framework, this chapter considers the following questions:

(1) What major changes characterize the evolution of the U.S. health-care field through the latter half of the twentieth century, from just before World War II when medical professionals had first solidified their dominant position within health care to the managed care revolution of the 1980s and 1990s?

(2) What have been recent trends and forces shaping the health-care field from the advent

of the era of managed care to today? How should we view our current era?

(3) What is the utility of a structuration framework for understanding these recent trends and forces?

(4) What are the implications of this perspective for understanding large-scale reform of the U.S. health-care system?

We argue that since the early 2000s, health care in the United States has moved into a period of incremental improvement characterized by several distinct mechanisms by which interests have endeavored to shape and reconstitute the field. What may appear to be institutional disarray during this time and, with respect to formation of policy, a process of "muddling through" (Lindblom 1959) can also be interpreted as a flurry of innovation in both models of organizing and attempts to reconcile or manage the plethora of competing actors, logics, and governance mechanisms spawned during earlier eras. Whether the past decade represents a discrete epoch in the evolution of the health-care field or is merely an extension of the previous era of managed care can be confirmed only from the vantage of greater historical distance—and even then assessments will not be devoid of contention.

In any case, the processes that distinguish the current period have implications for understanding potential future directions of health care in the United States, as well as for studying the structuration of organizational fields and organized social systems more generally. While it is difficult to predict from our current vantage point whether the present debate over comprehensive health-care reform in the United States will result in major systemic change, and what specific directions this reform may take, we can still learn from examining the nature of current developments and their underlying dynamics, since they will help chart the path to the future.

An Institutional Account of Profound Change: Three Eras in U.S. Health Care

We first briefly review the profound changes in U.S. health care from the 1940s to the 1990s based on our previous study (Scott et al. 2000), which chronicled the changes over the last half of the twentieth century in the field of health-care services in the San Francisco Bay area. Although by no means representative of the United States, this area was often on the leading edge of health-care change. Moreover, while the care-delivery systems we studied were limited to one geographic region, the organizational field approach we employed examined and incorporated the influence of wider state and national forces.

Utilizing the organization field framework just described, the study concluded that changes in the U.S. health-care field over this time are usefully partitioned into three periods or eras: professional dominance, federal involvement, and managed care (see Table 15.1). The era of professional dominance, commencing in the 1920s and extending until the mid-1960s, was marked by the growing number and influence of physicians in private practice, their professional associations (primarily, the American Medical Association), and independent nonprofit community hospitals (see also Freidson 1970a, b; Starr 1982). Health-care organizations were small and unspecialized. Doctors worked as independent providers or in small partnerships with other physicians. Connections among actors were sparse, primarily informal, and local. Governance structures were dominated by professional associations, their monopoly supported by state agencies that enforced licensure provisions at the behest of these associations. The primary institutional logics stressed professional authority and the quality of care—as defined by the physician—as well as a nonprofit, voluntary ethos that imparted a moral dimension to health services as a community benefit rather than a commercial enterprise.

It was during this period that many of the distinguishing organizational features of U.S. health care were established, such as the hierarchy of health professions that places physicians at the pinnacle, the "dual authority" structure of U.S. hospitals in which physicians are admitted to a medical staff that operates independently of hospital administration (with nurses and other health professionals reporting to the administrative structure but subject to dual control), and lack of formal bureaucratic controls—either by

Table 15.1. Institutional eras in U.S. health care: field actors, logics, and governance mechanisms

Era	Field actors	Institutional logics	Governance mechanisms
Professional dominance, 1940s to mid-1960s	*Independent physicians** Community hospitals Local/state governments Private insurance	*Professional authority* *Quality of care* Nonprofit, voluntary ethos	*Professional associations* State licensure of health occupations Voluntary health planning
Federal responsibility, mid-1960s to early 1980s	*Federal government* State governments Medical profession Multihospital systems	*Equity of access.* Consumer health movement Alternative conceptions of health	*Regulatory controls* Mandatory health planning Mandatory peer review Rate setting
Managed care, early 1980s through 1990s	*Health-care corporations* Purchasing groups Specialized health-care organizations Integrated health systems	*Managerial-market orientation* Cost containment Efficiency	*Market building* Selective contracting Prospective payment Risk-based contracting
Incremental improvement, 2000–present	*Health-care improvement movement* Standards-setting bodies Community-health coalitions	*Value-based services* Continuous quality improvement, patient safety Evidence-based medicine Partnership and collaboration	Pay for performance Voluntary standards setting Comparative effectiveness Collaborative networks

Source: Adapted from Scott et al. 2000

*Italics indicate the predominant actors, logics, or governance mechanisms for each era (except in the current era, in which no predominant governance mechanism has yet emerged)

administrators or third-party insurance carriers—over clinician discretion and provision of services.

A surge of growth in personnel and facilities occurred following World War II, responding to pent-up demand. Hospitals, with the help of federal funding, grew much larger and more differentiated, and physicians increasingly trained in medical specialties and organized themselves into specialty associations. Larger employers subsidized health-care coverage for their employees, and insurance companies became active and influential players in the field. After many failed attempts, the federal government in 1965 passed Medicare/Medicaid legislation covering hospital services for the elderly and the indigent. This significant political event marked the dramatic onset of the era of federal involvement. For the first time, the American nation-state was a major player in the field, purchasing more than half of all health services delivered (see also Stevens and Stevens 1974; Stevens 1971). Moreover, because of rising health-care costs, federal officials quickly

found themselves engaged in a variety of regulatory and planning activities to control costs in the field. Thus, governance structures that had been primarily private and professional were forced to share control with state and federal agencies. The prevailing institutional logics expanded to include equity and a moral dimension of access to health care as a right for all citizens. Patients began to assume a more active consumer orientation and to explore alternative and complementary forms of health care, including non-Western treatment modalities.

Early in the 1980s, a third era opened, that of managerial and market-based mechanisms, marked by rising concern with escalating costs and by efforts to increase efficiency. Hospitals increased in size as small hospitals were closed and others grew, often through merger or acquisition. Numerous specialized organizations appeared, including many freestanding organizations offering services such as renal dialysis or urgent care that had formerly been performed only within hospitals. For-profit hospitals and care units multi-plied. Physicians were increasingly organized into groups, both real and virtual, as insurance plans enlisted independent physicians for their panels. Relations among all players in the field became more dense and complex: employers formed groups to pressure for health-systems change and to negotiate rates with health-insurance plans; insurance companies contracted with physicians; and hospitals bought or contracted with physician groups and various specialized providers such as home-health services and extended-care facilities. Such combinations of health-care services yielded increasing numbers and varieties of so-called inte-grated health systems, ranging from formal con-solidation of firms under common ownership to arms-length integration based on contracts, stra-tegic alliances, and looser affiliations that allowed expanded production and market clout without the financial and operational investments that mergers entail. Managers of these systems and other health-care services now held MBAs and exercised broadened authority in health-care or-ganizations. To concerns for quality and access, a focus on efficiency and a faith in market-based solutions were added.

While these shifts point toward a consistent move during the 1980s and 1990s toward a managerial-market orientation, and related actors and governance structures inspired by these logics (see Table 15.1), they were the result not of an uncontested evolution of newer systems and log-ics replacing older, but of heated and disjointed struggle, debate, and contestation at various lev-els within health care—a process which arguably continues into the present. A host of intellectual champions, including economists and managerial professionals, developed and actively promoted the conceptual foundations justifying the ex-panded role of market logics and corporate actors in health care, while consolidation of health ser-vices was often motivated as much by concerns for market power, reputation, leverage over other system players, and even keeping up with the Joneses, as by concerns for economic efficiency, rationalization, and even profitability (Luke and Walston 2003; Wan, Ma, and Lin 2001; and see Light, this volume). Changes toward for-profit goals and forms of organization and management

met with staunch resistance from medical profes-sionals and community groups concerned with maintaining professional discretion and with health care as a social versus solely an economic good. New systems were layered on existing sys-tems rather than supplanting them.

Examining the dynamics of how these forces played out over time, time series analyses of the primary institutional logics across the three eras—professional authority, federal involvement, and managerial-market orientation—indicate that the decline of the medical profession's tradi-tional dominance was strongly influenced by the fragmentation of governance structures follow-ing passage of the Medicare/Medicaid programs in the 1960s, but was not associated with trends in the managerial-market logics underlying the advent of managed care (Scott et al. 2000, ch. 9).[1] These findings suggest that rather than be-ing responsible for dislodging professional power, corporate and managerial actors exploited this opportunity, bringing in their new procedures, ideologies, and structures. Conflicting logics and contending institutional regimes weaken the legitimacy of entrenched interests and provide openings for new actors and interests (Fligstein 1990; Greenwood and Hinings 1996; Deephouse and Suchman 2008).

In contrast to its stable history centered on a single dominant institutional regime, the health-care field by the 1990s harbored multiple relatively strong, frequently conflicting belief sys-tems, actors, and governance mechanisms. Such a cacophony of competing logics and divided regimes typically serves to delegitimate a system as a whole (Meyer and Scott 1983; Scott 1994), making it difficult for new arrangements to estab-lish themselves firmly.

Recent Trends and Forces

Backlash, Limits of Market-Managerial Strategies, and Institutional Impasse

Given this state of affairs, how have actors and interests in U.S. health care responded, and in what ways, if any, have these dynamics served to shape and reconstitute the field? The most widely noted reaction, building throughout the 1990s, was a strong, broad-scale backlash against managed care (Brodie, Brady, and Altman 1998; Blendon et al. 1998), which by early in the new century had begun to noticeably blunt the penetration of managed-care practices and forms of organization. Opponents of managed care, who were concerned that unchecked business interests in medical care were sacrificing quality and even endangering lives, were successful in passing legislation in a number of states to restrict the use of selective contracting and of closed provider panels (Anders 1996; Moran 1997; Marsteller et al. 1997).

The partial retreat of managed care was also attributable to generally perceived failures of the new arrangements to live up to their claimed potential to improve the efficiency and quality of health services. For instance, despite the seemingly unstoppable trend toward greater consolidation and ever-larger conglomeration of health-care organizations, integration met limits and challenges on a number of fronts. Hospital-centered and other health-care delivery networks based on looser forms of nonownership and virtual governance had become popular during the 1990s (Shortell et al. 2000; Bazzoli et al. 2001), but evidence showed they tended to underperform more tightly integrated systems based on common ownership in terms of costs, profitability, and other financial indicators (Bazzoli et al. 2000). Networks and systems both appeared to perform better with at least moderate levels of centralization in decision making, suggesting that consolidation without actual centralization and strategic reorganization of services might not yield the efficiency and other benefits expected of integrated health systems (Burns et al. 2005; Luke and Walston 2003; Shortell, Gillies, and Anderson 1994). Adequate centralization can be difficult to achieve as size of systems increase, and past a certain scale they may yield diminishing returns, making very large systems difficult to sustain.

Vertical integration, particularly of hospitals into upstream nonacute services such as home health and skilled-nursing facilities, have generally had negative effects on profit margins and negative or neutral effects on hospital efficiency

(Burns et al. 2005; Wan, Ma, and Lin 2001). Integration of health insurance with delivery systems has become less attractive as current competitive requirements within the insurance industry emphasize broad local networks of providers that necessitate including competing health services (Ginsburg 2005).

During the 1990s, hospitals also branched into acquisition of, and other strategic affiliations with, medical groups. Often termed physician-hospital organizations (PHOs), these arrangements were established partly to seek local market leverage against health plans, control community referrals into hospital services, and instigate risk contracting in which medical groups accepted capitated payments (i.e., a flat sum from health plans for all services a patient might need in a given period). Physicians thereby assumed greater financial risk for services but also might profit by controlling costs and encouraging preventive care and choice of appropriate treatments. But risk contracting proved fatal to many medical groups who lacked the size and capacity to adequately manage care. Interest in PHOs began to decline after a few years as the momentum toward risk contracting subsided and the benefits to hospitals of owning medical groups did not meet expectations (Lake et al. 2003; Casalino 2004; Terry 2005).

Medical groups themselves experienced a wave of merger and consolidation activity up through the mid-1990s, particularly strong in certain regions such as California (Robinson and Casalino 1996). Yet over the course of the decade, the average size of medical groups decreased, with very large practices remaining relatively rare and most growth occurring through the creation of groups of moderate size. Likewise, the share of physicians organized into group practices remained relatively modest at about a third of nonfederally employed MDs (Havlicek 1999), kept in check by a variety of factors. Constraints included the strong preference among physicians for autonomy, tensions in multispecialty groups between primary care and other specialists, and the increasing ability of solo and small practices to gain some of the benefits of scale of larger groups through coordinated contracting (e.g., Independent Practice Associations, or IPAs), collective on-call and purchasing arrangements, and information and communication technologies (Romano 2005; Crosson 2005). Multispecialty groups in particular had been hailed as a promising model to improve the delivery of medical care, given their potential for innovation, cross-fertilization, and coordination among primary care and specialist physicians. Nevertheless, single-specialty groups quickly became the predominant model of group practice, comprising over 70 percent of medical groups (Terry 2005). These groups often formed in order to provide the capital and patient volume to compete with hospitals in delivering the most profitable services, many of which had traditionally been provided in inpatient settings (Casalino, Pham, and Bazzoli 2004; Casalino et al. 2003).

Health plans and insurance carriers felt the managed care backlash even more forcefully. Health maintenance organizations (HMOs) retreated from methods of managing care that had been their defining features, such as capitated risk contracting, bureaucratic controls on utilization of services (e.g., preauthorization requirements), and restrictions on use of physicians and hospitals outside the plan. In this respect, HMOs increasingly resemble Preferred Provider Organizations (PPOs) in terms of the looseness with which they manage care and the breadth of their provider networks (Casalino 2004), blurring the line between these two forms of health plan that have dominated the managed-care insurance industry (Anthony and Banaszak-Holl 2003; Scott et al. 2000, ch. 3). Moreover, with the general decline of risk contracting, health insurers increasingly relied on selective contracting and negotiation of discounted fees-for-service with a narrower range of health-care providers. While producing short-term premium reductions for health plans able to exercise greater market leverage, these strategies tended to result in price shifting to public plans and other payers, rather than the reductions in longer-term costs of the system as a whole that had been the hope of managed care (Enthoven 1980).

Most tellingly, the continuing rise of health-care costs over the past two decades—regularly exceeding increases in the cost-of-living index and outpacing the general growth of the economy as measured by gross domestic product (Mitka 2009; Sisko et al. 2009)—strongly suggests that the managerial reforms and market-oriented strategies introduced since the 1980s have been ineffective in achieving their primary objectives: improving efficiency and containing costs for the health-care system as a whole. An argument that outcomes could have been worse if not for these strategies is a difficult sell to many stakeholders in health care, and in any case of little consolation, as public and private policy efforts have both failed to bend the curve of spending growth in health care, creating opportunities for sustained backlash to the managed-care revolution and an eventual state of impasse or gridlock in institutional interests and logics.

This impasse may well result from what Light (1997, 2004; and see this volume) views as an instance of "countervailing powers" in which one set of interests, such as the advocates of managerial and market approaches to organizing health care, overextends its attempts to dominate the field, prompting the regrouping and reaction of other interests, with swings back and forth as competing interests vie for control. But it is not simply a matter of contesting powers. The various types of players in health care—professionals, managers, regulators, consumer and public-interest advocates—have different identities and divergent interests, being committed to different goals and objectives. Such differences, which give rise to conflicting reform efforts and criteria for evaluating improvement, show up in the current contest over health-care quality.

New Tasks and Conflicting Jurisdictions: The Rise of Health-Care Improvement

Actors in social systems adopt roles that align them with particular worldviews, identities, and interests. In this vein, Casalino (2004) adapts a "tasks and jurisdiction" approach from the sociology of professions (Abbott 1988) to illuminate the tug-of-war over new and unfamiliar tasks in health care that have arisen with the institutional shifts of the past four decades—namely, the creation of organized processes to control costs and improve the quality of health care, and the oversight of the quality and cost performance of health-care organizations. We agree that the intensified contestations over the nature and control of the health-care improvement enterprise—and the up-to-now piecemeal application of these endeavors—have been a distinguishing characteristic of the current period, prompting our labeling it one of "incremental improvement" (see Table 15.1).

Fundamental to efforts to control these unfamiliar tasks within health care have been not only conflicting claims of jurisdiction by different groups, but also struggles over the definition of these tasks. The inability of any one perspective to achieve sufficiently general consensus in the framing of either quality or cost issues, or the priority of one versus the other, has created mounting pressures to reconcile these competing perspectives both at the ideological and practical levels.

For instance, quality in health care traditionally was defined as depending on the skill, judgment, and discretion of the individual physician. In contrast, the introduction of managerial approaches to the field brought with it innovations in quality improvement from commercial industries, often referred to as total quality management (TQM) or continuous quality improvement (CQI) (see also Zuiderent-Jerak and Berg, this volume). These newer-quality models stressed customer focus, continuous improvement, and teamwork, emphasizing the importance of contributions by the full range of participants in the health-care delivery system (Dean and Bowen 1994; Kimberly and Minvielle 2003). However, these conventional managerial approaches have consistently been troubled and stalled by several of the unique features of health care, including the uncertain and risky nature of the work, which predisposes against the experimentation required to implement innovations, and the highly hierarchical and segmented professional structure of the workforce, which creates strong professional and weak organizational identities and hinders the collaborative learning required for mastering increasingly interdisciplinary innovations in care. These problems are exacerbated by traditional perceived conflicts of goals between organizational management and the professional workforce—including the definition of quality and purposes of improvement initiatives—and by underdeveloped performance measurement and control systems, products of the divided authority

structure in health-care organizations and of persisting views of medical care as a craft profession (Nembhard et al. 2009).

Two landmark reports by the Institute of Medicine (IOM 1999, 2001) were instrumental in raising the salience of quality as a major issue and priority concern for the entire field, framing the problem in ways resonant with physicians and traditional health-care interests (e.g., as a reduction of medical errors that cause thousands of unnecessary patient deaths and violate the Hippocratic maxim to "first do no harm"), and providing endorsement by an authoritative voice of the medical establishment for industrial and systems-based approaches to solving the "quality chasm." These reports also arguably put the fledgling movement for quality and patient safety in health care on the map (Wachter 2004), spurring numerous health-care organizations to intensify the adoption of quality management and practices. The "improvement journeys" of leading health-care organizations demonstrated a number of successful strategies and principles, including creating opportunities for nonthreatening experimentation; fostering learning environments and cultures (through, for example, communities-of-practice) and encouraging new mindsets on how to implement change (e.g., from the customary clinical approach of full pilot tests to rapid-cycle "tests of change"); and anchoring the quality agenda in the existing values and self-image of the organization and of professional groups (Bate, Mendel, and Robert 2008; Nembhard et al. 2009).

Studies of these experiences also indicate that, in terms of its ability to control policies and institutions within the health-care field, the medical profession may be down, but it is far from out, particularly with regard to authority over clinical decisions and processes. Although physicians' justification of their clinical discretion as safeguarding the quality of patient care has frequently met with skepticism, professional self-interest and concern for client welfare can coexist (Scott 2008b). Moreover, as the pace of scientific and technical innovation continues to escalate, acceptance of physician control and authority over medical knowledge and expertise has only increased, affording doctors powerful structural positions in health-care organizations and systems despite having to share discretion over aspects of treatment with other health occupations and alternative providers. Individuals and occupations who can contend with the uncertainty in work processes are accorded power by others (Hickson et al. 1971; Scott et al. 2000, ch. 9). Nowhere is this more evident than in research that shows the importance of clinician involvement in quality improvement (QI) teams (Shortell et al. 2004) and clinicians' roles as "physician champions" whose clinical knowledge and credibility can determine support and buy-in for quality efforts among professional and other staff. Particularly effective in these roles are the increasing numbers of "hybrid physicians"—doctors who also acquire managerial training and thus more easily serve as "two-way windows" and boundary-spanners bridging the administrative and clinical worlds (Llewellan 2001; Mendel 2008; van het Loo, Bate, and Riley 2008).

The extent of these efforts notwithstanding, they still represent pockets of innovation within health-care organizations and the field, with great continuing variation in quality and performance (Fisher, Bynum, and Skinner 2009; Wennberg 2004; Fisher et al. 2003a, b). Moreover, while early adopters in health care appear to have customized total quality management (TQM) practices, adapting them to local circumstances to achieve efficiency gains, later adopters have tended to more blindly conform to off-the-shelf quality programs primarily to gain legitimacy rather than to enhance performance (Westphal, Gulati, and Shortell 1997). Other research has similarly found the adoption of new managerial innovations in health care, as in other fields, to be strongly influenced by pressures for conformity, especially given the uncertainty present in the health-care field, the ambiguity of how or when such innovations are supposed to have an effect, and the anticipatory actions of health-care organizations attempting to position themselves in a rapidly changing environment (Walston, Kimberly, and Burns 2001). Likewise, evidence indicates that whether such improvement activities significantly affect clinical quality and outcomes is conditioned on the degree to which these initiatives are implemented in practice, are used, and align with the health-care organization's strategic imperatives (Alexander et al. 2007).

Nevertheless, the quality movement in health care has gained urgency, attracting a range of new and reinvented organized actors. Recent research, including studies focused on health care, have emphasized the influence of social movements on organizations, as well as the utility of understanding the potential of social movement processes for change within organizations (Davis et al. 2005; Mendel 2002; Bate, Robert, and Bevan 2004; see also Brown et al., this volume). Movement scholars stress the structure of political opportunities, the mobilization of resources and people, and the framing of issues and emotional appeals, giving increased attention to the process by which these factors combine (and are combined), in the evolution of social movements. In particular, new actors, so-called social movement organizations (McCarthy and Zald 1977), arise mobilized specifically around reform objectives, such as furthering the cause of quality in health care. The most notable example is the Institute for Healthcare Improvement, led by a charismatic hybrid physician of the sort described earlier, which has launched a variety of national campaigns to catalyze improvements among health-care organizations (Kenney 2008). Similar improvement organizations that specialize in particular areas include the National Initiative for Children's Healthcare Quality (NICHQ), focused on improvement of pediatric services, and the Leapfrog Group, comprised of large-employer purchasers of health care primarily concerned with stimulating accountability and improvement in patient safety (NICHQ 2009; Scanlon, Christianson, and Ford 2008).

At the same time, a number of mainstream actors have refashioned themselves as part of the quality movement. The Joint Commission on the Accreditation of Healthcare Organizations (JCAHO), which has been accrediting hospitals and other provider organizations for more than a century, has restructured its certification process to emphasize quality, safety, and performance measurement, including a set of required "Core Measures." By all accounts, JCAHO's requirements have been a major catalyst for prioritizing quality and the adoption of improvement strategies throughout the hospital and other medical-care industries (Farley et al. 2009, ch. 2; Devers, Pham, and Liu 2004; Walshe and Shortell 2004). Even the state-level peer review organizations dating from the era of federal involvement have been repurposed into so-called Quality Improvement Organizations (QIOs), tasked with furthering the quality agenda of the federal Centers for Medicare and Medicaid Services (CMS), as well as branching out into facilitating QI projects for private clients (IOM 2006; Bradley et al. 2005; Sprague 2002). Recent entrants into the set of dedicated quality organizations have been disease-management companies—private services firms to whom health-insurance plans, payers, and others responsible for populations of patients can outsource the care coordination and quality improvement function for chronic diseases (Mattke, Seid, and Ma 2007; Buntin et al. 2009).

Reframing Old Debates and Devising New Approaches to Managing Interests

In addition to debate over definitions and perspectives on quality, the health-care improvement movement has struggled with the relationship between quality and costs, experimenting with alternatives to earlier conceptions that viewed the two in stark opposition. For example, there has been much resonance with the idea of a "business case" for quality that seeks to justify improvement efforts in terms of potential cost savings, including principal-agent problems when the party incurring the costs does not sufficiently share in the savings (Leatherman et al. 2003; Schoenbaum et al. 2004). More generally, this form of conceptual and rhetorical reorientation has been reflected in an ethos of value, the assertion that expenditures on health services should be consonant with benefits (Shortell 2004). Such a value-based logic has been at the heart of trials by CMS and various private parties of pay-for-performance reimbursement systems that seek to reward providers for quality care and to penalize providers for care considered subpar (Damberg et al. 2009; Mehrotra et al. 2009).

Another approach to confronting multiple conflicting interests and achieving consensus in the face of potentially politically charged issues is through voluntary standards setting, a distinct social form of coordination especially suited to domains in which other governance mechanisms such as markets and hierarchies (i.e., bureaucratic organization) are weak or fragmented (Brunsson 2000; Djelic and Sahlin-Andersson 2006). This process essentially delegates decision making to a body whose authority rests on assuring neutrality of outcome through the use of technical experts, or through decisions reached by democratic representativeness of affected stakeholders (Loya and Boli 1999; Tamm-Hallstrom 1996, 1998). The regulations or agreements reached are soft, in that compliance depends on voluntary cooperation augmented by mutually enforced, open methods of coordination and oversight (Mörth 2006). Examples in the health-care improvement movement include the National Committee for Quality Assurance (NCQA), which was formed primarily by health plans and has promoted a consensus set of quality standards and measures for assessing and reporting health-care performance (NCQA 2009; Casalino 2004). The National Quality Forum (NQF), with the motto "Achieving consensus, improving care," serves to set national consensus standards for measuring and publicly reporting on health-care performance and endorses thirty "safe practices" considered supported by evidence of reduced medical errors and improved patient safety (NQF 2007, 2009).[2]

This concern for evidence (of a particular variety) reflects a parallel emphasis in the medical profession on "evidence-based medicine," which insists that clinical treatments and interventions be scientifically proven, with the gold standard of assessment being the randomized controlled trial (see Timmermans, this volume). This logic now pervades the discourse on approaches to health-care quality, representing a successful instance of the medical profession's continuing influence on health-care matters. Indeed, most attempts to engage clinicians in quality improvement require repeated citation of empirical data of this sort (Bate 2008; Mendel 2008). This evidence-based logic has also spawned concern over the "research-to-practice gap" (Glasgow, Lichtenstein, and Marcus 2003; Lenfant 2003), the dissemination and implementation of scientifically validated QI interventions, from research-demonstration studies to community settings and wider scale-up efforts

(Mendel et al. 2008; Greenhalgh et al. 2004; Schoenwald and Hoagwood 2001), and a new discipline of "implementation science" in health services research (Eccles and Mittman 2006).

Recent and rising calls to base criteria for appropriate medical treatments on "comparative effectiveness" research (IOM 2007; Holve and Pittman 2009) favor a mechanism for oversight of quality and costs that combines elements of value-based and evidence-based logics, as well as voluntary standards setting. Cost effectiveness, a related approach long advocated by many health economists, directly compares the cost and benefits of a particular treatment—an unpalatable trade-off for many providers, patients, and policy makers, as well as for the public at large (Neumann 2005; Weinstein and Stason 1977). However, comparing the effectiveness of two treatments avoids this direct trade-off to focus on choosing treatments of equal or greater value—and how better to make this choice than to delegate the process to a body of putatively neutral technical experts? Of course, the more this body resembles a bureaucratic institute with binding decision-making authority such as the U.K.'s National Institute for Clinical Excellence (Chalkidou et al. 2009), the less enthusiasm is generated for these proposals in the U.S. political context (Fuchs and Emanuel 2005).

Yet another means for balancing multiple interests in the health-care field has centered on principles of partnering and collaboration, particularly reflected in the increasing development of local community-health coalitions and partnerships (Lasker, Weiss, and Miller 2001; Foster-Fishman, Berkowitz, et al. 2001). Although akin in some respects to the earlier-noted trend toward strategic partnerships and alliances among health-care organizations, these types of coalitions typically are intended to bring a diverse set of stakeholders and interest groups together to foster a communitywide orientation and perspective (Foster-Fishman, Salem, et al. 2001) and collective action to effect change in local health-care systems (Mitchell and Shortell 2000). Similar types of collaborative networks have also proliferated at the regional and national levels, focused on overcoming the fragmentation of health-care delivery and policy in the United States through

diffusing specific evidence-based practices (Sisk 1993) or addressing various facets of a more general cause, such as patient safety (Mendel et al. 2009). These kinds of diverse networks at local or higher levels can constitute "communities of practice" in which common understandings of best practices and collective learning take place (Bate and Robert 2002; Mendel 2008), as well as form the structural basis of conduits along which information, practices, and innovations can flow (Luke and Harris 2007; Valente 1995). Banaszak-Holl, Elms, and Grazman (2003) note that such networks represent distinct forms of governance that emphasize learning as an incentive for participation when, again, neither a market nor a hierarchy (i.e., bureaucratic organization) exists to sufficiently foster cooperation and ensure coordination.

Structuration Processes and the Health-Care Field

Several features characterize the structuration approach built upon here to understand large-scale institutional change in such an extensive sector as health care in the United States and to put recent trends in the context of earlier eras. The structuration approach is:

(1) context specific, recognizing that one type of organizational field differs from others in ways that require careful specification and examination.
(2) longitudinal, insisting on the value of examining the structure and functioning of social systems over longer rather than shorter spans of time. The importance of history—with the past shaping and constraining the present and future possibilities—is emphasized: institutional change is path dependent.
(3) multilayered, noting the ways in which broader national (and, increasingly, international) forces shape more localized systems, as well as the ways in which local actions and innovations shape and give rise to wider field changes.
(4) attentive to the interdependence of actors and logics, of activities and ideas. Concepts and

ideas have meaning only to the extent that they shape behavior, and behavior is mere motion unless it is informed by and interpreted to have meaning. In modern societies, collective actors (organizations) and the ideas embedded in their structures are of particular importance.

(5) attentive to governance structures, since these are the structures that define and enforce the rules of the game in a particular field of action. In examining governance structures, the question to ask is, Which classes of actors and what subset of logics are employed to coordinate and control actions within the field?

We have employed this structuration approach to review the evolving dynamics among field actors, governance mechanisms, and the logics that motivate them from earlier eras through the current period. We now comment on those trends, as well as the prospects and consequences of change on the horizon.

Incrementalism and Bricolage

We observe that earlier logics and governance mechanisms have not been replaced by later ones; rather the change processes in the health-care field have resulted in a multilayered, contested situation in which the professional, public, and private managerial now coexist in an uneasy configuration. Pure forms of managed care that include financial risk sharing by providers and controls over the use and provision of services have been difficult to sustain. The exceptions—including a few large, highly integrated systems such as Kaiser Permanente and the Veterans Health Administration—have shown notable progress over time in improving the quality of care (Asch et al. 2004), if not necessarily its costs. But these examples fall outside the mainstream of health-care organization in the United States The general failure of managerial and market orientations to deliver on their promise to remake health care during the initial era of managed care —particularly its overall cost and efficiency profile—has allowed the backlash to turn into impasse over the past decade. Managerial and market logics have been compelled to share the stage with competing actors and logics reflecting professional interests and political concerns for equity.

While this impasse may appear in many respects to reflect a condition of institutional disarray, it also has represented a period of considerable innovation in organizational forms and field-level arrangements. The existence of two or more strong, contending belief systems within a field is associated with greater variety of forms and complexity of structure, as organizations attempt to attend to multiple, sometimes conflicting, expectations and logics in their environments. In the era of managed care, the multiple competing institutional regimes were associated with new forms of health-service delivery, such as for-profit health-care corporations and specialized provider organizations, inspired by managerial and market orientations (Alexander and D'Aunno 2003; Scott et al. 2000, ch. 6). In the current period, the continuing strength of earlier logics and actors has resulted in innovative and hybrid forms focused on combining and counterbalancing competing interests and ideologies (rather than attempting to resolve or impose one over others).

Thus, we have many more hybrid physicians who assume dual managerial and clinical roles that often intersect in the pursuit of quality improvement. More generally, as Luke and Walston (2003, 310) note, "physicians function as employees, suppliers, buyers and partners for hospitals, often all at the same time." Similarly, traditional accreditation agencies have been substantially repurposed, joining a newer crop of movement organizations advocating the cause of health-care quality, which increasingly finds itself joined at the hip with costs in a formula of "value for the money" as a means to gain traction and justification in the current health-care environment. Where such synthesis has proved difficult, the field has emphasized forms of collaboration and standards making explicitly designed to facilitate mutual accommodation of multiple interests. As with the previous era, the development of many of these forms and arrangements reflect a process of bricolage: the piecing together and layering of seemingly distinct elements—some novel, some already in the field, others borrowed from elsewhere—to create models and sets of practices that appear both new and recognizable at the same time (Douglas 1986; Campbell 1997; Carruthers and Uzzi 2000).

But not all innovation is progress, and a multitude of improvement activity does not necessarily add up to improvement, especially for the field as a whole. Indeed, our characterization of the past decade in health care as one of incremental improvement may be misleading. Most innovative change efforts have been relatively small in scale—typically at the level of individual organizations or particular slices of the field—rather than broader systematic reforms. This emphasis has yielded many pockets of innovation and celebrated cases of improvement (McCarthy and Blumenthal 2006) but also great variation—as noted previously—in both practices and outcomes, as well as concern (and frustration) over how to disseminate, implement, and scale up innovations and best practices that appear effective (Berwick 2003).

In particular, while the movement for health-care improvement may have risen to prominence and value-based logics achieved widespread acceptance, governance mechanisms related to these newer logics and interests are fairly nascent and remain highly fragmented. The multiple demands and expectations produced by fragmented governance often result in superficial changes (or decoupling between pronouncements of reform and actual practice) (Meyer and Rowan 1977; Brunsson and Olsen 1993), difficulty in managing priorities, and greater complexity and transaction costs confronting organizations within the field (Meyer, Scott, and Strang 1987). Even well-intentioned health-care leaders report they are inundated with external quality and safety initiatives that claim to be "top priority," conflicting standards and guidelines, and fragmented reporting requirements that often ask for the same data but in varying formats—all of which depletes limited resources and impedes their ability to target efforts on high-impact areas and initiatives (Farley et al. 2009, ch. 2).

Certainly, looking at the overall performance of U.S. health care, it can be argued that incremental reform efforts have failed to substantially improve the system (Fuchs and Emanuel 2005). Despite spending substantially more per capita on health care than other developed nations, the U.S.

system consistently ranks in the middle to low range compared to these countries on mean levels of various outcome measures, including quality of care, population health, and satisfaction of different stakeholder groups (OECD 2005; WHO 2000; Hussey et al. 2004; Reinhardt, Hussey, and Anderson 2002; Blendon et al. 2003). This seemingly poor value for the dollar has drawn attention to the transaction costs and potential waste and duplication associated with such a complex system (Aaron 2003). Although debate has surrounded the best ways to quantify and interpret these costs, particularly compared to other countries, various studies have noted that administrative-personnel and overhead costs have increased substantially faster than have other components of health-care expenditures in the United States (Davis et al. 2007; Woolhandler, Campbell, and Himmelstein 2003), and that these are comprised in large part of billing, insurance, marketing, and other intermediary and interorganizational transaction costs of a fragmented, multilayered system (Bentley et al. 2008; Angrisano et al. 2007; Kahn et al. 2005).

Dynamics of Broader Reform

The major federal reform legislation winding its way through Congress at the moment appears to concentrate primarily on the issue of access: providing greater health insurance coverage for the millions of Americans currently lacking it. As discussed above, we see access as one of the three competing logics in the field, the others being cost-containment and quality. These latter are inherently more difficult to resolve, in part because health professions, private business interests, and consumers each have strong stakes at play.[3] The framework presented here highlights how these decisions and debates are embedded in the history and dynamics of actors, logics, and governance mechanisms. Reform at this level is about not only streamlining or rationalizing processes, but also bringing clarity to governance and helping define and resolve jurisdictions over tasks. With such reform, new tasks and jurisdictions encourage the entrance of new actors and the refashioning of existing roles and rationales.

Interests can also change. For example, one of the main differences between the current health-care debate and earlier major reform efforts has been a willingness of large employers to buck the health-care and insurance industries and embrace systemic changes as they struggle under the strain of health-insurance premiums for their employees. But employers, who have long suffered the effects of health-care inflation, traditionally did not recognize their interest in controlling health-care costs until they were organized, mobilized, and activated (Bergthold 1984). Rather than shifts and struggles between fixed sets of countervailing powers, systemic change involves the emergence of new kinds of actors as well as revised identities and reframed interests of other players.

Thornton, Jones, and Kury's (2005) comparison of three sectors—academic publishing, accounting, and architecture—suggests, similarly to our analysis, that fields gravitate away from governance mechanisms perceived to have failed in protecting the public or key stakeholder interests. The authors also postulate that fields with high public policy visibility in which professional control has been greatly displaced by private corporate bureaucracies (both of which have characterized health care since the mid-1980s) will experience expanded jurisdiction by the state in governance and exhibit a punctuated equilibrium, or a stepwise (as opposed to cyclical or linear) pattern of change. This would imply greater involvement by the state (particularly the federal government) in the health-care system, although given the strength of the multiple competing interests and the current trend toward institutional blending in health care, it is likely that any new arrangements that occur will incorporate a mixture of governance arrangements and multiple interests.

Whether or not major reform policies transpire, the present reform debate is proving to resemble a process of "muddling through," a phrase Lindblom (1959) used to evoke a world in which social problems of great complexity are not amenable to fully planned and modeled solutions. In this spirit, we have presented and extended a framework for comparing field dynamics over time to shed light on general processes of change, including hybridization and

bricolage; redefinition of roles, tasks, and logics; reframing of interests; and emergence of alternate forms of governance. Lindblom's classic essay also employed this conception of the policy world to argue for the supremacy of incremental change, given the limited applicability of existing knowledge and experience, unintended effects of large-scale change efforts, and enduring power of entrenched interests. Yet, for all its motion, the recent period of incremental improvement has cast serious doubt on the ability of continued tinkering around the edges to overcome the systemic problems of the health-care system in the United States (Fuchs and Emanuel 2005), especially in light of the distinct historical accretion of institutional forces and current institutional impasse characterizing the field. Old wisdom may be in need of revision, but like reform itself, the new wisdom, for the moment, remains elusive.

Notes

1. Of note, the same analyses indicated that the logics of federal involvement, which emphasized equity and access, were positively associated with professional dominance, after controlling for fragmentation in funding and governance (Scott et al. 2000, ch. 9). As other scholars of that period have noted, the federal Medicaid and Medicare programs were expressly fashioned to accommodate the interests of the medical profession (Starr 1982). The underlying logics of federal involvement were thus supportive of professional authority, with physicians not replaced but rather joined by public agencies and actors during the second era. However, the effect of federal involvement on the texture of governance regimes subverted the hegemony of the medical establishment through the development of diverse and generally uncoordinated entities that dispensed resources and exercised authority.

2. Similarly, many of the health-care standards set by the European Union involve regimes comprised of soft regulations (Mörth 2006).

3. A number of attempts to understand and disentangle these dynamics have centered on complexity theory, originally developed in the physical and natural sciences and increasingly applied in the social sciences and more recently to health care. Complexity theory offers a rich set of metaphors and concepts useful for describing complex adaptive systems, such as the massively entangled and interdependent nature of components; a focus on interactions rather than structure; and attention

to novelty and emergent, self-organizing behavior as components of the system adjust to each other (McDaniel, Lanham, and Anderson 2009). However, the ability of this approach to parse the complex dynamics of the health-care system or to identify system-level interventions is admittedly, even to some of its proponents, still in its infancy (Begun, Zimmerman, and Dooley 2003). Moreover, as others have noted, much of the current complexity within health care, rather than being an "emergent" property, has been built in by design, as a synonym or by-product of a desire to maintain "choice" (e.g., for patients to select their providers, and providers to exercise professional discretion) and "innovation" (e.g., the generation of new therapies and treatments, and methods for delivering services), no matter how meaningful or value-adding the choices or innovations are (or are not) in practice (Bate and Robert 2005).

References

Aaron, Henry J. 2003. "The Costs of Health Care Administration in the United States and Canada: Questionable Answers to a Questionable Question." *New England Journal of Medicine* 349:801–3.

Abbott, Andrew. 1988. *The System of the Professions: An Essay in the Division of Expert Labor.* Chicago: University of Chicago Press.

Alexander, Jeffrey A., and Thomas A. D'Aunno. 1990. "Transformation of Institutional Environments: Perspectives on the Corporatization of U.S. Health Care." In *Innovations in Health Care Delivery: Insights for Organization Theory,* ed. Stephen S. Mick, 53–85. San Francisco: Jossey-Bass.

———. 2003. "Alternative Perspectives on Institutional and Market Relationships in the U.S. Health Care Sector." In *Advances in Health Care Organization Theory,* ed. Stephen S. Mick and Mindy E. Wyttenbach, 45–77. San Francisco: Jossey-Bass.

Alexander, Jeffrey A., Bryan J. Weiner, Stephen M. Shortell, and Laurence C. Baker. 2007. "Does Quality Improvement Implementation Affect Hospital Quality of Care?" *Hospital Topics* 85(2): 3–12.

Alford, Robert R. 1972. "The Political Economy of Health Care: Dynamics without Change." *Politics and Society* 2 (winter): 127–64.

Anders, George. 1996. *Health against Wealth: HMOs and the Breakdown of Medical Trust.* Boston: Houghton Mifflin.

Angrisano, Carlos, Diana Farrell, Bob Kocher, Martha Laboissiere, and Sara Parker. 2007. *Accounting for the Cost of Health Care in the United States.* McKinsey Global Institute. mckinsey.com/mgi.

Anthony, Denise L., and Jane Banaszak-Holl. 2003. "Organizational Variation in the Managed Care Industry in the 1990s: Implications for Institutional Change." *Research in the Sociology of Health Care* 21:21–38.

Asch, Steven M., Elizabeth A. McGlynn, Mary M. Hogan, Rodney A. Hayward, Paul Shekelle, Lisa Rubenstein, Joan Keesey, John Adams, and Eve A. Kerr. 2004. "Comparison of Quality of Care for Patients in the Veterans Health Administration and Patients in a National Sample." *Annals of Internal Medicine* 141(12): 938–45.

Banaszak-Holl, Jane, Heather Elms, and David Grazman. 2002. "Sustaining Long-Term Change and Efficiency in Community Health Networks." In *Advances in Health Care Organization Theory,* ed. Stephen M. Mick and Mindy E. Wyttenback, 175–203. San Francisco: Jossey-Bass.

Barley, Stephen R. 2008. "Coalface Institutionalism." In *The Handbook of Organizational Institutionalism,* ed. Royston Greenwood, Christine Oliver, Kerstin Sahlin, and Roy Suddaby, 491–518. Thousand Oaks, Calif.: Sage.

Barley, Stephen R., and Pamela S. Tolbert. 1997. "Institutionalization and Structuration: Studying the Links between Action and Institution." *Organization Studies* 18(1): 93–117.

Bate, S. Paul. 2008. "The Art, the Science, and Sociology of Improvement: San Diego Children's Hospital." In *Organizing for Quality: Journeys of Improvement at Leading Hospitals and Health Care Systems in Europe and the United States,* by S. Paul Bate, Peter Mendel, and Glenn Robert, 15–34. Oxford: Radcliffe Publishers.

Bate, S. Paul, and Glenn Robert. 2002. "Knowledge Management and Communities of Practice in the Private Sector: Lessons for Modernizing the National Health Service in England and Wales." *Public Administration* 80(4): 643–63.

———. 2005. "Choice: More Can Mean Less." *British Medical Journal* 331:1488–89.

Bate, S. Paul, Glenn Robert, and Helen Bevan. 2004. "The Next Phase of Health Care Improvement: What Can We Learn from Social Movements?" *Quality and Safety in Health Care* 13(1): 62–66.

Bate, S. Paul, Peter Mendel, and Glenn Robert. 2008. *Organizing for Quality: The Improvement Journeys of Leading Hospitals in Europe and the United States.* Oxford: Radcliffe Publishers.

Bazzoli, Gloria J., Benjamin Chan, Stephen M. Shortell, and Thomas D'Aunno. 2000. "The Financial Performance of Hospitals Belonging to Health Networks and Systems." *Inquiry* 37(3): 234–52.

Bazzoli, Gloria J., Stephen M. Shortell, Federico Cilibreto, Peter D. Kralovec, and Nicole L. Dubbs.

2001. "Tracking the Changing Provider Landscape: Implications for Health Policy and Practice." *Health Affairs* 20(6): 188–96.

Begun, James W., Brenda Zimmerman, and Kevin J. Dooley. 2003. "Health Care Organizations as Complex Adaptive Systems." In *Advances in Health Care Organization Theory*, ed. Stephen S. Mick and Mindy E. Wyttenbach, 253–88. San Francisco: Jossey-Bass.

Bentley, Tanya G. K., Rachel M. Effros, Kartika Palar, and Emmett B. Keeler. 2008. "Waste in the U.S. Health Care System: A Conceptual Framework." *Milbank Quarterly* 86(4): 629–59.

Bergthold, Linda. 1984. "Crabs in a Bucket: The Politics of Health Care Reform in California." *Journal of Health Politics, Policy and Law* 9(2): 203–22.

Berwick, Donald M. 2003. "Disseminating Innovations in Health Care." *Journal of the American Medical Association* 289:1969–75.

Blendon, Robert J., Mollyann Brodie, John M. Benson, Drew E. Altman, Larry Levitt, Tina Hoff, and Larry Hugick. 1998. "Understanding the Managed Care Backlash." *Health Affairs* 17(4): 80–94.

Blendon, Robert J., Cathy Schoen, Catherine DesRoches, Robin Osborn, and Kinga Zapert. 2003. "Common Concerns amid Diverse Systems: Healthcare Experiences in Five Countries." *Health Affairs* (May/June): 106–21.

Bradley, Elizabeth H., Melissa D. A. Carlson, William T. Gallo, Jeanne Scinto, Miriam K. Campbell, and Harlan M. Krumholz. 2005. "From Adversary to Partner: Have Quality Improvement Organizations Made the Transition?" *Health Services Research* 40(2): 459–76.

Brodie, Mollyann, Lee Ann Brady, and Drew A. Altman. 1998. "Media Coverage of Managed Care: Is There a Negative Bias?" *Health Affairs* 7(1): 9–25.

Brunsson, Nils. 2000. "Standardization as a Social Form." In *A World of Standards*, ed. Nils Brunsson and Bengt Jacobsson, 52–70. Oxford: Oxford University Press.

Brunsson, Nils, and Johan P. Olsen. 1993. *The Reforming Organization*. London: Routledge.

Buntin, Melinda Beukes, A. K. Jain, S. Mattke, and Nicole Lurie. 2009. "Who Gets Disease Management?" *Journal of General Internal Medicine* 24(5): 649–55.

Burns, Lawton. 1990. "The Transformation of the American Hospital: From Community Institution toward Business Enterprise." In *Comparative Social Research*, vol. 12, ed. Craig Calhoun, 77–112. Greenwich, Conn.: JAI Press.

Burns, Lawton R., G. Gimm, S. Nicholson, and R. W. Muller. 2005. "The Financial Performance of Integrated Health Organizations." *Journal of Healthcare Management* 50(3): 191–212.

Campbell, John L. 1997. "Mechanisms of Evolutionary Change in Economic Governance: Interaction, Interpretation and Bricolage." In *Evolutionary Economics and Path Dependence*, ed. Lars Magnusson and Jan Ottosson, 10–31. Cheltenham, UK: Edward Elgar.

Caronna, Carol. 2004. "The Mis-alignment of Institutional 'Pillars.'" *Journal of Health and Social Behavior* 45, extra issue: 45–58.

Carruthers, Bruce G., and Brian Uzzi. 2000. "Economic Sociology in the New Millennium." *Contemporary Sociology* 29(3): 486–94.

Casalino, Lawrence P. 2004. "Unfamiliar Tasks, Contested Jurisdictions: The Changing Organization Field of Medical Practice in the United States." *Journal of Health and Social Behavior* 45, extra issue: 59–75.

Casalino, Lawrence P., Kelly J. Devers, Timothy K. Lake, Marie Reed, and Jeffrey J. Stoddard. 2003. "Benefits of and Barriers to Large Medical Group Practice in the United States." *Archives of Internal Medicine* 163(16): 1958–64.

Casalino, Lawrence P., Hoangmai Pham, and Gloria Bazzoli. 2004. "Growth of Single-Specialty Medical Groups." *Health Affairs* 23(2): 82–90.

Chalkidou, Kalipso, Sean Tunis, Ruth Lopert, Lise Rochaix, Peter Sawicki, Mona Nasser, and Bertrand Xerri. 2009. "Comparative Effectiveness Research and Evidence-Based Health Policy: Experience from Four Countries." *Milbank Quarterly* 87(2): 339–67.

Crosson, Francis J. 2005. "The Delivery System Matters." *Health Affairs* 24(6): 1543–48.

Damberg, Cheryl L., Kristiana Raube, Stephanie S. Teleki, and Erin dela Cruz. 2009. "Taking Stock of Pay-for-Performance: A Candid Assessment from the Front Lines." *Health Affairs* 28(2): 517–25.

Davis, Gerald F., Doug McAdam, W. Richard Scott, and Mayer N. Zald, eds. 2005. *Social Movements and Organization Theory*. New York: Cambridge University Press.

Davis, Karen, Cathy Shoen, Stuart Guterman, Tony Shi, Stephen C. Shoenbaum, and Ilana Weinbaum. 2007. *Slowing the Growth of U.S. Health Care Expenditures: What Are the Options?* Publication No. 989. New York: Commonwealth Fund.

Dean, James W., Jr., and David E. Bowen. 1994. "Management Theory and Total Quality: Improving Research and Practice through Theory Development." *Academy of Management Review* 19:392–418.

Deephouse, David L., and Mark Suchman. 2008. "Legitimacy in Organizational Institutionalism." In *The Handbook of Organizational Institutionalism*, ed. Royston Greenwood, Christine Oliver, Kerstin Sahlin, and Roy Suddaby, 49–77. Thousand Oaks, Calif.: Sage.

Devers, Kelly J., Hoangmai H. Pham, and Gigi Liu. 2004. "What Is Driving Hospitals' Patient-Safety Efforts?" *Health Affairs* 23(2): 103–15.

DiMaggio, Paul J. 1991. "Constructing an Organizational Field as a Professional Project: U.S. Art Museums, 1920–1940." In *The New Institutionalism in Organizational Analysis*, ed. Walter W. Powell and Paul J. DiMaggio, 267–92. Chicago: University of Chicago Press.

DiMaggio, Paul J., and Walter W. Powell. 1983. "The Iron Cage Revisited: Institutional Isomorphism and Collective Rationality in Organizational Fields." *American Sociological Review* 48:147–60.

Djelic, Marie-Laure, and Kerstin Sahlin-Andersson, eds. 2006. *Transnational Governance: Institutional Dynamics of Regulation*. Cambridge: Cambridge University Press.

Douglas, Mary. 1986. *How Institutions Think*. Syracuse, N.Y.: Syracuse University Press.

Eccles, Martin P., and Brian S. Mittman. 2006. "Welcome to Implementation Science." *Implementation Science* 1 (February): 1.

Enthoven, Alain C. 1980. *Health Plan: The Only Practical Solution to the Soaring Cost of Medical Care*. Reading, Mass.: Addison-Wesley.

Farley, Donna O., M. Susan Ridgely, Peter Mendel, Stephanie S. Teleki, Cheryl L. Damberg, Rebecca Shaw, Michael D. Greenberg, Amelia M. Haviland, Peter Hussey, Jake Dembosky, Hao Yu, Julie Brown, Chau Pham, and Scott Ashwood. 2009. *Assessing Patient Safety Practices and Outcomes in the U.S. Health Care System*. Technical Report TR-725AHRQ. Santa Monica, Calif.: RAND.

Ferlie, Ewan B., and Stephen M. Shortell. 2001. "Improving the Quality of Health Care in the United Kingdom and the United States: A Framework for Change." *Milbank Quarterly* 79(2): 281–315.

Fisher, Elliott S., Julie P. Bynum, and Jonathan S. Skinner. 2009. "Slowing the Growth of Health Care Costs: Lessons from Regional Variation." *New England Journal of Medicine* 360(9): 849–52.

Fisher, Elliott S., David E. Wennberg, Thérèse A. Stukel, Daniel J. Gottlieb, F. L. Lucas, and Étoile L. Pinder. 2003a. "The Implications of Regional Variations in Medicare Spending. Part 1: The Content, Quality, and Accessibility of Care." *Annals of Internal Medicine* 138(4): 273–87.

———. 2003b. "The Implications of Regional Variations in Medicare Spending. Part 2: Health Outcomes and Satisfaction with Care." *Annals of Internal Medicine* 138(4): 288–98.

Fligstein, Neil. 1990. *The Transformation of Corporate Control*. Cambridge, Mass.: Harvard University Press.

Flood, Ann B., and Mary L. Fennell. 1995. "Through the Lenses of Organizational Sociology: The Role of Organizational Theory and Research in Conceptualizing and Examining Our Health Care System." *Journal of Health and Social Behavior*, extra issue: 154–69.

Foster-Fishman, Pennie G., Shelby L. Berkowitz, David W. Lounsbury, Stephanie Jacobson, and Nicole A. Allen. 2001. "Building Collaborative Capacity in Community Coalitions: A Review and Integrative Framework." *American Journal of Community Psychology* 29(2): 241–61.

Foster-Fishman, Pennie G., Deborah A. Salem, Nicole A. Allen, and Kyle Fahrback. 2001. "Facilitating Interorganizational Collaboration: The Contributions of Interorganizational Alliances." *American Journal of Community Psychology* 29(6): 875–905.

Freidson, Eliot. 1970a. *Profession of Medicine: A Study in the Sociology of Applied Knowledge*. New York: Dodd, Mead.

———. 1970b. *Professional Dominance: The Social Structure of Medical Care*. Chicago: Aldine.

Fuchs, Victor R., and Ezekiel J. Emanuel. 2005. "Health Care Reform: Why? What? When? What It Might Take to Effect Comprehensive Change." *Health Affairs* 24(6): 1399–1414.

Ginsburg, Paul B. 2005. "Competition in Health Care: Its Evolution Over the Past Decade." *Health Affairs* 24(6): 1512–22.

Glasgow, Russell E., Edward Lichtenstein, and Alfred C. Marcus. 2003. "Why Don't We See More Translation of Health Promotion Research to Practice? Rethinking the Efficacy-to-Effectiveness Transition." *American Journal of Public Health* 93(8): 1261–67.

Greenhalgh, Trisha, Glenn Robert, Fraser Macfarlane, Paul Bate, and Olivia Kyriakidou. 2004. "Diffusion of Innovations in Service Organizations: Systematic Review and Recommendations." *Milbank Quarterly* 82(4): 581–629.

Greenwood, Royston, and C. R. Hinings 1996. "Understanding Radical Organizational Change: Bringing Together the Old and the New Institutionalism." *Academy of Management Review* 21:1022–54.

Havlicek, Penny. 1999. *Medical Group Practices in the U.S.: A Survey of Practice Characteristics*. Chicago: American Medical Association.

Hickson, David J., C. R. Hinings, C. A. Lee, R. E. Schneck, and J. M. Pennings. 1971. "A Strategic Contingencies' Theory of Intraorganizational Power." *Administrative Science Quarterly* 14:378–97.

Holve, Erin, and Patricia Pittman. 2009. "A First Look at the Volume and Cost of Comparative Effectiveness Research in the U.S." Monograph. academyhealth.org/files/FileDownloads/AH_Monograph_09FINAL7.pdf.

Hussey, Peter S., Gerard F. Anderson, Robin Osborn, Colin Feek, Vivienne McLaughlin, John Millar, and Arnold Epstein. 2004. "How Does the Quality of Care Compare in Five Countries?" *Health Affairs* 23(3): 89–99.

IOM [Institute of Medicine]. 1999. *To Err Is Human: Building a Safer Health Care System*, ed. L. T. Kohn, J. M. Corrigan, and M. S. Donaldson. Washington, D.C.: National Academies Press.

———. 2001. *Crossing the Quality Chasm: A New Health System for the Twenty-First Century*. Washington, D.C.: National Academies Press.

———. 2006. *Medicare's Quality Improvement Organization Program: Maximizing Potential*. Washington, D.C.: National Academies Press.

———. 2007. *Learning What Works Best: The Nation's Need for Evidence on Comparative Effectiveness in Health Care*. Washington, D.C.: National Academies Press. iom.edu/ebm-effectiveness.

Kahn, James G., Richard Kronick, Mary Kreger, and David N. Gans. 2005. "The Cost of Health Insurance Administration in California: Estimates for Insurers, Physicians and Hospitals." *Health Affairs* 24:1629–39.

Kenney, Charles. 2008. *The Best Practice: How the New Quality Movement Is Transforming Medicine*. New York: PublicAffairs.

Kimberly, John R., and Etienne Minvielle 2003. "Quality as an Organizational Problem." In *Advances in Health Care Organization Theory*, ed. Stephen S. Mick and Mindy E. Wyttenback, 205–22. San Francisco: Jossey-Bass.

Lake, Timothy, Kelly Devers, Linda Brewster, and Lawrence Casalino. 2003. "Something Old, Something New: Recent Developments in Hospital-Physician Relationships." *Health Services Research* 38(1, part 2): 471–88.

Lasker, Roz D., Elisa S. Weiss, and Rebecca Miller. 2001. "Partnership Synergy: A Practical Framework for Studying and Strengthening the Collaborative Advantage." *Milbank Quarterly* 79(2): 179–205.

Leatherman, Sheila, Donald Berwick, Debra Iles, Lawrence S. Lewin, Frank Davidoff, Thomas Nolan, and Maureen Bisognano. 2003. "The Business Case for Quality: Case Studies and an Analysis." *Health Affairs* 22(2): 17–30.

Lenfant, Claude. 2003. "Clinical Research to Clinical Practice—Lost in Translation?" *New England Journal of Medicine* 349:868–74.

Lindblom, Charles E. 1959. "The Science of 'Muddling Through.'" *Public Administration Review* 19(2): 79–88.

Light, Donald. 1997. "The Rhetorics and Realities of Community Health Care: The Limits of Countervailing Powers to Meet the Health Care Needs of the Twenty-First Century. *Journal of Health Politics, Policy and Law* 22(1): 105–45.

———. 2004. "Ironies of Success: A New History of the American Health Care System." *Journal of Health and Social Behavior* 45, extra issue: 1–24.

Llewellyn, Sue. 2001. "Two-Way Windows: Clinicians as Medical Managers." *Organization Studies* 22(4): 593–623.

Luke, Douglas A., and Jenine K. Harris. 2007. "Network Analysis in Public Health: History, Methods, and Applications." *Annual Review of Public Health* 28:16.1–16.25.

Luke, Roice D., and Stephen L. Walston. 2003. "Strategy in an Institutional Environment: Lessons Learned from the 1990s 'Revolution' in Health Care." In *Advances in Health Care Organization Theory*, ed. Stephen S. Mick and Mindy E. Wyttenbach, 289–323. San Francisco: Jossey-Bass.

Loya, Thomas, and John Boli. 1999. "Standardization in the World Polity: Technical Rationality over Power." In *Constructing World Culture: International Nongovernmental Organizations since 1875*, ed. John Boli and George M. Thomas, 169–97. Stanford, Calif.: Stanford University Press.

Marsteller, Jill A., Randall R. Bovbjerg, Len M. Nichols, and Diana K. Verrilli. 1997. "The Resurgence of Selective Contracting Restrictions." *Journal of Health Politics, Policy and Law* 22(5): 1133–89.

Mattke, Soeren, Michael Seid, and Sai Ma. 2007. "Evidence for the Effect of Disease Management: Is $1 Billion a Year a Good Investment?" *American Journal of Managed Care* 12(12): 670–76.

McCarthy, Douglas, and David Blumenthal 2006. "Stories from the Sharp End: Case Studies in Safety Improvement." *Milbank Quarterly* 84(1): 165–200.

McCarthy, John D., and Mayer N. Zald. 1977. "Resource Mobilization and Social Movements: A Partial Theory." *American Journal of Sociology* 82(6): 1212–41.

McDaniel, Reuben R., Holly J. Lanham, and Ruth A. Anderson. 2009. "Implications of Complex Adaptive Systems Theory for the Design of Research on Health Care Organizations." *Health Care Management Review* 34(3): 191–99.

Mechanic, David. 1994. "Managed Care: Rhetoric and Realities." *Inquiry* 31 (summer): 124–28.

Mehrotra, Ateev, Cheryl L. Damberg, Melony E. Sorbero, and Stephanie S. Teleki. 2009. "Pay for Performance in the Hospital Setting: What Is the State of the Evidence?" *American Journal of Medical Quality* 24(1): 19–28.

Mendel, Peter. 2002. "International Standardization and Global Governance: The Spread of Quality and Environmental Management Standards." In *Organizations, Policy, and the Natural Environment: Institutional and Strategic Perspectives*, ed. Andrew Hoffman and Marc Ventresca, 407–31. Stanford, Calif.: Stanford University Press.

———. 2008. "Organizational Learning and Sustained Improvement: The Quality Journey at Cedars-Sinai Medical Center." In *Organizing for Quality: Journeys of Improvement at Leading Hospitals and Health Care Systems in Europe and the United States*, by S. Paul Bate, Peter Mendel, and Glenn Robert, 57–82. Oxford: Radcliffe Publishers.

Mendel, Peter, Cheryl Damberg, Melony E. Sorbero, Danielle M. Varda, and Donna O. Farley. 2009. "The Growth of Partnerships to Support Safe Practice Adoption." *Health Services Research* 44 (2 part 2): 717–38.

Mendel, Peter, Lisa S. Meredith, Michael Schoenbaum, Cathy D. Sherbourne, and Kenneth B. Wells. 2008. "Interventions in Organizational and Community Context: A Framework for Building Evidence on Dissemination and Implementation in Health Services Research." *Administration and Policy in Mental Health and Mental Health Services Research* 35(1–2): 21–37.

Meyer John W., and Brian Rowan. 1977. "Institutionalized Organizations: Formal Structure as Myth and Ceremony." *American Journal of Sociology* 83:340–63.

Meyer, John W., and W. Richard Scott. 1983. *Organizational Environments: Ritual and Rationality.* Beverly Hills, Calif.: Sage.

Meyer, John W., W. Richard Scott, and David Strang. 1987. "Centralization, Fragmentation, and School District Complexity." *Administrative Science Quarterly* 32:186–201.

Mick, Stephen S., and Mindy E. Wyttenbach, eds. 2003. *Advances in Health Care Organization Theory.* San Francisco: Jossey-Bass.

Mitchell, Shannon M., and Stephen M. Shortell. 2000. "The Governance and Management of Effective Community Health Partnerships: A Typology for Research, Policy, and Practice." *Milbank Quarterly* 78(2): 241–89.

Mitka, Mike. 2009. "Growth in Health Care Spending Slows, but Still Outpaces Rate of Inflation." *Journal of the American Medical Association* 301(8): 815–16.

Moran, Donald W. 1997. "Federal Regulation of Managed Care: An Impulse in Search of a Theory?" *Health Affairs* 16(6): 7–21.

Mörth, Ulrika. 2006. "Soft Regulation and Global Democracy." In *Transnational Governance: Institutional Dynamics of Regulation*, ed. Marie-Laure Djelic and Kerstin Sahlin-Andersson, 119–37. Cambridge: Cambridge University Press.

NCQA [National Committee for Quality Assurance]. 2009. About NCQA. ncqa.org/. Accessed September 21, 2009.

Nembhard, Ingrid M., Jeffrey A. Alexander, Timothy J. Hoff, and Rangaraj Ramanujam. 2009. "Why Does the Quality of Health Care Continue to Lag? Insights from Management Research." *Academy of Management Perspectives* 23(1): 24–42.

Neumann, Peter J. 2005. *Using Cost-Effectiveness Analysis to Improve Health Care: Opportunities and Barriers.* New York: Oxford University Press.

NICHQ [National Initiative for Children's Healthcare Quality]. 2009. About Us. nichq.org/about/index .html. Accessed September 21, 2009.

NQF [National Quality Forum]. 2007. *Safe Practices for Better Healthcare—2006 Update: A Consensus Report.* No. NQFCR-17-07. Washington, D.C.: NQF.

———. 2009. About Us. qualityforum.org/About_ NQF/About_NQF.aspx. Accessed September 21, 2009.

OECD [Organisation for Economic Cooperation and Development]. 2005. *Health at a Glance—OECD Indicators 2005.* Paris: OECD.

Reinhardt, Uwe E., Peter S. Hussey, and Gerard F. Anderson. 2002. "Cross-National Comparisons of Health Systems using OECD Data, 1999." *Health Affairs* 21(3): 169–81.

Robinson, James C., and Lawrence P. Casalino. 1996. "Vertical Integration and Organizational Networks in Healthcare." *Health Affairs* 15(1): 7–22.

Romano, Michael. 2005. "'A Bigger Brood': As OB/ GYN Practices Grow Nationwide, What's Good News for the Docs Can Be Bad News for Hospitals and Health Plans." *Modern Healthcare* 25(43): 28–30.

Scanlon, Dennis P., Jon B. Christianson, and Eric W. Ford. 2008. "Hospital Responses to the Leapfrog Group in Local Markets." *Medical Care Research and Review* 65(2): 207–31.

Schneiberg, Marc, and Sarah A. Soule 2005. "Institutionalization as a Contested, Multilevel Process: The Case of Rate Regulation in American Fire Insurance." In *Social Movements and Organization Theory*, ed. Gerald F. Davis, Doug McAdam, W. Richard Scott, and Mayer N. Zald, 122–61. Cambridge: Cambridge University Press.

Schoenbaum, Michael, Kelly Kelleher, Judith R. Lave, Stephanie Green, Donna Keyser, and Harold Pincus. 2004. "Exploratory Evidence on the Market for Effective Depression Care in Pittsburgh." *Psychiatric Services* 55(4): 392–95.

Schoenwald, Sonja K., and Kimberly Hoagwood. 2001. "Effectiveness, Transportability, and Dissemination of Interventions: What Matters When?" *Psychiatric Services* 52:1190–97.

Scott, W. Richard. 1994. "Conceptualizing Organizational Fields: Linking Organizations and Societal Systems." In *Systemrationalitat und Partialinteresse*, ed. Hans-Ulrich Derlien, Uta Gerhardt, and Fritz W. Scharpf, 203–21. Baden Baden, Germany: Nomos Verlagsgesellschaft.

———. 2004. "Competing Logics in Health Care: Professional, State, and Managerial." In *The Sociology of the Economy*, ed. Frank Dobbin, 267–87. New York: Russell Sage Foundation.

———. 2008a. *Institutions and Organizations: Ideas and Interests*. 3rd ed. Thousands Oaks, Calif.: Sage.

———. 2008b. "Lords of the Dance: Professionals as Institutional Agents." *Organization Studies* 29:219–38.

———. Forthcoming. "Health Care Organization Theory." In *Encyclopedia of Health Services Research*, ed. Ross M. Mullner, Robert F. Rich, and Tricia J. Johnson. Thousand Oaks, Calif.: Sage.

Scott, W. Richard, Peter Mendel, and Seth Pollack. 1996. "Environments and Fields: Studying the Evolution of a Field of Medical Care Organizations." Invited paper presented at the Conference on Institutional Analysis, University of Arizona at Tucson, March 28–30.

Scott, W. Richard, Martin Ruef, Peter J. Mendel, and Carol A. Caronna. 2000. *Institutional Change and Healthcare Organizations: From Professional Dominance to Managed Care*. Chicago: University of Chicago Press.

Shortell, Stephen M. 2004. "Increasing Value: A Research Agenda for Addressing the Managerial and Organizational Challenges Facing Health Care Delivery in the United States." *Medical Care Research and Review* 61(3), suppl.: 12S–30S.

Shortell, Stephen M., Gloria J. Bazzoli, Nicole L. Dubbs, and Peter Kralovec. 2000. "Classifying Health Networks and Systems: Managerial and Policy Implications." *Health Care Management Review* 25(4): 9–17.

Shortell, Stephen M., Robin R. Gillies, and David A. Anderson. 1994. "The New World of Managed Care: Creating Organized Delivery Systems." *Health Affairs* 13(5): 46–64.

Shortell, Stephen M., Jill A. Marsteller, Michael K. Lin, Marjorie L. Pearson, Shin-Yi Wu, Peter Mendel, Shan Cretin, and Mayde Rosen. 2004. "The Role of Perceived Team Effectiveness in Improving Chronic Illness Care." *Medical Care* 42(11): 1040–48.

Sisk, Jane E. 1993. "Improving the Use of Research-Based Evidence in Policy-Making: Effective Care in Pregnancy and Childbirth in the United States." *Milbank Quarterly* 71(3): 477–96.

Sisko, Andrea, Christopher Truffer, Sheila Smith, Sean Keehan, Jonathan Cylus, John A. Poisal, M. Kent Clemens, and Joseph Lizonitz. 2009. "Health Spending Projections through 2018: Recession Effects Add Uncertainty to the Outlook." *Health Affairs* 28(2): w346–57.

Sprague, Lisa. 2002. *Contracting for Quality: Medicare's Quality Improvement Organizations*. Issue Brief No. 774. Washington, D.C.: National Health Policy Forum.

Starr, Paul. 1982. *The Social Transformation of American Medicine*. New York: Basic Books.

Stevens, Robert, and Rosemary Stevens. 1974. *Welfare Medicine in America: A Case Study of Medicaid*. New York: Free Press.

Stevens, Rosemary. 1971. *American Medicine and the Public Interest*. New Haven, Conn.: Yale University Press.

Tamm-Hallstrom, Kristina. 1996. "The Production of Management Standards." *Revue D'Economie Industrielle* 75(1): 61–76.

———. 1998. "Construction of Authority in Two International Standardization Bodies." Paper presented at the SCANCOR Conference on Organizations Research, Stanford University, Stanford, Calif., September 20–22.

Terry, Ken. 2005. "Pay for Performance: How Fast Is It Spreading?" *Medical Economics* 82(21): 30–34.

Thornton, Patricia H., Candace Jones, and Kenneth Kury. 2005. "Institutional Logics and Institutional Change in Organizations: Transformation in Accounting, Architecture, and Publishing." *Research in the Sociology of Organizations* 23:127–72.

Valente, Thomas W. 1995. *Network Models of the Diffusion of Innovations*. Cresskill, N.J.: Hampton.

van het Loo, Mirjam, Paul Bate, and Tony Riley. 2008. "Building a System of Leadership for Quality Improvement: A Dutch Hospital in Pursuit of Perfection." In *Organizing for Quality: Journeys of Improvement at Leading Hospitals and Health Care Systems in Europe and the United States*, by S. Paul Bate, Peter Mendel, and Glenn Robert, 83–100. Oxford: Radcliffe Publishers.

Wachter, Robert M. 2004. "The End of the Beginning: Patient Safety Five Years after *To Err Is Human*." *Health Affairs* (web exclusive), November 30. content.healthaffairs.org/cgi/content/full/hlthaff .w4.534/DC1.

Walshe, Kieran, and Stephen M. Shortell. 2004. "Social Regulation of Healthcare Organizations in the United States: Developing a Framework for Evaluation." *Health Services Management Research* 17(2): 79–99.

Walston, Stephen L., John R. Kimberly, and Lawton R. Burns. 2001. "Institutional and Economic Influences on the Adoption and Extensiveness of

Managerial Innovations in Hospitals: The Case of Reengineering." *Medical Care Research and Review* 58(2): 194–228.

Wan, Thomas T. H., Allen Ma, and Blossom Y. J. Lin. 2001. "Integration and the Performance of Healthcare Networks: A Growth Curve Modeling Approach." *International Journal of Integrated Care* 6(2): 117–24.

Weinstein, M. C., and W. B. Stason. 1977. "Foundations of Cost-Effectiveness Analysis for Health and Medical Practices." *New England Journal of Medicine* 296(13): 716–21.

Wells, Rebecca, and Jane Banaszak-Holl. 2000. "A Critical Review of Recent U.S. Market Level Health Care Strategy Literature." *Social Science and Medicine* 51(5): 639–56.

Wennberg, John E. 2004. "Practice Variations and Health Care Reform: Connecting the Dots." *Health Affairs* (web exclusive), October 7. pnhp.org/news/2004/october/practice_variations_.php.

Westphal, James D., Ranjay Gulati, and Stephen M. Shortell. 1997. "Customization or Conformity? An Institutional and Network Perspective on the Content and Consequences of TQM Adoption." *Administrative Science Quarterly* 42(2): 366–95.

WHO [World Health Organization]. 2000. *The World Health Report 2000—Health Systems: Improving Performance*. Geneva: World Health Organization.

Woolhandler, Steffie, Terry Campbell, and David U. Himmelstein. 2003. "Costs of Health Care Administration in the United States and Canada." *New England Journal of Medicine* 349(8): 768–75.

16

Health-Care Professions, Markets, and Countervailing Powers

Donald W. Light, University of Medicine and Dentistry of New Jersey

Professionalism is an Anglo-American disease.
—Eliot Freidson, 1983

Monopoly is essential to professionalism.
—Eliot Freidson, 2001

For more than two decades, an international crisis of professionalism has pervaded health care and weakened the grip of professional organizations over the training and oversight of professional work, especially in the United States and United Kingdom where professionalism is a preoccupation. Governments and other institutional payers have moved in to monitor professional behavior, control costs, and reduce large variations in the quality of clinical practice (Hafferty and Light 1995; UK Secretary of State for Health 2007). The unquestioned trust in the medical profession to apply the best scientific and technical information and skills to the needs of patients and fulfill a tacit social contract has been shaken.

I focus here on some aspects of the shaken trust in the medical profession that have to do with "markets," a term that refers to dynamically constructed arenas of economic exchange but also to the actors in those markets who have been challenging the elevated status of professions as state-protected monopolies that claim to provide complex and vital services to clients for their benefit in an impartial manner. For decades during the Gilded Age and into the twentieth century, professions were widely regarded by Durkheim and others as standing over against markets. By the 1970s, however, historical and contemporaneous evidence indicated that the medical profession was a kind of self-serving monopoly operating within protected markets (Berlant 1975; Burrow 1977; Freidson 1970a, b; Larson 1977). This radical recasting, as well as evidence of overtreatment, undertreatment, mistreatment, and excessive charges, led to a revolt by governments, businesses, and other payers that transformed them into active buyers demanding accountability and good value. (I described the dynamics and evidence of this transformation in previous editions of the handbook [Light 1989, 2000]). Since 2000, however, organized professional bodies have mounted campaigns to restore their professionalism and lost trust, with Eliot Freidson's last work (2001) as an intellectual beacon and inspiration to them. Yet as we will see, the professions-and-markets debate ignores a graver development of the commercial construction of medical categories, medical evidence, and clinical behavior that sociologists have largely overlooked in their research on risk, illness, and treatment.

The Countervailing Powers Framework

Single accounts of the rise of professions, while describing their relationships with the state, universities, and other bodies, tend to be what

Andrew Abbott (2005) wryly describes as the "historiography of imminent development," and they tend not to consider the wider ecological context. The framework of countervailing powers enables one to consider through historical periods the changing tensions, alliances, interests, rhetorics, and degrees of control among key stakeholders (Light 2000). They include organized professional groups, the state as legitimator and regulator, payers such as the state and insurers, clients as individuals or larger organized bodies, and corporations that make up the medical-industrial complex. This framework resonates with and expands on Elliott Krause's (1996) major comparative study in which he emphasizes three parties—the state, capitalism, and the professions—at the corners of a triangle. They vie to construct the reality of a domain, the structure of markets, the culture of professional work and its organization, status, and power. Jill Quadagno (2004) has made a valuable contribution by analyzing, with her theory of stakeholder mobilization, how these conflicts translate into decisions.

The countervailing powers framework first instructs researchers through the process of identifying the domain or field force, the major actors, and the nature of relations between them. Each in turn is made up of countervailing powers, such as the occupational competitors for professional status and greater jurisdictional control in a given domain (Abbott 1988). The professional constellation of countervailing forces ranges from the crucible of its academic and research segment, with strong ties to the medical-industrial complex, to competing providers both within medicine and in alternate paradigms of healing, to forms of clinically managed care that employ protocols to shape how professional work should be done. The state is a constellation in itself of countervailing power groups or divisions with different functions and priorities: the sponsor of health-care services and public health, the funder of most basic research to foster innovation and economic growth (Light 2006), the promoter of commerce at home and abroad, and the creator and enforcer of regulations. Clients or patients as a whole are composed of diverse, often conflicting groups of varied size and wealth. As Everett C. Hughes (1994 [1965], 46) pointed out, by the

1960s law and medicine were carried out in complex organized settings where "it becomes hard to say who is the client; . . . is it the insurance company or the patient?" If who the client is remains unclear, especially when one client (the patient) wants to have all their medical bills paid and the other client (the insurer) wants to pay as little as possible (Light 1992), can either patients or insurers trust how professionals will exercise their autonomy and discretionary expertise? A certain amount of the doctor as double agent seems unavoidable, even in a public health service (Angell 1993; Stone 1997).

A profession or professional cluster interacts with other countervailing powers in a political and cultural marketplace, as well as in the economic marketplace. Buyers and customers, often not the same persons in health care, are the key agents in markets. If they are lazy or uninformed or uninterested, sellers have more opportunities to exploit them. An occupation selling its services can claim it is expert and ethical and needs state protection from charlatans; the question is whether patients and politicians will buy the argument. A surgeon can claim that a twenty-minute cataract operation is worth $1200 for his time (plus the bills for everything else), but will payers agree? Patients have become an increasingly important countervailing power, in part through patient-advocacy groups for specific conditions (often sponsored by pharmaceutical companies to advocate for costly drugs), but also through increasingly rigorous patient-reported outcomes measures (PROMs) (Picker Institute Europe). Patients with chronic conditions also become expert at them, and the expert-patient movement mobilizes this knowledge for better care. Whether these developments constitute deprofessionalization depends on how paternalistic one's model of professionalism is.

Sometimes stakeholder dominance characterizes the relations among countervailing powers. This imbalance can last for years, but the countervailing powers framework requires one to examine how the other parties are reacting and how the stable state may hide unfolding tensions and countermoves. A central problem with professional-dominance theory was that it could explain only how dominance begets more dominance and not how countervailing powers organize against it to recast power relations (Light and Levine 1988). Any dominant party elaborates itself, offends other parties, and neglects important needs. Ironically, the launch of professional-dominance theory in 1970 (Freidson 1970a, b) coincided with the beginning of its demise, as physicians exploited every opportunity to raise fees and increase services, as corporations moved in to exploit the protected markets, and later as payers revolted against these excesses (Light 2004; Starr 1982). This is not the first time that sociologists theorize a historical trend as it is ending and a new era beginning.

An example of countervailing powers radically reframing what good professional health care meant and how it should be organized took place when President Richard Nixon in 1971 proposed universal access using a reorganization of health services based on market incentives that would turn the excesses and pathologies of Freidson's professional dominance on their head. Nixon proposed establishing a national network of health plans—based on rewarding prevention, primary care, and minimal use of hospitals or subspecialists—called health maintenance organizations, long regarded by the AMA as seditious hotbeds of socialism but now reconceived as enlightened business enterprises (Nixon 1972, item 63; Starr 1982). This proposal for well-managed, equitable, and universal health care did not happen, but one could see the countervailing powers in full force, contrary to professional dominance theory, reflecting a historic imbalance of power.

Besides the search for a wider analytic framework than theories of professional dominance or deprofessionalization, material for the countervailing powers framework came from a large comparative study of health professions in Germany that showed how the sharply countervailing relations with the state completely changed from Weimar to the Nazi period, and then again after 1945 under two contrasting visions of state and society (Light and Schuller 1986). By comparing in detail how professional-state relations altered mother-and-child care, abortion, psychotherapy, occupational health, drug supplies, ambulatory care, and hospital care in East and West Germany in the postwar decades, this large team project provided the materials for the countervailing powers framework.[1]

The internal elaboration of professional, state, or payer dominance can also result in unmanageable structures and neglect of vital needs. Backlashes occur, either overtly or surreptitiously, as they did in the first wave of market reforms of professional services in Europe (Light 2001). Success also has unintended consequences. In health care, a byproduct of clinical success is that more people live longer with chronic conditions and disabilities, changing the nature of professional work, clinician-patient relations, and the medical-industrial complex (Albrecht 1992; Mechanic 2006, ch. 6). Finally, larger external sociocultural movements can also change the entire domain of and relations among the countervailing powers, such as the civil rights movement and its manifestations in gay, disability, and women's rights.

As an organizing framework for research, the domains or arenas of countervailing powers benefit from Abbott's (2005) brilliant exposition of "linked ecologies," a systematic extension of formative Chicago-school studies of occupations by Hughes and in urban studies by Park, Burgess, and others. Just as each countervailing power in health-care markets is made up of its own countervailing powers in flux, so a given ecology is made up of other linked ecologies, "each of which acts as a (flexible) surround for others" (246). Thus jurisdictional claims by a profession have to succeed not only among other claimants for professional work but also with clients, insurers or health plans, and the state within the ecology of countervailing forces. The state itself "is itself an ecology, a complex interactional structure filled with competing subgroups and dominated by ecological forces quite similar to those driving the system of professions" (246). The same could be said for health plans or insurers and for clients or employers organizing their care.

Abbott provides a richly suggestive vocabulary for analyzing the sociological dynamics of professions and markets, such as actors, locations or arenas (the cluster of problems or areas of work), links, ties, claims, jurisdictions, settlements (arranged balances less exclusive or permanent than jurisdictions), bundles of political decisions and actions pertaining to a location, and hinges that reward actors in two or more ecologies. Abbott summarizes: "The concept of linked ecologies recognizes that events within any particular ecology are hostage in some sense to events in adjacent ecologies" (2005, 254). He illustrates this conceptual framework by examining medical licensing in the United States and England in the nineteenth century and disciplinary settlements in universities. These analytic tools can be used to understand historic changes at the intraprofessional level, the interprofessional level, and the level of health-care systems.

Professions as a Countervailing Power against Markets

At the turn of the twentieth century, leading social thinkers in Europe and America advocated the spread of professionalism as the antidote to rampant capitalism, the antimarket countervailing power. Political economists were claiming economics to be a science (and a profession) (Bledstein 1976). Thus their theory of how unfettered self-interest benefits society was promoted as scientific, not ideological. But Durkheim (1957) observed that pure self-interest destroyed society: "It is not possible for a social function to exist without moral discipline. Otherwise, nothing remains but individual appetites," which are boundless and unable to control themselves. Hope lay in occupations developing moral discipline and becoming professional communities: "Therefore, the true cure for the evil is to give the professional groups in the economic order a stability they so far do not possess," so they can flourish (10, 16). The moral development of professions comes from being a community, a collegium "within which these morals may be evolved, and whose business it is to see they be observed" (16). Within professional groups, members compete for respect and status among their peers by exhibiting their service to others and excellence in their work, not by seeing who can undercut or take over whom.

Durkheim hardly mentioned how specific professions work and offered no evidence for how professional ethics could rescue society from big business and amoral market forces. But he was convinced, as were other leading intellectuals, that occupations could be a countervailing force against the ruthless capitalism of the early twentieth century. Each could develop its own moral order and form of professional ethics and together they would function as "a kind of moral polymorphism" in which "the greater the strength of the group structure, the more numerous are the moral rules appropriate to it and the greater the authority they have over their members" (Durkheim 1957, 7). Haskell, an important historian of the professions, characterized this view of professions "as a 'countervailing market,' structuring a set of inducements and sanctions that can pull the path of self-interest up out of the rut of purely pecuniary advantage" (1984, 217).

In a similar vein, across the English Channel from Durkheim, R. H. Tawney mounted an influential critique of a society based on material self-interest and acquisitiveness. He also believed that the professionalization of occupations would infuse them with a principled, disinterested dedication to serving society that would counter relentless market forces. "A profession may be defined most simply as . . . a body of men who carry on their work in accordance with rules designed to enforce certain standards both for the better protection of its members and for the better service of the public," he wrote in *The Acquisitive Society*. "So, if they are doctors, they recognize that there are certain kinds of conduct which cannot be practiced, however large the fee offered for them; . . . it is wrong to make money by deliberately deceiving the public, as is done by makers of patent medicines, however much the public may clamor to be deceived" (1920, 94–95). What Tawney overlooked was how actively doctors participated in concocting and promoting cure-alls in Europe and the United States. While they no longer concoct them, physicians today play a central role in promoting and prescribing the latest drugs, even though most have no evidence of being superior to existing drugs (Brody 2007; Goozner 2004; Healy 2004).

Professions as a countervailing power to markets, or civic professionalism, also lay at the center of progressive reforms advocated in the United States by John Dewey, Jane Addams, and Herbert Croly. The moral ecology of communities was being destroyed by big business and the amoral pursuit of self-interest, they maintained. Croly (1965 [1909]) proposed that a new spirit of professionalism could become the moral salvation of U.S. society (see Sullivan 2005, ch. 3). A new citizenry would be responsible and enlightened by a new American hero, the civic professional. Jonathan Imber's 2008 study explores how the moral authority of physicians during this period was religiously infused.

Professionals were models of how to use expertise for social betterment by developing a scientific approach to crime, poverty, disease, bad food, dangerous drugs, poor housing, ineffective teaching, and many other spheres of life (Bledstein 1976). People would learn that self-fulfillment comes though mastery and dispassionate application of rigorous knowledge and skills along with others in a moral community. The cultural capital of professionalism was contrasted with economic capital, rather than regarding cultural capital as a complementary form of economic investment as we do today. The ethos of professional communities was the key attribute, not "autonomy," a term that then referred less to individual professionals than to the profession as a whole standing apart from amoral markets and ordinary occupations.

It may seem quaint to emphasize the degree to which big business in this earlier great era of raw market power regarded professions as communities of experts with a strong antimarket moral ethos. But a similar version of professions as a countervailing power to markets underlies the campaigns to restore professionalism today, as well as Eliot Freidson's (2001) construction of professionalism as an ideal type over against reliance on markets or bureaucracies as contrasting ideal types. An echo sounds in Sciulli's (2005) important review of professions, which emphasizes a fiduciary responsibility to advance client well-being, to apply services consistently to standards and to not tolerate opportunistic behaviors, to design institutions for governance and regulation of professional work, and to critically review their knowledge and practices. The strongest echo a century later is reflected in the work of the Carnegie Foundation for the Advancement of Teaching, a sustained assessment of U.S. professions aimed at restoring civic professionalism (Sullivan

2005). Freidson too emphasizes professionalism as an antidote to expert services being driven by consumers and profits, but more narrowly focused on those services and as a civilizing force and an exemplary community of service.

Are Professionals Altruistic?

Social scientists, even economists, so widely believed that professionals were altruistic while the rest of humankind pursued self-interest that when Haskell (1984) reviewed all articles in major social science journals from their inception through 1940, he could find no critique until Parsons's 1939 essay on the professions. Parsons found it implausible that different motives drive business executives than those that drive professionals, as if the two groups were cut from a different cloth or gene pool. He pointed out that professionals rationally apply universalistic knowledge and technical competence in value-neutral, functionally specific ways to all relevant clients. But so do business executives. Both provide services to customers. Both are egoistic. Both want to succeed. What differs is not their motives; rather, "the institutional patterns governing the two fields of action are radically different" (Parsons 1939, 465). These shape behavior and people's "motives" and define appropriate goals, actions, and rewards.

We cannot expect professionals to act too differently from the market structure and institutional framework in which they practice. Most will not be very altruistic or civic in a system focused on generating revenues and profits. Put them in a salary-based national health system like the Veterans Health Administration, however, and their motives will change. There seems little evidence that professions are a countervailing power against markets in a market-oriented system, and, as I argue later, professions have a natural affinity to markets and corporations that advance their interests. Still, a notable number of professionals since the mid-nineteenth century have dedicated themselves, against the market-oriented grain, to developing workers' health-care clinics, other mutual aid cooperatives, poverty medicine, and public health—all of which have played a critical role in changing institutional frameworks (Light and Schuller 1986; Schwartz 1965; Tudor Hart 2008).

Freidson's Case for Professionalism

In his final work, *Professionalism: The Third Logic*, Eliot Freidson echoed an avalanche of articles in the 1990s that argued against managed-care corporations and consumerism as inherently anathema to professionalism (Hafferty 2003, 137–38). Freidson aspired to establish professionalism as the third alternative or logic to Adam Smith's theory of markets and Max Weber's theory of bureaucracy for how social life can be organized.

At the heart of professionalism is discretionary specialization, the application of technical knowledge, skills, and tacit knowledge to problems that appear in various manifestations, guises, and contexts, Freidson theorized (2001, 23–25). Therefore, professionals must have "monopoly, or control over their own work" (32). Full-time dedication to this work over a lifetime enables them to build up tacit knowledge and skills. The profession must control the division of labor and work, specifically, "each specialization controls the work for which it is competent, negotiates its boundaries with other specializations, and by that method determines how the entire division

of labor is organized and coordinated" (55). The profession must determine the qualification of members and grant them permanent status in sheltered labor markets where they have the exclusive right to do certain kinds of work (73–78). Credentials provide clear market signals about who is competent and trustworthy.

Beneficial and Pernicious Competition

The neoclassical ideal type of market behavior assumes many buyers and sellers, clearly defined products or services, full information on prices and value, and other attributes in the first column of Table 16.1. By contrast, professional services are often characterized by uncertainties and contingencies, as professionals try something, see how well it works, and go from there. Information is often asymmetrical, incomplete, unreliable, and expensive. In health care there are often side effects from drugs, surgery, or other procedures that result in a large volume of iatrogenic harm (see Abraham, this volume; Light 2009). The patient's condition may also affect others when contagion is involved or may affect relations with others when mental or physical capacities are affected. In addition, medical markets usually have few hospitals or clinics, and institutional buyers

Table 16.1. Neoclassical markets versus markets for professional services

Conditions for beneficial competition	Conditions for pernicious competition
Product or service clearly defined; clear boundaries, property rights	Product or service needed uncertain and contingent; unclear boundaries
Buyers have full information on prices, quality, services	Buyers confront esoteric, complex, uncertain, and contingent information on services
Information cheap or free	Information and searching costly
No externalities. No harms or benefits to other parts of self or others in this transaction.	Externalities. Harms or benefits to other parts of self or others in this transaction.
Buyers rationally maximize clear preferences	Buyers scared, worried, vulnerable, conflicted
Many buyers and sellers, no relation to each other	Few sellers in a market; have historical, cultural, economic, political ties
No barriers to entry or exit	Barriers to entry and exit
Market signals quick; markets clear quickly	Market signals muddled and slow

Source: Adapted from Scott et al. 2000

*Italics indicate the predominant actors, logics, or governance mechanisms for each era (except in the current era, in which no predominant governance mechanism has yet emerged)

(insurance companies, health plans), creating a bilateral oligopoly, not a competitive market.

When one or more of the conditions necessary for beneficial market competition are lacking, the stage is set for pernicious competition, where the sellers or providers can exploit consumers and payers by charging a great deal for services or medicines of little value, and by delivering services of unknown quality or safety. Hospital and other service corporations have ties with suppliers in oligopolistic markets, and competition rewards inefficient fragmentation as each market player constructs niches to maximize profits (Geyman 2004; Lundberg 2000; Starr 1982). In sum, the failures in health care to meet the prerequisites of beneficial markets would seem to strengthen the case for professionalism to prevail instead, except that many physicians and their professional societies have demonstrated an affinity for commercial enterprises that enhance their repertoire of tools, equipment, devices, or drugs and that increase revenues—a prominent feature of the golden age of medicine (Light 2004; Starr 1982).

Professional Paternalism

It becomes clear in the chapters "The Assault on Professionalism" and "The Soul of Professionalism" of his book *Professionalism* that Freidson extends professional control to encompass "who is to perform what tasks and how much will be paid, on what terms." Still more broadly, in the development of the U.S. health-care system up to the 1960s, the profession "almost completely realized ideal-typical professionalism," he writes. "During the Golden Age, physicians had virtually complete control over the terms, conditions, and content of their work. They were free to charge all that the pockets of their patients could yield and to decide how much charity or free care to provide to whom" (2001, 180, 181, 184).

This remarkable characterization reflects a paternalistic ideal that leaves access and affordability up to each practitioner. It fails to take into account all the detail that Freidson himself provided thirty years earlier in his pathbreaking books *Profession of Medicine* (1970a) and *Professional Dominance* (1970b). Professionalization in the progressive

era involved converting hospitals from charitable institutions into fee-based "doctors' workshops"; elaborating specialization for greater control over a niche, more prestige, and higher fees; developing provider-based insurance that reinforced professional control over fees through passive reimbursement; and establishing relations with medical supply and pharmaceutical companies that enhanced professional power (Light 1989; Starr 1982). These changes served as ecological hinges and new jurisdictions among the profession, charitable institutions, manufacturers, and insurers.

These organizational features improved the quality of medical services but resulted in an inverse relationship between the availability of services and the need for them (Quadagno 2005), an "inverse care law" (Tudor Hart 1971) reflected in Part I of this volume (see Link and Phelan; Kawachi; and Dubowitz, Bates, and Acevedo-Garcia). This professional focus on treating sick patients also fits the conservative capitalist agenda to treat injured or sick workers and get them back on the job without addressing the upstream occupational risks, forms of exploitation or inequality, or issues of public health that led to their becoming injured or sick (Brown 1979; Navarro 1976; Navarro and Muntaner 2004; Waitzkin 1983, 2001). The great industrial fortunes of the nineteenth century bankrolled the campaign of the medical elite for a model of professionalism based on clinical intervention and for stopping broader efforts to improve occupational safety, reduce poverty, and improve public health for all (see references in Light 1989). Herein lies a fatal flaw in Freidson's ideal type: individual professional autonomy pays little attention to social causes of ill health, social injustices, or inequities. The organized profession has opposed universal health care in virtually every country that has attained it. Lacking a societal frame, as Parsons implies, professionals usually pursue their self-interests. If "monopoly is essential to professionalism," as Freidson claims, should we not be worried about possible abuses (2001, 3)?

Autonomy's Fallout: Dominance, Then Revolt

The autonomous exercise of discretionary specialism that lies at the heart of Freidson's third logic ironically led to the assault on professionalism that Freidson deplored. Freidson's own empirical studies of professional dominance were joined by an impressive number of studies by historians and sociologists summarized in the last edition of this handbook (Light 2000) and by more recent historical accounts (Gordon 2003; Light 2004). First, while the organized profession as a collectivity is granted autonomy, each professional claims this autonomy for him- or herself. This greatly weakens the possibility of collective autonomy in which professionals together monitor each other's practices and discuss better ways to treat certain kinds of cases. Individual professionals are protected from accountability and can cover up mistakes (Hughes 1958).

In a powerfully challenging review of Freidson's book, Fred Hafferty (2003, 140–41) cites numerous studies that document physicians missing a large number of clinical disorders, doing tests incorrectly, prescribing drugs for unproven indications, and ignoring dangerous side effects, which leads him to conclude: "I find it difficult to imagine how medicine can justify its calls for 'independence' and 'freedom of action,' given the prevalence of physician ineptitude and culpability." Individual autonomy leads to large variations in how individual clinicians diagnose and treat the same symptoms or problems, implying that the scientific basis for their decisions is thin or being selectively applied. Thus individual autonomy undermines the central claim of professionalism.

Second, these variations become amplified as autonomy leads to specialization, an extension of the "third logic" through internal segmentation, which gains for professionals greater autonomy, control over the scope of their work, capacity to do research, greater prestige, a competitive edge for patients, and income. Early specialization began, sometimes without any clear technical or therapeutic advance but often with advances based on professional rhetoric and theoretical models (see Stevens 1998; Halpern 1988; Scull 1979; Louden 2008; and Weisz 2006; Zetka 2008). Initial claims of expertise lead to—in Abbott's terms—settlements and, if successful, to jurisdictions. Specializing enables more detailed knowledge and research to develop, and certainly patients believe that specialty care is bet-ter, though considerable evidence questions how much better off many patients are. Structurally, specialization elaborates a linked ecology within clinical practice, with ties and hinges to terms of payment and commercial suppliers. It can also prompt "the erosion of medicine from within" (Zola and Miller 1973). Specialty societies erode the centralized power of the overall medical association, highlighting differences in agendas and priorities, and political control becomes more dissipated. Specialization also creates monopolistic niches and specialty societies that lobby for better pay for more elaborate care than for primary care (Light 2004; Stevens 1971). As a result, the market for primary care and family medicine is dying in the United States (McKinlay and Marceau 2008), even though integrated, nonprofit health systems like Kaiser-Permanente, the Veterans Health Administration, or the UK National Health Service find that primary-care teams can treat more than 90 percent of patient needs with greater continuity and at lower cost.

Freidson knew all this, wrote critically about it, yet hardly mentioned it as the dark, institutional side of his ideal type in *Professionalism: The Third Logic*, the side he researched with distinction for forty years (Halpern and Anspach 1993). "Where he concluded *Profession of Medicine* with concerns about a new tyranny of professionalism," Robert Dingwall observes, "*Third Logic* concludes with a call to sustain the independence of professions as a source of resistance to the greater tyrannies of markets and capital" (2008, 139). Freidson's chapter "The Assault on Professionalism" bemoans countervailing efforts by governments and employers, through insurers as their agents, to review and restrict tests, drugs, and procedures but does not cite the evidence that many of these are unnecessary and have harmful side effects. Freidson writes that peer review "created significant constraints on the freedom of physicians to do their work however they wished," but given the wide variations in quality of care, one might regard peer review as reinstating the social contract between the profession as a whole and society. Freidson describes the dismantling of legal protections of professions from antitrust strictures as tragic, without mentioning the self-serving forms of collusion and consumer exploitation that led to the removal of those protections (Havighurst 2003). The failure to describe the pathologies of unfettered autonomy and the reasons why countervailing powers have risen up to contain them keeps several recent works on professions and markets from being either accurate or realistic (Ameringer 2008; Leicht and Fennell 2001; Relman 2007; Sullivan 2005). Changes such as evidence-based medicine, clinical protocols, and clinical pathways are part of the buyers' revolt summarized in Table 16.2. These changes aim to improve quality and to reduce variation and unnecessary procedures resulting from professionalism based on individual autonomy, though they have their downsides. Targets and guidelines fragment care of the whole patient into bits and deflect attention both from what is not measured and from how what is measured may interact with aspects of a patient's situation. Nevertheless, this new focus represents a fundamental realignment of countervailing powers, and even of the knowledge base of medicine (Timmermans and Kolker 2004), in which the state and insurer/payers redefine their roles, the nature of oversight,

and the meaning of professionalism to base these on accountability (see Table 16.3).

The New Professionalism: Accountability and Value

Professionalism based on accountability is the outcome of countervailing powers today and a reconceptualization of medical science, practice, and profession. It represents a shift from a training-and-license model to a competency/performance model of professional work and thus to team models of care, like those that have been developing in the British National Health Service and elsewhere (Kuhlmann 2006). This shift lays the foundation for nonphysician clinicians to assume more professional work and even to replace physicians (McKinlay and Marceau 2008). What once was trust in the quality and integrity presumed of holders of medical degrees has become "enforceable trust" (Portes and Sensenbrenner 1993), or what Kuhlmann (2006) calls "justified trust," based on visible markers and measurable

Table 16.2. The buyer's revolt: axes of change

Dimensions	From provider driven	To buyer driven
Ideological	Sacred trust in doctors	Distrust of doctors' values, decisions, even competence
Clinical	Exclusive control of clinical decision making	Close monitoring of clinical decisions, their cost, and their efficacy
	Emphasis on state-of-the-art specialized interventions	Minimizing of high-tech and specialized interventions
	Lack of interest in prevention, primary care, and chronic care	Emphasis on prevention, primary care, and funding
Economic	Carte blanche to do what seems best; power to set fees; incentives to specialize	Fixed prepayment or contract with accountability for decisions and their efficacy
	Informal array of cross-subsidizations for teaching, research, charity care, community services	Elimination of "cost shifting"; pay only for services contracted
Political	Extensive legal and administrative power to define and carry out professional work without competition, and to shape the organization and economics of medicine	Extensive legal and administrative power to direct professional work and shape the organization and economics of services
Technical	Political and economic incentives to develop any new technology in protected markets	Political and economic restraints on developing new technologies
Organizational	Cottage industry	Corporate industry
Potential excesses and dislocations	Overtreatment, iatrogenesis, high cost, unnecessary treatment, fragmentation, depersonalization	Undertreatment, cuts in services, obstructed access, reduced quality, swamped in documentation of work

Table 16.3. Aspects of traditional versus new professionalism

Autonomy-based traditional professionalism	Accountability-based new professionalism
Quality focused on process and determined individually, so effectiveness and quality variable	Quality focused on outcomes established through clinical research, with guidelines, protocols, and care pathways
Subspecialization and hospital care as the center of power and prestige	Focus on primary care, prevention, and management; subspecialization and hospital care as backup New clinical research elite sets evidence-based standards and protocols
Physician-based practice and authority; delegated work to nurses, others	Team-based practice and collaboration
Oriented toward episodic treatment of acute problems	Oriented toward prevention and management of risks or problems to maximize functioning

outcomes. Demands for evidence of quality and value by countervailing powers are rescuing the medical profession from itself by hoisting it by its own petard, demanding it take science seriously (DeVries, Lemmens, and Bosk 2008). This effort can lead to new alliances among countervailing powers and also to the danger of commercial interests gaining unprecedented power by shaping clinical trials and evidence.

Despite the growth of evidence-based medicine, clinical guidelines, and systems for measuring quality, professional dominance is far from being reduced to "a historical curiosity," as a colleague put it to Robert Dingwall (2008). The managed-care backlash, encouraged by physicians, has forced employers and managed-care companies to become less assertive as a countervailing power and to shift the problem of cost containment to employees by making them pay increasing proportions of physician charges as well as insurance premiums (Robinson 2001). Since then, entrepreneurial specialist physicians have found myriad ways to increase tests, procedures, revenues, and profits.

Freidson ends his book on professionalism as the third logic with the chapter "The Soul of Professionalism," where he claims the worst scenario would be professionals turning into "merely technical experts in the service of the political and cultural economy," as in a national health service or universal health plan (2001, 212). Should this occur, he predicts, quality of service to clients will change as discretion is minimized. Line practi-

tioners will be less satisfied, and consumers (his word) will sense a perfunctory, standardized treatment of their problems. The spirit of ideal-typical professionals will be lost, as will be "their distinctive moral position that considers the use of their knowledge in light of values that transcend time and place" (213). What that moral position is, or what values transcend time and place besides a dedication to quality work, is not described but harkens back to Durkheim, Tawney, and Croly, who were equally vague and romantic about the moral ethos of professions in their day.

Hafferty (2003, 146–48) draws on his close observations and research to report that medical students often arrive with a desire to help and heal others but that training makes them more cynical, a pattern found repeatedly over the past forty years. Medical students come to disavow altruism and fear burnout and vulnerability to manipulative, demanding patients. They "reject the presumption that being a physician involves obligations" and assert "a healthy and cared-for self . . . as a precondition to helping others." The point of being a doctor is to have a good life and not work too hard, he reports from the field. Yet student leaders of the American Medical Student Association have for years been outspoken critics of commercialized medicine and a system that leaves forty-six million uninsured and millions of insured patients paying large sums for uncovered portions of their bills precisely when they can least afford it (AMSA 2009). They join a long tradition of public-spirited physicians working against the prevailing system. Thus the institutionalized ethos of most medical schools, residencies, and faculty weakens the "soul of professionalism," but an altruistic minority finds compatible places to practice on the margins, such as public hospitals, community health clinics, the National Health Service Corps, the Indian Health Service, some service-oriented nonprofits, and the Veterans Health Administration.

Besides ignoring decades of evidence on how autonomy undermines professionalism's promise to apply the best evidence, knowledge, and techniques to solve the problems of clients, Freidson and other champions of the medical profession do not acknowledge how much of medicine can be routinized around well-developed procedures, resulting in a level of quality higher than that produced by the variations of clinical autonomy. The best health-care systems, like Kaiser Permanente or the Veterans Health Administration, use protocols and standards of practice to attain high levels of quality, and England's National Health Service (NHS) has been working rapidly toward that end for the entire national system (Klein 2006; Oliver 2005). The NHS has steadily strengthened and broadened primary care into interprofessional teams, and the revolutionary new contract in 2003 builds in payments for realizing 146 population-based targets for prevention, diagnosis, treatment, and monitoring of chronic conditions that in effect define what the payer (the government) regards as good clinical practice. An important critique points out that paying in proportion to effort does not correlate well with paying in proportion to health gain, and vice versa (Fleetcroft and Cookson 2006). Further, payment for meeting clinical targets discourages providers from treating the more deprived and sicker patients who have more complex problems and take more time (Heath, Hippisley-Cox, and Smeeth 2007). Untargeted health needs also tend to become more neglected.

A protocol-driven contract like that of the new NHS embodies Freidson's vision of the worst that could happen to professionalism centered on autonomy: doctors and nurses reduced to mere technical workers told how to do their work by Big Brother. A new field study investigates this prediction by observing how the new

NHS contract's clinical targets are being implemented (McDonald, Checkland, Harrison, and Coleman 2009). Certain general-practice partners, designated "chasers," use detailed electronic clinical records shared by all to chase up those who are not performing to standard. Contrary to Freidson's predictions, the "chased" actively support the content of the targets and the goal of implementing a uniform high standard of care. The researchers found that the new system overcomes a central problem: lack of specific information on how individuals practice (Freidson 1975). The protocols enable both managers and providers to measure clinical performance. A GP commented: "I mean although I hate it, I do, you know, it's very paradoxical but I actually think it's a good idea and I think it makes things tangible and quantifies things and although I think it's a lot of hard work, I . . . the bottom line is I think patients benefit from it" (McDonald et al. 2009, 1202). The larger implication harkens back to Parsons's conclusion that the institutional framework defines the goals and rewards of work. Without a larger societal mandate to prevent illness, manage chronic conditions, and maximize a population's capacity to function, professionalism in an open field becomes the victim of its own excesses and deficiencies. With a societal mandate, the better qualities of professionals can be harnessed to beneficial societal ends (Light 1999).

Professionalism as Selfless Service to All?

At the end of his widely cited book on professionalism, Freidson turns away from his celebration of the golden age of medicine when physicians could treat whom they wanted, how they wanted, and for as much as they wanted to lay down moral mandates. "The ideology of professionalism asserts above all else devotion to the use of disciplined knowledge and skill for the public good," he declares. The profession should "declare social policies which deny equal access . . . to be professionally unethical" (2001, 217). Such policies would include much of the professionally constructed health-care system and the social policies of medical societies over the past fifty years.

Maximizing personal income at the expense

of quality, Freidson continues, should be declared unethical too. So should investing capital in professional services with the aim of maximizing returns on profit, a practice that turns attention from less profitable to more profitable procedures, regardless of benefit. (Yet it is the assertion of "professional autonomy" that underlies the expansion of physician-owned clinics and hospitals for profit.) Finally, "there can be no ethical justification for professionals who place personal gain above the obligation to do good work for all who need it, even at the expense of some potential income" (218). And professionals should not use patents to maximize profits.

If observed, these principles would turn health-care professions into a powerful countervailing force against the markets in medicine and the marketlike behavior that result from professional autonomy. Freidson's precepts offer greater moral clarity than anything Durkheim, Tawney, or Croly wrote. They are at such odds, however, with the rest of his argument that one does not know what to make of them. It is hard to imagine sociologically how these principles could be carried out except in a universal public health-care system or a national health service. Every one of them is violated every day in the U.S. health-care system as physicians profit from their incorporated specialty practices that undercut integrated care, and from the billions they accept from manufacturers to use new drugs or devices before their safety and added benefits are established (Angell 2009). If Freidson had built his model of professionalism on his strong ethic of public good and social justice, it would have been profoundly different. It would have taken into account his groundbreaking empirical studies, including the practices, limitations, and biases of professional work in early group and prepaid practices (see Freidson 1961, 1975).

Sources of Diminished Trust

If one examines the many accounts of diminished professionalism and trust, one finds four quite different sources: rare cases of bad-apple abusive or incompetent practitioners; widespread variations in treatment and cost for the same problem, which suggests that autonomous professionals do not apply a common body of expertise; self-commercialization; and corporate cooptation or colonialization.

Distrusting Self-Regulation

Reflecting a central institutional dynamic in the United Kingdom but oddly peripheral in the United States and elsewhere, the few bad apples among practitioners in that country led British leaders to conclude that professional bodies failed to monitor, investigate, and address serious cases of abuse, fraud, or incompetence and thus jeopardized the public's trust in practitioners (Yeung and Dixon-Woods 2009). Professional ethics—which Bledstein (1976) characterized as "professional etiquette" and Berlant (1975) as a vehicle for monopolization—were implicated in colleagues' failure to report suspicious behavior and protect their fellow professionals rather than patients. It seems that the social contract and the public's expectations that professionals will be honorable, ethical, and up-to-date were not honored on the occasions when the profession's assurances were not upheld.

Such cases exist everywhere, but in the United Kingdom, they have contributed to historic institutional changes among the countervailing powers that surround the profession as the government has subsumed traditional professional functions. British regulation no longer assumes that medical professionals are competent until found otherwise but rather that they must be examined as "fit to practice" through detailed reviews of work, "revalidation," and remediation when needed. The profession was given a chance to design these reforms of accountability, but its proposals were "scathingly rejected," and institutional redesign was turned over to government officials. The General Medical Council (GMC), responsible for education and registration, has been transformed from an organization based on a nineteenth-century model with most members selected by the profession to a model of public accountability, with parity of lay and professional members appointed through an independent commission. The power to adjudicate cases of professional misconduct has been transferred to the new Office of the Health Professions Adjudicator. All regulatory functions of the GMC are now overseen by an independent Council for Healthcare Regulatory Excellence accountable to Parliament (UK Secretary of State for Health 2007).

These new practices, standards, and institutions apply to all health professions in consistent ways that end the variable practices of professional organizations. Thus the autonomy of both individual clinicians and their professional bodies has been sharply curtailed, even though breaches of trust are rare. These new institutional arrangements in effect carry out parts of the mythic social contract that the organized profession did not monitor or enforce well. They aim to make professional work more trustworthy, and they provide a model for how state professional boards in other countries could assure the public that health professionals meet high standards. Few state boards in the United States measure up (Public Citizen 2008), yet similar cases of unethical or incompetent behavior have not led to significant U.S. reforms. Comparative research is needed on how the linked ecologies of countervailing powers operate in different countries.

Reining in Autonomous Market Behavior

The irony that autonomy leads to diminished trust by generating widespread variations in procedures, cost, and quality when specialists treat the same cases has led to evidence-based medicine and clinical guidelines (Hafferty and Light 1995; Timmermans and Berg 2003). Yet Americans receive care that meets established quality standards only about half the time (McGlynn et al. 2003). Quality varies considerably, not only by insurance status and other market variables, but even after controlling for them. Are quality and the application of professional expertise less variable elsewhere, in universal health-care systems that do not operate largely by economic markets? Historians maintain that medicine was ever thus—centuries of doctors running cottage practices based on charismatic and legal authority, marketing useless or harmful cures, and having little

systematic knowledge of which treatments work better (Imber 2008; Wootton 2006).[2]

A variety of measures have been taken to establish clinical standards. From a market perspective, these are analogous to measures to protect the public from unacceptable variations in other service industries, but they represent a revolution in medicine. For example, a cardiac team trying to decide how to treat a patient who has severe congestive heart failure can use comparative data to estimate his five-year survival chances based on tracked cases—medication 9.4 percent, angioplasty 26.5 percent, or bypass surgery 46.2 percent—and then review treatment choices with the patient (Millenson 1997). New Jersey, like several other states, publishes the risk-adjusted mortality rates of hospitals and surgeons so that patients can choose a surgeon with a proven track record (State of New Jersey 2009). A profit-seeking managed-care company, however, can use guidelines to squeeze time, tests, and treatments for profit (Burdi and Baker 1999). Researchers find that unless physicians choose and develop evidence-based guidelines themselves, as they do in large physician groups or physician-run organizations like Kaiser-Permanente, they resist them (Audet et al. 2005; Rittenhouse et al. 2004).

In the United Kingdom, particularly in England, the government as payer and governor of a national health service has developed National Service Frameworks that detail clinical standards for large clinical areas (e.g., cardiology) or kinds of patients (e.g., children). It established NICE, the National Institute for Clinical Excellence, to assess which of hundreds of new medicines, devices, and procedures meet criteria for effectiveness and value. Such efforts generate controversies about approaches or products not included, and about over- or underrating. Clinical governance has become a public rather than a self-governing professional function, overseen by the English Care Quality Commission. Pay now depends in part on meeting quality targets and leads to a certain amount of gaming and displays of compliance. These changes tacitly shift decisions about how to stay within a budget to doctors practicing evidence-based medicine and diffuse responsibility for rationing when it occurs (Harrison 1998). It changes the professional basis of work from the individual application of medical science to epidemiological evidence of effectiveness (Timmermans and Kolker 2004). Some observers may see this constellation of changes as professionalism destroyed; others regard it as professionalism finally realized (Millenson 1997). Still others in Scotland and Wales agree with the goals but not the particulars of the English approach. In the United States, there are many similar efforts to establish quality standards, one for each managed-care group or plan, specialty society, consulting firm, and government initiative, each with a somewhat different focus and approach.

Self-Commercialization

The third source of diminished trust, self-commercialization, although ever-present in medical practice, has shaped the large-scale institutionalization of practice and markets in the twentieth century (Larson 1977; Starr 1982). Contrary to the claims of Freidson and spokespersons for the profession, I contend that professionals have a considerable affinity for business and have embraced corporations that enhance their diagnostic and treatment capacities, even though new tests, devices, and drugs may not improve clinical results. Health-care corporations arose to exploit the protected markets the medical profession created in which margins were high and it was nearly impossible to lose. Calls to restore professionalism overlook the rapid escalation of costs, the unnecessary procedures, and the professional corporatization that occurred during the golden age of professional autonomy and dominance. Professions *as* markets and self-commercialization would characterize what led to the buyers' revolt (see Table 16.2).

William Sullivan, writing for the Carnegie Foundation's long-term project on restoring professionalism, misconstrues the decline of professional sovereignty as beginning when the profession partnered with government after Medicare and Medicaid were passed, resulting in "less room for autonomous maneuver" (2005, 57). Sullivan's account overlooks the history of Blue Cross and Blue Shield, a kind of nonprofit insurance that did not interfere with providers' freedom to

bill as they liked (Law 1974; Somers and Somers 1961). Later, as commercial insurers began to write health insurance, they emulated this model of passive reimbursement. As Medicare and Medicaid took shape in 1964, the profession threatened not to treat the elderly and the poor unless both programs were based on reimbursing what providers charge. Services and charges rapidly increased, and Congress has been trying to curb both ever since. By addressing neither self-commercialization among physicians who turned their practices into corporations during the golden age of medicine from 1945 to 1975 nor the implications of this process for the social contract (which is never described), the Carnegie Foundation project is likely to be strong on rhetoric but ineffective.

A new account of U.S. health-care professions and markets by Carl Ameringer (2008), sponsored by the Milbank Fund, likewise misses the extensive self-commercialization in the 1950s documented in the authoritative study by Somers and Somers (1961), as well as expanded forms in the 1960s documented by several studies cited in previous editions of this handbook. Ameringer's starting point—the Federal Trade Commission's attack on collusive and protectionist medical practices after 1975—makes it look as if neoconservatives attacked a noble profession. Ameringer mentions neither the self-serving ethics and practices that resulted in excessive tests, drugs, operations, hospital procedures, and charges (Berlant 1975), nor prior concerted efforts by Congress to regulate professional expansion (Starr 1982). Physicians and hospitals effectively sidelined or circumvented these efforts. Self-commercialization is especially prevalent in the United States, where physician practices incorporated in the 1970s and where specialists have invested in stand-alone clinics or diagnostic centers that siphon profitable cases from general hospitals, weakening them and fragmenting care. This trend led many leaders to conclude that only the market discipline of corporate managed care could bring professionally driven health care under control. Mahar (2006) describes the resulting "Hobbesian marketplace" that pits providers against each other and against payers in a "war of all against all" that wastes up to one of every three dollars on administrative complexity, profits, and unnecessary or unproven but overpriced procedures and products.

Corporate Co-optation

Beyond the long-standing ties between the profession and companies as countervailing powers, a more recent development involves the ways in which one commercial sector, the pharmaceutical industry, has succeeded in co-opting medical science, medical journals, and the creation of new risks or diseases. Pharmaceutical companies shape how physicians are trained, what they know about a given disease, how they think about alternate approaches to treatment, and what medications they have patients ingest (Abramson 2004; Brody 2007; Relman and Angell 2002). Models of pathology and risk are developed to sell drugs to treat them and often are based on synthetic or surrogate endpoints that eventually prove to have little clinical relevance, such as the serotonin model of major depression (Curtiss and Fairman 2008; Healy 2004; Horwitz and Wakefield 2007; Lacasse and Leo 2005; Moynihan and Cassels 2005).

Companies retain prominent clinical researchers and fund their work in order to create a commercialized science of heart disease, or menopause, or social anxiety disorder, or osteoporosis (Conrad 2007; Moynihan and Cassels 2005). Marcia Angell (2009), the former editor of the *New England Journal of Medicine*, summarizes the extensive investigations by the U.S. Senate into what she and Senator Charles Grassley call "the corruption" of universities, academic research, and prominent physicians through company grants, fees, and retainers that greatly increase psychiatric diagnoses, especially in children, and prescriptions for powerful drugs of unclear or unproven clinical benefit (see also Bass 2008; Lane 2007; Petersen 2008). These practices and institutional patterns of co-optation also appear to exist in other countries.

Commercial constructions of medical science are initially promoted through articles in medical journals, often written by hired ghostwriters and fronted by physicians who agree to be the authors of record for a fee (Ross et al. 2008). Articles on

sponsored research are three to four times more likely to find the results favorable to the sponsor's product than are articles based on research funded by independent sources (Lexchin et al. 2003; Turner et al. 2008). Salespersons then give the published articles to practicing physicians as proof that the sponsor's drug is better than the one they are prescribing. This pharmaceutically managed bias in medical science thus leads physicians, patients, and managers to inaccurate conclusions about the efficacy and safety of new drugs.

At the same time, companies sponsor invitational conferences on a new disease model to give heads of specialty services around the country the opportunity to meet the leading clinical researchers, all expenses paid, at a five-star resort, where attendees have a light schedule and the rest of each day off. Company-sponsored sessions at professional specialty meetings further establish the purported veracity of the new disease model, as do thousands of continuing medical education courses for practitioners, most of which are now sponsored by pharmaceutical companies as well (Relman 2007; U.S. Senate 2007). Over 90 percent of physicians report receiving gifts, perks, or money from drug companies, and they choose to get information about what to prescribe from sales reps who are required to spend their large monthly allowance in ways that will most effectively result in their doctors writing more prescriptions for new drugs (Lee 2007). Lakoff (2005) refers to the pharmaceutical companies' "sculpting" of doctor-patient interaction, as physicians' expertise is shaped by market-based science and the gift relationship established by their receiving samples of costly new drugs, which the doctors then bless and give to patients.

These clustered techniques of what Suddaby and Greenwood (2001) describe as "colonizing knowledge" begin by commodifying knowledge, honing complex volumes of test results down to a simple message and story, which are used to persuade physicians to prescribe and patients to want a new drug. About a hundred thousand sales reps in the United States alone are carefully trained in the social psychology of friendship with all their physician customers to sculpt their prescribing decisions (Fugh-Berman and Ahari

2007). Personal sales reps are supplemented by industry-funded patient groups, which lobby their physicians and legislators for new drugs that cost thousands a year. Other physicians, including three past editors-in-chief of the *New England Journal of Medicine*, have written books about the co-optation of medicine and physicians' clinical decisions by the pharmaceutical industry and how it endangers patients (Abramson 2004; Angell 2004; Avorn 2004; Breggin 1991; Brody 2007; Glenmullen 2000; Kassirer 2005; Relman and Angell 2002). Six out of every seven new drugs offer no or few clinical benefits over existing ones and yet bear greater risk for adverse side effects (Light, in press).

Concluding Comment

This review of the relations between the medical profession and markets has gone from professions against markets. to professions as markets, to professions marketed and colonized. Strangely, almost none of the policies to restore professionalism or of the sociological studies of the profession mention or address this most pervasive threat to professional knowledge and practice. For example, Susan Chimonas, Troyen A. Brennan, and David J. Rothman at the Center on Medicine as a Profession studied how physicians handled the conflicts of interest that arise from seeing drug sales representatives and were so struck by the physicians' forms of denial and rationalization that they concluded "only the prohibition of physician-detailer interactions will be effective" (2007, 189). They are part of a larger group that has called on academic medical centers to join members of Congress and state governments in eliminating commercial conflicts of interest (Brennan et al. 2006). They call for the prohibition of all gifts, free samples, company-sponsored professional education, and ghostwriting so that independent, trustworthy professionalism can be restored. Wider patterns of professional commercialization have led Arnold Relman (2007), a champion of professional integrity for the last thirty years and past editor-in-chief of the *New England Journal of Medicine*, to conclude that all medical practice must be completely decom-

mercialized under a salaried national health service. The physician-writer John Geyman (2008) summarizes the evidence and comes to a similar conclusion, with an emphasis on the profession serving the health needs of all, not just their patients. Durkheim and the later Freidson were wrong: the health-care professions do not embody a higher moral order for society but need to be rescued from market forces and from pursuing their own self-interests.

Notes

This essay has benefited from comments from Robert Dingwall, Mary Dixon-Woods, Allen Fremont, Fred Hafferty, Antonio Manturo, Daniel Menchik, and Arnold Relman, none of whom are responsible for its content.

1. One sees complete state dominance today in many dictatorships, usually to carry out internecine warfare and genocide, but sometimes to support population-based health care.
2. Imber (2008) notes that the basis for trust has shifted from medical professionals' moral integrity to their effective application of expert knowledge.

References

Abbott, Andrew. 1988. *The System of Professions.* Chicago: University of Chicago Press.

———. 2005. "Linked Ecologies: States and Universities as Environments for Professions." *Sociological Theory* 23:245–74.

Abramson, John. 2004. *Overdosed America: The Broken Promise of American Medicine.* New York: HarperCollins.

Albrecht, Gary L. 1992. *The Disability Business.* Thousand Oaks, Calif.: Sage.

AMSA [American Medical Students Association]. 2009. "AMSA's 60th Annual Convention: AMSA at 60! Celebrating Passion, Professionalism, Pride." amsa .org/conv/.

Ameringer, Carl F. 2008. *The Health Care Revolution: From Medical Monopoly to Market Competition.* Berkeley: University of California Press.

Angell, Marcia. 1993. "The Doctor as Double Agent." *Kennedy Institute of Ethics Journal* 3:279–86.

———. 2004. *The Truth about the Drug Companies: How They Deceive Us and What to Do about It.* New York: Random House.

———. 2009. "Drug Companies and Doctors: A Story of Corruption." *New York Review of Books*, January 15, 56.

Audet, Anne-Marie J., Michelle M. Doty, Jamil

Shamasdin, and Stephen C. Schoenbaum. 2005. "Measure, Learn, and Improve: Physicians' Involvement in Quality Improvement." *Health Affairs* 24:843–53.

Avorn, Jerry. 2004. *Powerful Medicines: The Benefits, Risks, and Costs of Prescription Drugs*. New York: Knopf.

Bass, Allison. 2008. *Side Effects: A Prosecutor, a Whistleblower, and a Bestselling Antidepressant on Trial*. Chapel Hill, N.C.: Algonquin Books.

Berlant, Jeffrey L. 1975. *Profession and Monopoly*. Berkeley: University of California Press.

Bledstein, Burton. 1976. *The Culture of Professionalism*. New York: W. W. Norton.

Breggin, Peter. 1991. *Toxic Psychiatry*. New York: St. Martin's Press.

Brennan, Troyen A., David J. Rothman, Linda Blank, David Blumenthal, Susan Chimonas, Jordon Cohen, Janlori Goldman, Jerome Kassirer, Harry Kimball, James Naughton, and Neil Smelser. 2006. "Health Industry Practices that Create Conflict of Interest." *Journal of American Medical Association* 295:429–33.

Brody, Howard. 2007. *Hooked: Ethics, the Medical Profession, and the Pharmaceutical Industry*. Lanham, Md.: Rowman and Littlefield.

Brown, E. Richard. 1979. *Rockefeller Medicine Men*. Berkeley: University of California Press.

Burdi, M. D. and L. C. Baker. 1999. "Physicians' Perceptions of Autonomy and Satisfaction in California." *Health Affairs* 18:134–45.

Burrow, James G. 1977. *Organized Medicine in the Progressive Era: The Move toward Monopoly*. Baltimore: Johns Hopkins University Press.

Chimonas, Susan, Troyen A. Brennan, and David J. Rothman. 2007. "Physicians and Drug Representatives: Exploring the Dynamics of the Relationship." *Journal of General Internal Medicine* 22:184–90.

Conrad, Peter. 2007. *The Medicalization of Society*. Baltimore: Johns Hopkins University Press.

Croly, Herbert. 1965 (1909). *The Promise of American Life*. Edited by A. R. Schlesinger. Cambridge: Belknap Press of Harvard University Press.

Curtiss, Frederic R., and Kathleen A. Fairman. 2008. "Looking for the Outcomes We Love in All the Wrong Places: The Questionable Value of Biomarkers and Investments in Chronic Care Disease Management Interventions." *Journal of Managed Care Pharmacy* 14:563–70.

DeVries, R. G., T. Lemmens, and C. L. Bosk. 2008. "The Subjectivity of Objectivity: The Social, Cultural, and Political Shaping of Evidence-Based Medicine." In *The Brave New World of Health*, ed. B. Bennett, T. Carney, and I. Karpin, 144–65. Sydney: Federation Press.

Dingwall, Robert. 2008. "In Memory of Eliot Freidson: Is 'Professional Dominance' an Obsolete Concept?" In *Essays on Professions*, ed. R. Dingwall, 127–41. Aldershot, UK: Ashgate.

Durkheim, Emile. 1957. *Professional Ethics and Civic Morals*. Translated by C. Brookfield. London: Routledge and Kegan Paul.

Fleetcroft, R., and R. Cookson. 2006. "Do the Incentives Payments in the New NHS Contract for Primary Care Reflect Likely Population Gains?" *Journal of Health Services Research Policy* 11:27–31.

Freidson, Eliot. 1961. *Patients' Views of Medical Practice*. Chicago: University of Chicago Press.

———. 1970a. *Profession of Medicine*. New York: Dodd, Mead.

———. 1970b. *Professional Dominance*. New York: Atherton.

———. 1975. *Doctoring Together: A Study of Professional Social Control*. New York: Elsevier.

———. 1983. "The Theory of Professions: State of the Art." In *The Sociology of the Professions*, ed. R. Dingwall and P. Lewis. New York: St. Martin's Press.

———. 2001. *Professionalism: The Third Logic*. Chicago: University of Chicago Press.

Fugh-Berman, Adrianne, and Shahram Ahari. 2007. "Following the Script: How Drug Reps Make Friends and Influence Doctors." *Public Library of Science Medicine* 4: e150.

Geyman, John. 2004. *The Corporate Transformation of Health Care: Can the Public Interest Still Be Served?* New York: Springer.

———. 2008. *The Corrosion of Medicine: Can the Profession Reclaim Its Moral Legacy?* Monroe, Me.: Common Courage Press.

Glenmullen, Joseph. 2000. *Prozac Backlash: Overcoming the Dangers of Prozac, Zoloft, Paxil, and Other Antidepressants with Safe, Effective Alternatives*. New York: Simon and Schuster.

Goozner, Merrill. 2004. *The $800 Million Pill: The Truth behind the Cost of New Drugs*. Berkeley: University of California Press.

Gordon, Colin. 2003. *Dead on Arrival: The Politics of Health Care in Twentieth-Century America*. Princeton, N.J.: Princeton University Press.

Hafferty, Fred. 2003. "Finding Soul in a 'Medical Profession of One.'" *Journal of Health Politics, Policy and Law* 28:133–58.

Hafferty, Fred, and D. W. Light. 1995. "Professional Dynamics and the Changing Nature of Medical Work." *Journal of Health and Social Behavior*, extra issue: 132–53.

Halpern, Sydney. 1988. *American Pediatrics: The Social Dynamics of Professionalism, 1880–1980*. Berkeley: University of California Press.

Halpern, Sydney, and Renee R. Anspach. 1993. "The

Study of Medical Institutions: Eliot Freidson's Legacy." *Work and Occupations* 20:279–95.

Harrison, Stephen. 1998. "The Politics of Evidence-Based Medicine in the United Kingdom." *Policy and Politics* 26:15–31.

Haskell, Thomas. 1984. "Professions versus Capitalism." In *The Authority of Experts: Studies in History and Theory*, ed. T. Haskell, 180–225. Bloomington: Indiana University Press.

Havighurst, Clark C. 2003. "An Apology for Professionalist Regimes." *Journal of Health Politics, Policy and Law* 28:159–63.

Healy, David. 2004. *Let Them Eat Prozac: The Unhealthy Relationship between the Pharmaceutical Industry and Depression.* New York: New York University Press.

Heath, I., J. Hippisley-Cox, and L. Smeeth. 2007. "Measuring Performance and Missing the Point?" *British Medical Journal* 335:1075–76.

Horwitz, Allan, and Jerome C. Wakefield. 2007. *The Loss of Sadness.* New York: Oxford University Press.

Hughes, Everett C. 1958 (1951). "Mistakes at Work." In *Men and Their Work*, ed. E. C. Hughes, 88–101. Glencoe, Ill.: Free Press.

———. 1994 (1965). "Professions." In *On Work, Race, and the Sociological Imagination*, ed. E. C. Hughes, 37–49. Chicago: University of Chicago Press.

Imber, Jonathan B. 2008. *Trusting Doctors: The Decline of Moral Authority in American Medicine.* Princeton, N.J.: Princeton University Press.

Kassirer, Jerome P. 2005. *On the Take: How Medicine's Complicity with Big Business Can Endanger Your Health.* New York: Oxford University Press.

Klein, Rudolf. 2006. *The New Politics of the NHS: From Creation to Reinvention.* Abingdon, UK: Radcliffe.

Krause, Elliott A. 1996. *Death of the Guilds: Professions, States, and the Advance of Capitalism, 1930 to the Present.* New Haven, Conn.: Yale University Press.

Kuhlmann, Ellen. 2006. *Modernizing Health Care: Reinventing Professions, the State and the Public.* Bristol, UK: Policy Press.

Lacasse, Jeffrey R., and Jonathan Leo. 2005. "Serotonin and Depression: A Disconnect between the Advertisements and the Scientific Literature." *Public Library of Science Medicine* 2:1212–16.

Lakoff, Andrew. 2005. "The Private Life of Numbers." In *Global Assemblages*, ed. A. Ong and S. J. Collier, 194–212. Oxford: Blackwell.

Lane, Christopher. 2007. *Shyness: How Normal Behavior Became a Sickness.* New Haven, Conn.: Yale University Press.

Larson, Magali Sarfatti. 1977. *The Rise of Professionalism: A Sociological Analysis.* Berkeley: University of California Press.

Law, S. A. 1974. *Blue Cross: What Went Wrong?* New Haven, Conn.: Yale University Press.

Lee, Christopher. 2007. "Drugmakers, Doctors Get Cozier: Gifts Continue, Contacts Increase Despite Guidelines." *Washington Post*, April 29.

Leicht, Kevin, and Mary L. Fennell. 2001. *Professional Work: A Sociological Approach.* Malden, Mass.: Blackwell.

Lexchin, Joel, Lisa A. Bero, Benjamin Djulbegovic, and Octavio Clark. 2003. "Pharmaceutical Industry Sponsorship and Research Outcome And Quality: Systematic Review." *British Medical Journal* 326:1167–70.

Light, Donald W. 1989. "Social Control and the American Health Care System." In *Handbook of Medical Sociology*, 4th ed., ed. H. E. Freeman and S. Levine, 456–74. Upper Saddle River, N.J.: Prentice Hall.

———. 1992. "The Practice and Ethics of Risk-Rated Health Insurance." *Journal of the American Medical Association* 267:2503–08.

———. 1999. "Good Managed Care Needs Universal Health Insurance." *Annals of Internal Medicine* 130:686–89.

———. 2000. "The Medical Profession and Organizational Change: From Professional Dominance to Countervailing Power." In *Handbook of Medical Sociology*, 5th ed., ed. C. Bird, P. Conrad, and A. Fremont, 201–16. Englewood Cliffs, N.J.: Prentice Hall.

———. 2001. "Comparative Institutional Response to Economic Policy, Managed Competition, and Governmentality." *Social Science and Medicine* 52(8): 1151–66.

———. 2004. "Ironies of Success: A New History of the American Health Care 'System.'" *Journal of Health and Social Behavior* 45, extra issue: 1–24.

———. 2006. "Basic Research Funds to Discover Important New Drugs: Who Contributes How Much?" In *Monitoring the Financial Flows for Health Research 2005: Behind the Global Numbers*, ed. M. A. Burke, 27–43. Geneva: Global Forum for Health Research.

———, ed. In press. *The Risks of Prescription Drugs.* New York: Columbia University Press.

Light, Donald W., and Sol Levine. 1988. "Changing Character of the Medical Profession: A Theoretical Overview." *Milbank Quarterly* 66, suppl. 2:1–23.

Light, Donald W., and Alexander Schuller. 1986. "Political Values and Health Care: The German Experience." Cambridge, Mass.: MIT Press.

Louden, Irving. 2008. "General Practice and Obstetrics: A Brief History." *Journal of the Royal Society of Medicine* 101:531–35.

Lundberg, George D. 2000. *Severed Trust.* New York: Basic.

Mahar, Maggie. 2006. *Money-Driven Medicine.* New York: Collins.

McDonald, Ruth, Kate Checkland, Stephen Harrison, and Anna Coleman. 2009. "Rethinking Collegiality: Restratification in English General Medical Practice 2004–2008." *Social Science and Medicine* 68(7): 1199–1205. Manchester, UK: University of Manchester.

McGlynn, Elizabeth A., Steven M. Asch, John Adams, and Joan Keesey. 2003. "The Quality of Health Care Delivered to Adults in the United States." *New England Journal of Medicine* 348:2635–45.

McKinlay, John, and Lisa Marceau. 2008. "When There Is No Doctor: Reasons for the Disappearance of Primary Care Physicians in the U.S. during the Early 21st Century." *Social Science and Medicine* 67(10): 1481–91.

Mechanic, David. 2006. *The Truth about Health Care: Why Reform Is Not Working in America.* New Brunswick, N.J.: Rutgers University Press.

Millenson, Michael L. 1997. *Demanding Medical Excellence.* Chicago: University of Chicago Press.

Moynihan, Ray, and Alan Cassels. 2005. *Selling Sickness: How the World's Biggest Pharmaceutical Companies Are Turning Us All into Patients.* New York: Nation Books.

Navarro, Vicente. 1976. *Medicine under Capitalism.* New York: Prodist.

Navarro, Vicente, and Carles Muntaner. 2004. "Political and Economic Determinants of Population Health and Well-Being." Amityville, N.Y.: Baywood.

Nixon, Richard M. 1972. *Public Papers of the Presidents of the United States: Richard Nixon 1971.* Washington D.C.: U.S. Government Printing Office.

Oliver, Adam. 2005. "The English National Health Service, 1979–2005." *Health Economics* 14, suppl.: S75–100.

Parsons, Talcott. 1939. "The Professions and Social Structure." *Social Forces* 17:457–67.

Petersen, Melody. 2008. "Our Daily Meds: How the Pharmaceutical Companies Transformed Themselves into Slick Marketing Machines and Hooked the Nation on Prescription Drugs." New York: Sarah Crichton/Farrar, Straus and Giroux.

Picker Institute Europe. pickereurope.org.

Portes, Alejandro, and Julia Sensenbrenner. 1993. "Embeddedness and Immigration: Notes on the Social Determinants of Economic Action." *American Journal of Sociology* 98:1320–50.

Public Citizen. 2008. "Public Citizen's Health Research Group Ranking of the Rate of the State Medical Boards Serious Disciplinary Actions 2005–07." Washington, D.C.: Public Citizen.

Quadagno, Jill. 2004. "Why the United States Has No National Health Insurance: Stakeholder Mobilization against the Welfare State, 1945–1996." *Journal of Health and Social Behavior* 45, extra issue: 25–44.

———. 2005. *One Nation, Uninsured: Why the U.S. Has No National Health Insurance.* New York: Oxford University Press.

Relman, Arnold S. 2007. *A Second Opinion: Rescuing America's Health Care.* New York: Public Affairs.

Relman, Arnold, and Marcia Angell. 2002. "America's Other Drug Problem: How the Drug Industry Distorts Medicine and Politics." *New Republic,* December 16, 27–36.

Rittenhouse, Diane R., Kevin Grumbach, Edward H. O'Neil, Catherine Dower, and Andrew Bindman. 2004. "Physician Organization and Care Management in California: From Cottage to Kaiser." *Health Affairs* 23:51–62.

Robinson, James C. 2001. "The End of Managed Care." *Journal of the American Medical Association* 285:2622–28.

Ross, Joseph S., Kevin P. Hill, David S. Egilman, and Harlan M. Krumholz. 2008. "Guest Authorship and Ghostwriting in Publications Related to Rofecoxib." *Journal of American Medical Association* 299:1800–1812.

Schwartz, Jerome I. 1965. "Early History of Prepaid Medical Care Plans." *Bulletin of the History of Medicine* 39:450–75.

Sciulli, David. 2005. "Continental Sociology of Professions Today: Conceptual Contributions." *Contemporary Sociology* 53:915–42.

Scull, Andrew. 1979. *Museums of Madness.* New York: St. Martin's Press.

Somers, Herman M., and Anne H. Somers. 1961. *Doctors, Patients, and Health Insurance.* Washington, D.C.: Brookings Institution.

Starr, Paul. 1982. *The Social Transformation of American Medicine.* New York: Basic.

State of New Jersey. Department of Health and Senior Services. 2009. "Cardiac Surgery." state.nj.us/health/healthcarequality/cardiacsurgery.shtml.

Stevens, Rosemary. 1971. *American Medicine and the Public Interest.* New Haven, Conn.: Yale University Press.

———. 1998. *American Medicine and the Public Interest.* Updated ed. Berkeley: University of California Press.

Stone, Deborah. 1997. "The Doctor as Businessman." *Journal of Health Politics, Policy and Law* 22:533–56.

Suddaby, Roy, and Rayston Greenwood. 2001. "Colonizing Knowledge: Commodification as a Dynamic of Jurisdictional Expansions in Professional Service Firms." *Human Relations* 54:933–53.

Sullivan, William M. 2005. *Work and Integrity: The Crisis and Promise of Professionalism in America.* 2nd ed. San Francisco: Jossey-Bass.

Tawney, R. H. 1920. *The Acquisitive Society*. London: Bell.

Timmermans, Stefan, and Marc Berg. 2003. *The Gold Standard: The Challenge of Evidence-Based Medicine and Standardization in Health Care*. Philadelphia: Temple University Press.

Timmermans, Stefan, and Emily Kolker. 2004. "Clinical Practice Guidelines and the Implications of Shifts in Knowledge for Sociological Accounts of Professional Power." *Journal of Health and Social Behavior* 45, extra issue: 177–93.

Tudor Hart, Julian. 1971. "The Inverse Care Law." *Lancet*, February 27, 405–12.

———. 2008. "A New Horizon for NHS Wales." *Bevan Foundation Review* 11 (autumn): 8–10.

Turner, Erick H., Annette M. Matthews, Eftihia Linardatos, Robert A. Tell, and Robert Rosenthal. 2008. "Selective Publication of Antidepressant Trials and Its Influence on Apparent Efficacy." *New England Journal of Medicine* 358:252–60.

UK Secretary of State for Health. 2007. "Trust, Assurance and Safety: The Regulation of Health Professionals in the 21st Century." London: Stationery Office.

U.S. Senate. Committee on Finance. 2007. "Use of Educational Grants by Pharmaceutical Manufacturers." Washington, D.C.: U.S. Government Printing Office.

Waitzkin, Howard. 1983. *The Second Sickness: Contradictions of Capitalist Health Care*. New York: Free Press.

———. 2001. *At the Front Lines of Medicine*. New York: Rowman and Littlefield.

Weisz, George. 2006. *Divide and Conquer: A Comparative History of Medical Specialization*. New York: Oxford University Press.

Wootton, David. 2006. *Bad Medicine: Doing Harm since Hippocrates*. Oxford: Oxford University Press.

Yeung, Karen, and Mary Dixon-Woods. 2009. "'Rotten Apples and Good Apples': Regulating the Medical Profession in the 21st Century." Leicester, UK: University of Leicester, Department of Sociology.

Zetka, James R., Jr. 2008. "The Making of the 'Women's Physician' in American Obstetrics and Gynecology: Reforging an Occupational Identity and a Division of Labor." *Journal of Health and Social Behavior* 49:335–51.

Zola, Irving Kenneth, and Stephen J. Miller. 1973. "The Erosion of Medicine from Within." In *The Professions and Their Prospects*, ed. E. Freidson, 153–72. Beverly Hills, Calif.: Sage.

17

The Sociological Concomitants of the Pharmaceutical Industry and Medications

John Abraham, University of Sussex

Pharmaceuticals are pervasive in medicine and society. The transnational industrial nature and scale of pharmaceutical markets and the level of technoscientific sophistication in pharmaceutical development in the last twenty to twenty-five years are unprecedented. Between 1960 and the early 1980s, prescription-drug sales were almost static as a percentage of GDP in most of the major Western economies, including the United States, which alone makes up about half the world's prescription-drug sales.[1] However, from the early 1980s to 2002, prescription-drug sales tripled to nearly US$400 billion worldwide, and almost US$200 billion in the United States (Angell 2004, 1–5). By 2007, global sales were approaching US$600 billion (IMS Health 2008). Pharmaceuticals also seem to be more pervasive in public discourse and media outlets than in previous decades (Applbaum 2006). Many who speak for the pharmaceutical industry in drug companies, the scientific community, or within the media assert or give the impression that the expansion of pharmaceutical markets and prescribing over the last few decades is best understood as the innovative responses of biomedical science to growing and new health needs. I refer to this as the "biomedicalism thesis," which has long been a deep-seated part of the popular, commercial, and scientistic discourse about drug products.

Conventionally, the biomedicalism thesis has been challenged by the well-established sociological concept of medicalization—the making of the

social medical. The medicalization thesis asserts that the growth in medical conditions partly reflects medical dominance in society and the significance of the "sick role" in redefining social deviance or dysfunctionality (Conrad and Schneider 1992; Parsons 1951). One can envisage such medicalization leading to growth in drug treatment, but medicalization theorists focused primarily on interactions between the medical professions, patients, and health-care organizations. Until very recently, medicalization theorists paid very little attention to the pharmaceutical industry, the drug regulatory state, or patients as organized interests.

I contend that, while medicalization can account for some of the growth in pharmaceutical markets, it is only one of a constellation of sociological factors. To compensate for this, I introduce the new concept of "pharmaceuticalization," which I define as the process by which social, behavioral, or bodily conditions are treated, or deemed to be in need of treatment/intervention, with pharmaceuticals by doctors, patients, or both. For example, the treatment of mood with anxiolytics (tranquilizers and sleeping pills) or antidepressants; treatment of behavior such as attention deficit hyperactivity disorder (ADHD) with methylphenidate (Ritalin); treatment of erectile dysfunction with sildenafil (Viagra); or even treatment of heart-disease risk factors with cholesterol-lowering drugs, such as statins. Notably, not all pharmaceuticalization involves making the social medical. The appropriate treatment of bacterial infections, previously without effective drug remedies, with new antibiotics involves pharmaceuticalization, but not medicalization.

In this chapter I suggest that, in addition to medicalization, one needs to appreciate the salience of other sociological factors to explain pharmaceuticalization—specifically, the political economy of the pharmaceutical industry, consumerism, and deregulatory state ideology. I argue that these factors, while conceptually distinct, are empirically mutually interrelated, particularly by the pharmaceutical industry's power and influence in promoting its commercial interests. Overall, I conclude that these mutually interacting sociological factors almost certainly provide a better explanation for growing pharmaceuticalization than does the biomedicalism thesis.

Biomedicalism, Medicalization, and the Pharmaceuticalization of Medicine: Response to Need or Creation of Markets?

There is evidence that pharmaceuticalization is increasing along with the expansion of pharmaceutical markets. Between 1993 and 2002, National Health Service (NHS) prescriptions in England for the antidepressant drugs known as selective serotonin reuptake inhibitors (SSRIs) grew from 1,884,571 to 15,500,000; for Ritalin to treat ADHD, they grew from 3,500 to 161,800 (Department of Health 1994, 2003). In the United States, sales of the SSRI fluoxetine (Prozac) more than doubled between 1994 and 2000, sales of Viagra nearly doubled within four years of market release in 1998, and sales of Ritalin multiplied fivefold in the ten years after 1992 (Scripnews 1999, 1995; Drug Enforcement Administration 2001; Eli Lilly 2000; Timmerman 2003). In Canada, prescription of Ritalin grew fivefold between 1990 and 1995, while in New South Wales (Australia), treatment of children with drugs in 2000 was nine times the rate in 1990 (Phillips 2006, 433).

Some argue that growing pharmaceuticalization reflects advances in medical science which enable people with, say, ADHD, depression, or erectile dysfunction, who would previously have

gone undiagnosed, to be treated (Castellanos 2002; Harding 2001). On this biomedicalist view, pharmaceuticalization corresponds to meeting health needs. For example, treatment of ADHD with Ritalin (and other drugs) depends on diagnosis of an identifiable condition amenable to *biochemical* intervention. ADHD is regarded as an organic brain dysfunction—either due to reduced metabolism and inhibition in regions of the brain associated with attention and motor activity, or due to dopamine deficiency (Barkley 1997, 2003; Castellanos 2002; Couvoisie and Hooper 2003; Diller 1998; Krause et al. 2003; Zametkin et al. 1990). Additionally or alternatively, other proponents of biomedicalism contend that increasing pharmaceuticalization is the result of more sophisticated *clinical* diagnostics.

Yet, these technoscientific advances declared by biomedicalism exhibited many uncertainties within the scientific literature itself. In the case of ADHD, the brain-imaging studies have lacked replicability and suffered from problems of small sample size and experimental rigor in matching the ages of the children in control and test groups (DeGrandpre 2000; Thambirajah 1998). The hypothesis that ADHD is caused by dopamine deficiency is derived from post hoc pharmaceutical intervention, because Ritalin has been observed to help some children with ADHD while it is simultaneously believed to increase dopamine levels in the brain. However, direct measurement of dopamine levels in the brain cannot be sampled from living people, so they have to be inferred from dopamine metabolites in the blood, urine, or cerebrospinal fluid. The validity of such measurement is questionable given the existence of dopamine in other parts of the body. For similar reasons, the setting of normal levels of dopamine in the brain, from which people diagnosed with ADHD are supposed to deviate, is also problematic (Yuwiler, Brammer, and Yuwiler 1994). Indeed, it is quite possible that Ritalin's effects on some ADHD children are via some mechanism other than dopamine increase (Glenmullen 2000). Thus, the biomedicalism claim that rising pharmaceuticalization, with respect to ADHD, is due to increased identification of people with biological markers of the disease is not convincing.

Nor is it compelling that pharmaceuticalization

has been spreading because increasingly sensitive clinical diagnostics have discovered more people in need of drug treatment. For ADHD, diagnosis is based on nine criteria, of which six need to be present. Over the last forty years, the diagnostic criteria for ADHD have been consistently widened, making it virtually impossible to disentangle increased identification of ADHD sufferers from increased medicalization, and leading to concern that the threshold between normal behavior and ADHD has been set too low. For example, Goldman, Genel, and Bezman (1998) have estimated that the official diagnostic criteria for ADHD apply to almost 20 percent of school-age children in the United States. More fundamentally, the diagnostic criteria are problematic because of their overlap with normal experience or other psychiatric diagnoses. A large-scale epidemiological study found that nearly 50 percent of U.S. children satisfied the symptom-criteria for official ADHD diagnosis (Bird et al. 1990). Indeed, up to 70 percent of children in the United States diagnosed with ADHD are also diagnosed with "conduct disorder" or "oppositional defiant disorder" (Sharma, Halpern, and Newcorn 2000).

Furthermore, research in medical sociology and medicines policy over the last fifteen years has suggested that there is an alternative explanation to biomedicalism for pharmaceuticalization, namely socioinstitutional processes involving the marketing strategies of the pharmaceutical industry. Indeed, pharmaceuticalization may go hand in hand with the more established sociological concept of medicalization to form the "pharmaceuticalization-medicalization" complex, one aspect of the medical-industrial complex (Abraham 1995a). Doctors' prescribing of pharmaceuticals may increase because of widening diagnostic criteria of conditions for which new drugs are emerging or for which existing drugs may be repackaged for a new market (Conrad and Potter 2000). For example, the growth in prescriptions for antipsychotics in the West in recent decades is due to those drugs being redefined to also treat bipolar disorder—a condition whose medicalization is claimed to have increased fiftyfold since it first entered the *Diagnostic and Statistical Manual of Mental Disorders* (*DSM*) in 1980 (Healy 2006a). Simultaneously, the apparent clinical effects of a

drug combined with a hypothesized mode of action may give rise to a medical diagnosis, such as "dopamine deficiency."

It should be recognized, however, that pharmaceutical firms can achieve much of this pharmaceuticalization only with the collaboration of key parts of the medical profession.

For example, the International Obesity Task Force is a group of medical experts who work with the World Health Organization (WHO) and was widely regarded as an independent think-tank on how to define, prevent, and manage obesity. The group was one of the driving forces behind boundary changes that broadened the definitions of childhood overweight and obesity. Yet this group allowed itself to be funded by up to £1 million by pharmaceutical companies, including major manufacturers of obesity drugs, such as Roche and Abbot (Moynihan 2006).

Similarly, the UK Defeat Depression Campaign (1992–1997), which was run through the Royal College of Psychiatrists and the Royal College of General Practitioners, was sponsored by the manufacturers of antidepressants, who provided about a third of the funding. The campaign targeted doctors to emphasize in particular that these drugs did not cause addiction or dependence. Those claims have since been disputed and warnings about withdrawal symptoms are now included on the labels of those antidepressants (HCHC 2005b, 70). These disease-awareness campaigns, involving an alliance between pharmaceutical manufacturers and the medical establishment, are vital to the process of pharmaceuticalization. That such pharmaceuticalization is merely a reflection of medical need is highly questionable given that major case studies from sociology and other policy research suggest that industry-sponsored disease-awareness campaigns aimed at doctors have exaggerated the benefits and neglected serious adverse effects of tranquilizers in the 1970s and 1980s, and of antidepressants since the early 1990s (Abraham and Sheppard 1999; Healy 2004; HCHC 2005b, 69–70; Medawar 1992; Medawar and Hardon 2004).

Disease-awareness campaigns are supported by the pharmaceutical industry because they invent, develop, and sustain markets for whole classes of drugs. However, pharmaceuticalization is also driven by the promotion and advertising of individual drug products by their manufacturers to the medical profession, which might involve little or no medicalization (e.g., the promotion of painkillers). Pharmaceutical advertising and promotion are huge enterprises, and growing at a much faster rate than are pharmaceutical research and development (R&D) in most Western industrialized countries. Between 1995 and 2005, research staff numbers in the UK pharmaceutical industry actually *fell* by 2 percent, while marketing staff numbers increased dramatically, by perhaps as much as 59 percent (HCHC 2005b, 58). Similarly, in the United States, industry expenditure on marketing is about double that on R&D—US$54 billion and US$26 billion in 2000, respectively (Angell 2004, 40, 120). Such findings cast further doubt on the veracity of the biomedicalism thesis, because if the major drivers of pharmaceuticalization were scientific discoveries that meet new medical needs, rather than socioeconomic forces, then one would expect clearer evidence of growth in R&D relative to marketing activities.

Subtle aspects of drug promotion include the integration of senior members of the medical profession and medical science into pharmaceutical marketing strategies by first paying them through grants or consultancies to be involved in the development of company products and then funding them to act as "opinion leaders" who speak favorably about the drug at various symposia attended by doctors. This assimilation of allies may be combined with publication via special supplements of journals, the editors of which are company sponsored and known to be sympathetic to the product (HCHC 2005b, 56–57). Before publication, significant editorial changes may be made to scientists' manuscripts with a view to portraying the drug more positively than the author intended (Abraham 1994b). Indeed, many industry-sponsored medical articles might be written not by the researchers under whose names they appear in publication, but rather by professional medical writers working for the manufacturer—so-called ghostwriters (HCHC 2005b; Healy 2006b). Ostensibly to save the time of busy medical experts, such ghostwriting may extend market size by promoting the off-label

use of new drugs, as is believed to have occurred with the prescribing of SSRIs to children in some countries (HCHC 2005b, 54).[2]

After an article showing their drug in a positive light reaches publication, pharmaceutical companies may hire public relations firms to create an exaggerated, favorable media and professional reception. Conversely, they may delay publication of findings that reveal problems with their drug by demanding much higher standards of proof for "negative" results, such as "confirmatory" repeat studies by loyal internal company scientists (Abraham 1994a, 1995a). Frequently, negative findings about a drug are not published at all, leading to a systematic bias in the medical literature prescribing doctors read about that drug. This is mainly due to drug companies' reluctance to submit articles showing their products in an unfavorable light, though it is also partly due to journals' preference to publish positive results (HCHC 2005b, 55–56; Lexchin et al. 2003).

Doctors' continued prescribing of pharmaceutical products, and hence pharmaceuticalization, is also maintained by drug companies' strategies to contain criticism of their products as unsafe or ineffective. This may involve withdrawing funding from institutions that provide platforms for the critics' views; attempting to prevent further publication of critics' data; or using experts supportive of the company to undermine critics' concerns about the product (Abraham and Sheppard 1999; Healy 2004). For instance, internal memos of the pharmaceutical manufacturer Upjohn, released in open court, revealed that the company was willing to use what the judge called "cut-throat commercial tactics" to prevent doctors such as van der Kroef and Oswald from publicizing concerns about the dangers posed by the benzodiazepine sleeping pill triazolam (Halcion): "We [Upjohn] must stop further publication by van der Kroef in major journals. . . . We must learn everything possible about van der Kroef, and be prepared to use the evidence. It should be clear that someone is going to get hurt and this is going to be a long and tough battle. . . . Oswald paper indicated high percentage of Halcion users have problems. So far we have been successful in having it stopped" (cited in Abraham 2002, 1677, 1679).

Pharmaceuticalization and Consumerism

Alongside the growth in pharmaceuticalization has emerged rising consumerism characterized by greater reflexivity, expertise, and activism among patients. Two distinct types of consumerism vis-à-vis the medical-industrial complex can be identified: injury-oriented adversary, and access-oriented collaborator.[3] The former involves patients (or their surviving relatives, or both) who believe they have been harmed by particular drugs and who embark on campaigns and litigation against the pharmaceutical manufacturers of those drugs. Such adversarial consumerism has been more extensive and more successful in the United States than in any other country. For example, in the 1980s, plaintiffs claiming compensation against Eli Lilly for alleged injury from the antiarthritis drug benoxaprofen (marketed as Oraflex in the United States) were awarded many millions of dollars by the U.S. courts in punitive damages against the company. One plaintiff alone received US$6 million for the death of his wife from Oraflex (Abraham 1995b). Twenty years later, some U.S. plaintiffs received tens of millions of dollars of compensation in punitive damages against Merck for fatal and severe injuries allegedly caused by an antiarthritis drug marketed as Vioxx, though Merck's final payment of US$4.85 billion to settle 27,000 lawsuits claiming injury from Vioxx is generally regarded as a better outcome for the company than first expected (Berenson 2007). Even in the United States, there have been plenty of failed alleged injury cases against pharmaceutical companies. Eli Lilly won most of the cases (mostly suicide or homicide related) brought against it concerning Prozac, for instance (Cornwall 1996).

In Europe, there has been much less injury-oriented adversarial consumerism. When it has occurred, it has enjoyed much less success. For example, during the late 1980s, UK plaintiffs also embarked on extensive legal actions against Eli Lilly and the UK drug regulators following injuries associated with benoxaprofen (marketed as Opren in the UK). Similarly, patients took large-scale legal action in the early 1990s against the manufacturers of benzodiazepines, and a BBC TV *Panorama* documentary featured patients and medical experts attacking Upjohn for its handling of safety problems with Halcion. However, the Opren litigation dissipated into a low-cost out-of-court settlement offered by the company, with no blame attached to either the manufacturer or the regulators, and the legal action against benzodiazepine manufacturers collapsed, leaving many users of the drugs still without compensation, while Upjohn *won* a major libel action against the BBC regarding its documentary on Halcion (Abraham 1994b; Abraham and Sheppard 1999; HCHC 2005b, 65–66).

There are several reasons for the different fortunes of adversarial consumerism in the United States and the UK (and much of Europe). The United States is a much more litigious society with an established no-win no-fees consumer-friendly legal philosophy, while plaintiffs must pay legal fees up front in the UK or seek legal aid, which is generally not substantial enough to support complex and extensive litigation against a colossal transnational company. Moreover, U.S. lawyers are much more likely to take on a case, because of the much greater freedom of information in the United States, which enables them to see more clearly at an early stage how they could build a prosecution. This is to be contrasted with the long-standing government secrecy in the UK, which has prevented British plaintiffs from realizing that there might even be a case to answer.[4] The landscape of consumer politics is also different. The United States is home to the largest public-health advocacy group on pharmaceuticals (Public Citizen) and the largest drug-industry regulator (FDA, the Food and Drug Administration) in the world. Public Citizen has its own legal staff with regular experience using the 1967 U.S. Freedom of Information Act (FOIA) to obtain detailed information about the safety of pharmaceuticals approved by the FDA and can help plaintiffs and lawyers taking action against pharmaceutical firms (Abraham 1995b). In some cases, such as the Oraflex litigation, FDA scientists testified on behalf of the plaintiffs. By contrast, public-health advocacy organizations concerned with pharmaceuticals in the UK (and other European countries) are tiny, and the UK regulatory authorities, traditionally much closer to the pharmaceutical industry than is the FDA, sided with Eli Lilly during the Opren litigation (Abraham and Lewis 2002).

While injury-oriented adversarial consumerism occasions the presence of pharmaceutical controversies in the courts and the mass media, it does not increase pharmaceuticalization. If anything, it is likely to raise doubts in the minds of doctors and prospective patients about the safety of drug products and hence reduce pharmaceutical prescription and use. Hence, there is generally an inverse relationship between pharmaceuticalization and injury-oriented adversarial consumerism. Access-oriented collaborative consumerism, however, increases pharmaceuticalization because it involves patient groups, often in alliance with pharmaceutical firms, who seek faster access to new drugs via accelerated marketing and cost-effectiveness approval by regulators. The main focus of this type of consumerism is generally not safety but expectations about the therapeutic efficacy of a new drug. Access-oriented consumerism has also often involved public campaigns and litigation, but in collaboration with pharmaceutical manufacturers and against the government. Unlike injury-oriented adversarial consumerism, access-oriented consumerism has enjoyed considerable success on both sides of the Atlantic.

In the United States, the recent growth in access-oriented consumerism probably has its roots in the activism of HIV/AIDS patients in the late 1980s. Significant numbers of people diagnosed with HIV/AIDS organized themselves into an effective social movement, which aggressively lobbied the FDA to allow patients faster access to HIV/AIDS drugs either by accelerating approval of such drugs for the market or permitting the drugs still in development to be made more widely available, despite more limited knowledge about safety and efficacy than FDA standards had previously required (Epstein 1996). Several authors have mistakenly pointed to this AIDS activism as the principal or sole cause of major subsequent changes in FDA policies that made provisions for accelerated approval of drugs for life-threatening diseases based on less data and less thorough testing (Carpenter 2004; Daemmrich and Krucken 2000; Edgar and Rothman 1990).[5] Rather, the crucial point is that the activism had considerable support from the pharmaceutical industry, who saw it as a way to reduce the FDA's regulatory barriers to pharmaceutical markets and to induce the regulatory agency to accelerate its approval of new drugs generally, not only for HIV/AIDS or life-threatening conditions. The activists also had the support of the Reagan and Bush Senior administrations, whose deregulatory political proclivities were already putting pressure on the FDA to reduce its regulatory "burden" on industry and "innovation" (Scripnews 1988).

Since the late 1980s, the FDA has introduced many policies designed to hasten regulatory review of all types of new drugs. Between 1993 and 2003, FDA cut regulatory review times by half, and these were based on cuts made in the very early 1990s (FDA 2004). Also, from 1992, the FDA established "accelerated-approval regulations," which permit the marketing approval of particular drug products that, compared with existing treatments, appear to provide meaningful therapeutic benefits to patients with serious or life-threatening illnesses on the basis of clinical trials demonstrating that the drug product has an effect on a surrogate endpoint (i.e., nonclinical measure) that is "reasonably likely" to predict clinical benefit (Code of Federal Regulations 1992). In these respects, U.S. access-oriented collaborative consumerism has been largely successful in making drug products available to patients sooner, though it is doubtful that such haste and fast-tracking development, which involve fewer regulatory checks on drug safety and efficacy, are in the interests of public health.

For example, tumor shrinkage by anticancer drugs is a surrogate endpoint for the clinical endpoints/benefits of decreased mortality or morbidity of cancer patients, but tumor shrinkage does not necessarily deliver these clinical benefits. Thus the standard of efficacy for accelerated approval is lower than that for regular approval (Roberts and Chabner 2004). The consequence of fast tracking and accelerated approvals based on surrogate endpoints for some pharmaceuticals is a lack of data comparing the efficacy of the drugs with alternatives in relation to the relevant clinical conditions, such as mortality and morbidity. This has made it very difficult for physicians to know whether, or how, to use the drugs. The problem of not having this knowledge has been hugely compounded because some of these drugs have had serious adverse effects in some patients and, like the cancer drug Iressa, have had to be withdrawn from the market (HCHC 2005b). As Gale (2001) puts it: "Clinicians trade a known risk for an unknown risk only when there is reasonable expectation that the new therapy is better."

As the true effect on morbidity and mortality of products granted accelerated approval is unknown, approval under these regulations requires that companies must conduct postmarketing studies of the drug "to validate the surrogate endpoint or otherwise confirm the effect on the clinical endpoint" (FDA 1997). However, there is evidence that such confirmatory postmarketing studies, which are supposed to provide vital data to determine whether these new drugs do in fact have a positive benefit-risk profile, frequently have not been done. In 2004, it was reported that the FDA's Division of Oncology Drug Products had approved twenty-three new drug products or applications for new indications under the accelerated-approval legislation, but companies had completed postmarketing confirmatory studies for only six of them (Roberts and Chabner 2004). According to Fleming (2005), the average projected time for completion of these confirmatory studies for cancer drugs is ten years. This problem has not been confined to cancer drugs. According to Mitka (2003), only half of all accelerated-approval drugs had completed postmarketing confirmatory studies in the United States by May 2003.

In the UK, access-oriented collaborative consumerism has also enjoyed considerable victories in alliance with pharmaceutical firms. Much of the focus has been on patient access to new drugs on the NHS, which pays the full cost of drug treatment in the UK provided that the appropriate NHS authorities approve funding. A crucial body in this respect is the National Institute for Health and Clinical Excellence (NICE), which assesses the cost-effectiveness of many new drugs for use in the NHS after they have received marketing approval from UK drug-regulatory authorities, the Medicines and Healthcare products Regulatory Agency (MHRA). Access-oriented collaborative consumerism is a more recent phenomenon in the UK than in the United States but has grown significantly since the late 1990s.

For example, NICE recommended the use of the drug Herceptin on the NHS for advanced breast cancer in March 2002, but there was no such advice for its use to treat early-stage breast cancer. Indeed, at that time the manufacturer, Roche, had not even submitted data to the MHRA in support of a licensing application to have the drug approved to treat early-stage breast cancer in the UK. However, in May 2005, a U.S. trial of the drug with women suffering from early-stage breast cancer reported promising results. A few months later, when a woman with early-stage breast cancer in England was refused Herceptin on the NHS, she threatened litigation in the national media. After publication of the promising U.S. trial, Roche hired a public relations firm to contact some women in the UK with breast cancer to ask them if they would be willing to help to get the drug funded on the NHS before NICE, or even MHRA, approval (BBC News 24 2006b). In October 2005, the secretary of state for health, Patricia Hewitt, responded to the increasingly public controversy by stating on national television that all breast-cancer sufferers should have access to the drug, even though Roche had still not made a licensing application for full regulatory review of Herceptin for such use. After Hewitt's intervention, the NHS reversed its decision, obviating the need for a very public court case. However, when the NHS withheld Herceptin from another woman with early-stage breast cancer, its decision was overruled in a high-profile court case in April 2006 (BBC News 24 2006a). In June 2006, after Herceptin had been licensed for treatment of early-stage breast cancer by the MHRA, NICE speedily recommended it for such use on the NHS under a cloud of suspicion that it had been rushed into doing so by patient pressure (BBC News 24 2006b).

Further evidence of the significance of access-oriented collaborative consumerism may be observed regarding drugs for Alzheimer's disease. In March 2005, NICE recommended that the NHS not fund four drug treatments licensed for Alzheimer's (Aricept, Exelon, Reminyl, and Ebixa) because they were not cost-effective. However, following a high-profile campaign in the media and a formal appeal involving patient groups such as the Alzheimer's Society, NICE revised its guidance to allow NHS funding of the drugs for people in moderate stages of the disease, but still not those with early-stage Alzheimer's. The Alzheimer's Society then took NICE to the courts, which ultimately insisted that NICE should investigate ways of making the drugs available to all those with the disease (BBC News 24 2007). Notably, the manufacturers of these Alzheimer's drugs were the lead claimants in the court case and centrally involved in the formal appeal to NICE—a form of collaborative activism that also occurred with the Multiple Sclerosis Society's campaign for access to beta-interferon on the NHS (BBC News 24 2007).

The evidence suggests that the apparent power of consumer/patient activism to achieve its objectives in pharmaceutical controversies depends significantly on whether it is supporting or contravening the fundamental interests of the pharmaceutical industry. Failure is not inevitable when opposing the industry, as some adversarial consumerism in the United States has shown, but success is much more likely with industry support. More germane to the analysis here, the failures of injury-oriented adversarial consumerism and the successes of access-oriented collaborative consumerism almost certainly combine to produce pro-pharmaceuticalization consequences that outweigh the countervailing effects of the less pervasive successes of adversarial consumerism.

Moreover, collaborative consumerism is likely to become a permanent feature of the pharmaceutical landscape, because many patient organizations that campaign for availability of better treatments for various medical conditions not only have formed alliances with drug manufacturers when tactically advantageous but also, in the last decade, have become increasingly *funded* by pharmaceutical companies (O'Donovan 2007). For example, in the United States, the preeminent advocacy group for people with ADHD is Children and Adults with Attention Deficit/Hyperactivity Disorder (CHADD), 22 percent of whose revenue in 2004–2005 came from the pharmaceutical industry (Phillips 2006, 434). While the precise effects of pharmaceutical firms' financial support on patient groups are difficult to gauge, such close associations are clearly important to the industry as an additional pathway,

beyond doctors, for creating consumer demand for their products (Herxheimer 2003). In a survey of U.S. executives from fourteen pharmaceutical companies, 75 percent of respondents cited "patient education" as the top-ranked marketing activity necessary to bring a brand to "the number one spot" (HCHC 2005b, 74–76).

The interaction between pharmaceuticalization and consumerism is even more complex if one includes debates about patient education and direct-to-consumer advertising (DTCA) of prescription drugs. In Europe and most other Western industrialized countries, pharmaceutical companies are not allowed to advertise or promote their prescription medicinal products directly to patients or the general public, but such DTCA is legal in the United States and New Zealand. In the United States, many physicians at the FDA and even many pharmaceutical companies believed that DTCA of prescription drugs was inappropriate when it first entered FDA policy debate in the early 1980s (U.S. House Subcommittee 1984). Indeed, historically, the claim by the research-based firms that they produced solely medical drugs for the medical profession and did not flirt with the fancies of the general public was how that part of the industry defined itself as "ethical" (Abraham 1995b, 39). However, when the FDA lifted its moratorium on DTCA in 1985, the industry could not resist the lure of sales and profits, and U.S. pharmaceutical companies spent US$12 billion on (mostly print) DTCA in 1989 (Conrad and Leiter 2009, 17).[6] However, the FDA retained cumbersome "fair balance" and "brief summary" regulations for *broadcast* DTCA, which greatly limited the industry's use of that media. In 1997 the FDA markedly relaxed these regulations in line with demands from the pharmaceutical industry and the Republican-dominated antiregulation Congress, now keen to expand DTCA. The extent of patient demand for extensive broadcast DTCA is unclear, though consumer expectations were often cited by the industry, Congress, and FDA as the justification for relaxing the regulations. Broadcast DTCA in the United States grew from US$55 million in 1991 to US$4.2 billion in 2005 with a 330 percent growth in DTCA from 1996 to 2005 (Conrad and Leiter 2009).

The experience of print, and especially broadcast, DTCA in the United States since 1997 is that it has contributed to the growth in medicalization and pharmaceuticalization because it has encouraged consumers to self-diagnose and then increasingly to ask doctors for advertised pharmaceutical products, which, in turn, has led to increased prescribing of those products (Mintzes et al. 2003). To a much greater extent than before, physicians have become gatekeepers for drugs advertised directly to consumers, rather than initiators of pharmaceutical treatment. The health informational value of DTCA for patients has proved questionable, as most U.S. physicians believe that the advertisements do not provide balanced information. Moreover, there is evidence that patients prompted by DTCA to request drugs from their doctors are much more likely to receive prescriptions for those drugs than are patients who make no such requests, even though, in some cases, as many as half of those prescriptions might be for drugs without evidence to support therapeutic efficacy in treating the condition (Conrad and Leiter 2009, 21).

Meanwhile, in Europe during the last decade, the pharmaceutical industry, with support from the European Commission's director-general for enterprise, has campaigned vigorously but so far unsuccessfully for the legalization of DTCA of prescription drugs in the European Union (EU).[7] This campaign characterized patients as consumers able to decide which drugs are best for them without doctors' supervision. It utilized a discourse of "the informed patient" and the "expert patient," which was subsequently adopted uncritically by some national European governments, including the UK Department of Health (2001). Doctors' failure to adequately inform patients about prescription medicines is a significant problem (Britten 2008). However, as the U.S. experience has shown, while DTCA can sometimes raise awareness about illnesses and availability of medical treatments, it is a considerable leap of faith to embrace a policy based on the assumption that pharmaceutical companies will fill the gap left by doctors in this respect. Furthermore, that assumption lacks any analysis of the interests involved and remarkably ignores the evidence of widespread problems for public health and

health-care resources posed by misleading advertisements to doctors, let alone patients.

The expert-patient discourse can be put in its proper sociological context by relating it to the interests of those planning to provide the information intended to construct patient expertise and to the ideological nature of its emergence. The UK research-based pharmaceutical industry led the way, probably because London is home to the EU's drug-regulatory agency, the European Medicines Evaluation Agency (EMEA). Quoting from a speech by the director-general of the Association of the British Pharmaceutical Industry (ABPI), Medawar and Hardon (2004, 121) report that the 1998 "Informed Patient Initiative" was the first part of the industry's "battle plan," while the second part was the ABPI's publication "The Expert Patient," which according to the director-general was "part of a softening-up assault to be mounted through those interested parties and opinion leaders by stimulating debate." Evidently, the purpose of the campaign was to promote a consumerist ideology of patient self-care and self-medication in order to create a basis for arguing that patients are sufficiently knowledgeable to evaluate advertising claims about powerful prescription drugs. As the following passage from an article published in *Pharmaceutical Marketing* suggests, the industry hoped that the creation of such consumerist ideology would be sufficient to compel European regulators and governments to legalize DTCA throughout the EU:

> The ABPI battle plan is to employ ground troops in the form of patient support groups, sympathetic medical opinion and healthcare professionals which will lead the debate on the informed patient issue. This will have the effect of weakening political, ideological and professional defences. . . . Then the ABPI will follow through with high-level precision strikes on specific regulatory enclaves in both Whitehall and Brussels. (Jeffries 2000, quoted in Medawar and Hardon 2004, 121)

To date, the European Parliament has refused complete legalization of DTCA. It has concluded that it would not be in the interests of patients' health. Nevertheless, the consumerist ideology surrounding the campaign left its mark on European pharmaceutical policy frameworks. For example, after consultation with the pharmaceutical industry, and following the extensive opposition to complete legalization of DTCA, the EU Commission proposed new legislation in 2008 that would maintain the general ban on DTCA but would allow industry to provide "additional information" to the public via the media (Richards 2008). Many EU public-health organizations, medical professionals, and some national government health agencies have opposed relaxation of the ban, underlining the crucial role of health professionals in the provision of tailored information to patients, and pointing to the practical difficulties of regulating and enforcing the distinction between "information" and "advertisement" (Association Internationale de la Mutualité et al. 2008).

Specifically, DTCA might encourage doctors to prescribe obesity drugs (recommended only after patients' lifestyle modifications are unsuccessful) when a change in diet, exercise, or some other lifestyle change is more appropriate (Padwal and Majumdar 2007). In highly prevalent conditions such as obesity, this could create major problems for public health (McCarthy 2004). In the UK, between 1980 and 1996, the prevalence of obesity increased from 6 to 17 percent of the population, and between 1993 and 2002 the percentage of overweight and obese adults rose from 59 to 65 (Ferriman 1999; Kopelman 2005, 65). With the number of obese adults in England predicted to exceed twelve million by 2010, the cost to the NHS just to treat all those people clinically defined as obese with drugs is estimated at £750 million per year (BBC News 24 1999; O'Dowd 2006).

Biomedicalism, Pharmaceutical Innovation, and Deregulatory Ideology

By looking at case studies and macro-organizational factors, I suggested in the previous sections that the sociological processes of medicalization, industry promotion, deregulatory ideology, and consumerism are much more likely explanations for growing pharmaceuticalization than the biomedicalism thesis that such growth simply reflects advances in science to meet medical need.

However, it is clearly possible that, while such sociological processes might be significant, the biomedicalism thesis could still be correct, because *most* of the explanation for increased pharmaceuticalization lies in technoscientific advances in drug therapy. For instance, if a new antibiotic that could kill previously resistant strains of TB were discovered, then one would not readily attribute its uptake by doctors and patients to medicalization, industry promotion, deregulatory ideology, or consumerism. This could be because TB is already a well-recognized medical condition, the drug has been shown to eliminate the relevant bacterial strain by the most rigorous regulatory standards, irrespective of industry promotion, and patients really get better by any measure of respiratory condition. Thus, to obtain a more comprehensive characterization of pharmaceuticalization, sociological analysis must also examine the extent to which pharmaceutical product innovation contributes new medical drugs that are really needed by doctors and patients (therapeutic advance).

Such an analysis is conceptually intricate and empirically imperfect because of the incomplete nature of databases. Nevertheless, one begins by noting that, in all conventional pharmaceutical-policy literature, a drug product innovation is defined as a new molecular entity (NME) that is brought to the market. An NME is defined as a patentable *technical* novelty—it has a unique molecular structure (Vos 1991). Thus, a patent is awarded to protect commercially the intellectual property embedded in the discovery of the NME, and the transformation of an NME into a drug innovation depends only on meeting the commercial criterion of advance into the marketplace. It follows that the conventional definition of pharmaceutical product innovation is based on technological and commercial criteria, but does not necessarily imply that a new drug innovation offers any therapeutic advance *unless that is a requirement for marketing approval imposed by regulatory agencies*. However, regulatory agencies in the EU, North America, Australasia, and most other industrialized countries have never imposed such a requirement.[8] Pharmaceuticals legislation requires only that manufacturers demonstrate the quality, safety, and efficacy of their products. It does not require that those new products deliver therapeutic advance over drugs already available (Abraham 2004; Abraham and Lewis 2000).

A distinction, therefore, has to be drawn between pharmaceutical innovation and therapeutic advance—the latter necessarily involving a product that provides some therapeutic advantage in relation to efficacy, safety, or ease of administration and use over existing therapies (International Society of Drug Bulletins 2001). For example, many NMEs do not represent any (significant) therapeutic advance, no matter how novel in technological terms or how extensive their entrance into the marketplace. Conversely, new indications or new dosing schedules for, and new combinations of, already marketed products may well offer a therapeutic advantage for patients, no matter how old the products (HCHC 2005b). While product innovation retains commercial significance for pharmaceutical manufacturers, irrespective of therapeutic advance, it is generally the latter that satisfies the medical needs of patients, public health, and health professionals.

Thus, a major challenge for the sociology of pharmaceuticals is to untangle the dominant policy and popular discourse on innovation, which conflates technological novelty and commercial viability with therapeutic progress, and to refocus attention on innovations that offer therapeutic advance, rather than on innovation per se. Before considering the contentious issue of trends in therapeutic advance, it is worth noting that data from the FDA and the UK-based, ABPI-funded Centre for Medicines Research show that pharmaceutical product innovation in the United States and globally has been declining over the same period in which growing pharmaceuticalization has been witnessed (Figures 17.1 and 17.2). Between 2004 and 2008, FDA data show that the number of NMEs continued to decline at an annual average of twenty per year. Of course, these data do not reveal whether the number of NMEs, which offer significant therapeutic advance, has also been falling, but it is highly suggestive that the biomedicalism thesis is unlikely to explain most of the growth in pharmaceuticalization.

Remarkably, neither the MHRA nor the EMEA even collect data on the subset of NMEs that offer significant therapeutic advance, and the MHRA testified in 2005 that they saw no need to do so (HCHC 2005a). Nor does the Japanese drug-regulatory agency provide any English-language data on the proportion of NMEs offering therapeutic advance.[9] Consequently, there is no quantitative official government data on the extent to which the pharmaceutical industry is producing new drugs that offer therapeutic advance in the second- and third-largest pharmaceutical markets in the world, namely the EU and Japan, respectively. This demonstrates the influence of the dominant technical and commercial discourses on pharmaceutical innovation within governments and policy making, even though the primary objective of new drugs, which governments represent to citizens in public discourse, is to meet health needs.

Nevertheless, in the United States, the world's largest pharmaceutical market, the FDA does distinguish between NMEs that offer significant therapeutic advance and those that do not as part of its drug-regulatory review process. Those that do are given "priority" review status, while the others receive "standard" review status. Table 17.1 shows that between 1993 and 2003, only 152 of the total 359 (42 percent) NMEs were judged to offer significant therapeutic advance. From 2004 to 2008, the figure rose slightly but remained below 50 percent (FDA 2009). Each year typically more than half the drugs, conventionally defined as innovations and submitted to the FDA, offered little or no therapeutic advantage over the drugs already on the market. More importantly to my concerns in this chapter, the number of NMEs offering significant therapeutic advance has also been declining in this period of growth in pharmaceuticalization. The situation may be worse than the FDA figures imply, because when the French organization of medical and pharmaceutical professionals, La Revue Prescrire (2005), reviewed 3,100 new drugs or new indications for existing drugs in the period 1981 to 2004 (most of which were on the French, EU, or U.S. markets), they concluded that only 10 percent offered moderate to significant therapeutic advance. From the perspective of therapeutic contribution to global health needs, the picture is stark. Of the 1,393 NMEs approved between 1975 and 1999, only 13 drugs (less than 1 percent)

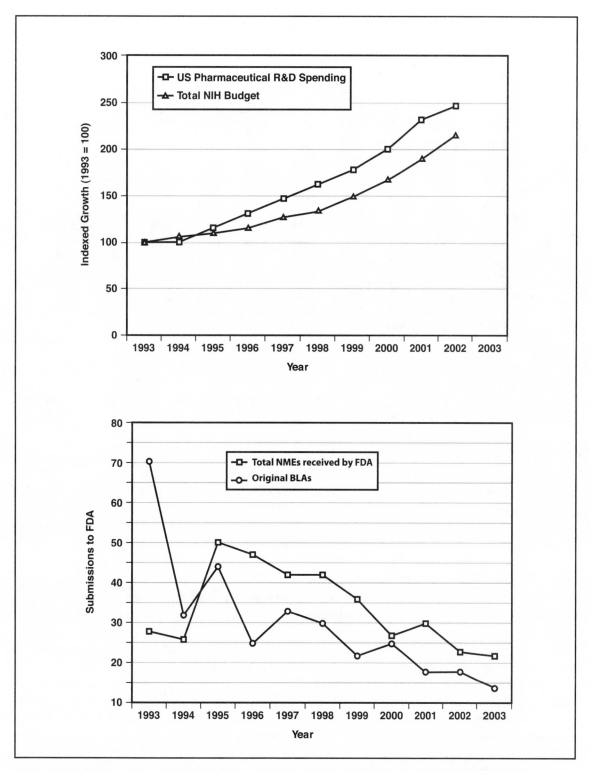

Figure 17.1. Ten-year trends in major drug and biological product submissions to FDA (fda.gov/oc/initiatives/criticalpath/nwoodcodk0602.html). NMEs are new molecular entities; BLAs are biologics license applications.

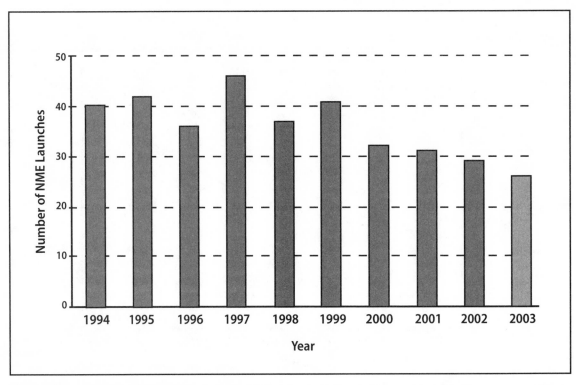

Figure 17.2. Number of new molecular entities first launched onto the world market between 1994 and 2003 (Center for Medicines Research 2005)

were specifically indicated for much-needed treatment of tropical diseases (Selgelid and Sepers 2006, 156).

Thus, there is no convincing evidence to support the biomedicalism thesis that, overall, most of the growth in pharmaceuticalization in the last fifteen years is the result of scientific discoveries producing a plethora of new medicines addressing unmet health needs. On the contrary, the evidence suggests that, while pharmaceuticalization has been growing, the contribution from scientific R&D to deliver drugs that are really needed to treat illnesses has been declining. These findings also signify that a much more complex sociological analysis of pharmaceutical innovation and markets is required than the conventional wisdom among industry and governments that if the sector is less regulated, then the potential of biomedicine can be released to produce therapeutically valuable innovations. That conventional wisdom may be regarded as a policy

ally of the biomedicalism thesis because, like the biomedicalism thesis, it tends to deny the enormous importance of sociological factors such as medicalization, industry promotion, deregulatory ideology, and consumerism.

In fact, by examining trends in both drug-regulatory policies and innovation in Europe and the United States, one finds that deregulatory policies during the 1980s and 1990s (e.g., of Reagan and Bush Senior administrations and the Republican Congress in the United States, and the Thatcher, Major, and Blair governments in the UK) have been followed by *declines* in innovation. As I noted earlier, from 1990 the FDA drastically cut its time to review and approve both priority *and* standard NMEs largely in response to complaints by the pharmaceutical industry and anti-regulation think tanks that overregulation was inhibiting innovation (Kaitin and DiMasi 2000; Kessler et al. 1996). The industry-funded American Enterprise Institute and the Tufts Centre had at-

Table 17.1. FDA review and approval times (in months) for priority and standard new molecular entities, 1993–2003

Calendar Year	Priority			Standard		
	Number approved	Median FDA review time	Median total approval time	Number approved	Median FDA review time	Median total approval time
1993	13	13.9	14.9	12	27.2	27.2
1994	12	13.9	14.0	9	22.2	23.7
1995	10	7.9	7.9	19	15.9	17.8
1996	18	7.7	9.6	35	14.6	15.1
1997	9	6.4	6.7	30	14.4	15.0
1998	16	6.2	6.2	14	12.3	13.4
1999	19	6.3	6.9	16	14.0	16.3
2000	9	6.0	6.0	18	15.4	19.9
2001	7	6.0	6.0	17	15.7	19.0
2002	7	13.8	16.3	10	12.5	15.9
2003	9	6.7	6.7	12	13.8	23.1

Source: fda.gov/AboutFDA/ReportsManualsForms/Reports/UserFeeReports/PerformanceReports/PDUFA/default.htm

tacked the FDA for depriving U.S. doctors and patients of innovations because the agency was relatively cautious about approving new drugs compared with the UK and some other European countries (Grabowski, Vernon, and Thomas 1978; Wardell 1973). For these U.S. critics, whose views became influential during the Reagan–Bush Senior era, the UK's lighter-touch regulation was superior to the FDA's approach because, they argued, it delivered in a more timely manner more pharmaceutical innovations that patients and doctors needed.

It is true that during the 1970s and 1980s, the FDA was slower in approving NMEs overall than were regulatory authorities in the UK and many other European countries. However, Schweitzer, Schweitzer, and Sourty-Le Guellec (1996) analyzed the approval dates of thirty-four pharmaceuticals marketed in the G-7 countries plus Switzerland between 1970 and 1988 and designated especially therapeutically significant by panels of doctors and pharmacists in the United States and France. The FDA was found to have approved *more* of these drugs *before* the UK regulatory authorities had and ranked third out of the eight countries in approving these drugs onto the market. This suggests that the FDA's comparative slowness in approving NMEs as a whole, during the 1970s and 1980s, may be largely irrelevant

to a discussion about the crucial subset of NMEs that are of significant therapeutic value to patients, medical professionals, and public health.

Similar trends have occurred in Europe. For example, the average net in-house review times of the UK regulatory agency for new drugs fell from 154 working days in 1989 to just 44 days by 1998. The regulatory review times of Germany, Sweden, and many other EU countries also fell dramatically in this period (Abraham and Lewis 2000, 20). It is generally acknowledged that there is a ten-year lag between a regulatory reform and its effects on pharmaceutical innovation, so the declines in innovation between 1995 and 2005 are associated with the deregulatory reforms between the early 1980s and early 1990s in the United States and Europe. Hence, it appears that deregulatory ideology (and associated policies) were drivers of growing pharmaceuticalization *not* primarily by releasing many more innovations needed by patients and medical professionals, as the biomedicalism thesis would have it, but rather mainly by allowing the industry to expand its markets for drugs that offer little or no therapeutic advance in a sea of declining innovation.

Nowhere is this more evident than in the case of antibiotics. By the late 1980s and early 1990s, it was known to biomedical scientists that bacterial resistance to existing antibiotics was becoming a significant health problem in both developed and developing countries (Blumberg, Carroll, and Wachsmuth 1991; Mastro et al. 1991; O'Neill and McIntosh 1987; Vallejo, Kaplan, and Mason 1991; van Klingeren, Dessens-Kroon, and Verheuvel 1989). This problem has grown steadily since. By 2004, the World Health Organization ranked infections caused by drug-resistant bacteria as the area of medical need where there was the largest "pharmaceutical gap," above even AIDS and malaria (WHO 2004). Clearly, then, between the late 1980s and 2004, there was a real health need for the development of new antibiotics to which bacteria would not be resistant. This was also a period of growing pharmaceuticalization and deregulatory-reform policies and ideology.

Yet, between 1983 and 2004, the development of antibiotics declined steadily: the FDA approved 16 between 1983 and 1987; 14 between 1988 and 1992; 10 between 1993 and 1997; 7 between 1998 and 2002; and just 3 in 2003 and 2004 (Infectious Diseases Society of America 2004, 15). Regarding antibiotics under development that might be approved after 2004, Spellberg et al. (2004) found that of 506 molecules under development in 2002 at twenty-two major pharmaceutical and biotechnology companies, only 6 were antibiotics. Despite this, Bradley and colleagues (2007, 68), from the Antimicrobial Availability Task Force of IDSA, find that "two years later, very little has changed." Talbot and colleagues (2006) identified six resistant pathogens posing serious threats to patients for which there are few or no drugs in late-stage development. To explain this, Bradley and colleagues (2007, 68) conclude: "Anti-infective drug products are less profitable than other types of medicines, particularly those for chronic conditions. . . . As a result, many major pharmaceutical companies have decided to focus their research and development efforts elsewhere, leaving the pipeline in this essential field dangerously dry." Evidently, pharmaceuticalization and the production of new drugs that are needed for world health are quite different, and only loosely related, phenomena, because the political economy of the pharmaceutical industry as currently constituted, not therapeutic value, tends to determine the nature and direction of innovation.

Conclusion

Overall, pharmaceutical markets have expanded in the last few decades in many societies. While this may partly result from general economic growth, there is considerable evidence that it is largely due to increased pharmaceuticalization of our societies. The biomedicalism thesis, popular among many scientists and media discourses, that growing pharmaceuticalization simply reflects discoveries in biomedical science that correspond to health needs is not plausible. Some pharmaceuticalization may fall into this category, but there is no good reason to support the thesis that most of it can be explained in this way. Indeed, there is evidence to suggest that, while pharmaceuticalization has increased, the number of medications needed by patients and public health is actually decreasing, along with pharmaceutical innovation.

Growing pharmaceuticalization seems to be best explained by sociological factors such as the political economy of the pharmaceutical industry and associated medicalization (especially promotion and advertising activities involving physicians and clinicians), deregulatory ideology toward drug development and innovation, and access-oriented collaborative consumerism, which outweighs the countervailing effects of adversarial consumerism. The sociological analysis required to explain pharmaceuticalization is complex because those factors are not mutually independent; rather they interact with each other. Medicalization can facilitate, even stimulate, pharmaceutical development and promotion, but it can also be shaped by industry-driven technoscience and marketing strategies. Furthermore, medicalization can be encouraged as an interim stage toward pharmaceuticalization by patients' self-diagnoses and demands for medications. Yet, such demands may themselves be strongly influenced, sustained, or even created by industry promotion, advertising, and financial support. While industry promotion, medicalization, and consumerism can all encourage the growth of pharmaceuticalization, such growth is substantially, though not entirely, dependent on a regulatory state that is willing to grant marketing approval to drugs that offer no therapeutic advance, to lower regulatory standards of efficacy in order to accelerate more NMEs on to the market, and indeed to relax restrictions or prohibitions on DTCA of prescription medications.

The pharmaceutical industry has proved versatile. Its presence is notable in all the areas contributing to the growth of pharmaceuticalization. Drug firms work with (and undermine when necessary) members of the medical profession in order to secure the viability of products while simultaneously supporting DTCA and the discourse of "expert patient," which are generally opposed by medical and health professionals. The industry encourages consumerism when it is about patients' access to medications but vigorously contests the relevance and expertise of consumerism when it condemns the safety problems of some pharmaceutical products. Perhaps most importantly, the industry has persuaded government drug-regulatory agencies that the economic performance of the industry is so important that state intervention should become involved in fostering its commercial success, rather than give unambiguous and unrivalled priority to the protection of public health, irrespective of the private interests of industry.

One may conclude that pharmaceuticalization has expanded largely because the drug industry has used its power to have a central influence on all the key sociological factors driving the phenomenon. Consequently, pharmaceuticalization has increased mainly in accordance with the commercial interests of the pharmaceutical industry. However, contrary to what would follow from the biomedicalism thesis, a pharmaceuticalization process driven by the interests of the industry has not to a very significant extent delivered drug products in response to medical and health needs.

Notes

1. For the purposes of brevity and focus, this chapter is almost exclusively concerned with prescription pharmaceuticals in Europe and North America.
2. Off-label use occurs when a doctor prescribes a medication for a condition not sanctioned by the regulatory authorities, and hence not stipulated on the label.

3. Arguably, there is a third type, namely access-oriented adversary, which has been particularly relevant to some developing countries where patient activists have campaigned against pharmaceutical firms in order to force them to sell their drugs at affordable prices, especially antiretroviral medications for HIV/AIDS.
4. In 2005, the UK introduced a Freedom of Information Act, but it is very weak compared with its U.S. counterpart and has made only a tiny dent in the conventional secrecy of British pharmaceutical regulation.
5. This activism may not have been in the interests of HIV/AIDS patients, because subsequent research has suggested that the early drugs that were rushed on to the market, such as AZT, may have offered little or no therapeutic benefit, were highly toxic, and may even have weakened patients' immune systems (WTO 2006).
6. The FDA represented this shift as a response to inferred patient demand, but it may have been influenced by the deregulatory ideology of the Reagan administration.
7. A proposal to relax the ban on DTCA in the EU is currently under consideration by the European Parliament. If passed, then from 2010 the industry would be permitted to provide some "information" about their products directly to consumers via some media.
8. Norway had a "needs" clause (requiring new drugs to demonstrate therapeutic advance over existing products on the market) in its pharmaceutical regulation until 1994, when the national government abandoned it in expectation of joining the EU and hence of conforming to the EU's supranational rules of "fair competition."
9. I have been unable to ascertain data availability in Japanese.

References

Abraham, John. 1994a. "Bias in Science and Medical Knowledge: The Opren Controversy." *Sociology* 28:717–36.

———. 1994b. "Distributing the Benefit of the Doubt: Scientists, Regulators and Drug Safety." *Science, Technology and Human Values* 19:493–522.

———. 1995a. "The Production and Reception of Scientific Papers in the Medical-Industrial Complex: Clinical Evaluation of New Medicines." *British Journal of Sociology* 46:167–90.

———. 1995b. *Science, Politics and the Pharmaceutical Industry*. London and New York: UCL/St. Martin's Press/Routledge.

———. 2002. "Transnational Industrial Power, the

Medical Profession and the Regulatory State: Adverse Drug Reactions and the Crisis over the Safety of Halcion in the Netherlands and the UK." *Social Science and Medicine* 55:1671–90.

———. 2004. "Pharmaceuticals, the State and the Global Harmonisation Process." *Australian Health Review* 28:150–61.

Abraham, John, and Graham Lewis. 2000. *Regulating Medicines in Europe: Competition, Expertise and Public Health*. London: Routledge.

———. 2002. "Citizenship, Medical Expertise and the Capitalist Regulatory State in Europe." *Sociology* 36:67–88.

Abraham, John, and Julie Sheppard. 1999. *The Therapeutic Nightmare: The Battle over the World's Most Controversial Sleeping Pill*. London: Earthscan.

Angell, Marci. 2004. *The Truth about Drug Companies*. New York: Random House.

Applbaum, K. 2006. "Pharmaceutical Marketing and the Invention of the Medical Consumer." *Public Library of Science Medicine* 3:445–47.

Association Internationale de la Mutualité (AIM), European Social Insurance Platform (ESIP), Health Action International (HAI), International Society of Drug Bulletins (ISDB), and Medicines in Europe Forum (MiEF). 2008. "Legal Proposals on 'Information' to Patients by Pharmaceutical Companies: A Threat to Public Health." Joint briefing paper. March 6. prescrire.org/docus/LegalProposalsInfoPatient_JointPaper_March2009.pdf.

Barkley, Russell. 1997. "Behavioral Inhibition, Sustained Attention, and Executive Functions: Constructing a Unifying Theory of ADHD." *Psychological Bulletin* 121:65–94.

———. 2003. "Attention-Deficit/Hyperactivity Disorder." In *Child Psychopathology*, ed. Russell Barkley and Eric Mash, 75–143. New York: Guildford Press.

BBC News 24. 1999. "Tough Guidance on Obesity Drugs." January 13. news.bbc.co.uk.

———. 2006a. "Herceptin: Was Patient Power Key?" June 9. news.bbc.co.uk.

———. 2006b. "Woman Wins Herceptin Court Fight." April 12. news.bbc.co.uk.

———. 2007. "Alzheimer's Drugs Remain Limited." August 10. news.bbc.co.uk.

Berenson, A. 2007. "Analysts See Merck Victory in Vioxx Deal." *New York Times*, November 10.

Bird, H., T. J. Yager, B. Staghezza, and M. S. Gould. 1990. "Impairment in the Epidemiological Measurement of Childhood Psychopathology in the Community." *Journal of the American Academy of Childhood and Adolescent Psychiatry* 29:796–803.

Blumberg, H. M., D. J. Carroll, and I. K. Wachsmuth.

1991. "Rapid Development of Ciprofloxacin Resistance in Methicillin-Susceptible and -Resistant Staphylococcus Aureus." *Journal of Infectious Diseases* 163:1279–85.

Bradley, J. S., R. Guidos, S. Baragona, and J. G. Bartlett. 2007. "Anti-Infective Research and Development—Problems, Challenges, and Solutions." *Lancet Infectious Diseases* 7:68–69.

Britten, Nicola. 2008. *Medicines and Society*. Basingstoke, Eng.: Palgrave.

Carpenter, Daniel P. 2004. "The Political Economy of FDA Drug Review: Processing, Politics and Lessons for Policy." *Health Affairs* 23:52–63.

Castellanos, X. 2002. "Development Trajectories of Brain Volume Abnormalities in Children and Adults with ADHD." *Journal of the American Medical Association* 288:1740–48.

Centre for Medicines Research. 2005. "Innovation on the Wane?" Latest News. www.cmr.org.

Code of Federal Regulations. 1992. "Accelerated Approval of New Drugs for Serious or Life-Threatening Illnesses." CFR Part 314, Subpart H.

Conrad, Peter, and Valerie Leiter. 2009. "From Lydia Pinkham to Queen Levitra: Direct-to-Consumer Advertising and Medicalization." In *Pharmaceuticals and Society: Critical Discourses and Debates*, ed. Simon J. Williams, Jonathon Gabe, and Peter Davis, 12–24. Chichester, Eng.: Wiley-Blackwell.

Conrad, Peter, and D. Potter. 2000. "From Hyperactive Children to ADHD Adults." *Social Problems* 47:559–82.

Conrad, Peter, and J. W. Schneider. 1992. *Deviance and Medicalization: From Badness to Sickness*. Philadelphia: Temple University Press.

Cornwall, John. 1996. *The Power to Harm: Mind, Murder and Drugs on Trial*. Harmondsworth, Eng.: Penguin.

Couvoisie, H., and S. R. Hooper. 2003. "Neurometabolic Functioning and Neuro-Psychological Correlates in Children with ADHD: Preliminary Findings." *Journal of Neuro-Psychiatry and Clinical Neuro-Sciences* 16:63–69.

Daemmrich, Arthur, and Georg Krucken. 2000. "Risk versus Risk: Decision-Making Dilemmas of Drug Regulation in the U.S. and Germany." *Science as Culture* 9:505–34.

DeGrandpre, R. 2000. *Ritalin Nation: Rapid-Fire Culture and the Transformation of Human Consciousness*. New York: W. W. Norton.

Diller, L. 1998. *Running on Ritalin: A Physician Reflects on Children, Society and Performance in a Pill*. New York: Bantam Books.

Drug Enforcement Administration. 2001. *Aggregate Production Quota History, 1992–2002*. Washington, D.C.: Department of Justice.

Edgar, H., and D. J. Rothman. 1990. "New Rules for New Drugs: The Challenge of AIDS to the Regulatory Process." *Milbank Quarterly* 68, suppl. 1:111–42.

Eli Lilly. 2000. *Eli Lilly Annual Report 2000*.

Epstein, Steven. 1996. *Impure Science: AIDS, Activism, and the Politics of Knowledge*. Berkeley: University of California Press.

FDA [Food and Drug Administration]. 1997. Modernization Act. Section 506(b)(3) of the Food, Drug and Cosmetic Act (as amended by Section 112 of FDAMA). Washington, D.C.: GPO.

———. 2004. "Review and Approval Times for Priority and Standards NMEs." www.fda.gov.

———. 2009. "CDER Approval Times for Priority and Standard NMEs, 1993–2008." www.fda.gov/cder/rdmt/default.htm.

Ferriman, A. 1999. "Fat Is a Medical Issue." *British Medical Journal* 318:144.

Fleming, T. R. 2005. "Surrogate Endpoints and FDA's Accelerated Approval Process." *Health Affairs* 24:67–78.

Gale, E. A. M. 2001. "Lessons from the Glitazones." *Lancet* 357:1871.

Glenmullen, J. 2000. *Prozac Backlash: Overcoming the Dangers of Prozac, Zoloft and Paxil and Other Antidepressants with Safe, Effective Alternatives*. New York: Simon and Schuster.

Goldman, L. S., M. Genel, and R. J. Bezman. 1998. "Diagnosis and Treatment of ADHD in Children and Adolescents." *Journal of the American Medical Association* 279:1100–1107.

Grabowski, H., J. Vernon, and L. Thomas. 1978. "Estimating the Effects of Regulation on Innovation: An International Comparative Analysis of the Pharmaceutical Industry." *Journal of Law and Economics* 21:133–63.

Harding, R. 2001. "Unlocking the Brain's Secrets." *Family Circle*, November 20, 10–11.

Healy, David. 2004. *Let Them Eat Prozac*. London: New York University Press.

———. 2006a. "The Latest Mania: Selling Bipolar Disorder." *Public Library of Science Medicine* 3:441–44.

———. 2006b. "The New Medical Oikumene." In *Global Pharmaceuticals*, ed. Adriana Petryna, Andrew Lakoff, and Arthur Kleinman, 61–84. Durham, N.C.: Duke University Press.

Herxheimer, Andrew. 2003. "Relationships between the Pharmaceutical Industry and Patients' Organizations." *British Medical Journal* 326:1208–10.

HCHC [House of Commons Health Committee]. 2005a. "Evidence" Nos. 354–56 in *Proceedings of the Health Select Committee Hearings on Inquiry into the Influence of the Pharmaceutical Industry*, January 20. London: TSO.

———. 2005b. *Inquiry into the Influence of the Pharmaceutical Industry: Health Select Committee Report*. London: TSO.

IMS Health. 2008. "Global Pharmaceutical Sales 2000–2007." imshealth.com/deployedfiles/imshealth/global/content/statcfile.pdf.

Infectious Diseases Society of America. 2004. *Bad Bugs, No Drugs: As Antibiotic Discovery Stagnates, a Public Health Crisis Brews*. Alexandria, Va.: ISDA.

International Society of Drug Bulletins. 2001. *ISDB Declaration on Therapeutic Advance in the Use of Medicines*, Paris, November 15–16.

Jeffries, M. 2000. "The Mark of Zorro." *Pharmaceutical Marketing*, May, 4–5.

Kaitin, Kenneth I., and J. DiMasi. 2000. "Measuring the Pace of New Drug Development in the User Fee Era." *Drug Information Journal* 24:673–80.

Kessler, David A., A. E. Hass, K. L. Feiden, M. Lumpkin, and R. Temple. 1996. "Approval of New Drugs in the U.S.: Comparison with the UK, Germany and Japan." *Journal of the American Medical Association* 276:1826–31.

Kopelman, P. G. 2005. "Clinical Treatment of Obesity: Are Drugs and Surgery the Answer?" *Proceedings of the Nutrition Society* 64:65–71.

Krause, K-H., S. H. Dresel, J. Krause, C. La Fougere, and M. Ackervell. 2003. "The Dopamine Transporter and Neuro-Imaging in ADHD." *Neuro-Science Bio-Behavioral Review* 27:605–13.

La Revue Prescrire. 2005. "A Review of New Drugs in 2004: Floundering Innovation and Increased Risk-Taking." *Prescrire International* 14:68–73.

Lexchin, Joel, L. A. Bero, B. Djulbegovic, and O. Clark. 2003. "Pharmaceutical Industry Sponsorship and Research Outcomes and Quality." *British Medical Journal* 326:1167–70.

Mastro, T. D., J. S. Spika, R. R. Facklam, C. Thornberry, A. Ghafoor, N. K. Nomani, Z. Ishaq, F. Anwar, and D. M. Granoff. 1991. "Antimicrobial Resistance of Pneumococci in Children with Acute Lower Respiratory Tract Infection in Pakistan." *Lancet* 337:156–59.

McCarthy, M. 2004. "The Economics of Obesity." *Lancet* 364:2169–70.

Medawar, Charles. 1992. *Power and Dependence: Social Audit on the Safety of Medicines*. London: Social Audit.

Medawar, Charles, and Anita Hardon. 2004. *Medicines out of Control? Antidepressants and the Conspiracy of Goodwill*. Amsterdam: Askant.

Mintzes, Barbara, M. L. Barer, R. L. Kravitz, K. Bassett, J. Lexchin, A. Kazanjian, R. G. Evans, R. Pan and S. A. Marion. 2003. "How Does Direct-to-Consumer

Advertising (DTCA) Affect Prescribing? A Survey in Primary Care Environments with and without Legal DTCA." *Canadian Medical Association Journal* 169:405–12.

Mitka, M. 2003. "Accelerated Approval Scrutinized—Confirmatory Phase 4 Studies on New Drugs Languish." *Journal of the American Medical Association* 289:3227–29.

Moynihan, Raymond. 2006. "Obesity Task Force Linked to WHO Takes 'Millions' from Drug Firms." *British Medical Journal* 332:1412.

O'Donovan, Orla. 2007. "Corporate Colonization of Health Activism?" *International Journal of Health Services* 37:711–33.

O'Dowd, A. 2006. "More Than 12 Million Adults in England Will Be Obese by 2010." *British Medical Journal* 333:463.

O'Neill, P., and S. McIntosh. 1987. "Bacteria Resistant to Antibiotics Spread Concern." *New Scientist*, August 27, 16.

Parsons, Talcott. 1951. *The Social System*. New York: Free Press.

Padwal, R. S., and S. R. Majumdar. 2007. "Drug Treatments for Obesity." *Lancet* 369:71–77.

Phillips, C. B. 2006. "Medicine Goes to School: Teachers as Sickness Brokers for ADHD." *Public Library of Science Medicine* 3:433–35.

Richards, T. 2008. "Border Crossing: Purely Medicinal?" *British Medical Journal* 336:693.

Roberts, T. G., and B. A. Chabner. 2004. "Beyond Fast Track for Drug Approvals." *New England Journal of Medicine* 351:501–3.

Schweitzer, S. O., M. E. Schweitzer and M-J. Sourty-Le Guellec. 1996. "Is There a U.S. Drug Lag? The Timing of New Pharmaceutical Approvals in the G-7 Countries and Switzerland." *Medical Care Research and Review* 53:162–78.

Scrip News. 1988. "Bush Calls for Speedier U.S. Approvals." Scripnews 1335:16.

———. 1995. "SSRIs—Unprecedented U.S. Growth." Scripnews 2020:23.

———. 1999. "Pfizer's Pharma Sales Soar 28%." Scripnews 2405:8.

Selgelid, M. J., and E. M. Sepers. 2006. "Patents, Profits, and the Price of Pills: Implications for Access and Availability." In *The Power of Pills*, ed. Jillian Clare Cohen, Patricia Illingworth, and Udo Schuklenk, 153–63. London: Pluto Press.

Sharma, V., J. M. Halpern, and J. H. Newcorn. 2000. "Diagnostic Co-morbidity, Attentional Measures, and Neuro-Chemistry in Children with ADHD." In *Ritalin: Theory and Practice*, ed. L. Greenhill and B. Osman, 15–24. Larchmont, Md.: Liebert.

Spellberg, B., J. H. Powers, E. P. Brass, L. G. Miller, and J. E. Edwards. 2004. "Trends in Antimicrobial Drug Development: Implications for the Future." *Clinical Infectious Diseases* 38:1279–86.

Talbot, G. H., J. Bradley, J. E. Edwards, D. Gilbert, M. Scheld, and J. G. Bartlett. 2006. "Bad Bugs Need Drugs: An Update on the Development Pipeline from the Anti-Microbial Availability Task Force of IDSA." *Clinical Infectious Diseases* 42:657–68.

Thambirajah, M. 1998. "Attention Deficit Hyperactivity Disorder in Children: Danger Is One of Over-Diagnosis." *British Medical Journal* 317:1250.

Timmerman, L. 2003. "Impotence Drug *Cialis* Gets OK for Sales in U.S." *Seattle Times*, November 22.

UK Department of Health. 1994. *Prescription Cost Analysis*. London: Government Statistical Service.

———. 2001. *The Expert Patient—A New Approach to Chronic Disease Management for the 21st Century*. London: HMSO.

———. 2003. *Prescription Cost Analysis*. London: Government Statistical Service.

U.S. Congress. House. Committee on Energy and Commerce. Subcommittee on Oversight and Investigations. 1984. *Prescription Advertising to Consumers*. Washington, D.C.: GPO.

Vallejo, J. G., S. L. Kaplan, and E. O. Mason. 1991. "Treatment of Meningitis and Other Infections due to Ampicillin-Resistant Haemophilus Influenzae Type B in Children." *Reviews of Infectious Diseases* 13:197–200.

Van Klingeren, B., M. Dessens-Kroon, and M. Verheuvel. 1989. "Increased Tetracycline Resistance in Gonococci in The Netherlands." *Lancet* 334:1278.

Vos, Rein. 1991. *Drugs Looking for Diseases: Innovative Drug Research and the Development of the Beta Blockers*. Dordrecht, Netherlands: Kluwer.

Wardell, William. 1973. "Introduction of New Therapeutic Drugs in the U.S. and Great Britain: An International Comparison. *Clinical Pharmacology and Therapeutics* 14:773–90.

WHO [World Health Organization]. 2004. *Priority Medicines for Europe and the World*. Geneva: WHO.

———. 2006. "TRIPs and Pharmaceutical Patents." WTO Fact Sheet, 1–8. wto.org/english/tratop_E/TRIPS_e/factsheet_pharm00_e.htm.

Yuwiler, A., G. L. Brammer, and K. C. Yuwiler. 1994. "The Basics of Serotonin Neuro-Chemistry." In *The Neuro-Transmitter Revolution: Serotonin, Social Behavior, and the Law*, ed. R. Masters and M. McGuire, 37–46. Carbondale: Southern Illinois University Press.

Zametkin, A. J., T. E. Nordhal, M. Gross, A. C. King, W. E. Semple, J. Rumsey, S. Hamburger, and R. M. Cohen. 1990. "Cerebral Glucose Metabolism in Adults with Hyperactivity of Childhood Onset." *New England Journal of Medicine* 323:1361–66.

18

Evidence-Based Medicine
Sociological Explorations

Stefan Timmermans, University of California–Los Angeles

Evidence-based medicine (EBM) refers to a process of evaluating and incorporating research evidence into medical decision making. It is commonly defined as "the conscientious, explicit, and judicious use of current best evidence in making decisions about the care of individual patients" (Sackett et al. 1996, 71). The term is rather loosely employed and can refer to anything from conducting a statistical meta-analysis of accumulated research, promoting randomized clinical trials, or supporting uniform reporting styles for research to a personal orientation toward critical self-evaluation. Initially, EBM was defined in opposition to clinical experience but later definitions emphasized its complementary character and aimed to improve clinical experience with better scientific evidence (Sackett et al. 2000).

For many clinicians, medicine has always been evidence based (Dopson et al. 2003). For others, the current turn to EBM privileges specific kinds of evidence that have been less emphasized. EBM represents a break with the past, when the most reliable evidence in medicine was pathophysiological, to augur a time where epidemiological evidence prevails (EBM Working Group 1992). Since the late 1980s, the goal of EBM has been to inform clinical decision making with an evaluation of a clearly defined hierarchy of available evidence. EBM elevated population-based, epidemiological studies with randomized controlled double-blind clinical trials to the apex of the "hierarchy of evidence" (Sackett et al. 1996). Less

convincing are nonrandomized trials and single-group cohort studies, and least authoritative are nonexperimental and descriptive studies. The new knowledge was disseminated through formalized tools such as utilization reviews, clinical practice guidelines, risk assessment tools (Will 2005), and metareviews (Moreira 2007).

This reshuffling of epistemics came after various high-profile researchers in Canada, the UK, and the United States expressed dissatisfaction with the basis of medical decision making, noting that many common medical interventions and therapies lack a scientific foundation of their efficacy (Daly 2005; Eddy 2005). Medical interventions, these observers argued, were authority based rather than evidence based. Their dissatisfaction gained notoriety in the seventies in the small-area variation studies that showed that clinicians vary tremendously in the kind of care they provide over geographical units. In some areas of the United States, prostate surgeries were eight times as common as in others (Wennberg and Cooper 1999). The high degree of variation for almost any intervention could not be explained by chance but was born out of inadequate medical knowledge, different physician practice styles, patient preferences, overreliance on inadequately verified diagnostic tools, and basic inequities in the health-care system. In the eighties, a group at RAND showed that large proportions of routinely used medical procedures were considered inappropriate by professional standards (Chassin et al.

1987). In a policy environment with strong external pressure on clinicians to reign in climbing health-care costs, practice variation is professionally embarrassing because it throws into question the financial basis for reimbursement, the therapeutic acumen of clinicians, and the scientific foundation of contemporary medicine. EBM was embraced by medical professional groups concerned that practice variation may lead to a loss of trust, by payers in the health-care system looking to reform clinical practice, by allied professionals aiming to capture medical jurisdictions, and by educators looking for a stronger curriculum (Timmermans and Mauck 2005).

It is difficult to exaggerate the resonance of EBM in contemporary health care. Advocates have elevated EBM to a new international health-care "paradigm" (EBM Working Group 1992). Some indications of this new paradigm are the appearance of new national and international research institutions concerned with EBM (e.g., the National Institute for Health and Clinical Excellence in the UK and the National Guideline Clearinghouse in the United States), the centrality of EBM at the U.S. Agency for Healthcare Research and Quality, new journals and recurring editorials discussing the importance of evidence-based medicine, innovations in methodologies and criteria for gathering and evaluating data, the surge of randomized clinical trials in medical research, and the rise of "causal pathways," "care plans," and "outcome research" to streamline and evaluate every aspect of health care. In addition, EBM-based curricula have changed medical education, while EBM journal clubs have sprung up in hospitals. Evidence-based thinking has also been tied to nursing and allied health professions, nutrition, public health (McGuire 2005), justice, policy (Gordon 2006), and even hospital chaplaincy.

Social scientists have studied the emergence and consequences of this epistemic turn in medicine. The journals *Health, Social Science and Medicine*; *Health Affairs*; *Biosocieties*; and *Perspectives in Biology and Medicine* have devoted special issues to the phenomenon of EBM. This literature can be roughly divided into three major areas. First, science studies scholars have examined the epistemological qualities of randomized clinical trials (RCTs) and what constitutes evidence in EBM.

These scholars particularly take issue with the elevation of RCTs to the pinnacle of biomedical knowledge. A second strong theme in the social science literature is the role of EBM as a professional strategy to maintain authority in health care and keep competitors and externally imposed reforms at bay. This literature situates EBM as a medical response to buttress medicine's authority among countervailing forces such as consumer movements, payer's dissatisfaction with exploding health-care costs, and increased state regulation. The third major theme in the literature is the effect of EBM in clinical encounters, including in teaching medical students. Here I review these three areas of scholarship and conclude with a research agenda for medical sociology.

Counting Evidence

Along with critical medical observers, social scientists have documented the many ways in which evidence is constrained in EBM. This body of literature is highly critical of EBM in general and its presumptions in particular. The critique questions the logic and wisdom of an EBM. Philosophers have taken aim at the positivist underpinnings of EBM, particularly "the understanding of evidence as 'facts' about the world in the assumption that scientific beliefs stand or fall in light of the evidence." In light of postpositivist feminist and phenomenological critiques, EBM is viewed as a reincarnation of scientism, "modernity's rationalist dream that science can produce the knowledge required to emancipate us from scarcity, ignorance, and error" (Goldenberg 2006, 2622, 2630). Others have located EBM as the next installment in a continuous history to render medicine more scientific through quantification (Marks 1997; Porter 1995; Berg 1997). EBM purports to provide the science behind the art of medicine but historians have viewed EBM as one more instance of a mathematical differentiation of spaces, bodies, populations, and diseases (Armstrong 1997).

A second target has been randomized clinical trials' elevation to the preferred method for health-related questions. For critics, the preference of RCTs in all circumstances leads to the elevation of a study's research design over its quality. Thus, a bad RCT is preferred over a good observational study (Grossman and MacKenzie 2005). In fact, examples abound of the recall of drugs whose efficacy was shown in randomized clinical trials insufficiently powered to find serious side effects. Methodologists have argued that RCTs are good for answering some questions but that their benefits may be squandered if certain conditions regarding treatment modality, blinding, time frame, sample size, and so on are not met. RCTs' presumed superiority lies in the use of a concurrent control group and randomization, yet philosophers of science have argued that there is nothing about randomization that secures scientific integrity. Randomization avoids selection bias, but causal inference is similar to other methods and selection bias can be addressed through different means (Worrall 2002).

Evidence-based medicine depends on the availability of published materials, but the literature is itself commercially stratified, as Greene (2007, 232–33) explains:

> Perhaps the greatest risk in the practice of evidence-based medicine lies in treating the available pool of medical knowledge as a balanced reservoir of facts that emerge from dedicated scientists and circulate solely through the convective currents of peer-reviewed journals and enlightened discussion. . . . In the fluid dynamics of medical knowledge there are deep, undisturbed trenches and there are continually pumping vents of activity, such as pharmaceutical corporations, which act as engines for the development and promotion of forms of knowledge they find useful.

These commercial interests are pursued through clinical trials (Brody, Miller, and Bogdan-Lovis 2005). Such trials do not necessarily constitute bad science—in fact, many of the trials are methodologically exemplary and much better funded than academic trials—but pharmaceutical companies cultivate the commercial potential and legitimacy that a positive trial may produce. Pharmaceutical representatives and company-paid clinicians often distribute the findings directly to practicing physicians and place company-funded research scientists on guideline panels (Prosser and Walley 2006). In addition, there is a publication bias against negative trials (de Vries and Lemmens 2006).

Doing a content analysis of critics of EBM in the medical literature, Helen Lambert (2006) lists the incommensurability of population evidence and individual patient needs, bias toward individualized interventions, exclusion of clinical skills in EBM, production of formulaic guidelines, failure to consider patient views, and difficulties in translating evidence into practice. A major problem for EBM is that evidence is generated from patients very different from the ones on which the knowledge is applied. Patients with extensive comorbidities are typically excluded from clinical trials but are regularly encountered in clinical settings (Upshur 2005).

Advocates of EBM have noted that most of these problems are not unique to EBM but are part of any kind of medicine. Considering that a true individualized medicine is impossible, EBM is not more or less dehumanizing or objectifying than a medicine based in pathology (Straus and McAlister 2000). Particularly galling for many social scientists is EBM's implication that social science methodologies do not register as legitimate, giving rise to proposals to expand EBM to incorporate these methods as well (Bluhm 2005; Landsman 2006). Here, social scientists aim to counter the "decontextualization" (Moreira 2005) on which standardization rests with context-sensitive methodologies. The clinical payoff of this contextualization, however, remains unclear.

Evidence-Based Medicine as a Professional Project

Various commentators have viewed EBM as a move in the chess game of countervailing powers vying for dominance in the health-care market (Rappolt 1997; Traynor 2000; Denny 1999; Timmermans and Kolker 2004; Pope 2003). Health policy makers agree that at least some of the variation in health care stems from overuse, underuse, and misuse of medical care, leading to iatrogenesis and escalating costs. In this context, EBM emerged as a professional answer to the pressure from government agencies and insurance companies to render medicine more efficient and cost-effective. Evidence-based medicine can be viewed as an intraprofessional attempt to replace disciplinary with mechanical objectivity or as the shift of a reliance on peer consensus to decisions based on algorithms, protocols, and numbers (Daston and Galison 1992; Porter 1995). The turn to evidence offers a dominant and sweeping social mechanism to control unruly individual professionals, regain the public's trust, keep out competitors, and shore up the scientific quality of the professional medical project. One way to safeguard the professions' position in this system of countervailing powers is to standardize the scientific foundation of one's work.

In the sociology of professions, a move toward standardization is a two-edged sword: what begins as a tool for greater rationality and autonomy may ultimately undermine the foundations of the market shelter. Already in the 1960s, Crozier predicted that "the rationalization process gives [experts] power, but the end results of rationalization curtail this power. As soon as a field is well-covered, as soon as the first institutions and innovations can be translated into rules and programs, the expert's power disappears" (Crozier 1964, 164). Clinicians eye evidence-based medicine warily because the technologies may undermine the profession from within. Greater transparency through protocols and standards may lead to outsourcing, cost-control measures, or professional downsizing based on protocols. Reed explains that "the trick seems to be to strike the right— i.e., inevitably shifting—political balance between indeterminacy and formalization of knowledge and skill as a prerequisite to constructing expert power bases and action domains that will stand the test of time" (Reed 1996, 583). The danger for professions is that formal tools will be used as cost-cutting devices. Indeed, Light postulates that much of the attraction of evidence-based medicine in contemporary health care resides in its money-saving potential (Light 1988). Third parties such as insurers, government payers, and the courts wield practice guidelines and other standards to hold clinicians financially accountable for their actions (Light 2000). Rather than strengthening their professional base, professions may then have surrendered their expert knowledge to outsiders, even if these outsiders have an MD degree but have now joined management (Hoff 1999). Medical observers refer to this danger by the shorthand "cookbook medicine": EBM may turn professional autonomy into a mindless process of following recipes.

The main suppliers of clinical-practice guidelines are medical colleges and academies (Timmermans and Kolker 2004). If third parties can seize evidence-based medicine to use it against professional interests, why would these professional organizations expose their members to this risk (Pope 2003)? Here, it is useful to distinguish between, on the one side, the actual effects of introducing guidelines and other evidence-based instruments in clinical settings and, on the other, the political and educational value of evidence-based medicine on the organizational level. In the clinics, a decade of experience with evidence-based medicine shows, with some notable exceptions (Timmermans and Mauck 2005), that clinical-practice guidelines are limited in their ability to change clinical behavior. Evaluation studies show that practice variation continues after the introduction of evidence-based medicine (McGlynn et al. 2003), leading to articles with titles such as "Why Don't Physicians Follow Clinical Practice Guidelines?" (Cabana et al. 1999), and the field has focused on the problem of implementing guidelines (Grimshaw et al. 2001). Professional organizations produce guidelines but they do not enforce their implementation, leaving such decisions up to their individual members. Instead, these organizations count on the intrinsic rationality of superior science to trigger behavioral changes, with mixed success (Dopson et al. 2003). It is very difficult to make professionals voluntarily change their practices, precisely because they have autonomy over their work (Freidson 2001; Timmermans and Kolker 2004).

The difficulty EBM has in affecting clinical care is clear in EBM's effect on clinical autonomy, the hallmark of medical professionalism. Evidence-based medicine promises to preserve the professional autonomy of clinicians by committing to high scientific standards of care. Yet, this same autonomy may be under attack, since EBM aims to restrict clinical discretion on scientific grounds. Whether individual discretion gives way to standardization depends on how clinicians learn and modify their behavior. In a study of how primary-care clinicians determine what kind of drugs to use for treatment of depression, David Armstrong (2000) found that clinicians conducted personalized "clinical trials" with individual patients to check the effectiveness of new drugs and to match drugs with particular groups of patients, and remained attentive to patient choice and to their general relationship with patients. He noted that "a formalized approach to patient care, especially one based on trial evidence derived from populations of patients, was far removed from the individualized clinical decisions being made by these doctors" (Armstrong 2002, 1775). General practitioners also relied on senior academic colleagues for the most up-to-date information, but the information exchange followed a particular etiquette by which seniors made suggestions without undermining the professional autonomy of the first-line practitioners (Armstrong and Ogden 2006; see also Prosser and Walley 2006).

At the larger organizational level, medical colleges and academies view the creation and publication of clinical-practice guidelines as an informational service to their members, providing a set of authoritative scientific tools to be used in education and training. The guidelines also help to stalk out areas of professional responsibility and stimulate further research. Even when third parties such as insurance companies or government agencies have attempted to link clinical-practice guidelines to financial incentives and performance indicators, the results have been modest—largely because the required high-quality population-based evidence drawn from randomized clinical trials is often not available (Rowe 2006; Guggenheim 2005). Evidence-based medicine has lost some of its luster as a policy solution for the ailments of contemporary health care, and the U.S. government and third parties have focused on distributing rather than creating EBM (Gray, Gusmano, and Collins 2003).

One example of third-party engagement with EBM lies in the use of clinical-practice guidelines in tort law to establish liability, deter future harmful conduct, and compensate injured victims (see also Timmermans and Berg 2003, ch. 3). In theory, clinical-practice guidelines could strengthen the medical profession by shifting to it the regulatory powers of the legal tort system.

For example, clinical-practice guidelines could be interpreted as contracts between physicians and patients and become the standard of care (Havighurst 1995). In practice, the courts have been gradually accepting clinical-practice guidelines as one element of evidence to establish a standard of care. The consequence is that clinical-practice guidelines are incorporated in the tort system but their status is still ambiguous. No conclusive pattern has emerged in the way courts regard clinical-practice guidelines, but it is likely that guidelines may gain importance if widely adopted and followed by the medical community. If the court finds a guideline definitive as a standard of care, the guideline becomes the yardstick against which a physician's practice is judged. Clinical-practice guidelines can be used to immunize physicians from malpractice liability, but failure to comply with guidelines can expose them to liability, rendering guidelines "two-way streets" (Hyams et al. 1995). Physicians might, for example, be able to dismiss lawsuits when they can document adherence to clinical-practice guidelines, but the burden of persuasion might also shift from the plaintiff to the physician who did not adhere to existing practice guidelines.

Although plaintiffs and defendant physicians can use clinical guidelines, there is evidence that these are used more for inculpatory purposes (by plaintiffs) than for exculpatory purposes (by defendant physicians) (Hyams et al. 1995). To complicate the matter, courts have also issued policy statements that physicians bear the responsibility of medical treatment decisions. This means that if a physician follows professional practice guidelines but those guidelines are not accepted as the standard of care, the physician could still be considered negligent. In addition, legislators in states such as Maine and Minnesota use clinical guidelines in a way favorable to defendant physicians in a malpractice liability lawsuit. The court's attitude is still marred with ambiguity regarding whether clinical-practice guidelines are definitive of standards of care. Most observers anticipate that "courts will treat clinical-practice guidelines as one piece of evidence in establishing the standard of care, rather than as the primary determinant of the appropriate standard of care" (Jacobson 1997, 74H).

Clinical medicine's experience with EBM demonstrates the field's ability to turn an engagement with third parties to its advantage. While professional organizations under pressure from third parties initially embraced EBM as a solution for the problem of unwanted practice variation, they have largely been able to neutralize the danger to clinical autonomy by claiming ownership over the formulation of guidelines and neutralizing the enforcement and incentive mechanisms for guideline following. Clinical-practice guidelines are used as guidelines rather than as absolute, strictly enforced rules. Evidence-based medicine has not solved the problem of practice variation, but it also has not been responsible for a loss of professional economic, cultural, or political power. Evidence-based medicine shows medical professions willing to critically engage with the current highest-valued level of scientific evidence and claim procedures and interventions as their jurisdiction.

The most durable effect of EBM on clinical care may be its ability to restratify medical knowledge production, a reformulation of what counts as scientific knowledge (e.g., the ascent of RCT and population measures at the expense of physiopathology and individual health outcomes). In this context, the confrontation of alternative medicine with EBM and RCTs is interesting because it underscores EBM's potential to keep out competitors. Critics in the alternative medicine community have regarded the ascent of EBM as a political act to exclude complementary and alternative medicine (CAM) from the health-care market (Borgerson 2005; Barry 2006). They argue that the nature of alternative therapies precludes a straightforward measurement of benefits in individual patients. For example, in acupuncture or homeopathy the same condition may be treated very differently in different individuals based on their personality picture, and the spiritual impacts are impossible to measure in RCTs (Jackson and Scambler 2007; Barry 2006). In reality, the effects have not been dramatic: CAM has been flourishing rather than disappearing, but different factions within the CAM community have seized EBM to advance their own professional agenda.

Chiropractic medicine originated in the early twentieth century as a metaphysical epistemology in reaction to the "mechanistic" and empirical elements of orthodox medicine (Starr 1982). Chiropractors were committed to "vitalism," a body's ability to heal itself through an equilibrium of vital forces. They helped patients remove subluxations through adjustments—quick, forceful thrusts by hand to the spinal vertebrae. With a much shorter medical education and an avoidance of scientific proof, chiropractic efficacy was measured simply: patients got better or they didn't. From the beginning of its history, chiropractic medicine was split between straight chiropractors and mixers, who combined spinal adjustments with other forms of medicine and who during the 1960s and 1970s attempted to professionalize the discipline by strengthening educational requirements and claiming a subject matter.

After chiropractic plaintiffs prevailed in a lawsuit against the American Medical Association and other defendants for trying to destroy chiropractic practice by disallowing free competition and violating the Sherman Anti-Trust Act, some leaders in the chiropractic community saw EBM as a means to elevate their professional standing and validate chiropractic procedures. EBCAM—evidence-based complementary and alternative medicine—could bridge allopathic and alternative medicine. Consequently, a consensus conference established standards of chiropractic care in 1993. This step sent tremors through the chiropractic community. While professional leaders considered the practice guidelines a step to protect their jurisdiction against orthodox medicine, the move also bolstered the mixers in the community: "EBM not only privileges positivism, but then becomes skewed in favor of the agenda of mixer chiropractors, who aspire for chiropractic to become a mechanistic and therapeutic discipline that complements or is on-par to orthodox medicine" (Villanueva-Russell 2005, 551). A related problem was that a guideline of the federal Agency for Health Care Policy and Research indeed showed that "manipulation" (the medical term for what chiropractors call "adjustment") is beneficial for acute low-back pain. Critics of EBM feared that orthodox physicians might appropriate the technique. In spite of highly charged rhetoric, EBM did not make a huge impact upon the clinical practices of chiropractors. The first set of guidelines was followed by two other sets and "the three sets of practice guidelines were never really integrated into the day-to-day reality of individual chiropractors, the delivery of care, or reimbursement by third party payers" (557).

Other borderline CAM disciplines such as midwifery may have the evidence on their side but have difficulty translating superior epistemics into professional currency (Bogdan-Lovis and Sousa 2006). Among certified nurse-midwives, not only does the evidence validate the safety and effectiveness of midwifery but the field of obstetrics was an early adopter of EBM. Still, the uptake of EBM by midwifery was confounded by a consumerist movement to request extra interventions and by EBM's tendency to study the benefits of intervention rather than of inaction. Finally, the uptake of EBM in midwifery circles is hampered by the fact that certified nurse-midwives work under supervision of a physician and reimbursement follows interventions. This occupational vulnerability negates many of the advantages of a well-established knowledge base. Rather than validating strong midwifery knowledge, the financial pressures increasingly lead midwives to mimic physician's medicalized birth management (ibid.).

EBM fits into various professional agendas. Clinical disciplines look at EBM as a means to shore up scientific practice, third-parties see in EBM a promising tool to install accountability, while the CAM community eyes EBM warily as an incompatible set of standards. However, better science in the form of guidelines has limited effect on everyday clinical practice, and its ability to maintain or conquer professional jurisdictions is similarly limited. Two decades of EBM show that unless guidelines and other protocols are part of comprehensive social, political, and economic reform efforts in which relevant stakeholders participate, little changes on an organizational or professional level (Timmermans and Mauck 2005).

Evidence-Based Medicine and Medical Education

Since EBM was initially developed at McMaster University, Ontario, as a pedagogical innovation to strengthen a residency program, it makes sense to examine the impact of EBM on medical education. In medical education, the role of EBM is to encourage students to ask, "What's the evidence?" when contemplating therapeutic interventions (Eisenberg 1999, 1868). This question is further split into five key components: translation of uncertainty into an answerable question; systematic retrieval of the best evidence available; critical appraisal of evidence for validity, clinical relevance, and applicability; application of the results into practice; and evaluation of performance—ask, acquire, appraise, apply, and assess (Sackett et al. 2000). Proponents of evidence-based medicine suggest that learning EBM skills will allow practitioners to deal more directly and effectively with gaps in their knowledge and to develop an approach that is more self-directed and patient-centered (Bordley, Fagan, and Theige 1997).

Current medical literature describes a range of methods and formats for teaching these skills: required coursework in EBM, journal clubs, faculty development and training in EBM, work groups, use of the Internet and laptops in clinical settings, use of PDAs (personal digital assistants) or smartphones, electronic medical records, research mentors, EBM clerkships or rotations, grand rounds, peer discussion groups, use of the librarian or medical school/library partnerships, and organizational and infrastructural support for EBM on an institutional level. The Internet is a fundamental component of both teaching and practicing EBM principles in clinical settings, and the many information sources available online include: MEDLINE, Cochrane Database of Systematic Reviews, Best Evidence, ACP Journal Club, Ovid Technologies, PubMed, and the National Guideline Clearinghouse. In addition, technologies such as smartphones (Leon et al. 2007)—hybrid devices that combine mobile phones with PDA devices and the electronic medical record (Stewart et al. 2007)—filled with reminders to use guidelines or indicate contraindications for medications have been used in teaching EBM.

Implementation

Because students form a captive audience for the best available medical knowledge, implementing

EBM in educational settings should be less complicated than trying to transfer its principles to hospital settings or private clinics. Even in education, however, the implementation of EBM has run into barriers, including infrastructural and personnel obstacles. In a study with 417 program directors of U.S. internal medicine residency programs, Green, Ciampi, and Ellis (2000) found that the primary barriers to incorporating EBM principles into practice were that only about half (51–64 percent) the programs had onsite electronic information and only about one-third (31–45 percent) had site-specific faculty development. Fewer than half the curricula incorporated evaluations, and many did not include important sources of medical information such as well-regarded EBM databases. Furthermore, the authors cited the lack of documentation of actual EBM behaviors among residents for all major areas, particularly in the emergency departments, weekly rounds led by attending, and interdisciplinary daily bedside rounds. Limited information exists on the effectiveness of existing faculty-training programs, including computing capacity.

Other obstacles to implementation of evidence-based medicine can be broadly categorized as lack of evidence and cognitive barriers. Many clinical outcomes in medicine are uncertain or do not have current research to direct clinical decision making. Furthermore, several researchers have questioned the worth of the evidence in current medical research, given issues such as publication bias, poor validity and reliability of studies, and unclear recommendations for practical application. In clinically uncertain circumstances with little, poor, or no evidence to guide clinical decision making, physicians will likely turn to their own clinical experience or gut reactions to resolve clinical problems (Porzsolt et al. 2003).

In the opposite situation, where there is extensive evidence, cognitive barriers exist in the form of the massive volume of literature students and practitioners of EBM must master. Extensive literature for common conditions such as heart disease may overwhelm students sifting through it to determine which studies constitute the best evidence. Several studies have also indicated that medical students and residents experience difficulty in understanding and applying prin-

ciples of biostatistics and epidemiology in order to critically appraise research articles. Windish, Huot, and Green (2007) evaluated the ability of residents to understand statistical principles and interpret research findings. They administered a survey to 277 residents and found that only 41 percent could correctly understand statistical concepts and research results and that 75 percent did not understand all statistics they read in journal articles, though 95 percent felt it was important to understand these concepts to intelligently navigate the literature.

Even if infrastructural problems are overcome and the necessary skills are acquired, the implementation of EBM still faces the barrier of being simply one concern in a very hectic and high-stakes educational environment. Green and Ruff (2005) explored reasons behind the failure of residents to pursue answers to their clinical questions, using focus groups of thirty-four internal medicine residents. The predominant barriers included access to medical information, skills for searching, time, clinical question tracking and priority, personal initiative, team dynamics, and institutional culture. The authors concluded that educators should pay increased attention to attitudes toward learning EBM and the influence of institutional cultures. In a different study also exploring unanswered clinical questions by residents, Green, Ciampi, and Ellis (2000) interviewed sixty-four residents after 401 patient encounters. In this study, authors found that residents had approximately two questions for every three patients but pursued answers only 29 percent of the time. Questions were typically related to therapy (38 percent) or diagnosis (27 percent). The most common reasons for failure to pursue answers was lack of time (60 percent) and forgetting the question (29 percent). In order to answer questions, residents typically turned to textbooks, original articles, or attending physicians.

Uncertainty

A good way to assess how this influx of technology and sensitivity to new forms of knowledge has affected the educational experience is to revisit the sociological topic of uncertainty in medical education. Based on research in Cornell's medical school during the early fifties, Renée Fox argued that medical knowledge is inherently uncertain because it is riddled with gaps and unknowns and because the amount of medical facts is ever expanding and impossible to completely master (Fox 1957). The dilemma for students in medical school consists of managing the limitations of their own cognitive ability in the face of the vast medical literature. During the clinical training years, medical uncertainty emerges when students apply textbook knowledge to clinical situations and handle both the physiological and psychological aspects of patient care. Fox's sociology of knowledge consists of a gradual socialization in medical confidence; instead of blaming oneself for clinical mistakes, the aspiring doctor learns to manage successfully the limitations of medicine. Training for uncertainty serves to imprint a professional attitude of objective expertise and detached concern on the next generation of physicians. Other authors have questioned the primacy of uncertainty and stressed that "training for control" closely follows "training for uncertainty" (Atkinson 1984; Katz 1984; Light 1979). Instead of medical students imbued with scientific skepticism, for example, Atkinson portrays medical students as pragmatists, "content to work within the conceptual bounds of a given 'paradigm'" (Atkinson 1984, 954). In her most recent update of the uncertainty literature, Fox (2000) addresses the surge of EBM and contends that EBM reinforces collective-oriented approaches in medicine at the expense of individualized patient-doctor interactions. Siding with the critics of EBM, she remains apprehensive of EBM's narrow biomedical positivism and its threat to clinical expertise. Extrapolating from these general predictions to education, we can examine whether EBM reduces or enhances uncertainty.

Timmermans and Angell (2001) studied how residents in two pediatric programs used EBM to manage the uncertainty of medical knowledge and to weigh EBM knowledge against firsthand experience. They found that residents were exposed to EBM but engaged with this scientific evidence in different ways. About two-thirds of the residents interviewed (designated by Timmermans and Angell as "librarians") interpreted EBM as equiva-lent to consulting the medical literature, while for the remaining third, EBM required an active evaluation of the research literature ("researchers"). Timmermans and Angell found that EBM foremost created a new source of uncertainty to be mastered by medical residents: research-based uncertainty, or learning the skills to retrieve and evaluate the research literature. Whether EBM installed an attitude of scientific skepticism or of increasing medical dogmatism depended on the way the researcher used scientific evidence. To inform clinical decision making, "librarian" residents tended to become frustrated with evaluating individual studies and used summaries of the medical literature to gain confidence. They may become more dogmatic from their uncritical and instrumentalist take on the literature or avoid consulting the literature for a lack of clear answers. "Researcher" residents, in contrast, appreciated the contradictions and uncertainties of the medical knowledge base and learned when not to follow guidelines or published recommendations. They turned the critical attitude fostered by EBM on EBM itself, sharpening their discriminatory powers in decision making. Even these researchers, however, ran into trouble if they attempted to contradict superiors based on EBM. Attending physicians' understanding of the literature and scientific evidence prevailed in training situations, and every resident agreed that it was more important to know what your supervisor expected than to be familiar with the latest literature.

How does EBM mediate the tension between firsthand experience and external (book) knowledge? Timmermans and Angell (2001) argue that the difference between these two realms of experience is exaggerated, because any consultation of the literature is already influenced by clinical observations, while any observation is steeped in book knowledge. They came to this conclusion because no resident seemed to be able to implement EBM unproblematically. At each point, they all ran into problems with attending physicians, patient preferences, allied professionals, and organizational constraints. Clinicians in training are faced with evidence-based clinical judgment, an inevitable mixture of hard-won experience from watching others; personal tryouts, mistakes, and admonishments; and evidence gathered from lectures, written sources, and their own attempts to summarize the literature. Over time, the knowledge base of both experience and published evidence expands and may shift when, for example, residents move from consumers to producers of knowledge over their careers.

Impact on Medical Care

While EBM may have been one factor in an ongoing stream of factors that reshaped the uncertainties of learning medicine and professional autonomy, what have been its effects on how and what physicians learn? Evidence-based medicine supports and presumes a positivistic science of behavior modification: if physicians knew about the best evidence, they would be compelled to implement this knowledge. The literature on outcomes of EBM in medical education and the overall biomedical literature suffer from similar gaps, biases, and weaknesses. EBM is generally accepted as effective, but precious little research supports this presumption (Green 2006). Ironically, many of the evaluation studies do not meet the highest evidentiary standards of EBM because RCTs are notoriously difficult to run in educational settings (Hatala and Guyatt 2002). Yet, EBM advocates have turned to RCTs to grapple with the implementation gap of EBM in education and clinical practice in general.

In the last five years, educators and biomedical researchers have aimed to improve the available methodology and evidence. One of the few studies with a control group of an EBM educational intervention showed a statistically significant increase in awareness of EBM principles and their use in the experimental group (Ross and Verdieck 2003). Yet, the researchers were unable to demonstrate changes in patient care or improved health outcomes, and this research may thus lack face validity. The same problem occurred in a study where residents were asked about their familiarity with recent journal articles relevant to primary care (Stevermer, Chambliss, and Hoekzema 1999). More promising may be the attempt to have medical students maintain evidence-based learning portfolios, representing a student's addressing of clinical problems. Studies have shown

that working on these portfolios leads to greater "self-directed learning readiness" (Crowley et al. 2003; Fung et al. 2000).

These evaluation studies reflect the distinction between Timmermans and Angell's (2001) "researchers" and "librarians." Studies where students are tested on their familiarity with formal EBM tools and databases interpret EBM in the librarian mode, while studies where students are evaluated on their ability to put a research portfolio together are more likely to check for critical appraisal researcher skills. The studies thus contain different conceptual models of learning centered on EBM and of EBM itself (see also Straus et al. 2004). An observational study by McCord and colleagues (2007, 301) of how residents use EBM after receiving training showed that librarians are more numerous than researchers: residents are most likely to consult summarized EBM sources to answer clinical questions. The study's authors noted that "residents operated more as information managers within the constraints of time limitations and job responsibilities." The most important information resource remained consulting their superiors. Launching a critical appraisal of the literature was often not performed because of simple logistical barriers such as having to go to a different room to access a computer. Other studies have confirmed that residents pursue only about a quarter of their clinical questions, often consulting non-evidence-based information sources (Green, Ciampi, and Ellis 2000).

The key question is whether this influx of EBM has resulted in improved patient outcomes. This question should be easy to measure because researchers can review therapeutic decisions based on chart reviews by assigning primary diagnoses and interventions and determine whether the resident reached a decision backed by the best available evidence. Ellis et al. (1995) introduced this methodology by classifying the evidence in three broad categories: intervention with evidence from RCTs, intervention with convincing nonexperimental evidence, and intervention without substantial evidence. While this method has indeed been employed in medical subspecialties such as surgery, anesthesiology, and other fields (Green 2006), it has been used only sporadically in medical education. In one study (Straus et al. 2005), patients were significantly more likely to receive EBM-derived therapy than were those treated before the intervention (82 versus 74 percent; P = .046). Even in this study, the researchers focused on process outcomes rather than on clinical outcomes such as mortality.

We have thus some evidence that EBM teaching modules may change some clinical decision making, but physicians in training are more likely to rely on authoritative EBM sources than to conduct their own critical appraisal of the literature. While some decisions seem to have a stronger scientific foundation as defined by EBM proponents, the question is still open as to whether training in EBM-saturated environments benefits patients.

Research Agenda

Evidence-based medicine is everywhere in contemporary health care. In one decade, the number of articles in PubMed with evidence-based medicine as a MeSH term increased sevenfold—from 648 in 1997 to 4,340 in 2007 (as of September 12, 2008)—with a total of more than 30,000 articles over the decade. It is difficult to argue against the basic premise that health-care interventions should be based on scientific evidence. Still, social scientists have questioned whether RCTs constitute the best possible evidence under all circumstances and whether standardization will lead to better clinical care. They situated the emergence of EBM as a professional response to offset the likelihood of reforms enforced by government agencies and insurance companies. EBM is embraced as a solution for the problem of practice variation due to physicians following traditional authority or anecdote. An industry of conducting RCTs and reviewing evidence in consensus conferences and specialized organizations helped disseminate EBM across the medical spectrum, yet as the experience in medical education shows, it is still unclear what effect EBM has on the behavior of clinicians. While EBM may have sensitized the current generation of health-care providers to research methodology and epidemiology, logistical and cognitive barriers have

created an implementation gap in medical decision making. In the ongoing struggles between medical subdisciplines and between alternative and allopathic medicine, the commodification of the pharmaceutical industry, and the power hierarchy of medical schools, EBM has not infused medicine with scientific rationality but has been mobilized as a political tool to stake out an advantageous position.

Where does this leave a social science analysis? Social scientists have often taken the role of external critic, extrapolating about what would happen if EBM was implemented rather than examining what has actually happened. This attitude gave way to hyperbole while the actual effects of EBM on professional power and clinical care are either difficult to measure or negligible. First, there is a need for a much more solid research base of what EBM actually is and how it matters for whom. As the discussion of researchers and librarians hinted, even among health-care providers EBM is many things to many people: everyone seems to be doing EBM, but tremendous differences exist in how clinicians engage with evidence. Within the social science literature, the absence of patient perspectives is glaring, although some social scientists have advanced theoretical arguments about the kind of experiences patients can bring up in an EBM-infused care context (May et al. 2006). Most of the EBM literature still follows a professional "extract and apply" approach to patient relationships in which clinicians view patients as objects of information gathering, care providers make decisions, and the presumption is that the patient relationship does not change but that patients simply receive better care (Upshur 2005). With clinical-practice guidelines only a Website away, direct-to-consumer advertising, and vocal patient health movements actively involved in the production of scientific knowledge (Epstein 1997), the patient-provider relationship under EBM is likely more dialogical and complicated. In fact, patient preferences are often cited as a reason for the EBM implementation gap (Upshur 2005).

A related set of projects takes aim at the epistemic consequences of EBM. Here, the role of EBM in global biomedicalization (Clarke et al. 2003) is ripe for deeper exploration: how does the flow of trials, protocols, personnel, and guidelines across national borders affect local caregiving and care priorities? EBM seems remarkably insensitive to national contexts, although EBM defenders have charged that critics mistake the excesses of, for example, managed care with the characteristics of EBM (Brody, Miller, and Bogdan-Lovis 2005). Such a defense imbues EBM with political neutrality, while the professional perspective established convincingly that EBM is politically attractive for many parties aiming to defend or expand economic and professional interests. This raises questions about the generation of knowledge on a global scale, in countries with different health-care systems and evolving policy and political priorities.

A different set of research projects shifts the focus from EBM to the initial problem of practice variation. Two decades into EBM, practice variation has not diminished and patients continue to be over- or undertreated based on physician idiosyncratic preferences (Fisher et al. 2008). The difficulty of EBM to affect clinical care raises the issue of how to change clinical behavior individually, organizationally, and professionally. Evidence-based medicine's implementation gap shows that health-care providers easily resist attempts to diminish their autonomy, even if these initiatives originate from their own professional organizations. At the same time, contemporary health care is continuously under pressure to change. The art of changing clinical behavior has been fine-tuned by the representatives of pharmaceutical companies armed with weekly updated prescription data who target individual practitioners (Lakoff 2005). Pursuing the latest quality-improvement strategies, organization scientists have proposed a redesign of health-care delivery, usually centered around information technologies, to change clinical decision making (Shojania and Grimshaw 2005). Drawing from well-established user studies in the information field, social scientists have an opportunity to examine how change occurs and can be stimulated among workers with great autonomy. The issue of changing clinical behavior is not specific to EBM or practice variation but relates to issues as mundane as the difficulty of making physicians wash their hands and as large as the persistence of gender and race health disparities.

Finally, the basic, unresolved question is whether EBM makes a difference for patient outcomes—and, if so, under what kind of conditions for what kind of disorders. To address this question, social scientists may want to team up with health researchers and merge their expertise in social contextualization with the intricacies of clinical outcome research.

Note

This review draws extensively from earlier reviews I have written about evidence-based medicine.

References

Armstrong, David. 1997. "Foucault and the Sociology of Health and Illness: A Prismatic Reading." In *Foucault, Health and Medicine*, ed. A. Petersen and R. Bunton, 15–30. London and New York: Routledge.

———. 2002. "Clinical Autonomy, Individual and Collective: The Problem of Changing Doctors' Behaviour." *Social Science and Medicine* 55(10): 1771–77.

Armstrong, David, and Jane Ogden. 2006. "The Role of Etiquette and Experimentation in Explaining How Doctors Change Behavior: A Qualitative Study." *Sociology of Health and Illness* 28(7): 951–68.

Atkinson, Paul. 1984. "Training for Certainty." *Social Science and Medicine* 19(9): 949–56.

Barry, Christine Ann. 2006. "The Role of Evidence in Alternative Medicine: Contrasting Biomedical and Anthropological Approaches." *Social Science and Medicine* 62(11): 2646–57.

Berg, Marc. 1997. *Rationalizing Medical Work: Decision Support Techniques and Medical Practices*. Cambridge, Mass.: MIT Press.

Bluhm, Robyn. 2005. "From Hierarchy to Network: A Richer View of Evidence for Evidence-Based Medicine." *Perspectives in Biology and Medicine* 48(4): 535–48.

Bogdan-Lovis, Elisabeth A., and Aron Sousa. 2006. "The Contextual Influence of Professional Culture: Certified Nurse-Midwives' Knowledge of and Reliance on Evidence-Based Practice." *Social Science and Medicine* 62 (11): 2681–93.

Bordley, Donald R., Mark Fagan, and David Theige. 1997. "Evidence-Based Medicine: A Powerful Educational Tool for Clerkship Education." *American Journal of Medicine* 102 (May): 427–32.

Borgerson, Kristin. 2005. "Evidence-Based Alternative Medicine?" *Perspectives in Biology and Medicine* 48(4): 502–15.

Brody, Howard, Franklin G. Miller, and Elisabeth A. Bogdan-Lovis. 2005. "Evidence-Based Medicine: Watching Out for Its Friends." *Perspectives in Biology and Medicine* 48(4): 570–84.

Cabana, Michael D., Cynthia S. Rand, Neil R. Power, and Albert W. Wu. 1999. "Why Don't Physicians Follow Clinical Practice Guidelines? A Framework for Improvement." *Journal of the American Medical Association* 282(15): 1458–65.

Chassin, Mark R., Jacqueline Kosecoff, David H. Solomon, and Robert H. Brook. 1987. "How Coronary Angiography Is Used. Clinical Determinants of Appropriateness." *Journal of the American Medical Association* 258(18): 2543–47.

Clarke, Adele E., Janet K. Shim, Laura Mamo, Jennifer R. Fosket, and Jennifer R. Fishman. 2003. "Biomedicalization: Technoscientific Transformations of Health, Illness, and U.S. Biomedicine." *American Sociological Review* 68 (April): 161–94.

Crowley, Steven D., Thomas A. Owens, Connie M. Schardt, Sarah I. Wardell, Josh Peterson, Scott Garrison, and Sheri A. Keitz. 2003. "A Web-Based Compendium of Clinical Questions and Medical Evidence to Educate Internal Medicine Residents." *Academic Medicine* 78(3): 270–74.

Crozier, Michel 1964. *The Bureaucratic Phenomenon.* Chicago: University of Chicago Press.

Daly, Jeanne. 2005. *Evidence-Based Medicine and the Search for a Science of Clinical Care.* Berkeley: University of California Press.

Daston, Lorraine, and Peter Galison. 1992. "The Image of Objectivity." *Representations* 40:81–128.

de Vries, Raymond, and Trudo Lemmens. 2006. "The Social and Cultural Shaping of Medical Evidence: Case Studies from Pharmaceutical Research and Obstetric Science." *Social Science and Medicine* 62(11): 2694–2706.

Denny, Keith. 1999. "Evidence-Based Medicine and Medical Authority." *Journal of Medical Humanities* 20(4): 247–63.

Dopson, Sue, Louise Locock, John Gabbay, Ewqan Ferlie, and Louise Fitzgerald. 2003. "Evidence-Based Medicine and the Implementation Gap." *Health* 7(3): 311–30.

Eddy, David M. 2005. "Evidence-Based Medicine: A Unified Approach." *Health Affairs* 24(1): 9–18.

Eisenberg, John M. 1999. "Ten Lessons for Evidence-Based Technology Assessment." *Journal of the American Medical Association* 282(19): 1865–69.

Ellis, J., I. Mulligan, J. Rowe, and D. L. Sackett. 1995. "Inpatient General Medicine Is Evidence Based." *Lancet* 346:407–10.

Epstein, Steven. 1997. "Activism, Drug Regulation, and the Politics of Therapeutic Evaluating in the AIDS Era: A Case Study of ddC and the 'Surrogate Markers' Debate." *Social Studies of Science* 27(3): 691–726.

Evidence-Based Medicine [EBM] Working Group. 1992. "Evidence-Based Medicine: A New Approach to Teaching the Practice of Medicine." *Journal of the American Medical Association* 268:2420–25.

Fisher, Elliott S., David C. Goodman, Jonathan S. Skinner, and John E. Wennberg. 2008. *Tracking the Care of Patients with Severe Chronic Illness: The Darthmouth Atlas of Health Care 2008.* Lebanon, N.H.: Darthmouth Institute for Health Policy and Clinical Practice.

Fox, Renée C. 1957. "Training for Uncertainty." In *The Student Physician*, ed. R. K. Merton, G. Reader, and P. L. Kendall, 207–40. Cambridge, Mass.: Harvard University Press.

———. 2000. "Medical Uncertainty Revisited." In *The Handbook of Social Studies in Health and Medicine*, ed. G. L. Albrecht, R. Fitzpatrick, and S. C. Scrimshaw, 409–25. London: Sage Publications.

Freidson, Eliot. 2001. *Professionalism: The Third Logic.* Cambridge: Polity Press.

Fung, Michael F., Mark Walker, K. F. Fung, Lora Temple, Francois Lajoie, Guy Bellemare, and S. C. Bryson. 2000. "An Internet-Based Learning Portfolio in Resident Education: The KOALA Multicentre Programme." *Medical Education* 34(6): 474–79.

Goldenberg, Maya J. 2006. "On Evidence and Evidence-Based Medicine: Lessons from the Philosophy of Science." *Social Science and Medicine* 62:2621–32.

Gordon, Elisa J. 2006. "The Political Contexts of Evidence-Based Medicine: Policymaking for Daily Hemodialysis." *Social Science and Medicine* 62(11): 2707–19.

Gray, Bradford H., Michael K. Gusmano, and Sara R. Collins. 2003. "AHCPR and the Changing Politics of Health Services Research." *Health Affairs* Suppl Web:W3–283–307.

Green, Michael L. 2006. "Evaluating Evidence-Based Practice Performance." *Evidence Based Medicine* 11(4): 99–101.

Green, Michael L., Marc A. Ciampi, and Peter J. Ellis. 2000. "Residents' Medical Information Needs in Clinic: Are They Being Met?" *American Journal of Medicine* 109(3): 218–23.

Green, Michael L., and Tanya R. Ruff. 2005. "Why Do Residents Fail to Answer Their Clinical Questions? A Qualitative Study of Barriers to Practicing Evidence-Based Medicine." *Academic Medicine* 80(2): 176–82.

Greene, Jeremy A. 2007. *Prescribing by Numbers.* Baltimore: Johns Hopkins University Press.

Grimshaw, Jeremy M., Liz Shirran, Ruth Thomas, Graham Mowatt, Cynthia Fraser, Lisa Bero, Roberto Grilli, Emma Harvey, Andy Oxman, and Mary Ann

O'Brien. 2001. "Changing Provider Behavior: An Overview of Systematic Reviews of Interventions." *Medical Care* 39, 8 Supplement 2: II2–45.

Grossman, Jason, and Fiona J. MacKenzie. 2005. "The Randomized Controlled Trial: Gold Standard or Merely Standard." *Perspectives in Biology and Medicine* 48(4): 516–34.

Guggenheim, Ricardo. 2005. "Putting EBM to Work (Easier Said Than Done)." *Managed Care* 14(12): 33–43.

Hatala, Rose, and Gordon Guyatt. 2002. "Evaluating the Teaching of Evidence-Based Medicine." *Journal of the American Medical Association* 288(9): 1110–12.

Havighurst, Clark C. 1995. *Health Care Choices: Private Contracts as Instruments of Health Reform.* Washington, D.C.: AEI Press.

Hoff, Timothy J. 1999. "The Social Organization of Physician-Managers in a Changing HMO." *Work and Occupations* 26(3): 324–51.

Hyams, Andrew L., Jennifer A. Brandenburg, Stuart R. Lipsitz, David W. Shapiro, and Troyen A. Brennan. 1995. "Practice Guidelines and Malpractice Litigation: A Two-Way Street." *Annals of Internal Medicine* 122(6): 450–55.

Jackson, Sue, and Graham Scambler. 2007. "Perceptions of Evidence-Based Medicine: Traditional Acupuncturists in the UK and Resistance to Biomedical Modes of Evaluation." *Sociology of Health and Illness* 29(3): 412–29.

Jacobson, Peter D. 1997. "Legal and Policy Considerations in Using Clinical Practice Guidelines." *American Journal of Cardiology* 80(8B): 74H–79H.

Katz, Jay. 1984. *The Silent World of Doctor and Patient.* New York: Free Press.

Lakoff, Andrew. 2005. *Pharmaceutical Reason: Knowledge and Value in Global Psychiatry.* Cambridge: Cambridge University Press.

Lambert, Helen. 2006. "Accounting for EBM: Notions of Evidence in Medicine. *Social Science and Medicine* 62(11): 2633–45.

Landsman, Gail H. 2006. What Evidence, Whose Evidence? Physical Therapy in New York State's Clinical Practice Guideline and in the Lives of Mothers of Disabled Children." *Social Science and Medicine* 62(11): 2670–80.

Leon, Sergio A., Paul Fontelo, Linda Green, Michael Ackerman, and Fang Liu. 2007. "Evidence-Based Medicine among Internal Medicine Residents in a Community Hospital Program Using Smart Phones." *BMC Medical Informatics and Decision Making* 7(5).

Light, Donald W. 1979. "Uncertainty and Control in Professional Training." *Journal of Health and Social Behavior* 20(4): 310–22.

———. 1988. "Towards a New Sociology of Medical Education." *Journal of Health and Social Behavior* 29:307–22.

———. 2000. "The Medical Profession and Organizational Change: From Professional Dominance to Countervailing Power." In *The Handbook of Medical Sociology*, 5th ed., ed. C. E. Bird, P. Conrad, and A. M. Fremont, 201–16. Upper Saddle River, N.J: Prentice Hall.

Marks, Harry. 1997. *The Progress of Experiment: Science and Therapeutic Reform in the United States, 1900–1990.* Cambridge: Cambridge University Press.

May, Carl, Tim Rapley, Tiago Moreira, Tracy Finch, and Ben Heaven. 2006. "Technogovernance: Evidence, Subjectivity, and the Clinical Encounter in Primary Care Medicine." *Social Science and Medicine* 62(4): 1022–30.

McCord, Gary, William D. Smucker, Brian A. Selius, Scott Hannan, Elliot Davidson, Susan L. Schrop, Vinod Rao, and Paula Albrecht. 2007. "Answering Questions at the Point of Care: Do Residents Practice EBM or Manage Information Sources?" *Academic Medicine* 82(3): 298–303.

McGlynn, Elisabeth A., Steven M. Asch, John Adams, Joan Keesey, Jennifer Hicks, Alison DeCristofaro, and Eve A. Kerr. 2003. "The Quality of Health Care Delivered to Adults in the United States." *New England Journal of Medicine* 348(26): 2635–45.

McGuire, Wendy L. 2005. "Beyond EBM: New Directions for Evidence-Based Public Health." *Perpectives in Biology and Medicine* 48(4): 557–69.

Moreira, Tiago. 2005. "Diversity in Clinical Guidelines: The Role of Repertoires of Evaluation." *Social Science and Medicine* 60(9): 1975–85.

———. 2007. "Entangled Evidence: Knowledge Making in Systematic Reviews in Healthcare." *Sociology of Health and Illness* 29(2): 180–97.

Pope, Catherine. 2003. "Resisting Evidence: The Study of Evidence-Based Medicine as a Contemporary Social Movement." *Health* 7(3): 267–82.

Porter, Theodore. 1995. *Trust in Numbers: Objectivity in Science and Public Life.* Princeton, N.J.: Princeton University Press.

Porzsolt, Franz, Andrea Ohletz, Anke Thim, David Gardner, Helmuth Ruatti, Horand Meier, Nicole Schlotz-Gorton, and Laura Schrott. 2003. "Evidence-Based Decision Making—The 6-Step approach." *ACP Journal Club* 139(3): A11–12.

Prosser, Helen, and Tom Walley. 2006. "New Drug Prescribing by Hospital Doctors: The Nature and Meaning of Knowledge." *Social Science and Medicine* 62:1565–78.

Rappolt, Susan M. 1997. "Clinical Guidelines and the Fate of Medical Autonomy in Ontario." *Social Science and Medicine* 44(7): 977–87.

Reed, Michael I. 1996. "Expert Power and Control in Late Modernity: An Empirical Review and Theoretical Synthesis." *Organization Studies* 17(4): 573–97.

Ross, Robert, and Alex Verdieck. 2003. "Introducing an Evidence-Based Medicine Curriculum into a Family Practice Residency—Is It Effective?" *Academic Medicine* 78(4): 412–17.

Rowe, John W. 2006. "Pay-for-Performance and Accountability: Related Themes in Improving Health Care." *Annals of Internal Medicine* 145:695–99.

Sackett, David L., William M. C. Rosenberg, J. A. Gray, Brian R. Haynes, and W. Scott Richardson. 1996. "Evidence Based Medicine: What It Is and What It Isn't." *British Medical Journal* 312 (January 13): 71–72.

Sackett, David L., Sharon E. Straus, W. Scott Richardson, William Rosenberg, and Brian R. Haynes. 2000. *Evidence-Based Medicine: How to Practice and Teach EBM.* 2nd ed. Edinburgh: Churchill Livingstone.

Shojania, Kaveh G., and Jeremy Grimshaw. 2005. "Evidence-Based Quality Improvement: The State of the Science." *Health Affairs* 24(1): 138–50.

Starr, Paul. 1982. *The Social Transformation of Medicine.* New York: Basic Books.

Stevermer, James J., Mark L. Chambliss, and G. S. Hoekzema. 1999. "Distilling the Literature: A Randomized, Controlled Trial Testing an Intervention to Improve Selection of Medical Articles for Reading." *Academic Medicine* 74(1): 70–72.

Stewart, Walter F., Nirah R. Shah, Mark J. Selna, Ronald A. Paulus, and James M. Walker. 2007. "Bridging the Inferential Gap: The Electronic Health Record and Clinical Evidence." *Health Affairs* 26(2): w181–91.

Straus, Sharon E., Chris Ball, Nick Balcombe, Jonathan Sheldon, and Finlay A. McAlister. 2005. "Teaching Evidence-Based Medicine Skills Can Change Practice in a Community Hospital." *Journal of General and Internal Medicine* 20(4): 340–43.

Straus, Sharon E., Michael L. Green, Douglas S. Bell, Robert Badgett, Dave Davis, Marta Gerrity, Eduarado Ortiz, Terrence M. Shaneyfelt, Chad Whelan, and Rajesh Mangrulkar. 2004. "Evaluating the Teaching of Evidence Based Medicine: Conceptual Framework." *British Medical Journal* 329:1029–32.

Straus, Sharon E., and Finlay A. McAlister. 2000. "Evidence-Based Medicine: A Commentary on Common Criticisms." *Canadian Medical Association Journal* 163:837–41.

Timmermans, Stefan, and Alison Angell. 2001. "Evidence-Based Medicine, Clinical Uncertainty, and Learning to Doctor," *Journal of Health and Social Behavior* 42 (4): 342–59.

Timmermans, Stefan, and Marc Berg. 2003. *The Gold Standard: The Challenge of Evidence-Based Medicine and Standardization in Health Care.* Philadelphia: Temple University Press.

Timmermans, Stefan, and Emily Kolker. 2004. "Evidence-Based Medicine and the Reconfiguration of Medical Knowledge." *Journal of Health and Social Behavior* 45, extra issue: 177–93.

Timmermans, Stefan, and Aaron Mauck. 2005. "The Promises and Pitfalls of Evidence-Based Medicine." *Health Affairs* 24(1): 18–28.

Traynor, Michael. 2000. "Purity, Conversion and the Evidence-Based Movements." *Health* 4(2): 139–58.

Upshur, Ross E. G. 2005. "Looking for Rules in a World of Exceptions." *Perpectives in Biology and Medicine* 48(4): 477–89.

Villanueva-Russell, Yvonne 2005. "Evidence-Based Medicine and Its Implications for the Profession of Chiropractic." *Social Science and Medicine* 60(3): 545–61.

Wennberg, John E., and M. M. Cooper, eds. 1999. *The Quality of Medical Care in the United States: A Report on the Medicare Program; The Dartmouth Atlas of Health Care 1999.* Chicago: American Hospital Publishing.

Will, Catherine M. 2005. "Arguing about the Evidence: Readers, Writers, and Inscription Devices in Coronary Heart Disease Risk Assessment." *Sociology of Health and Illness* 27(6): 780–801.

Windish, Donna M., Stephen J. Huot, and Michael L. Green. 2007. "Medicine Residents' Understanding of the Biostatistics and Results in the Medical Literature." *Journal of the American Medical Association* 298:1010–22.

Worrall, John. 2002. What Evidence in Evidence-Based Medicine? *Philosophy of Science* 69:S316–30.

19

The Sociology of Quality and Safety in Health Care
Studying a Movement and Moving Sociology

Teun Zuiderent-Jerak, Erasmus University Rotterdam

Marc Berg, Plexus Medical Group and Erasmus University Rotterdam

In the last decade the emerging activities in the field of quality and safety improvement in health care are resulting in new practices of governing medicine and posing challenges to prevailing notions of what it means to be a good doctor, patient, manager, or even health-care system. Following the seminal work of Wennberg and Gittelsohn (1973), who analyzed high variation in treatment patterns in neighboring communities in New England that could not be explained by clinical differences or "case mix" (Wennberg 1984), and based on reported adherence rates to clinical guidelines by medical professionals of approximately 50 percent, institutions for health-care improvement have created an awareness among patients, policy makers, and clinicians that receiving treatment is actually a risky business.[1] Health care is not simply a domain where patients are cured or cared for: it is a field full of dangers, and hospitals in particular are increasingly seen as risky places.

When the Institute of Medicine published its report *To Err Is Human: Building a Safer Health System* (CQHCA 2000), major newspapers including the *Wall Street Journal* and the *Washington Post* led with front-page articles citing the conclusion that between forty-four thousand and ninety-eight thousand Americans died each

year as a consequence not of the diseases they were being treated for, but of errors that occurred during hospital treatment (Kenney 2008, 87). Besides the strength of these large numbers, there were shocking individual cases that further indicated problems with the health-care system. One of these cases was the dreadful death of Betsy Lehman, chief medical columnist of the *Boston Globe*, who received a massive overdose of experimental chemotherapy during her cancer treatment in one of the most renowned cancer institutes in the United States, the Dana-Farber Cancer Institute in Boston. Her doctor had prescribed "cyclophosphamide dose 4 grams/square meter (of body surface area) over 4 days" (ibid., 6), but where this was intended to be the *total* dose that should be administered over a period of four days, it was taken by the fellow administering the medication to signify the *daily* dose of medication over a four-day period. After strong reactions to the medication, which were classified by care professionals as "normal" responses to this form of experimental treatment, Lehman died in the hospital at age thirty-nine.

Quality and safety in health care are by no means completely new topics in medical sociology. Discussions on the quality and safety of care practices have been discussed as part of the sociology of professions, for example. As Donald Light wrote in his critical reading of authors like Freidson and Abbott in the previous edition of the *Handbook of Medical Sociology*:

> To wistfully remember "the Golden Age of Doctoring" (McKinlay 1999) is to forget that it was also the age of gold (Rodwin 1993), the age of unjustified large variations of hospitalization and surgery caused by autonomy and lack of accountable standards (Wennberg and Gittelsohn 1973), the age of large portions of tests, prescriptions, operations, and hospitalizations judged to be unnecessary by clinical researchers (Greenberg 1971), the age of medicalizing social problems (Conrad and Schneider 1992), the age of irresponsibly fragmented care in the name of "autonomy," the age of escalating prices and overcharging to a degree unknown anywhere else in the West (Navarro 1976; Waitzkin 1983; White 1991), the age of provider-structured insurance that paid for almost any mistake or poor investment anyone happened to make, and the age of corporations moving in to reap the no-lose profits of such a world by exploiting the profession on its own terms. (Light 2000, 202).

In this sense it has long been clear to medical sociologists that quality and safety in health care should never be assumed. However, the discussion on countervailing powers that Light presents as a solution to the problem of the excesses of professional autonomy implies that quality and safety is lacking because of failing institutional arrangements that should "help the profession be as trustworthy as it would like to be, but cannot be on its own" (ibid., 212). Having countervailing powers in place may suffice to counter *intentional* flaws in the systems of health care, but not to address errors and problems in medical practice that stem from more systemic properties.

The quality and safety improvement movement that is emerging in response to the problems in the delivery of health care is highly involved in a practice that medical sociology has for many decades been exploring: analyzing and problematizing medical practice in substantial and increasingly influential ways. Yet this movement also is involved in this practice in different ways than medical sociologists have been. What is particularly interesting about the problematization that comes from health-care improvement agents is that this critique on the one hand comes from

within influential institutions like the Institute for Healthcare Improvement, and on the other hand is coupled to a strong agenda for change—which seems to force outsiders like medical sociologists to respecify what exactly they are doing.

In this chapter we explore these developments in the quality and safety movement in health care, analyze how a topology of this field produces new and interesting areas for sociological enquiry, and explore the reflexive discussions the movement is triggering within the field of medical sociology. Developments in quality and safety in health care provide an interesting domain for doing medical sociology as well as an opportunity for respecifying what the role of medical sociology might entail in the problematization of medical practice. We also propose that the quality and safety movement can be seen as an inspiriting field to sociologically address one of the aspects that has largely been denied in medical sociology: the study of clinical outcomes and effective health care as an integral part of medical sociology (Timmermans and Haas 2008). Such a sociology of effectiveness is likely to take into account the normative purpose of quality and safety improvement, while rendering many of the prevailing notions of clinical outcomes in quality and safety improvement practices much more complex and problematizing present conceptualizations of much improvement work. A sociology of effectiveness therefore by no means needs to become subservient to quality improvement agendas, but neither will it fall back into merely critiquing quality and safety improvement initiatives. We propose that the aim of sociologically scrutinizing effectiveness in healthcare (improvement) practices should be, to paraphrase Latour (2004, 231), not to get away from outcomes but to get closer to them, not to fight effectiveness but, on the contrary, to renew it.

Dissecting the Quality and Safety Movement

Though there are tendencies to present a wide range of quality and safety improvement initiatives as a uniform movement (Kenney 2008) or as a social movement (Bate, Robert, and Bevan 2004), such categorizations seem to gloss over crucial differences within the field of improving health care. These differences are not merely due to the large variety of medical domains that is targeted by improvement initiatives. More importantly, they seem to stem from different ontologies about what it means to do quality improvement in health care. These differences lead to a wide range of practices within quality and safety improvement that both afford and warrant different medical sociological analyses. We propose that one of the difficulties in studying the quality and safety movement is that it is theoretically and empirically much more fragmented than is often assumed (Zuger 2008). Dissecting this movement in terms of its subfields may be helpful for developing the social study of this emerging field. To this end, we suggest four prominent themes that are theoretically and empirically rather distinct: (1) the improvement of patient safety through safety science and the systems approach; (2) the approach of quality improvement collaboratives with their focus on shared knowledge development and learning; (3) the introduction of performance management practices with their focus on indicators as drivers of improvement; and (4) practices of standardizing health-care practices with the aim of designing reliable health-care systems. These themes not only provide a (partial) overview of the field of quality and safety improvement but also indicate different sociological questions regarding issues of effective improvement that one can ask in relation to these subfields, and thus are helpful for exploring various strands of the sociology of effectiveness.

Safety and Systems: Dissolving the Human in Care Practices

One of the most important and well-researched strands within health-care improvement initiatives focuses on the improvement of patient safety through safety science and the systems approach. Following the report *To Err Is Human* and a series of other reports and white papers, health-care improvement advocates have redefined health-care institutions in two ways: first, these institutions are unsafe due to the many human errors that occur when providing care, and second,

this lack of safety can be fixed, since these institutions are systems in which safety can be built in as a nonhuman property. This definition has proven highly consequential for improvement and research agendas that deal with patient safety in many (inter)national health-care settings. It has, for example, resulted in additional funding for safety improvement programs in the United States (Aspden et al. 2004), provided a substantial boost for the importance of incident-monitoring systems in Australia (Runciman 2002), and led to the development of a safety management system in the Netherlands aiming at "attacking medical errors" (van Geenen 2005) in health-care systems.

One of the most striking aspects of the development of the focus on safety improvement is the definition of (un)safety as a system property. On the one hand, this definition is an attempt to shift the problem of unsafe care from the individual practitioner to the system in which such a practitioner is working (Perrow 1999; Vaughan 1997); on the other hand, this way of conceptualizing safety makes self-regulation of the medical profession problematic, in that medical professionals are not experts on designing complex organizational systems. Therefore, the connection of safety improvement to safety science with its own expertise, institutions, and journals such as *Human Factors* provides what Justin Waring has called "a non-medical knowledge-base from which to regulate medical performance" (Waring 2007, 164). The introduction of safety science to health-care improvement thus has interesting epistemological consequences as it reclassifies clinical expertise as just one of the forms of knowledge needed to organize good care.

Medical sociologists have realized for some time that this was an interesting field for studying safety improvement practices. Medical professionals had to find ways to deal with situations where, for example, root cause analysis (RCA) techniques developed in industry and in defense were deployed to analyze errors in clinical practice. Interestingly, RCA in industry was initially modeled on a biomedical image—having to diagnose the root of the problem before coming up with the right cure for the disease. This model of medical practice has been problematized within medical sociology, as empirical studies show that medical work often is more iterative, that is, starting a treatment with only a general notion of what the diagnosis may be and using the response to the treatment to find out, in part, what needs to be done and what the disease is (Berg 1997). Yet this textbook version of good medical practice took a detour via industry and is now presented back to medical practice to improve the safety of healthcare work. In RCA sessions, medical professionals have to scrutinize the errors of their colleagues according to the model of diagnosis before treatment, a practice that David Armstrong has conceptualized as the medical gaze being turned in on itself (Armstrong 2002).

Medical sociologists studying such RCA practices empirically have mainly focused on the questions this development raises for the governance of medicine. Rick Iedema and colleagues (2006, 1605), for example, have asked whether the reflexivity imposed on doctors through RCAs leads to a specific type of root causes being defined, and they are particularly interested in "whether this reflexivity will lock the clinical gaze into a microsociology of error, or whether it will enable this gaze to influence . . . the over-arching governance and structuring of hospital care." Raising a similar question, Waring (2007) has found that doctors do try to circumvent the managerial implications of the inclusion of new forms of expertise in defining what good medical work is, for example, by refusing to report clinical errors. As other aspects of the new safety science practices are adopted, Waring terms as "adaptive regulation" the way "doctors seek to maintain their regulatory monopoly and limit managerial encroachment" (ibid., 163). Drawing on the Foucauldian notion of governmentality (Foucault 1991), Waring states that the adaptations doctors make in their regulatory practice allow them to include safety science in their self-surveillance practices. Hereby they seem to serve the policy aims but no longer need to provide access to more management or external surveillance of medical work.

These interesting findings within the debate on professional autonomy and self-regulation of the medical profession should be related to the issue that was the reason for introducing safety improvement practices and different expertise into clinical practice. To mainly view these activities to build safe systems as attempts to control professionals would be a cynical reading, in light of the safety problems encountered in medical practice. It is therefore relevant to ask *why* care professionals are "resistively compliant" (Timmons 2003) to these practices. As Waring (2005) claims, it may be that doctors see error as an integral and unavoidable part of medical work, which reduces the relevance of RCA practices and turns them into an extra and pointless administrative burden. If this analysis is correct, conceptualizing the limited adoption by clinicians of RCA as "anti-bureaucratic sentiment" (ibid., 1927) is not an end point but the point at which to start looking for the instances where errors do seem unavoidable in complex practices (Law 2000) and separating those from routinized errors that may easily be prevented by other organizational routines. As medical sociologists have shown, medical professionals who are training new professionals are deemed highly able to both "control mistakes" and allow for "honest errors of the inexperienced" (Bosk 2003). Such discriminatory skills may also be relevant for the analysis of routinized errors by *experienced* professionals. By bringing such processes of separating harmful from fruitful errors into the analysis of the construction of "safe systems," sociological discussions on professionalism remain connected to the effectiveness of safety improvement and of clinical work. In this light it becomes important not only to understand how errors occur as gaps in the safety net but also to understand how safe systems are already achieved in practice—and which errors are part of such systems. If this is not studied, any attempt to build safe systems might actually lead to a reduction of safety, as it may interfere with the resilience of care practices to prevent errors in the complexity of medical work. These are exactly the questions that Mesman (2007, 2008, forthcoming) raises in her work on safety practices in the high-risk environment of the neonatal intensive care unit. From the perspective of a sociology of effectiveness, the question on avoiding errors can thereby draw upon a differentiation between errors that are to be avoided and errors that are to be accepted, and can learn how to make this difference partly by studying how safety is achieved in practice.

Quality Improvement Collaboratives: Tensions between Learning and Best Practices

As a second substrand in our topology, one of the main approaches for quality improvement developed since the late 1980s is the quality improvement collaborative in which improvement teams from different institutions meet to work on a particular domain of care provision, like reducing pressure sores or the number of medication errors. Such collaboratives are characterized by a strong focus on rapid learning cycles of trial and error and a can-do attitude that values creative ideas by care professionals and patients about ways to redesign care practices. This focus on learning within a collaborative setting is combined with a thorough belief in the importance of *measuring* in quality improvement. This aspect of the quality movement thereby combines a focus on learning environments and bottom-up organizational change with a strong conviction in progress and the notion that learning leads all organizations ultimately in the same direction, i.e., toward a best practice (Kilo 1998; Mittman 2004).

The tensions between bottom-up improvement in local settings and measuring performance to ensure that all involved organizations develop toward the standard set by the single best practice raise interesting questions about how these seemingly incommensurable requirements are aligned in practice. When studying quality improvement collaboratives, this tension seems to be resolved during working conferences partly by familiarizing improvement teams from participating care institutions with notions that form part of the grammar of quality improvement, such as the distinction between structure indicators, process indicators, and outcome indicators (Donabedian 2005) and by introducing them to the practicalities of making run-charts in Excel to monitor their results. Performance measurement is generally presented as a core element of improvement practices and yet, in order not to scare off participating care workers with this quite new and technical world of performance measurement, the work that is implied in measuring improvement is generally presented as doable and easy (Zuiderent-Jerak et al., 2009).

Through these two notions—improvement requires measurement, and measuring performance is simple—the teams are introduced to a conceptualization of performance management that is similar to, as Thomas Kuhn critically phrased it, "our most prevalent notions both about the function of measurement and about the source of its special efficacy [which] are derived largely from myth" (1977, 179). The resulting difficulty for collaborative improvement projects is that they try to reconcile the wish for finding simple measurement structures with the immensely complex improvement practices of bottom-up quality and safety improvement. More complex measurement infrastructures are often—though not always—shunned out of fear of frustrating local improvement practices, although for these measurements to be relevant for these practices, they would need to be much more specific. The mythological strength of simple performance measurement and the singularized notion of "effectiveness" in complex practices has been discussed and critiqued over the last decades in general terms (Kuhn 1977; Porter 1995, 1997; Power 1997, 2004) and in specific relation to quality and safety improvement in health care (May et al. 2006; Tanenbaum 1994, 2005). However, within the world of health-care improvement collaboratives, this myth of the unproblematic nature of performance management is kept alive to reconcile measuring the so-called objective performance of improvement with the complexity of sites where such improvement takes place and with very different experiences by local improvement teams.

In those cases where indicators *were* productive in coordinating quality improvement initiatives, achieving this productive relationship seemed far from easy or natural. In a collaborative improvement project with the aim of improving the flow of patient trajectories through Dutch hospitals (Zuiderent-Jerak 2009), we found that the indicator of "throughput time" of patients from the moment of referral until the moment of ending the follow up was able to coordinate efforts to reduce many forms of suffering: the suffering of patients who had to wait long times before their diagnosis was known, the suffering of professionals who were unable to deliver the quality of care they were hoping to deliver due to long waits at the radiology department, for example, and the suffering of managers who had to face the high costs not only in terms of quality but also in terms of financial losses due to inefficiencies. This only became clear, however, through enormous amounts of extra work by various improvement actors. Therefore, the issue we wish to address here is not that indicators cannot be productively aligned with collaborative quality improvement initiatives, but that the notion that such productive relations emerge self-evidently and are in any sense easy is largely derived from myth and managerial daydreaming about "steering" improvement based on the often-used metaphor of "dashboards" of performance indicators. Such assumptions are unproductive, as they desensitize improvement agents for all the forms of often "invisible work" (Star and Strauss 1999; Suchman 1995) that need to be done by IT departments, nurses, quality managers in care institutions, and quality improvement agents in collaboratives to make this seemingly simple work possible.

Analyzing these complexities of measuring effective improvement and bottom-up organizational development on domains in quality and safety produces a number of questions that a sociology of effectiveness could aim to address: How are learning and measuring aligned in the practice of collaborative quality improvement? Which forms of invisible work need to be carried out to enact this alignment? What is the relationship between the content and complexity of an improvement initiative and the ease with which quality indicators can be used as generic measures of "effectiveness"? What other forms of articulating improvement— e.g., more narrative forms of sharing local improvement experiences with other organizations—could be explored and how would these create different opportunities for learning? How would a different conceptualization of a best practice that is not attached to the highest measured performance but that draws upon a more processual notion of "best suiting a local improvement initiative" generate other possibilities for sharing relevant insights across improvement teams? And what can such studies of improvement contribute to the exploration of the relation between aggregates and their particulars in health-care improvement and also in more general terms (Stinchcombe 2001)?

This last question brings us to the next subdomain of the quality improvement movement:

the development of quality and safety indicators in health care.

Indicators of Quality and Safety: Incentives for Improvement?

This third subsphere of the quality and safety movement has an equally high trust in measuring, but rather than aligning measurement to bottom-up improvement initiatives, this sphere focuses on the strength of performance indicators to *generate* potential for improvement. The performance management initiatives within quality improvement suppose that by measuring performance, health-care practices are typically first inspired and later forced to improve their quality. The introduction of indicator systems is related to the idea that the autonomy of professionals can no longer be decoupled from the outcomes of their work, as it has been by the classical medical sociological focus on self-regulation (Freidson 1970). Though starting as externally imposed governance infrastructures, these indicators have been conceptualized as attempts to incorporate health-care professionals in more managerial agendas (Harrison and Pollitt 1994). Such a conceptualization however often seems to produce an illusive distinction between managers and professionals when studying the ways in which professional work involves organizational aspects and managerial work focusing on coordinating care trajectories (Noordergraaf 2007). Another way to analyze the introduction of indicators is to see them as experimental devices that allow for an empirical exploration of the consequences of such externally imposed structures for quality and safety of health care (Berg et al. 2005). In that sense, quality indicators as performance management infrastructures could be seen as attempts to refigure the notion of autonomy toward what Pieter Degeling and colleagues have coined "responsible autonomy" (Degeling, Maxwell, and Iedema 2004). This is a form of autonomy that is not disjoined from quality in terms of the clinical outcomes that professionals achieve.

Yet, though the study of clinical indicators has led to such interesting reconceptualizations of long-standing discussions on professional autonomy and on the role of indicators as experiments in health-care practices, most of these discussions have been programmatic rather than empirical. The pragmatic study of performance management practices has largely been carried out by policy scientists (see, for example, Bevan 2004, Bevan and Hood 2006) rather than by medical sociologists. The rare examples that are there, however, show that the social study of performance indicators generates interesting findings about the role such indicators play in quality improvement and the difficulties improvement agents face when trying to align the need for good scores with prevailing improvement practices. In their empirical study of the consequences of the introduction of a national set of performance indicators for Dutch hospital care, Sonja Jerak-Zuiderent and Roland Bal (forthcoming) indicate, for example, that the inclusion of the glucose value HbA1c of diabetes patients in the set of indicators that hospitals need to deliver each year to the Netherlands Health Care Inspectorate provided a logic of improvement that was hard to reconcile with the prevailing logic of improvement that had mainly focused on providing integrated care for diabetes patients across care institutions. Due to the initial focus on good integration of the care provided by the general practitioners (GPs) and the hospital, most of the patients with lower HbA1c values were receiving their treatment from their general practitioner, which had been considered good care before the introduction of the performance indicators: the hospital could then focus on the clinically harder cases, while the GPs could serve the patients who mainly needed coaching in reconciling their roles as patients with the other social worlds they were inhabiting (Clark 1997; Zuiderent-Jerak, in press). But as this hospital had been quite successful in dividing the care among the GPs and their physicians, the majority of these good patients were not seen in the hospital and the score on HbA1c value for their remaining patients therefore was bound to be poor. This situation left the quality manager and care workers with the question of which logic of improvement to follow: the logic of improvement as integrated care or the logic of improvement as a good HbA1c score at the hospital level?

What this study shows is that programmatic claims about the strength of logics of improvement that are based on incentives for improving care are in need of a reality check to see with which prevailing improvement practices and incentives they may be conflicting. Such analyses can of course lead to insights for improving sets of performance indicators by highlighting, for, example the need for case-mix correction, adjusting the HbA1c score per hospital for the type of diabetes patients treated there. With this correction alone, however, a sociology of effectiveness could get caught in the "repair metaphor" (Markussen and Olesen 2007) of infrastructures that do not perform as expected. This would also lead to a role for medical sociologists as improvement agents of quality improvement initiatives. Another possibility is to object to the creation of accountability structures in care practices, as these would merely frustrate the actual care work (Wiener 2000). Yet this would lead to a sociology of effectiveness that is merely critical and that bypasses the substantial problems that health-care systems are facing in producing safe and reliable care. Though it may be possible to critique all forms of indicator-driven accountability and improvement initiatives, the stakes of some of those initiatives seem to be too high to justify such a one-sided analysis. Included in the Dutch set of indicators, for example, is a volume indicator for surgeons performing esophagus resections that is based on clinical evidence which shows that surgeons performing less than fifteen such operations a year have substantially higher mortality rates than do their colleagues for whom such surgery is more routine (Birkmeyer et al. 2003). Since the introduction of this indicator, surgeons who are unable to do at least fifteen such operations a year are no longer allowed to perform them, which should be an immediate livesaver for a number of patients. Though this indicator may lead to registering more cases as esophagus resections—a practice that health economists call "upcoding" (Steinbusch et al. 2007)—and to other unforeseen consequences for quality improvement, medical sociologists will have some explaining to do if they want to claim that such accountability structures merely frustrate clinical work rather than rightly shape care practices.

We therefore rather think that such empirical

studies of performance indicators should lead to sociological reflection on both the productive potential of their coordinating strength and on the limitations and tricky nature (Haraway 1991) of accountability systems in clinical practice. Such sensitivity to these different aspects of performance indicators prevents what Sheila Jasanoff has called "peripheral blindness toward uncertainty and ambiguity" without losing track of the potential gains that accountability practices may produce. Such analyses can also help prevent what Jasanoff has called "technologies of hubris" and contribute to the experimental development of "technologies of humility" that are highly specific of their actual consequences for quality and safety in care practices (Jasanoff 2003, 238–39). In the case of performance indicators, this would further highlight the importance not only of studying the unforeseen consequences that emerge when indicators are introduced to care practices but also of analyzing the performance regimes in which such indicators are used and how much space those regimes provide for the explanations of a possible bad outcome (Bal 2008; Jerak-Zuiderent and Bal, forthcoming).

Within this study of performance indicators in health care, the insight that the quantitative format tends to lead to a process of purification (Latour 1987) in which the space for the story behind the outcomes quickly gets lost (Zuiderent-Jerak 2009) may help remind quality and safety improvement agents of the *predictable* unexpected consequences of performance measurement infrastructures, such as the ranking that often follows from indicators that were produced for internal use. Such a study of the probabilities produced through certain forms of improvement will produce highly interesting research (Thévenot 2002).

Standardizing Health-Care Practices: Clinical Pathways as Process or Product

The attempt to standardize health-care practices, a fourth theme of quality and safety improvement, is strongly related to the development of integrated care pathways that sway between the evidence-based medicine focus on reducing practice variation and the more processual approaches to standardization as a political process. The aim of such practices often is to *design for reliability* (Nolan et al. 2004) and to ensure that health care is organized in care processes that allow organizations and professionals to deliver care that is of better quality in the sense that it is more coordinated.

Since the early 1950s, standardization and patient-centered care have been strongly contrasted in the medical sociological literature (Freidson 1960; Parsons 1951; Strauss et al. 1997). Standardization has generally been conceptualized as an ally of the biomedical model of medicine that was criticized to make way for patient-centered care delivery (Benzing 2000; Mead and Bower 2000), which is thus generally positioned as a response to the proliferation of evidence-based medicine. Proponents of this dichotomy claim that in "the conventional way of doing medicine, often labeled the 'biomedical model,' . . . the patient's illness is reduced to a set of signs and symptoms which are investigated and interpreted within a positivist biomedical framework" (Mead and Bower 2000, 1088), whereas patient-centered medicine requires a "willingness to become involved in the full range of difficulties patients bring to their doctors, and not just their biomedical problems" (Stewart et al. 1995).[2] In this discussion, a rather interesting actor is introduced: the "patient-centered doctor" (Mead and Bower 2000). This unusual and compassionate being of course makes all other doctors seem like awkward medical professionals who set the wrong priorities in what otherwise could be a noble profession.

The dichotomy between patient-centered care and standardization has been brought to the fore in the analysis of the development of all kinds of integrated care pathways (ICPs), a trend very much in vogue over the last few years (Pinder et al. 2005). Whereas proponents tend to ascribe almost mythical powers to care pathways, claiming, for example, that standardization of health-care practices can provide impressive increases in efficiency (Evans 1997), effectiveness (Berdick and Humphries 1994), and patient and professional satisfaction (Ford and Fottler 2000), standardization of care practices has mainly been critically analyzed by (medical) sociologists who warn of the creation of "assembly-line medicine" that will ultimately lead to the "dehumanization and depersonalization of medical practice" (Ritzer 1992, 43).

However, such claims about patient-centered doctors and general sociological critiques of standardizing care practices can be maintained only by excluding from the sociological analysis the study of effectiveness. To overcome the analytical gridlock created by proponents and critics of standardization, it would be important to study standardization in health care in a less antagonistic way and to include the study of effectiveness of care. To do so, Timmermans and Berg have proposed "a study of the *politics of standardization in practice*" (2003, 21, emphasis in the original), that focuses on the actual changes in medical practice as a result of standardization and on the perceivable renegotiations of orders, autonomies, and, we would add, outcomes that come with the standards. Focusing on standardization as, "paradoxically, *a dynamic process of change*" (ibid., 23, emphasis in the original) may change the value of pathways from "Taylorist devices for standardizing care and treating each individual in precisely the same way" to "means of affording individualistic treatment, while simultaneously creating organizational efficiency by 'tayloring' the organisation to the patient (rather than the other way round)" (Pinder et al. 2005, 774–75). With this shift it is no longer the pathway but the pathwaying that is put center stage, and this opens up new spaces for differentiating between forms of standardization and their consequences.

When we studied the development of integrated care pathways in a Dutch university hospital (Zuiderent-Jerak 2007), the aim of improving the patient-centeredness of care was pursued through the development of standardized care trajectories. This practice invoked the question of how the dichotomy between standardization and patient-centeredness could be refigured. It turned out that including effectiveness in the sociological analysis problematized the classical opposition of these two concepts. We soon discovered that one of the oncologists in this hospital neatly fit the description of a patient-centered doctor, taking all the time a patient could ask for and even advising on personal matters that other doctors would immediately classify as outside their expertise and at

best problems for the medical psychologist. Perhaps unsurprisingly, she also strongly opposed the initiative to standardize certain aspects of the care work that would allow some parts of her work to be carried out by specialized nurses. She claimed that the so-called efficiency gains this shift promised would in fact lead to more work for her, as she would have to check all the work of nurses, who, she stated, were actually unable to give psychosocial care. Later, one of the nurses informed us that this oncologist was deviating widely from the protocols of the treatment trials her patients were going through, continuing with treatment for much longer than clinically advised. Interestingly, her patient-centered approach gave her almost full control over patients at their weakest moments, when they would have to accept that there were no further treatment options—a situation nurses administering the extended treatment could hardly bear. Standardizing certain aspects of the work would lead to shared responsibility among professionals and would make this oncologist accountable for clinical decisions in ways that challenged her present care practices. She successfully refused these initiatives, partly by mobilizing patients to send letters of complaint to the professor of oncology indicating they were upset that their doctor was no longer allowed to spend more time with them. What this study indicates is that by focusing primarily on patient-centered care as situated in the interpersonal encounter between two human beings—a doctor and a patient—*patient-centered care* is completely decoupled from notions of *effective care*. So though classical definitions of patient-centeredness may at first look very sympathetic, justifying critiques of standardization, connecting notions of patient centeredness to the sociology of effectiveness shows how such care can turn out to be highly coercive (Silverman 1987). A more processual approach to the development and the study of standardizing health-care practices leads to opening up both concepts—patient-centered care and standardization—and allows more specific analysis of the effectiveness of these different forms. In this sense a sociological critique of standardization initiatives is able to take into account the normative consequences not only of standardizing care but also of *not* standardizing particular care trajectories, thereby also elucidating the normative purchase of standardization initiatives.

With this topology of various subspheres of quality and safety improvement in health care, and by drawing on the very different debates that the social study of improvement generates, we have shown that these themes afford specific analyses of the consequences of quality and safety improvement on the relationship between professionals and managers, on the governance of medical work, and on the types of implementation problems these initiatives face. We also have made the case that including the sociological analysis of the effectiveness of quality improvement enriches the debates that sociologists engage with and ignores the normative purpose of quality and safety improvement initiatives when studying them. We now return to the question of how the sociology of effectiveness is helpful for reflecting on the role of medical sociologists in relation to the practices of quality and safety they may want to study.

Sociological Contributions to Quality and Safety

Now that medical sociology has been joined by the health-care improvement movement in the work of problematizing medical practice, a discussion is emerging about how the initiatives of the quality and safety movement are compatible with the task medical sociologists set themselves— the analysis and refiguring of medical practices. Some medical sociologists have proposed that similarities between sociologists and improvement agents present opportunities for coming to a more engaged medical sociology dedicated to the improvement of health care. Others have argued that these initiatives confine the conceptual space of sociological enquiry in ways that make medical sociologists weary of their association with quality improvement agendas. However, when exploring how sociologists can relate to quality and safety improvement practices, we may want to draw upon the long debate on the relation of medical sociology to medicine. This debate, which has run since the late fifties, has been characterized by the fear that "the sociology of medicine runs the risk of losing its professional

identity if it engages too closely with medicine" (Timmermans and Haas 2008, 661, referring to Straus 1957). The risk of loss of identity seems to resurface in the recent debate on the role of medical sociology in relation to quality and safety improvement. When Timmermans and Berg (2003, epilogue) proposed that the study of quality and safety improvement provided refreshing opportunities for various strands of the social sciences to gain societal relevance, Bruun Jensen responded that allowing the patient-safety agenda to be set solely by institutions like the Institute of Medicine leaves medical sociologists to either take "the critical stance" that Timmermans and Berg (2003, 216) depict as "deadly stale" or enter "a vibrant future, in which medical sociologists are reconfigured as system designers" (Jensen 2008, 321), which Jensen finds equally unattractive. The risk of identity loss seems to be mainly a risk that, if medical sociology is subsumed into improvement agendas, medical sociologists will be confined to realizing better systems design, even when their research shows interesting complexities rather than clear answers (Barry et al. 1999; Jensen 2007; Riley, Hawe, and Shiell 2005).

If medical sociology is to contribute to improvement practices in a way that neither makes the social investigator stand "with his or her back to the heart of [quality and safety improvement in] medicine" while studying "the 'social phenomena' surrounding it" (Casper and Berg 1995, 397), nor forces medical sociologists to "enthusiastic[ally] endorse . . . existing agendas" (Jensen 2008, 322) in this field, including the study of effectiveness in the sociological analysis may be crucial. If this is done, the challenge for medical sociology seems to become how to take the normative purpose of quality and safety improvement into account without becoming subservient to quality improvement agendas by buying into a simplified and monolithic notion of effectiveness that is often deployed by improvement agents. The ability to analyze the complexities involved in taken-for-granted notions of effectiveness and to unpack how these notions were constructed may be one of the most useful contributions that medical sociology has to make to the study of quality and safety improvement— though this is a type of usefulness that is bound to be perceived as problematic and frustrating when social scientists are expected merely to elucidate the factors that support or hamper safety (Grol, Baker, and Moss 2002).

Yet by confronting the issue of effectiveness head-on—not merely criticizing the improvement movement's focus on effectiveness but analyzing its complexities and renewing notions of effectiveness that are deployed in improvement practices—medical sociologists seem to have a fruitful opportunity to critically engage with patient safety improvement without cutting off all connections to clinical outcomes and denying the normative purpose of quality improvement. Stressing the ambivalences and ambiguities that emerge during practices of quality and safety improvement may of course still be seen as frustrating the actual work of quality improvement. It will therefore be a daunting challenge to medical sociologists to study effectiveness in a way that is productive sociologically without bracketing the normative purpose of improvement work. Yet, as the studies we refer to in this chapter show, it is exactly this challenge that seems to produce highly interesting sociological findings and that may at times be able to contribute to more humble improvement practices that are more precise about what "effective improvement" actually means.

Notes

1. For the 50 percent adherence rate, Timmermans and Mauck (2005) cite Burstin et al. 1999 and Grilli and Lomas 1994.
2. Quoted in Mead and Bower 2000.

References

Armstrong, David. 2002. *A New History of Identity: A Sociology of Medical Knowledge*. Basingstoke, Eng.: Palgrave.

Aspden, Philip, Janet M. Corrigan, Julie Wolcott, and Shari M. Erickson. 2004. *Patient Safety: Achieving a New Standard for Care*. Washington, D.C.: National Academy Press.

Bal, Roland. 2008. "De Nieuwe Zichtbaarheid: Sturing in Tijden van Marktwerking" [The new visibility: Steering in times of marketization]. Inaugural lecture presented at Erasmus University, Rotterdam. oldwww.bmg.eur.nl/personal/r.bal/oratie.pdf. Accessed January 14, 2010.

Barry, Christine, Nicky Britten, Nick Barber, Colin Bradley, and Fiona Stevenson. 1999. "Using Reflexivity to Optimize Teamwork in Qualitative Research." *Qualitatve Health Research* 9:26–44.

Bate, Paul, Glen Robert, and Helen Bevan. 2004. "The Next Phase of Healthcare Improvement: What Can We Learn from Social Movements?" *Quality and Safety in Health Care* 13:62–66.

Benzing, Jozien. 2000. "Bridging the Gap: The Separate Worlds of Evidence-Based Medicine and Patient-Centered Medicine." *Patient Education and Counceling* 39:17–25.

Berdick, Edward L., and Vicky W. Humphries. 1994. "Hospital Re-engineers to Improve Patient Care." *Health Care Strategic Management* 12:13–14.

Berg, Marc. 1997. *Rationalizing Medical Work: Decision-Support Techniques and Medical Practices*. Cambridge, Mass.: Massachusetts Institute of Technology.

Berg, Marc, Yvonne Meijerink, Marit Gras, Anne Goossensen, Wim Schellekens, Jan Haeck, Marjon Kallewaart, and Herre Kingma. 2005. "Feasibility First: Developing Public Performance Indicators on Patient Safety and Clinical Effectiveness for Dutch Hospitals." *Health Policy* 75:59–73.

Bevan, Gwyn. 2004. "Targets, Inspections, and Transparency: Too Much Predictability in the Name of Transparency Weakens Control." *British Medical Journal* 328:598.

Bevan, Gwyn, and Christopher Hood. 2006. "What's Measured Is What Matters: Targets and Gaming in the English Public Health Care System." *Public Administration* 84:517–38.

Birkmeyer, John D., Therese A. Stukel, Andrea E. Siewers, Philip P. Goodney, David E. Wennberg, and F. Lee Lucas. 2003. "Surgeon Volume and Operative Mortality in the United States." *New England Journal of Medicine* 349:2117–27.

Bosk, Charles L. 2003. *Forgive and Remember: Managing Medical Failure*. Reprint. Chicago: University of Chicago Press.

Burstin, Helen R., Alasdair Conn, Gary Setnik, Donald W. Rucker, Paul D. Cleary, Anne C. O'Neil, E. John Orav, Colin M. Sox, and Troyen A. Brennan. 1999. "Benchmarking and Quality Improvement: The Harvard Emergency Department Quality Study." *American Journal of Medicine* 107:437–49.

Casper, Monica, and Marc Berg. 1995. "Constructivist Perspectives on Medical Work: Medical Practices and Science and Technology Studies." *Science, Technology, and Human Values* 20:395–407.

Clark, Adele. 1997. "A Social Worlds Research Adventure: The Case of Reproductive Science." In *Grounded Theory in Practice*, ed. A. L. Strauss, and J. M. Corbin, 63–94. Thousand Oaks, London, New Delhi: Sage Publications.

Conrad, Peter, and Joseph W. Schneider. 1992. *Deviance and Medicalization: From Badness to Sickness*. Philadelphia: Temple University Press.

CQHCA [Committee on Quality of Health Care in America]. 2000. *To Err Is Human: Building a Safer Health System*. Washington, D.C.: National Academy Press.

Degeling, Pieter, Sharyn Maxwell, and Rick Iedema. 2004. "Restructuring Clinical Governance to Maximize Its Developmental Potential." In *Governing Medicine: Theory and Practice*, ed. A. Gray and S. Harrison, 163–79. Berkshire, N.Y.: McGraw-Hill.

Donabedian, Avedis. 2005. "Evaluating the Quality of Medical Care." *Milbank Quarterly* 83:691–729.

Evans, John H., III, Yuhchang Hwang, and Nandu J. Nagarajan. 1997. "Cost Reduction and Process Reengineering in Hospitals." *Journal of Cost Management* 11(3): 20–27.

Ford, Robert C., and Myron D. Fottler. 2000. "Creating Customer-Focused Health Care Organizations." *Health Care Management Review* 25:18–33.

Foucault, Michel. 1991. "Governmentality." In *The Foucault Effect: Studies in Governmentality*, ed. G. Burchell, C. Gordon, and P. Miller, 87–104. Chicago: University of Chicago Press.

Freidson, Eliot. 1960. "Client Control and Medical Practice." *American Journal of Sociology* 65:374–82.

———. 1970. *Profession of Medicine*. New York: Harper and Row.

van Geenen, Ronald. 2005. "Aanval Op Medische Missers" [Attack of Medical Failures]. *Algemeen Dagblad*, November 24.

Greenberg, Selig. 1971. *The Quality of Mercy: A Report on the Critical Condition of Hospital and Medical Care in America*. New York: Atheneum.

Grilli, Roberto, and Jonathan Lomas. 1994. "Evaluating the Message: The Relationship between Compliance Rate and the Subject of a Practice Guideline." *Medical Care* 32:202–13.

Grol, R., R. Baker, and F. Moss. 2002. "Quality Improvement Research: Understanding the Science of Change in Health Care." *Quality and Safety in Health Care* 11:110–11.

Haraway, Donna J. 1991. *Simians, Cyborgs and Women: The Reinvention of Nature*. New York: Routledge.

Harrison, Stephen, and Christopher Pollitt. 1994. *Controlling Health Professionals*. Buckingham, Eng.: Open University Press.

Iedema, Rick, Christine Jorm, Debby Long, Jeffrey Braithwaite, Jo Travaglia, and Mary Westbrook. 2006. "Turning the Medical Gaze upon Itself: Root Cause Analysis and the Investigation of Clinical Error." *Social Science and Medicine* 62:1605–15.

Jasanoff, Sheila. 2003. "Technologies of Humility: Citizen Participation in Governing Science." *Minerva* 41:223–44.

Jensen, Casper Bruun. 2007. "Sorting Attachments: On Intervention and Usefulness in STS and Health Policy." *Science as Culture* 16:237–51.

———. 2008. "Sociology, Systems and (Patient) Safety: Knowledge Translations in Healthcare Policy." *Sociology of Health and Illness* 30:309–24.

Jerak-Zuiderent, Sonja, and Roland Bal. 2010. "Locating the Worths of Performance Indicators: Performing Transparencies and Accountabilities in Health Care." In *The Mutual Construction of Statistics and Society*, ed. Ann Rudinow Saetnan, Heidi Mork Lomell, and Svein Hammer, 224–42. London and New York: Routledge.

Kenney, Charles. 2008. *The Best Practice: How the New Quality Movement Is Transforming Medicine*. New York: Public Affairs.

Kilo, Charles M. 1998. "A Framework for Collaborative Improvement: Lessons from the Institute for Healthcare Improvement's Breakthrough Series." *Quality Management in Health Care* 6:1–13.

Kuhn, Thomas S. 1977. "The Function of Measurement in Modern Physical Science." In *The Essential Tension: Selected Studies in Scientific Tradition and Change*, ed. T. S. Kuhn, 178–224. Chicago: University of Chicago Press.

Latour, Bruno. 1987. *Science in Action: How to Follow Scientists and Engineers through Society*. Cambridge, Mass.: Harvard University Press.

———. 2004. "Why Has Critique Run Out of Steam? From Matters of Fact to Matters of Concern." *Critical Inquiry* 30:225–48.

Law, John. 2000. "Ladbroke Grove, or How to Think about Failing Systems." Center for Science Studies, Lancaster University. lancs.ac.uk/fass/sociology/papers/law-ladbroke-grove-failing-systems.pdf. Accessed September 2005.

Light, Donald W. 2000. "The Medical Profession and Organizational Change: From Professional Dominance to Countervailing Power." In *Handbook of Medical Sociology*, 5th ed., ed. Chloe E. Bird, Peter Conrad, and Allen M. Fremont, 201–16. Upper Saddle River, N.J.: Prentice Hall.

Markussen, Randi, and Finn Olesen. 2007. "Rhetorical Authority in STS—Studies of Information Technology: Reflections on a Study of Implementation of IT at a Hospital Ward." *Science as Culture* 16:267–79.

May, Carl, Tim Rapley, Tiago Moreira, Tracy Finch, and Ben Heaven. 2006. "Technogovernance: Evidence, Subjectivity, and the Clinical Encounter in Primary Care Medicine." *Social Science and Medicine* 62:1022–30.

McKinlay, John B. 1999. "The End of the Golden Age of

Doctoring." *New England Research Institutes Network* (summer). Later published as J. B. McKinlay and L. D. Marceau. 2002. "The End of the Golden Age of Doctoring." *International Journal of Health Services* 32:379–416.

Mead, Nicola, and Peter Bower. 2000. "Patient-Centredness: A Conceptual Framework and a Review of the Empirical Literature." *Social Science and Medicine* 51:1087–1110.

Mesman, Jessica. 2007. "Disturbing Observations as a Basis for Collaborative Research." *Science as Culture* 16:281–95.

———. 2008. *Uncertainty in Medical Innovation: Experienced Pioneers in Neonatal Care.* Hampshire, Eng.: Palgrave MacMillan.

———. Forthcoming. "The Relocation of Vulnerability in Critical Care Medicine." In *The Vulnerability of Technological Culture,* ed. A. Hommels, J. Mesman, and W. Bijker. Cambridge, Mass.: MIT Press.

Mittman, Brian S. 2004. "Creating the Evidence Base for Quality Improvement Collaboratives." *Annals of Internal Medicine* 140:897–901.

Navarro, Vincente. 1976. *Medicine under Capitalism.* New York: Prodist.

Nolan, Thomas, Roger Resar, Carol Haraden, and Frances A. Griffin. 2004. *Improving the Reliability of Healthcare.* Boston: Institute for Healthcare Improvement.

Noordergraaf, Mirko. 2007. "From 'Pure' to 'Hybrid' Professionalism: Present-Day Professionalism in Ambiguous Public Domains." *Administration and Society* 39:761–85.

Parsons, Talcott. 1951. *The Social System.* Glencoe, Ill.: Free Press.

Perrow, Charles. 1999. *Normal Accidents: Living with High-Risk Technologies.* Princeton, N.J.: Princeton University Press.

Pinder, Ruth, Roland Petchey, Sara Shaw, and Yvonne Carter. 2005. "What's in a Care Pathway? Towards a Cultural Cartography of the New NHS." *Sociology of Health and Illness* 27:759–79.

Porter, Theodore M. 1995. *Trust in Numbers: The Pursuit of Objectivity in Science and Public Life.* Princeton, N.J.: Princeton University Press.

———. 1997. "The Management of Society by Numbers." In *Science in the Twentieth Century,* ed. J. Krige and D. Pestre, 97–110. Amsterdam: Harwood Academic Publishers.

Power, Michael. 1997. *The Audit Society: Rituals of Verification.* Oxford: Oxford University Press.

———. 2004. "Counting, Control and Calculation: Reflections on Measuring and Management." *Human Relations* 57:765–83.

Riley, Therese, Penelope Hawe, and Alan Shiell. 2005. "Contested Ground: How Should Qualitative Evidence Inform the Conduct of a Community Intervention Trial?" *Journal of Health Services Research and Policy* 10:103–10.

Ritzer, George. 1992. *The McDonaldization of Society: An Investigation into the Changing Character of Contemporary Social Life.* Thousand Oaks, Calif.: Pine Forge.

Rodwin, Marc A. 1993. *Medicine, Money and Morals.* New York: Oxford University Press.

Runciman, W. B. 2002. "Lessons from the Australian Patient Safety Foundation: Setting up a National Patient Safety Surveillance System—Is This the Right Model?" *Quality and Safety in Health Care* 11:246–51.

Silverman, David. 1987. *Communication and Medical Practice: Social Relations in the Clinic.* London: Sage Publications.

Star, Susan Leigh, and Anselm Strauss. 1999. "Layers of Silence, Arenas of Voice: The Ecology of Visible and Invisible Work." *Computer Supported Cooperative Work* 8:9–30.

Steinbusch, Paul J. M., Jan B. Oostenbrink, Joost J. Zuurbier, and Frans J. M. Schaepkens. 2007. "The Risk of Upcoding in Casemix Systems: A Comparative Study." *Health Policy* 81:289–99.

Stewart, Moira, Judith Belle Brown, W. Wayne Weston, Ian R. McWhinney, Carol L. McWilliam, and Thomas R. Freeman Sage. 1995. *Patient-Centred Medicine: Transforming the Clinical Method.* London: Sage Publications.

Stinchcombe, Arthur L. 2001. *When Formality Works: Authority and Abstraction in Law and Organizations.* Chicago: University of Chicago Press.

Straus, Robert. 1957. "The Nature and Status of Medical Sociology." *American Sociological Review* 22:200–204.

Strauss, Anselm, Shizuko Fagerhaugh, Barbara Suczek, and Carolyn Wiener. 1997. *Social Organization of Medical Work.* New Brunswick and London: Transaction.

Suchman, Lucy. 1995. "Representations of Work: Making Work Visible." *Communications of the ACM* 38:56–64.

Tanenbaum, Sandra J. 1994. "Knowing and Acting in Medical Practice: The Epistemological Politics of Outcomes Research." *Journal of Health Politics, Policy and Law* 19:27–44.

———. 2005. "Evidence-Based Practice as Mental Health Policy: Three Controversies and a Caveat." *Health Affairs* 24:163–74.

Thévenot, Laurent. 2002. "Which Road to Follow? The Moral Complexity of an 'Equipped' Humanity." In *Complexities: Social Studies of Knowledge Practices,* ed. John Law and Annemarie Mol, 53–87. Durham: Duke University Press.

Timmermans, Stefan, and Marc Berg. 2003. *The Gold Standard: An Exploration of Evidence-Based Medicine and Standardization in Health Care*. Philadelphia: Temple University Press.

Timmermans, Stefan, and Steven Haas. 2008. "Towards a Sociology of Disease." *Sociology of Health and Illness* 30:659–76.

Timmermans, Stefan, and Aaron Mauck. 2005. "The Promises and Pitfalls of Evidence-Based Medicine." *Health Affairs* 24:18–29.

Timmons, Stephen. 2003. "Resistance to Computerized Care Planning Systems by Qualified Nurses Working in the UK NHS." *Methods of Information in Medicine* 42:471–76.

Vaughan, Diana. 1997. *The Challenger Launch Decision: Risky Technology, Culture, and Deviance at NASA*. Chicago: University of Chicago Press.

Waitzkin, Howard. 1983. *The Second Sickness: Contradictions of Capitalist Health Care*. New York: Free Press.

Waring, Justin. 2005. "Beyond Blame: Cultural Barriers to Medical Incident Reporting." *Social Science and Medicine* 60:1927–35.

———. 2007. "Adaptive Regulation or Governmentality: Patient Safety and the Changing Regulation of Medicine." *Sociology of Health and Illness* 29:163–79.

Wennberg, John E. 1984. "Dealing with Medical Practice Variations: A Proposal for Action." *Health Affairs* 3:6–32.

Wennberg, John E., and Alan Gittelsohn. 1973. "Small-Area Variations in Health Care Delivery." *Science* 183:1102.

White, Joseph. 1991. *Competitive Solutions: American Health Care Proposals and International Experience*. Washington, D.C.: Brookings Institution.

Wiener, Carolyn L. 2000. *The Elusive Quest: Accountability in Hospitals*. New York: Aldine de Gruyter.

Zuger, Abigail. 2008. "Crusaders for Quality, a Health-Care Intangible." *New York Times*, July 29.

Zuiderent-Jerak, Teun. 2007. "Standardizing Healthcare Practices: Experimental Interventions in Medicine and Science and Technology Studies." PhD thesis, Erasmus University, Rotterdam.

———. 2009. "Competition in the Wild: Configuring Healthcare Markets." *Social Studies of Science* 39:765–92.

———. In press. "Embodied Interventions— Interventions on Bodies: Experiments in Practices of Science and Technology Studies and Hemophilia Care." *Science, Technology, and Human Values*.

Zuiderent-Jerak, Teun, Mathilde Strating, Anna Nieboer, and Roland Bal. 2009. "Sociological Refigurations of Patient Safety: Ontologies of Improvement and 'Acting with' Quality Collaboratives in Healthcare." *Social Science and Medicine* 69:1713–21.

PART IV

Crosscutting Issues

20

Religion, Spirituality, Health, and Medicine
Sociological Intersections

Wendy Cadge, Brandeis University

Brian Fair, Brandeis University

When Michelle Bird, a white woman in her early forties, developed a rare form of cancer several years ago, she sought treatment at the Dana-Farber Cancer Institute in Boston. There she was cared for by Dr. George Demetri, an expert in the field. In addition to standard biomedical treatments, Michelle, a Catholic, received reiki and acupuncture at Dana-Farber and attended services and readings in the small interfaith chapel there. She met monthly with a priest to receive his blessings and carried books like Jerome Groopman's *The Anatomy of Hope: How People Prevail in the Face of Illness* with her to medical appointments. She described talking daily with God as a way of keeping up her strength and spirits: "I pray for strength, faith, and a cure, and I know that God is listening. . . . I've always believed in an afterlife, but I feel I've grown spiritually as a result of my cancer experience. . . . Without my faith, I don't think I would be making it through this" (Wisnia 2004, 15).

Michelle and the Dana-Farber Cancer Institute are not alone in thinking about the relationships between religion, spirituality, health, and medical care in the United States. Many of the nation's first hospitals were founded by religious organizations, and religion/spirituality has long been a source of support for people when they are ill. National surveys report that 80 percent of Americans think personal religious/spiritual practices including prayer can help with medical treatments, and close to 25 percent say they have been cured of an illness through prayer or another religious/spiritual practice.[1] In a recent study, 60 percent of the public and 20 percent of medical professionals said they think it possible for an individual in a persistent vegetative state to be saved by a miracle (Jacobs, Burns, and Jacobs 2008). Just over 60 percent of Americans say they want physicians to ask about their spiritual histories if they become ill, and two-thirds of hospitals have chaplains (Cadge, Freese, and Christakis 2008).[2] Prayer chains on the Internet connect people with a wide range of medical conditions, and religious groups regularly hold services for health and healing in small towns and large cities across the United States (Barnes and Sered 2005).

These examples point to intersections among religion, spirituality, health, and medicine that are further evident in conversations taking place in newspapers, magazines, books, and scholarly journals. Some of this conversation is about religion, spirituality, and medical care, like whether pharmacists are obliged to dispense birth control when it conflicts with their personal religious values, or how medical teams should respond to families who are waiting for a miracle for a loved one the health-care team believes is terminal. Other pieces focus on the human condition more broadly through ethical questions about genetic technologies, assisted reproduction, euthanasia, medical decision making, and especially the social processes of birth and death. Medical and religious professionals, journalists, and members of the public contribute distinctive voices to these conversations, tapping into core questions about what it means to be human, and how we as a collective value life and make difficult decisions about birth and death in the process.

Sociologists have been involved in discussions about religion, spirituality, health, and medicine more from the periphery than from the center of academic and public debates. Handbooks of medical sociology rarely include chapters about religion, and handbooks in the sociology of religion have only recently started to include chapters on health. While Max Weber, Emile Durkheim, Georg Simmel, and other early sociologists inquired about the role of religion in the development of modern societies, their narratives of secularization combined with the secularization of the academy partly explain these silences. The compartmentalization of topics within sociology as a discipline is also responsible, as questions at the intersections between religion/spirituality and health/medicine were left on the fringes of two subfields and failed to develop into a robust sociological literature. Outside a relatively narrow set of questions about whether religion/spirituality influences the health of individuals and a broader set of bioethical concerns, sociologists have paid little sustained attention to the intersections between religion/spirituality and health/medicine in the lives of individuals or institutions (Fox and Swazey 2008).

This chapter responds to these silences by identifying central sociological questions about religion, spirituality, health, and medicine, summarizing available research about these questions, and outlining several directions for future sociological thinking. We highlight the work of sociologists but also draw from other disciplines. Following Geertz (1973, 90), we conceive of religion/spirituality broadly as a "system of symbols which act to establish powerful, pervasive, and long-lasting moods and motivations in men by formulating conceptions of a general order of existence and clothing these conceptions with such an aura of factuality that the moods and mo-

tivations seem uniquely realistic." While scholars and the public tend to define religion in terms of institutions structured around the worship of sacred beings, and spirituality as related to the wider range of ways people find meaning in their lives, we use the terms interchangeably in this chapter because they are not used consistently in the research literature.[3] We also focus primarily on biomedically informed conceptions of health and the presence of religion/spirituality in biomedical institutions in the United States.[4]

After a brief social history of religion and medicine in the United States and some basic descriptive information about contemporary Americans' religious beliefs and practices, we review the existing literature about the question sociologists working in this area have spent the most time investigating: whether religion/spirituality influences the health of individuals. We go on to highlight several promising lines of research at the institutional level and conclude by outlining directions for future research and pointing to the theoretical benefits of sociological approaches that consider multiple levels of analysis.[5]

A Social History of Religion and Medicine

Conceptions of "holiness" and "healing" share an etymology rooted in notions of wholeness and related to shifting distinctions between the body and the soul, mind, or spirit (Turner 1987). In the Christian context, people of faith were taught to offer charity to those in need, most especially the sick, through hospitals that emerged during the Middle Ages from houses of Christian charity (Mollat 1986). These medieval hospitals, which provided more solace and shelter than treatment, first institutionalized public care for the sick, which expanded dramatically in eighteenth- and nineteenth-century England and then through European, North American, and overseas Christian missions (Porter 1993; Risse 1999). Started as what some called "houses of God," it was not religious/spiritual concern but biomedicine that was new to hospitals as they developed in the modern context (Lee 2002).

The model of the physician emerged from the ecclesiastical form and content of higher education based in the Middle Ages and developed over subsequent centuries. Scientifically trained physicians evolved from physicians trained in religious universities, as physicians and religious leaders gradually mapped out separate spheres (Porter 1993). In the early American colonies, clergy provided much of the medical care, particularly in New England. This changed in the nineteenth century as scientific medicine and medical education emerged, and states enacted laws prohibiting clergy without medical training from practicing medicine (Numbers and Sawyer 1982). Formal training for nurses also emerged in the United States in the late nineteenth century following much informal nursing done by women in the home. Orders of religious or vowed nurses were gradually replaced by secular nurses over the next century (Reverby 1987; Coburn and Smith 1999; Nelson 2001).

Early U.S. hospitals were charity institutions for the poor, the gravely ill, and the desperate; everyone else was cared for in their homes (Starr 1982; Rosenberg 1987; Kauffman 1995; Kaufman 2005). When hospitals began to develop and expand numerically in the mid-nineteenth century, religion influenced the process. Catholic and Jewish hospitals were started for patients not treated well in other facilities, and for Catholic and Jewish doctors and nurses who could not find work in them (Vogel 1980; Lazarus 1991). Catholic hospitals offered not only ethnic identity but also the privilege of being treated as a paying patient rather than a charity case (McCauley 2005). Similarly, Jewish hospitals were started by members of the Jewish community to meet the needs of Jewish patients (Levitan 1964; Sarna 1987). Religious-affiliated hospitals were open to everyone and until the mid-twentieth century cared for more than one quarter of all hospitalized patients (Numbers and Sawyer 1982).

In the past century and a half, the formal organizational distance between religion and biomedical organizations has increased. Scientific developments and professional sectarian battles led to medicine's greater technological foci (Starr 1982; Stevens 1989).[6] Religious ownership of hospitals has become less common and a source of contention, particularly when religious and secular hospitals consider merging (Uttley 2000).[7]

Despite the formal institutional secularization of medical care, some religiously based healthcare organizations remain, and others have been started. Immigrants who arrived in the United States after 1965 have opened medical centers in a range of traditions. A Cambodian Buddhist temple began to offer Western counseling services supported by Buddhist healing practices in the 1980s, and in the 1990s the University Muslim Medical Association Free Clinic was established in Los Angeles, and other Muslim health-care organizations followed to offer free health care to all in the Muslim tradition of compassion (Aswad and Gray 1996; Orr and May 2000; Laird and Cadge 2007). Buddhist hospices have opened on the West Coast and many Christian congregations have started parish nursing programs (Garces-Foley 2003).

Despite the formal secularization of medical institutions, some indicators suggest that attention to religion/spirituality is stable or increasing in the medical community.[8] The number of publications catalogued in the main biomedical search engine, PubMed, with "religion" or "spirituality" in the title or key word has increased, and elective courses about these topics are offered at many medical schools (Levin, Larson, and Pulchalski 1997; Barnes 2006). A growing number of assessment tools encourage physicians and other health-care professionals to ask patients about spirituality/religion, and institutional centers of religion, spirituality, and medicine exist at several prominent medical schools (Fosarelli 2008). While medical institutions have formally secularized, survey data show that many members of the U.S. public, including those who are treated and work in medical institutions, retain religious/spiritual beliefs and practices (Curlin et al. 2005).

Current Contours of Religion/ Spirituality in America

A 2007 national survey conducted by the Pew Forum for Religion and Public Life reported that 51.3 percent of Americans are Protestant, 23.9 percent Catholic, 1.7 percent Jewish, 1.7 percent Mormon, and less than 1 percent each Orthodox,

Muslim, Buddhist, Hindu, Jehovah's Witness, and other world religions. Just over 16 percent are unaffiliated. Among the 51.3 percent who are Protestant, 26.3 percent identify with evangelical denominations (the Southern Baptist Convention, Assemblies of God, Church of Christ, and various Pentecostal, Holiness, and independent churches), while 18.1 percent identify with mainline Protestant denominations (United Methodist, Evangelical Lutheran Church in America, Presbyterian Church USA, Episcopal, United Church of Christ, and American Baptist) and 6.9 percent are members of historically black denominations (such as the African Methodist Episcopal, National Baptist Convention, and Churches of God in Christ) (Pew Forum 2007). Surveys do not reliably estimate membership in small religious groups, which may include as many as six million Muslims, four million Buddhists, and more than one million Hindus (Smith 2002; Wuthnow and Cadge 2004). Since 1965, immigration has reshaped the U.S. religious landscape, particularly through large influxes of Catholics from Mexico and Central and South America (Jasso et al. 2003).

Two-thirds of Americans claim to be members of local religious organizations, a figure that has remained roughly constant since the 1970s (Gallup and Lindsay 1999). Membership tends to be higher among women than men, among blacks than whites, and in the South and Midwest than in the Northeast and West. According to the 1998 National Congregations Study, the median congregation had seventy-five regular participants and the median person attended a congregation with four hundred regular participants (Chaves 2004). The fraction of Americans that regularly attends religious services is smaller than the fraction that claims membership (Hout and Greeley 1998; Woodberry 1998; Hadaway and Marler 2005). The 2007 U.S. Religion Landscape Survey conducted by the Pew Forum reports that 54 percent of Americans attend religious services once or twice per month and 39 percent attend every week, with evangelical Protestants, black Protestants, Mormons, and Jehovah's Witnesses attending more frequently than members of other religious groups (Pew Forum 2007).

In addition to service attendance, many Americans have religious/spiritual beliefs and practices. According to surveys conducted by the Gallup organization, 95 percent of U.S. adults claim belief in God or a higher power, 79 percent believe in miracles, and 67 percent believe in life after death (Gallup and Lindsay 1999). According to the General Social Survey (1998), 50 percent of Americans feel God's love for them daily and 52 percent feel at least daily that they want to be closer to God. The U.S. Religion Landscape Survey reports that 58 percent of Americans pray at least daily, and close to half of all Americans report receiving answers to their prayers several times a year or more. Just over 80 percent of Americans say religion is very or somewhat important in their lives (Pew Forum 2007).

The ways in which religion/spirituality influences the health beliefs of medical professionals and laypeople represent an important area for future sustained sociological consideration. It is only recently that demographic information about religion/spirituality has been gathered among a representative sample of physicians (Curlin et al. 2005). One study demonstrates that more than half of physicians believe religion/spirituality influences people's health by helping them cope, giving them a positive state of mind, and providing emotional and practical support (Curlin, Lawrence, et al. 2007). Other articles show that religiously committed physicians are less likely than others to believe that when they oppose a medical procedure for moral reasons, they must refer patients to another physician or disclose their opposition to patients (Curlin, Sellergren, et al. 2007). Studies also suggest that religion/spirituality influences physicians' decision making about a range of topics (Imber 1986; Christakis and Asch 1995; Aiyer et al. 1999; Abdel-Aziz, Arch, and Al-Taher 2004). Among nurses, a recent survey conducted at a large academic medical center reported that 91 percent consider themselves spiritual and more than 80 percent think there is something spiritual about the care they provide. Almost none believe that promoting spirituality is at odds with medicine (Cavendish et al. 2004; Grant, O'Neil, and Stephens 2004).

Survey data suggests that religion/spirituality also shapes some Americans' health beliefs (e.g., Mansfield, Mitchell, and King 2002; Baker 2008). Conservative and moderate Protestants, for example, are less accepting than others of the practice of physician-assisted suicide and terminal palliative care, according to the General Social Survey (Burdette, Hill, and Moulton 2005). Differences among religious traditions are also evident in public opinion about euthanasia, family planning, and beliefs about the appropriate use of clergy as a source of mental health assistance (Ellison and Goodson 1997; Hamil-Luker and Smith 1998; Abrums 2000; Ellison et al. 2006; Moulton, Hill, and Burdette 2006). These studies are yet to be pulled into a synthesized body of research that clearly outlines how religion/spirituality influences health beliefs across religious/spiritual traditions, age, geography, issue, and so on. Glimpses of these relationships are further evident in studies of patient satisfaction and medical decision making, but attention is needed to systematically delineate precise relationships.

Does Religion/Spirituality Influence Health at the Individual Level?

Sociologists who have studied the relationship between religion/spirituality and health/medicine in the past twenty years have focused almost exclusively on epidemiological questions about whether religion/spirituality influences physical and mental health, based on quantitative indicators of health. These studies generally suggest a positive relationship but are limited by their reliance on survey data, their attention to individuals outside their institutional contexts, and their tendency to make causal arguments in the absence of longitudinal data, which raises concerns about reverse causality. Theoretically, they draw from Durkheim's classic insights about the "regulative" and "integrative" functions of religion. Scholars argue that healthy behaviors, social support within religious communities, psychosocial resources, and belief structures which give meaning to life are the mechanisms through which religion/spirituality may lead people to have better

health. We focus primarily on meta-analyses and overview articles written by sociologists to outline three main lines of research in this area.

Mortality

One line of research investigates the relationship between religion/spirituality and mortality, with particular attention to religious service attendance. Two large-scale longitudinal studies of healthy adult populations, the Tecumseh Community Health Study and the Alameda County Study, examine the frequency of people's religious services attendance in the context of other social activities and find it to be negatively associated with their mortality, particularly for women (House, Robbins, and Metzner 1982; Strawbridge et al. 1997). These findings are reinforced by studies by Hummer and colleagues and Musick and colleagues, who find self-reported rates of religious service attendance in a large nationally representative sample of adults to be negatively related to mortality in follow-up studies (Hummer et al. 1999; Musick, House, and Williams 2004). Likewise, a smaller but often-cited study of nearly four thousand older people in Piedmont, North Carolina, over a six-year period found that frequency of religious service attendance was related to lower mortality rates (Koenig et al. 1999).

Two recent meta-analyses consider the relationship between religious service attendance and mortality. After locating all relevant published and unpublished studies, McCullough and Smith (2003:197) estimated the association between mortality and religious participation based on over 120,000 respondents. They concluded that "religious people had, on average, a 29 percent higher chance of survival during any follow-up period than did less-religious people." Powell and colleagues conducted a similar analysis, concluding that church attendance reduced the risk of mortality by 25 percent after adjusting for appropriate confounders (Powell, Shahabi, and Thoresen 2003).

A less conclusive body of research focuses on the relationship between religion/spirituality and timing of death. For example, a popular study by

Idler and Kasl (1992) found that religious group membership influenced the timing of death for elderly people, with Christians and Jews less likely to die in the month before important religious holidays. Subsequent studies in the medical literature, however, raise questions about these relationships based on mixed empirical results.

Physical and Mental Health

A second line of empirical work investigates how religion/spirituality influences people's physical and mental health over the life course. While some researchers posit biological and physiological mechanisms, sociologists tend to focus on how religion/spirituality, variously defined, influences health measured in multiple ways. In a review of epidemiological research on religion and blood pressure, for example, Levin and Vanderpool (1989) found people who are religiously committed likely to have lower blood pressure than those with no religious affiliation. Religious teachings/communities inform some people's behaviors around alcohol and tobacco use, for example, which accounts for significantly lower rates of cancer morbidity and mortality in areas where there are high concentrations of members of particular religious groups (Troyer 1988; Dwyer, Clarke, and Miller 1990). A study of women in Utah found that Mormon women who attended church regularly had lower risks of cervical cancer than did non-Mormons (Gardner, Sanborn, and Slattery 1995). Similarly, studies investigate how religious factors protect adolescents from experimenting with smoking, drug use, and alcohol consumption through personal religiosity and public participation in religious social activities with religious peers (Wallace and Williams 1997; Wallace and Forman 1998; Nonnemaker, McNeely, and Blum 2006). Similar findings are evident in studies of virginity pledges among young people (Bearman and Bruckner 2001). A large interdisciplinary body of literature also investigates the relationship between personal religion/spirituality and recovery from alcohol, drug, and other addictions (e.g., Booth and Martin 1998).

Another large literature addresses the relationship between religion/spirituality and psychological or mental health, as well as how these concepts should be measured.[9] In one study, Ellison (1991) found a significant connection between religiousness and existential certainty, a concept associated with a sense of coherence known to promote psychological health. Following Durkheim's classic work in *Suicide*, much of this research focuses on how religion/spirituality influences depressive symptoms, including hopelessness and thoughts of suicide (Schieman, van Gundy, and Taylor 2001; Eliassen, Taylor, and Lloyd 2005). McCullough and Smith (2003) conducted a meta-analysis of the relationship between religion/spirituality and depression, concluding that people with higher levels of religiousness have slightly lower levels of depressive symptoms.

In addition to establishing relationships between religion/spirituality and psychological health, scholars are exploring mechanisms that may explain these connections. George, Ellison, and Larson (2002) present evidence connecting participation in religious organizations to psychosocial mechanisms such as self-esteem, self-efficacy, and mastery that are linked to aspects of mental health. Commerford and Reznikoff (1996), for example, found that people's feelings of mastery influenced the effect of religious service attendance and personal faith on their experiences of psychological distress. Other research has examined how the belief structure provided by religion and spirituality contributes to mental health (Bjarnason 1998; Ellison et al. 2001). For example, a study by Pollner (1989) suggests that a personal relationship with a deity is related to subjective well-being, which influences people's senses of coherence and emotional management. A study by Maton (1989) demonstrates how perceived spiritual support serves as a buffer against stress, which in turn promotes mental health.

Coping

A third line of research, closely related to the second, focuses on religious/spiritual coping, or the process through which individuals use religious/spirituality-based strategies to deal with physical and psychological illness. In some studies, religious/spiritual coping is seen as mediating the effects of illnesses on the body, potentially limiting the physical and emotional distress caused by illnesses and disability (Pargament et al. 1990; Kendler, Gardner, and Prescott 1997; Pargament 1997; Pargament et al. 1998; Poindexter, Linsk, and Warner 1999; Chatters 2000; Nooney and Woodrum 2002; Pargament et al. 2005; Thune-Boyle et al. 2006; Klemmack et al. 2007). A central study in this area of research is Idler and Kasl's (1992) on elderly people in New Haven, Connecticut. Over a three-year period they found public religious involvement to protect men and women against physical disability, and private religiousness to protect recently disabled men against depression. The authors highlight how religion's ritualistic and symbolic aspects may influence health among the elderly more than do secular sources of support. In a related study, the spirituality of individuals born in San Francisco in the 1920s that resulted from adherence to non-institutionalized religious beliefs and practices did not have the same buffering or protective effects against depression in older age that traditional religious memberships had (Wink, Dillon, and Larsen 2005).

Populations Studied and Limitations

When considering research about the relationship between religion/spirituality and individual health, it is important to note that approximately half the studies in this area focus on people over the age of sixty.[10] As a result, much of the religion/spirituality research relates to physical health issues often associated with old age, such as chronic illness, physical disability, and pain management (Idler and Kasl 1992; Levin and Vanderpool 1992; Krause 1993; Svetkey et al. 1993; Wachholtz, Pearce, and Koenig 2007). Similarly, studies of mental health ask how religion/spirituality buffers the psychological distress that can accompany decreased physical abilities and personal independence among older people (Idler 1987, 1995; Blazer, Hughes, and George 1987; Broyles and Drenovsky 1992; Krause, Ellison, and Wulff 1998; Murphy et al. 2000; Barkan and Greenwood 2003; Krause 2003, 2006; Jacobs, Burns, and Jacobs 2008). While older people are more

likely to have the physical and mental health experiences these studies investigate, the focus on older individuals limits the generalizability of study findings.

Although they do not regularly explore variation by age, these three lines of research do investigate variation across racial and ethnic categories, focusing especially on the health of black and white Americans and the historical centrality of the church in African American communities (Ellison 1993, 1995; Caldwell et al. 1995; Levin, Chatters, and Taylor 1995; Musick 1996, 2000; Krause 2004). A study by Ferraro and Koch (1994) suggests that black Americans are more likely than whites to turn to religion when having health problems and generally receive greater health benefits from religious practices (but not from social support) than do whites. A later study by Drevenstedt (1998) finds that higher rates of religious service attendance by blacks and Latinos does not fully dissipate the negative health effects associated with sociodemographic factors, such as lower levels of social support, income, and education. Other research shows that church attendance, and ministers in particular, serve as key psychological health resources for African Americans (Neighbors, Musick, and Williams 1998; Bierman 2006). Black Americans whose parents encouraged religiosity have also been found to have higher levels of personal religiousness and self-esteem at older ages (Krause and Ellison 2007).

There are few studies of religion/spirituality and health linkages among members of other racial/ethnic minorities (for recent studies of Mexican Americans, see Levin, Markides, and Ray 1996; Reyes-Ortiz et al. 2008). Likewise, little research has examined how the conceptualization of religion/spirituality itself may vary across race and ethnicity (Neff 2006). But contemporary research has become more attentive to the gendered dynamics of religion and health (Mirola 1999; Ferraro and Kelley-Moore 2002; Krause, Ellison, and Marcum 2002; Idler 2003).

When reading and evaluating studies about the relationship between religion/spirituality and health among individuals, it is important to keep several key limitations in mind. First, almost all of this research is epidemiological, based on the analysis of survey data about individuals outside of their familial, religious/spiritual, and other institutional contexts. While indicators of these contexts can be gathered in surveys, they are only indicators and not representative of the detailed information about social processes and intersecting causal factors that can be gathered in interviews, participant observation, or multimethod projects. Second, with few exceptions (see Pargament et al. 1998; Krause and Wulff 2004; Krause 2006; Bjorck and Thurman 2007), researchers generally frame their questions in terms of the positive effects of religion/spirituality, likely leading this literature to underrepresent the negative effects of religion/spirituality on health.

In addition, this body of research has numerous methodological weaknesses, as pointed out by other researchers, including inconsistent definitions/conceptualizations of religion and spirituality, the use of self-reports of key measures, reliance on cross-sectional data, and a tendency to make causal arguments in the absence of longitudinal data and without attention to issues of reverse causation, which raises significant questions about the findings (Levin and Vanderpool 1987; Levin 1994, 1996; George et al. 2002; Flannelly, Ellison, and Strock 2004; Hall, Koenig, and Meador 2004; Regnerus and Smith 2005; Vaillant et al. 2008). Researchers rarely recognize variation within religious traditions in these studies or include members of non-Christian or non-Jewish traditions in their studies. Expanding conceptions of spirituality and religion to include meditation, yoga, and other spiritual practices would also reshape and challenge many of the assumptions underlying these studies.

The Individual in Organizational and Institutional Contexts

The focus on individuals apart from the social contexts and institutions that shape them in the studies reviewed in the previous section leaves several distinctly sociological contributions to conversations about religion, spirituality, health, and medicine to be made. Specifically, we know little about the relationship between religion/spirituality and medicine as institutions, such as how religion/

spirituality is currently present in medical organizations and how health and medicine are present and significant in religious and spiritual organizations. We highlight several promising lines of research, among many possibilities, at the institutional level, focusing on policies of the Joint Commission, the work of hospital chaplains, and the way local religious organizations address health issues, including through public health initiatives.

Joint Commission Policies

Started in 1910, the Joint Commission establishes guidelines to ensure the provision of safe and quality health care at hospitals, nursing homes, and other health-care organizations across the United States. These organizations are required to meet Joint Commission guidelines in order to receive federal funding through Medicare and Medicaid programs.[11] To understand how religion/spirituality is present and significant in medical institutions, it is helpful to start with the Joint Commission's first statement about religion in hospitals, made in 1969 and yet to be explored by sociologists: "Patients' spiritual needs may be met through hospital resources and/or through an arrangement with appropriate individuals from the community." During the 1970s and 1980s, this guideline was expanded to state that religion had to be assessed in patients being treated in hospitals for alcoholism and drug dependence. In the 1990s, issues around religion and spirituality were reframed in the guidelines as a "right," treated primarily under the heading "Patients Rights." The Commission replaced the language of "religion" with the more inclusive language of "spirituality" and expanded the range of topics for which spirituality could be relevant to include end-of-life issues. In 1995 the guidelines incorporated the rights of hospital staff related to spirituality and religion by directing hospitals to address conflicts between staff members' cultural or religious beliefs and their work.

In the 1990s there was discussion and transition in the standards for hospitals about what the spiritual care of patients should be called and who specifically might provide it. In 1996, the Joint Commission stated that hospitals were to demonstrate respect for "pastoral counseling," a phrase replaced with "pastoral care and other spiritual services" in 1999 after leaders in hospital chaplaincy argued this phrase better reflects what they do. While the Joint Commission has not established specific guidelines or licensing requirements about who should or can provide spiritual care, in the late 1990s pastoral services departments and pastoral personnel from outside the facility are mentioned as possibilities. For example, small hospitals could "maintain a list of clergy who have consented to be available to the hospital's patients in addition to visiting their own parishioners," while larger hospitals could "employ qualified chaplains who have graduated from an accredited Master of Divinity degree program" (CDC 1999). Following similar discussions in the medical and nursing literatures, the Joint Commission also described "spiritual assessments" that, in the words of the Joint Commission's associate director of standards interpretation, "determine how a patient's religion or spiritual outlook might affect the care he or she receives. . . . At minimum the spiritual assessment should determine the patient's religious denomination, beliefs, and what spiritual practices are important to the patient" (Staten 2003, 55).

The 2008 Joint Commission standards for hospitals state: "Patients deserve care, treatment, and services that safeguard their personal dignity and respect their cultural, psychosocial and spiritual values," and hospitals need to accommodate the "right to pastoral and other spiritual services for patients." The Commission provided additional guidelines about religion and spirituality in relation to dietary options, pain concerns, resolving dilemmas about patient care issues, end-of-life issues, and the treatment and responsibilities of staff. Little to no research charts these policy developments, examines how hospitals and other health-care organizations have responded to changing policies, or considers how spiritual assessments take place in hospitals across the country. While health-care providers have developed a range of templates for conducting spiritual assessments that could be analyzed by sociologists, little is known about how they are actually used and responded to by health-care providers and patients (LaPierre 2003).

Health-Care Chaplains

At some hospitals, religious and spiritual issues are addressed primarily by hospital chaplains. Data collected by the American Hospital Association in its annual survey of hospitals suggest that 54–64 percent of hospitals had chaplaincy services between 1980 and 2003, with no systematic trend during the period. As in smaller studies, larger hospitals, those in more urban areas, and hospitals that are church affiliated were more likely to have chaplains in 1993 and 2003 than were others (Flannelly, Handzo, and Weaver 2004; Cadge, Freese, and Christakis 2008). Researchers estimate there are more than ten thousand hospital chaplains in the United States, many of whom belong to professional organizations, including the Association of Professional Chaplains, the National Association of Catholic Chaplains, the National Association of Jewish Chaplains, and the Association of Clinical Pastoral Education (Weaver et al. 2004). Chaplains include women and men who are laypeople and ordained leaders in their religious traditions.

Despite chaplains' positions at the intersections of medical and religious organizations, sociologists have devoted almost no attention to their work and professional evolution. Hospital chaplaincy developed in the late nineteenth and early twentieth century through the work of Richard Cabot, Anton T. Boisen, Helen Flanders Dunbar, and others in parallel with Clinical Pastoral Education (CPE), an initially Protestant-based movement designed to train theological students in the work of bedside ministry, which remains centrally present at many large academic hospitals (Hall 1992; Lee 2002; Angrosino 2006). CPE students likely provide a fair amount of care to patients at hospitals where they are trained because federal Medicare funds will reimburse hospitals for a portion of the students' work, a form of graduate medical education (McSherry and Nelson 1987; White 2003). Otherwise, chaplains' work is not reimbursed by health insurance or other groups and is paid for from a hospital's bottom line (for more on financing see VandeCreek and Lyon 1994–1995).

Glimpses of chaplains are evident in some hospital-based ethnographies, but sociologists know very little about who they are and how they work with other medical and religious professionals (Kudler 2007). Limited social science research conducted by chaplains themselves suggests that at some hospitals, chaplains are employed directly by the hospital, while at others they are exclusively volunteers or are employed by local Catholic dioceses, churches, or Jewish social service organizations. In some cases, particularly in New York City through the work of the Healthcare Chaplaincy, outside organizations hire and supervise hospital chaplains (VandeCreek et al. 2001; Flannelly et al. 2003).

The daily work of chaplains at individual hospitals may include providing emotional, practical, ritual, and crisis intervention services to patients, families, and staff individually or as members of health-care teams (Carey 1973; Bassett 1976; Barrows 1993; Rodrigues, Rodrigues, and Casey 2000; Flannelly et al. 2005; Sakurai 2005). Increasingly, hospitals are working on multi- or interfaith models where individual chaplains work with people across traditions rather than only with those who share their religious/spiritual backgrounds. In a study of chaplains working at Memorial Sloan-Kettering Cancer Center, researchers found that chaplains worked with family members and friends in addition to patients; received referrals, particularly from nurses; and spent more time with patients after surgeries than before (Flannelly, Weaver, and Handzo 2003). At a community hospital, chaplains were most often called for patients with anxiety, depression, or pregnancy loss (Fogg et al. 2004). Various hospital constituencies perceive chaplains' roles and importance differently, with the largest number of referrals to chaplains often coming from nurses and social workers (Thiel and Robinson 1997; Bryant 1993; Fogg et al. 2004).

As a group, hospital chaplains have become professionalized in recent years, a process perhaps best described through Freidson's famous work on professions (Freidson 1970; De Vries, Berlinger, and Cadge 2008). As chaplains shift from the subjective to the official labor market, they develop and redevelop certification processes and outline criteria for "board certification," which currently includes the certification of a faith tradition, a graduate level theological degree, and four units of clinical pastoral education.[12] Related to efforts to professionalize and the emergence of evidence-based medicine, studies have begun to assess the relationship between patients' visits with hospital chaplains and patient satisfaction with the overall hospital experience (Parkum 1985; VandeCreek and Connell 1991; VandeCreek and Lyon 1997; Clark, Drain, and Malone 2003; Fitchett, Thomason, and Lyndes 2008), as well as to describe how chaplains work differently with different populations depending on age of the patient, severity of illness, religious/spiritual tradition, presence of family, or availability of local clergy (VandeCreek and Lyon 1997). Evolving relationships between medical and religious organizations and professionals set the backdrop for chaplains' daily work and professionalizing processes in hospitals and other health-care organizations, a case and example of the kinds of insights sociologists could bring to questions at the institutional level.

Local Religious Organizations

In addition to biomedical institutions, health concerns are often addressed in local religious congregations in regular services and special gatherings. Some congregations regularly act around health and healing in communal prayers and rituals. A primary prayer for spiritual healing and physical cure in Judaism, the *Mi Sheberakh*, is often recited in synagogue by an individual or a family member of someone who is ill. Similarly in many Christian congregations, sick individuals are publicly named during prayers and rituals in the context of weekly services.

Across traditions, groups also have separate gatherings and rituals for health and healing. Many Episcopal congregations, for example, have healing services that include anointing people who are ill with oil, laying hands on them, and praying with them. These rituals create spaces in which those who are ill can speak publicly about their illnesses and receive support. Health and healing is rarely restricted to physical health in these contexts, and instead encompasses emotional and spiritual processes not limited to the body (Hollis 2005). Similar kinds of specialized communal services for health take place across religious contexts in the contemporary United States (Barnes and Sered 2005; Jacobs 2005).

Along with communal gatherings, individuals in some traditions address health concerns privately with their spiritual and religious leaders. Thai Buddhist monks in the United States, for example, offer chants, amulets, and herbal remedies intended to effect cures. Others encourage practitioners to obtain a treatment and diagnosis plan from a physician and then work with the individual around meditation and other trainings for the mind that make it easier to follow the doctor's instructions (Numrich 2005). Private rituals in the Thai Buddhist tradition and others take place in religious centers, individuals' homes, and hospitals. These rituals supplement the regular visiting and counseling many religious leaders do with their congregants (Chalfant et al. 1990; Moran et al. 2005).

In addition to working with their congregations, some religious leaders actively facilitate relationships with biomedical health programs. Individuals often seek such assistance from religious leaders, who refer congregants to health-care providers (Daaleman and Frey 1998). Religious leaders also bring health-care services to religious centers in the form of information, public health screenings, health promotion efforts, and religiously based health centers (Djupe and Westberg 1995; Chatters, Levin, and Ellison 1998). A smoking-cessation program facilitated through local congregations in Baltimore, for example, proved more successful than self-help models (Voorhees et al. 1996). Blood pressure screenings, blood drives, and healthy eating and exercise programs also regularly take place in religious centers (Griffith 2004). Such efforts may influence health behaviors inside and outside religious organizations; some studies show that highly religious individuals may be more likely to privately seek out care from biomedical institutions. For example, studies by Benjamins and colleagues find, across denominations, frequent service attendance associated with increased use of preventative health services, such as mammograms, pap smears, and prostate and cholesterol screenings (Benjamins and Brown 2004; Benjamins 2006; Benjamins, Trinitapoli, and Ellison 2006).

Health efforts in African American congregations have been the subject of particular research attention. Studies point to the importance of fostering relationships between black churches and a range of physical and mental health providers (Moore 1992; Caldwell et al. 1995; Adkison-Bradley et al. 2005). Clergy are often a first contact point for African Americans, particularly for people with mental health concerns (Neighbors, Musick, and Williams 1998). Substantial numbers of African American congregations also have programs that offer assistance with family, health, or social service needs (Taylor et al. 2000). The size of a congregation and the educational attainment of its clergy were found to be the most significant predictors of whether it has church-sponsored community health outreach programs (Thomas et al. 1994).

Parish nursing is another way that religious organizations address public health issues. Started by Granger Westberg in the mid-1980s, parish nursing programs in Protestant and Catholic contexts attempt to combine the work of physicians, nurses, and religious leaders by providing limited health-care services through local congregations. The first parish nurses were employed at Lutheran General Hospital in Chicago and also began to care for people at local churches. Today parish nurses are employed or volunteer within local churches or hospitals to provide health-care services ranging from routine screenings and immunizations to more involved medical follow-up and coordination. The American Nursing Association recognized parish nursing as a specialty in the late 1990s. No sociological research has been conducted about its history, demographics, practices, or organizational models (Solari-Twadell and McDermott 1999; Orr and May 2000; Vandecreek and Mooney 2002).

Directions for Future Research

Given the variety of ways religion, spirituality, health, and medicine intersect in the contemporary United States, existing sociological studies have just begun to map the terrain. To better understand how religion and spirituality influence health and medicine, and vice versa, sociologists of medicine and religion need only look around and turn their observations into sociological research questions.

At the individual level, sociologists might begin to develop a robust qualitative literature about the relationship between specific religious/spiritual beliefs and practices and individuals' health beliefs and behaviors. Rather than starting with existing survey data that furthers the epidemiological questions researchers have investigated, sociologists might begin with individual interviews embedding those individuals in the familial, religious, work, and other institutional contexts that shape the ways they think about health and religion/spirituality. Researchers might ask about the extent to which religion/spirituality influences health, as well as how health events, particularly seriously illness, influence people's religious/spiritual beliefs and behaviors (e.g., Ferraro and Kelley-Moore 2002). Such studies could also explore in more detail how individuals combine religious/spiritual practices and biomedicine (as in McGuire 1988; Eisenberg et al. 1993). In addition to generating new insights about the relationships between religion/spirituality and health, such interviews might generate theoretically grounded testable hypotheses about the relationships explored in existing epidemiological studies. Research designs that systematically compare people across religious/spiritual traditions, health experiences, professional backgrounds, and so on would further develop this literature analytically.

In addition to embedding individuals within their social institutions, researchers might further consider how different medical and religious institutions relate to one another organizationally as modeled in the examples here. In individual cities, they might ask how leadership overlaps and religious/spiritual and medical professionals play roles in both sets of organizations. More detailed attention could be paid to the processes by which medical organizations secularize, the ways mergers between religious and secular health-care organizations happen, and the ways religious/spiritual organizations from Buddhist groups to African American congregations address health concerns in the day to day. Such studies could be conducted at the city or state level of analysis or at the national level, as modeled by Blanchard and colleagues (2008) in their work about the relationships between religious ecology and population health. Similar approaches might compare how religion/spirituality is present formally and informally in different types of medical institutions through Joint Commission policies, the work of hospital chaplains, the presence of hospital chapels, and the formal and informal conversations that take place between medical staff, patients, and families (e.g., Cadge and Catlin 2006; Cadge and Daglian 2008; Cadge, Ecklund, and Short 2009; Cadge and Ecklund 2009). While some of this research has been conducted around end-of-life issues, recent survey data about medical professionals' and laypeople's beliefs about miracles call for further investigation.

Perhaps more important than specifically focusing on individuals or institutions, however, sociologists might best follow the examples of journalists and anthropologists by investigating topics and issues at the intersections of religion, spirituality, health, and medicine that are often in the news, aiming to speak to a broader audience in the process (e.g., Fadiman 1998; Rapp 1999; Kaufman 2005, Cadge 2009). While some of these topics are explicitly about religion/spirituality, such as questions about whether pharmacists are obliged to dispense birth control and whether intercessory prayer heals, many others are about broad ethical issues with strong moral undertones. When Terry Schiavo's case brought end-of-life issues and decision making into the public view, for example, sociologists could have asked how people's religious/spiritual backgrounds shaped their opinions about the case, their own actions around living wills and health-care proxies, and their reactions to the religious leaders often shown on television praying in front of the hospice where she was cared for. Responding to public debates about stem-cell issues, sociologists might consider the underlying factors that lead these issues to come into and out of the public view. And in response to post-1965 immigrants, sociologists might further explore the range of new religious-inspired health organizations these immigrants are starting and the ways their religious beliefs and organizations mediate their access to health care, especially in refugee communities.

Regardless of the specific topics sociologists decide to investigate, a generative and robust sociological literature about religion, spirituality, health, and medicine needs to consider the interactions among these concepts at multiple levels of analysis. Studies need to be designed around analytically based comparative questions, including comparisons between religious traditions and countries whenever possible, that privilege multiple ways of knowing (epidemiologic, ethnographic, etc.). Throughout, sociologists need to be aware of how religion/spirituality and health are conceptualized and measured and whom their conceptualizations include and exclude (see, e.g., Laird, de Marrais, and Barnes 2007).

Notes

Research for this chapter was supported by the Theodore and Jane Norman Fund for Faculty Research at Brandeis University. Portions of this chapter also appear in "Religion, Spirituality, and Health: An Institutional Approach" in the *Oxford Handbook of the Sociology of Religion*, edited by Peter Clarke (Oxford: Oxford University Press, 2009).

1. Survey by CBS/New York Times, April 29, 1998. iPOLL Databank, the Roper Center for Public Opinion Research, University of Connecticut. ropercenter.uconn.edu/ipoll.html. Retrieved August 6, 2008.
2. Survey by Princeton Survey Research Associates/ Newsweek, October 30–31, 2003. iPOLL Databank, the Roper Center for Public Opinion Research, University of Connecticut. ropercenter.uconn.edu/ ipoll.html. Accessed August 6, 2008. For details about this debate in the medical literature see Ehman et al. 1999.
3. The distinctions between the terms "religion" and "spirituality" and the emergence of the category "spiritual" in the medical literature deserves its own article following the example of Roof (2003).
4. Readers interested in accounts of religious healing, studies focused outside the United States, or both should refer to the work of anthropologists, religious studies scholars, and public health researchers in these areas (such as Marty and Vaux 1982; Fox 1984; Numbers and Amundsen 1986; Gevitz 1988; Hufford 1988; Dole 2004; Barnes and Sered 2005; Porterfield 2005; Barnes 2006). Similarly, studies of complementary and alternative medicine (CAM) in the social science and medical literatures inconsistently include prayer and other spiritual/ religious practices, leading to fragmented overlap

between the literatures we leave for other scholars to delineate (Ruggie 2004).
5. For additional interdisciplinary review articles on the relationships between religion, spirituality, health, and medicine, please see Ellison 1998; Ellison and Levin 1998; Sherkat and Ellison 1999; Chatters 2000; George et al. 2000; Koenig, McCullough, and Larson 2001; Miller and Thoresen 2003; Weaver and Ellison 2004.
6. Interestingly, however, the American Medical Association established a Committee on Medicine and Religion in the mid-1960s, which included a column in the *Journal of the American Medical Association* (*JAMA*) to facilitate work between physicians and religious leaders (Rhoads 1967; O'Donnell 1970). *JAMA* has continued to address questions about religion and medicine, though they are clearly peripheral to the journal's other emphases (Rosner 2001).
7. A small body of research considers other differences between Catholic and non-Catholic hospitals in terms of compassionate care, services available, etc. (White and Begun 1998–1999; White 2000; White, Begun, and Tian 2006; Prince 1994).
8. The process of secularization is also not without its critics (Bull 1990; Grant, O'Neil, and Stephens 2003).
9. For interdisciplinary reviews, see Ellison 1991; Payne et al. 1991; Levav et al. 1997; Scott, Agresti, and Fitchett 1998; Weaver, Kline, et al. 1998; Weaver, Samford, et al. 1998; Leventhal, Idler, and Leventhal 1999; Hackney and Sanders 2003; Salsman and Carlson 2005; Nonnemaker et al. 2006.
10. For interdisciplinary overviews of the religion-health relationship among older adults, see Chatters and Taylor 1994; Idler 1994; Koenig 1995; Krause 2005.
11. For more information, see jointcommission.org/ AboutUs/joint_commission_history.htm.
12. For more information, see acpe.edu/acroread/ Common percent20Standards percent20for percent20Professional percent20Chaplaincy percent20Revised percent20March percent202005 .pdf.

References

Abdel-Aziz, E., B. N. Arch, and H. Al-Taher. 2004. "The Influence of Religious Beliefs on General Practitioners' Attitudes towards Termination of Pregnancy—A Pilot Study." *Journal of Obstetrics and Gynaecology* 24(5): 557–61.

Abrums, Mary. 2000. "'Jesus Will Fix It after Awhile': Meanings and Health." *Social Science and Medicine* 50(1): 89–105.

Adkison-Bradley, Carla, Darrell Johnson, JoAnn Lipford

Sanders, Lonnie Duncan, and Cheryl Holcomb-McCoy. 2005. "Forging a Collaborative Relationship between the Black Church and the Counseling Profession." *Counseling and Values* 49(2): 147–54.

Aiyer, Aryan N., George Ruiz, Allegra Steinman, and Gloria Y. F. Ho. 1999. "Influence of Physician Attitudes on Willingness to Perform Abortion." *Obstetrics and Gynecology* 93(4): 576–80.

Angrosino, Michael. 2006. *Blessed with Enough Foolishness: Pastoral Care in a Modern Hospital.* West Conshohocken, Pa.: Infinity Publishing.

Aswad, Barbara, and Nancy Gray. 1996. "Challenges to the Arab-American Family and ACCESS." In *Family and Gender among American Muslims*, ed. Barbara Aswad and Barbara Bilge, 223–40. Philadelphia: Temple University Press.

Baker, Joseph O. 2008. "An Investigation of the Sociological Patterns of Prayer Frequency and Content." *Sociology of Religion* 69(2): 169–85.

Barkan, Steven E., and Susan F. Greenwood. 2003. "Religious Attendance and Subjective Well-Being among Older Americans: Evidence from the General Social Survey." *Review of Religious Research* 45(2): 116–29.

Barnes, Linda L. 2006. "A Medical School Curriculum on Religion and Healing." In *Teaching Religion and Healing*, ed. Linda L. Barnes and Ines M. Talamantez, 307–25. New York: Oxford University Press.

Barnes, Linda L., and Susan S. Sered, eds. 2005. *Religion and Healing in America.* New York: Oxford University Press.

Barrows, David C. 1993. "'A Whole Different Thing'—The Hospital Chaplaincy: The Emergence of the Occupation and the Work of the Chaplain." Ph.D. diss., University of California, San Francisco.

Bassett, S. Denton. 1976. *Public Religious Services in the Hospital.* Springfield, Ill.: Charles C. Thomas.

Bearman, Peter S., and Hannah Bruckner. 2001. "Promising the Future: Virginity Pledges and First Intercourse." *American Journal of Sociology* 106(4): 859–912.

Benjamins, Maureen R. 2006. "Religious Influences on Female Preventive Service Utilization in a Nationally Representative Sample of Older Women." *Journal of Behavioral Medicine* 29(1): 1–16.

Benjamins, Maureen R., and Carolyn Brown. 2004. "Religion and Preventative Care Utilization among the Elderly." *Social Science and Medicine* 58:109–18.

Benjamins, Maureen R., Jenny A. Trinitapoli, and Christopher G. Ellison. 2006. "Religious Attendance, Health Maintenance Beliefs, and Mammography Utilization: Findings from a Nationwide Survey of Presbyterian Women." *Journal for the Scientific Study of Religion* 45(4): 597–607.

Bierman, Alex. 2006. "Does Religion Buffer the Effects of Discrimination on Mental Health? Differing Effects by Race." *Journal for the Scientific Study of Religion* 45(4): 551–65.

Bjarnason, Thoroddur. 1998. "Parents, Religion and Perceived Social Coherence: A Durkheimian Framework of Adolescent Anomie." *Journal for the Scientific Study of Religion* 37(4): 742–54.

Bjorck, Jeffrey, and John W. Thurman. 2007. "Negative Life Events, Patterns of Positive and Negative Religious Coping, and Psychological Functioning." *Journal for the Scientific Study of Religion* 46(2): 159–67.

Blanchard, Troy C., John R. Bartkowski, Todd L. Matthews, and Kent R. Kerley. 2008. "Faith, Morality and Mortality: The Ecological Impact of Religion on Population Health." *Social Forces* 86(4): 1591–1620.

Blazer, Dan G., Dana C. Hughes, and Linda K. George. 1987. "The Epidemiology of Depression in an Elderly Community Population." *Gerontologist* 27(3): 281–87.

Booth, Jennifer, and John E. Martin. 1998. "Spiritual and Religious Factors in Substance Use, Dependence, and Recovery." In *Handbook of Religion and Mental Health*, ed. Harold G. Koenig, 175–200. San Diego: Academic Press.

Broyles, Philip A., and Cynthia K. Drenovsky. 1992. "Religious Attendance and the Subjective Health of the Elderly." *Review of Religious Research* 34(2): 1992.

Bryant, Cullene. 1993. "Role Clarification: A Quality Improvement Survey of Hospital Chaplain Customers." *Journal for Healthcare Quality* 15(4): 18–20.

Bull, Malcolm. 1990. "Secularization and Medicalization." *British Journal of Sociology* 41(2): 245–61.

Burdette, Amy M., Terrence D. Hill, and Benjamin E. Moulton. 2005. "Religion and Attitudes toward Physician-Assisted Suicide and Terminal Palliative Care." *Journal for the Scientific Study of Religion* 44(1): 79–93.

Cadge, Wendy. 2009. "Saying Your Prayers, Constructing Your Religions: Medical Studies of Intercessory Prayer." *Journal of Religion* 89:299–327.

Cadge, Wendy, and Elizabeth A. Catlin. 2006. "Making Sense of Suffering and Death: How Health Care Providers Construct Meanings in a Neonatal Intensive Care Unit." *Journal of Religion and Health* 45(2): 248–63.

Cadge, Wendy, and M. Daglian. 2008. "Blessings, Strength, and Guidance: Prayer Frames in a Hospital Prayer Book." *Poetics* 36:358–73.

Cadge, Wendy, and Elaine Howard Ecklund. 2009. "Prayers in the Clinic: How Pediatricians and

Pediatric Oncologists Respond." *Southern Medical Journal* 102(12): 1218–21.

Cadge, Wendy, Elaine Howard Ecklund, and Nicholas Short. 2009. "Religion and Spirituality: A Barrier and a Bridge in the Everyday Professional Work of Pediatric Physicians." *Social Problems* 56(4): 702–21.

Cadge, Wendy, Jeremy Freese, and Nicholas Christakis. 2008. "Hospital Chaplaincy in the United States: A National Overview." *Southern Medical Journal* 101(6): 626–30.

Caldwell, Cleopatra H., Linda M. Chatters, Andrew Billingsley, and Robert J. Taylor. 1995. "Church-Based Support Programs for Elderly Black Adults: Congregational and Clergy Statistics." In *Aging, Spirituality and Religion*, ed. Mel Kimble, Susan H. McFadden, James W. Ellor, and James J. Seeber, 306–24. Minneapolis: Fortress Press.

Carey, Raymond G. 1973. "Chaplaincy: Component of Total Patient Care?" *Hospitals: The Journal of the American Hospital Association* 47(14): 166–72.

Cavendish, Roberta, Barbara Kraynyak Luise, Donna Russo, Claudia Mitzeliotis, Maria Bauer, Mary Ann McPartlan Bajo, Carmen Calvino, Karen Horne, and Judith Medefindt. 2004. "Spiritual Perspectives of Nurses in the United States Relevant for Education and Practice." *Western Journal of Nursing Research* 26(2): 196–212.

CDC [Centers for Disease Control and Prevention.] Public Health Practice Program Office. 1999. "Engaging Faith Communities as Partners in Improving Community Health: 1999. Highlights from a CDC/ATSDR Forum. Atlanta: CDC.

Chalfant, Paul H., Peter L. Heller, Alden Roberts, David Briones, Salvador Aguirre-Hochbaum, and Walter Fan. 1990. "The Clergy as a Resource for Those Encountering Psychological Distress." *Review of Religious Research* 31(3): 305–13.

Chatters, Linda M. 2000. "Religion and Health: Public Health Research and Practice." *Annual Review of Public Health* 21:335–67.

Chatters, Linda M., Jeffrey S. Levin, and Christopher G. Ellison. 1998. "Public Health and Health Education in Faith Communities." *Health Education and Behavior* 25(6): 689–99.

Chatters, Linda M., and Robert J. Taylor. 1994. "Religious Involvement among Older African Americans." *Religion in Aging and Health: Theoretical Foundations and Methodological Frontiers*, ed. Jeffrey S. Levin, 196–230. Newbury Park, Calif.: Sage.

Chaves, Mark. 2004. *Congregations in America*. Cambridge, Mass.: Harvard University Press.

Christakis, Nicholas A., and David A. Asch. 1995. "Physician Characteristics Associated with Decisions to Withdraw Life Support." *American Journal of Public Health* 85(3): 367–72.

Clark, Paul A., Maxwell Drain, and Mary P. Malone. 2003. "Addressing Patients' Emotional and Spiritual Needs." *Joint Commission Journal on Quality and Safety* 29(12): 659–70.

Coburn, Carol K., and Martha Smith. 1999. *Spirited Lives: How Nuns Shaped Catholic Culture and American Life, 1836–1920*. Chapel Hill: University of North Carolina Press.

Commerford, Mary C., and Marvin Reznikoff. 1996. "Relationship of Religion and Perceived Social Support to Self-Esteem and Depression in Nursing Home Residents." *Journal of Psychology* 130(1): 35–50.

Curlin, Farr A., John D. Lantos, Chad J. Roach, Sarah A. Sellergren, and Marshall H. Chin. 2005. "Religious Characteristics of U.S. Physicians: A National Survey." *Journal of General Internal Medicine* 20(7): 629–34.

Curlin, Farr A., Ryan E. Lawrence, Marshall H. Chin, and John D. Lantos. 2007. "Religion, Conscience, and Controversial Clinical Practices." *New England Journal of Medicine* 356(6): 593–600.

Curlin, Farr A., Sarah A. Sellergren, John D. Lantos, and Marshall H. Chin. 2007. "Physicians' Observations and Interpretations of the Influence of Religion and Spirituality on Health." *Archives of Internal Medicine* 167(7): 649–54.

Daaleman, Timothy P., and Bruce Frey. 1998. "Prevalence and Patterns of Physician Referral to Clergy and Pastoral Care." *Archives of Family Medicine* 7(6): 548–53.

De Vries, Raymond, Nancy Berlinger, and Wendy Cadge. 2008. "Lost in Translation? Sociological Observations and Reflections on the Practice of Hospital Chaplaincy." *Hastings Center Report*, November–December.

Djupe, Anne M., and Granger Westberg. 1995. "Congregation-Based Health Programs." In *Aging, Spirituality and Religion*, ed. Mel Kimble, Susan H. McFadden, James W. Ellor, and James J. Seeber, 325–34. Minneapolis: Fortress Press.

Dole, Christopher. 2004. "In the Shadows of Medicine and Modernity: Medical Integration and Secular Histories of Religious Healing in Turkey." *Culture, Medicine and Psychiatry* 28(3): 255–80.

Drevenstedt, Greg L. 1998. "Race and Ethnic Differences in the Effects of Religious Attendance on Subjective Health." *Review of Religious Research* 39(3): 245–63.

Dwyer, Jeffrey, Leslie Clarke, and Michael Miller. 1990. "The Effect of Religious Concentration and Affiliation on County Cancer Mortality Rates." *Journal of Health and Social Behavior* 3:185–202.

Ehman, John W., Barbara B. Ott, Thomas H. Short, Ralph C. Ciampa, and John Hansen-Flaschen.

1999. "Do Patients Want Physicians to Inquire about Their Spiritual or Religious Beliefs If They Become Gravely Ill?" *Archives of Internal Medicine* 159(15): 1803–6.

Eisenberg, David M., Ronald C. Kessler, Cindy Foster, Francis E. Norlock, David R. Calkins, and Thomas L. Delbanco. 1993. "Unconventional Medicine in the United States: Prevalence, Costs, and Patterns of Use." *New England Journal of Medicine* 328(4): 246–52.

Eliassen, A. Henry, John Taylor, and Donald A. Lloyd. 2005. "Subjective Religiosity and Depression in the Transition to Adulthood." *Journal for the Scientific Study of Religion* 44(2): 187–99.

Ellison, Christopher G. 1991. "Religious Involvement and Subjective Well-Being." *Journal of Health and Social Behavior* 32(1): 80–99.

———. 1993. "Religious Involvement and Self-Perception among Black Americans." *Social Forces* 71:1027–55.

———. 1995. "Race, Religious Involvement and Depressive Symptomatology in a Southeastern U. S. Community." *Social Science and Medicine* 40(11): 1561–72.

———. 1998. "Introduction to Symposium: Religion, Health, and Well-Being." *Journal for the Scientific Study of Religion* 37(4): 692–94.

Ellison, Christopher G., Jason D. Boardman, David R. Williams, and James S. Jackson. 2001. "Religious Involvement, Stress, and Mental Health: Findings from the 1995 Detroit Area Study." *Social Forces* 80(1): 215–49.

Ellison, Christopher G., Kevin J. Flannelly, Kevin J. Vaaler, and Andrew J. Weaver. 2006. "The Clergy as a Source of Mental Health Assistance: What Americans Believe." *Review of Religious Research* 48(2): 190–211.

Ellison, Christopher G., and Patricia Goodson. 1997. "Conservative Protestantism and Attitudes toward Family Planning in a Sample of Seminarians." *Journal for the Scientific Study of Religion* 36(4): 512–29.

Ellison, Christopher G., and Jeffrey S. Levin. 1998. "The Religion-Health Connection: Evidence, Theory, and Future Directions." *Health Education and Behavior* 25(6): 700–720.

Fadiman, Anne. 1998. *The Spirit Catches You and You Fall Down*. New York: Noonday Press.

Ferraro, Kenneth F., and Jessica A. Kelley-Moore. 2002. "Religious Consolation among Men and Women: Do Health Problems Spur Seeking?" *Journal for the Scientific Study of Religion* 39(2): 220–34.

Ferraro, Kenneth F., and Jerome R. Koch. 1994. "Religion and Health among Black and White Adults: Examining Social Support and Consolation."

Journal for the Scientific Study of Religion 33(4): 362–75.

Fitchett, George, Clayton Thomason, and Kathryn A. Lyndes. 2008. "What Health Care Chaplains Think about Quality Improvement." *Hastings Center Report* November–December.

Flannelly, Kevin J., Christopher G. Ellison, and Adrienne L. Strock. 2004. "Methodologic Issues in Research on Religion and Health." *Southern Medical Journal* 97(12): 1231–41.

Flannelly, Kevin J., George F. Handzo, and Andrew J. Weaver. 2004. "Factors Affecting Healthcare Chaplaincy and the Provision of Pastoral Care in the United States." *Journal of Pastoral Care and Counseling* 58(1–2): 127–30.

Flannelly, Kevin J., George F. Handzo, Andrew J. Weaver, and Walter J. Smith. 2005. "A National Survey of Health Care Administrators' Views on the Importance of Various Chaplain Roles." *Journal of Pastoral Care and Counseling* 59(1–2): 87–96.

Flannelly, Kevin J., Andrew J. Weaver, and George F. Handzo. 2003. "A Three-Year Study of Chaplains' Professional Activities at Memorial Sloan-Kettering Cancer Center in New York City." *Psycho-Oncology* 12(8): 760–68.

Flannelly, Kevin J., Andrew J. Weaver, Walter J. Smith, and George F. Handzo. 2003. "Psychologists and Health Care Chaplains Doing Research Together." *Journal of Psychology and Christianity* 22(4): 327–32.

Fogg, Sarah L., Andrew J. Weaver, Kevin J. Flannelly, and George F. Handzo. 2004. "An Analysis of Referrals to Chaplains in a Community Hospital in New York over a Seven Year Period." *Journal of Pastoral Care and Counseling* 58(3): 225–35.

Fosarelli, Pat. 2008. "Medicine, Spirituality, and Patient Care." *Journal of the American Medical Association* 300(7): 836–38.

Fox, Margery. 1984. "Conflict to Coexistence: Christian Science and Medicine." *Medical Anthropology* 8(1): 292–301.

Fox, Renée C., and Judith P. Swazey. 2008. *Observing Bioethics*. New York: Oxford University Press.

Freidson, Eliot. 1970. *Profession of Medicine: A Study of the Sociology of Applied Knowledge*. Chicago: University of Chicago Press.

Gallup, George, Jr., and D. Michael Lindsay. 1999. *Surveying the Religious Landscape: Trends in U.S. Beliefs*. Harrisburg, Pa.: Morehouse Publishing.

Garces-Foley, Kathleen. 2003. "Buddhism, Hospice, and the American Way of Dying." *Review of Religious Research* 44(4): 341–53.

Gardner, John W., Jill S. Sanborn, and Martha L. Slattery. 1995. "Behavioral Factors Explaining the Low Risk for Cervical Carcinoma in Utah Mormon Women." *Epidemiology* 6(2): 187–89.

Geertz, Clifford. 1973. *The Interpretation of Cultures: Selected Essays.* New York: Basic Books.

General Social Survey. 1998. thearda.com/.

George, Linda K., Christopher G. Ellison, and David B. Larson. 2002. "Explaining the Relationships between Religious Involvement and Health." *Psychological Inquiry* 13(3): 190–200.

George, Linda K., David B. Larson, Harold G. Koenig, and Michael McCullough. 2000. "Spirituality and Health: State of the Evidence." *Journal of Social and Clinical Psychology* 19:102–16.

Gevitz, Norman. 1988. *Other Healers: Unorthodox Medicine in America.* Baltimore: Johns Hopkins University Press.

Grant, Don, Kathleen M. O'Neil, and Laura S. Stephens. 2003. "Neosecularization and Craft versus Professional Religious Authority in a Nonreligious Organization." *Journal for the Scientific Study of Religion* 42(3): 479–87.

———. 2004. "Spirituality in the Workplace: New Empirical Directions in the Study of the Sacred." *Sociology of Religion* 65(3): 265–83.

Griffith, R. Marie. 2004. *Born Again Bodies: Flesh and Spirit in American Christianity.* Berkeley: University of California Press.

Hackney, Charles H., and Glenn S. Sanders. 2003. "Religiosity and Mental Health: A Meta-Analysis of Recent Studies." *Journal for the Scientific Study of Religion* 42(1): 43–55.

Hadaway, C. Kirk, and Penny Long Marler. 2005. "How Many Americans Attend Worship Each Week? An Alternative Approach to Measurement." *Journal for the Scientific Study of Religion* 44(3): 307–22.

Hall, Charles. 1992. *Head and Heart: The Story of the Clinical Pastoral Education Movement.* Decatur, Ga.: Journal of Pastoral Care Publications.

Hall, Daniel E., Harold G. Koenig, and Keith G. Meador. 2004. "Conceptualizing 'Religion': How Language Shapes and Constrains Knowledge in the Study of Religion and Health." *Perspectives in Biology and Medicine* 47(3): 386–401.

Hamil-Luker, Jenifer, and Christian Smith. 1998. "Religious Authority and Public Opinion on the Right to Die." *Sociology of Religion* 59(4): 373–91.

Hollis, Jennifer L. 2005. "Healing into Wholeness in the Episcopal Church." In *Religion and Healing in America*, ed. Linda L. Barnes and Susan S. Sered, 89–102. New York: Oxford University Press.

House, James S., Cynthia Robbins, and Helen L. Metzner. 1982. "The Association of Social Relationships and Activities with Mortality: Prospective Evidence from the Tecumseh Community Health Study." *American Journal of Epidemiology* 116(1): 123–40.

Hout, Michael, and Andrew Greeley. 1998. "What Church Officials' Reports Don't Show: Another Look at Church Attendance Data." *American Sociological Review* 63(1): 113–19.

Hufford, David. 1988. "Contemporary Folk Medicine." In *Other Healers: Unorthodox Medicine in America*, ed. Norman Gevitz, 228–64. Baltimore: Johns Hopkins University Press.

Hummer, Robert A., Richard G. Rogers, Charles B. Nam, and Christopher G. Ellison. 1999. "Religious Involvement and U.S. Adult Mortality." *Demography* 36(2): 273–85.

Idler, Ellen L. 1987. "Religious Involvement and the Health of the Elderly: Some Hypotheses and an Initial Test." *Social Forces* 66:226–38.

———. 1994. *Cohesiveness and Coherence: Religion and the Health of the Elderly.* New York: Garland.

———. 1995. "Religion, Health, and Non-Physical Senses of Self." *Social Forces* 74:683–704.

———. 2003. "Gender Differences in Self-Rated Health, in Mortality, and in the Relationship between the Two." *Gerontologist* 43(3): 372–75.

Idler, Ellen L., and Stanislav V. Kasl. 1992. "Religion, Disability, Depression, and the Timing of Death." *American Journal of Sociology* 97(4): 1052–79.

Imber, Jonathan B. 1986. *Abortion and the Private Practice of Medicine.* New Haven, Conn.: Yale University Press.

Jacobs, Claude F. 2005. "Rituals of Healing in African American Spiritual Churches." In *Religion and Healing in America*, ed. Linda L. Barnes and Susan S. Sered, 333–41. New York: Oxford University Press.

Jacobs, Lenworth M., Karyl Burns, and Barbara Bennett Jacobs. 2008. "Views of the Public and Trauma Professionals on Death and Dying from Injuries." *Archives of Surgery* 143(8): 730–35.

Jasso, Guillermina, Douglas S. Massey, Mark R. Rosenzweig, and James P. Smith. 2003. "Exploring the Religious Preference of Recent Immigrants to the United States: Evidence from the New Immigrant Survey Pilot." In *Religion and Immigration: Christian, Jewish, and Muslim Experiences in the United States*, ed. Yvonne Yazbeck Haddad, Jane I. Smith, and John L. Esposito, 217–53. Walnut Creek, Calif.: AltaMira Press.

Kauffman, Christopher J. 1995. *Ministry and Meaning: A Religious History of Catholic Health Care in the United States.* New York: Crossroad.

Kaufman, Sharon R. 2005. *And a Time to Die: How American Hospitals Shape the End of Life.* New York: Scribner.

Kendler, Kenneth S., Charles O. Gardner, and Carol A. Prescott. 1997. "Religion, Psychopathology, and Substance Use and Abuse: A Multi-Measure, Genetic-Epidemiologic Study." *American Journal of Psychiatry* 154(3): 322–29.

Klemmack, David L., Lucinda Lee Roff, Michael W. Parker, Harold G. Koenig, Patricia Sawyer, and Richard M. Allman. 2007. "Cluster Analysis Typology of Religiousness/Spirituality among Older Adults." *Research on Aging* 29(2): 163–83.

Koenig, Harold G. 1995. *Research on Religion and Aging.* Westport, Conn.: Greenwood Press.

Koenig, Harold G., Judith C. Hays, David B. Larson, Linda K. George, Harvey J. Cohen, Michael E. McCullough, Keith G. Meador, and Dan G. Blazer. 1999. "Does Religious Attendance Prolong Survival? A Six-Year Follow-Up Study of 3,968 Older Adults." *Journal of Gerontology Series A: Biological and Medical Sciences* 54A: M370–77.

Koenig, Harold G., Michael E. McCullough, and David B. Larson. 2001. *Handbook of Religion and Health.* New York: Oxford University Press.

Krause, Neal. 1993. "Race Differences in Life Satisfaction among the Aged." *Journal of Gerontology Series B: Psychological and Social Sciences* 48: S235–44.

———. 2003. "Religious Meaning and Subjective Well-Being in Late Life." *Journal of Gerontology Series B: Psychological and Social Sciences*: 58B: S160–70.

———. 2004. "Assessing the Relationships among Prayer Expectancies, Race, and Self-Esteem in Later Life." *Journal for the Scientific Study of Religion* 43(3): 395–408.

———. 2005. "Aging." In *Handbook of Religion and Social Institutions*, ed. Helen R. Ebaugh, 139–60. New York: Springer.

———. 2006. "Religious Doubt and Psychological Well-Being: A Longitudinal Investigation." *Review of Religious Research* 47(3): 287–302.

Krause, Neal, and Christopher G. Ellison. 2007. "Parental Religious Socialization Practices and Self-Esteem in Late Life." *Review of Religious Research* 49(2): 109–27.

Krause, Neal, Christopher G. Ellison, and Jack P. Marcum. 2002. "The Effects of Church-Based Emotional Support on Health: Do They Vary by Gender?" *Sociology of Religion* 63(1): 21–47.

Krause, Neal, Christopher G. Ellison, and Keith Wulff. 1998. "Church-Based Support, Negative Interaction, and Psychological Well-Being: Findings from a National Sample of Presbyterians." *Journal for the Scientific Study of Religion* 37(4): 725–41.

Krause, Neal, and Keith Wulff. 2004. "Religious Doubt and Health: Exploring the Potential Dark Side of Religion." *Sociology of Religion* 65(1): 35–56.

Kudler, Taryn. 2007. "Providing Spiritual Care." *Contexts* 6(4): 60–61.

Laird, Lance, and Wendy Cadge. 2007. "Caring for Our Neighbors: How Muslim Community-Based Health Organizations Are Bridging the Health Care Gap in America." *A Report oby the Institute for Social Policy and Understanding.* ispu.org/files/PDFs/mcbho.pdf.

Laird, Lance D., Justine de Marrais, and Linda L. Barnes. 2007. "Portraying Islam and Muslims in MEDLINE: A Content Analysis." *Social Science and Medicine* 65(12): 2425–39.

LaPierre, Lawrence L. 2003. "JCAHO Safeguards Spiritual Care." *Holistic Nursing Practice* 17(4): 219.

Lazarus, Barry. 1991. "The Practice of Medicine and Prejudice in a New England Town: The Founding of Mount Sinai Hospital, Hartford, Connecticut." *Journal of American Ethnic History* 10(3): 21–42.

Lee, Simon J. Craddock. 2002. "In a Secular Spirit: Strategies of Clinical Pastoral Education." *Health Care Analysis* 10(4): 339–56.

Levav, Itzhak, Robert Kohn, Jacqueline M. Golding, and Myrna M. Weissmen. 1997. "Vulnerability of Jews to Affective Disorder." *American Journal of Psychiatry* 154:941–47.

Leventhal, Howard, Ellen L. Idler, and Elaine L. Leventhal. 1999. "The Impact of Chronic Illness on the Self System." In *Self, Social Identity, and Physical Health: Interdisciplinary Explorations*, ed. Richard D. Ashmore and Richard J. Contrada, 185–208. New York: Oxford University Press.

Levin, Jeffrey S. 1994. "Religion and Health: Is There an Association, Is It Valid, and Is It Causal?" *Social Science and Medicine* 38(11): 1475–82.

———. 1996. "How Religion Influences Morbidity and Health: Reflections on Natural History, Salutogenesis and Host Resistance." *Social Science and Medicine* 43(5): 849–64.

Levin, Jeffrey S., Linda M. Chatters, and Robert. J. Taylor. 1995. "Religious Effects on Health Status and Life Satisfaction among Black Americans." *Journal of Gerontology Series B: Psychological and Social Sciences* 50(3): S154–63.

Levin, Jeffrey S., Kyriakos S. Markides, and Laura A. Ray. 1996. "Religious Attendance and Psychological Well-Being in Mexican Americans: A Panel Analysis of Three-Generations Data." *Gerontologist* 36:454–63.

Levin, Jeffrey S., David B. Larson, and Christina M. Pulchalski. 1997. "Religion and Spirituality in Medicine: Research and Education." *Journal of the American Medical Association* 278(3): 782–93.

Levin, Jeffrey S., and Harold Y. Vanderpool. 1987. "Is Frequent Religious Attendance Really Conducive to Better Health: Toward an Epidemiology of Religion." *Social Science and Medicine* 24(7): 589–600.

———. 1989. "Is Religion Therapeutically Significant for Hypertension?" *Social Science and Medicine* 29(1): 69–78.

———. 1992. "Religious Factors in Physical Health and the Prevention of Illness." In *Religion and Prevention in Mental Health: Research, Vision, and Action*, ed. Robert Hess, Kenneth I. Maton, and Kenneth I. Pargament, 83–103. New York: Haworth.

Levitan, Tina. 1964. *Islands of Compassion: A History of the Jewish Hospitals of New York*. New York: Twayne.

Mansfield, Christopher J., Jim Mitchell, and Dana E. King. 2002. "The Doctor as God's Mechanic? Beliefs in the Southeastern United States." *Social Science and Medicine* 54(3): 399–409.

Marty, Martin E., and Kenneth L. Vaux. 1982. *Health/ Medicine and the Faith Traditions: An Inquiry into Religion and Medicine*. Philadelphia: Fortress Press.

Maton, Kenneth I. 1989. "The Stress-Buffering Role of Spiritual Support: Cross-Sectional and Prospective Investigations." *Journal for the Scientific Study of Religion* 28(3): 310–23.

McCauley, Bernadette. 2005. *Who Shall Take Care of Our Sick? Roman Catholic Sisters and the Development of Catholic Hospitals in New York City*. Baltimore: Johns Hopkins University Press.

McCullough, Michael E., and Timothy B. Smith. 2003. "Religion and Health: Depressive Symptoms and Mortality as Case Studies." In *Handbook of the Sociology of Religion*, ed. Michele Dillon, 190–204. Cambridge: Cambridge University Press.

McGuire, Meredith B. 1988. *Ritual Healing in Suburban America*. New Brunswick, N.J.: Rutgers University Press.

McSherry, Elisabeth, and William A. Nelson. 1987. "The DRG Era: A Major Opportunity for Increased Pastoral Care Impact or a Crisis for Survival." *Journal of Pastoral Care* 41(3): 201–11.

Miller, William R., and Carl E. Thoresen. 2003. "Spirituality, Religion, and Health: An Emerging Research Field." *American Psychologist* 58(11): 24–35.

Mirola, William A. 1999. "A Refuge for Some: Gender Differences in the Relationship between Religious Involvement and Depression." *Sociology of Religion* 60(4): 419–37.

Mollat, Michel. 1986. *The Poor in the Middle Ages: An Essay in Social History*. Translated by Arthur Goldhammer. New Haven, Conn.: Yale University Press.

Moore, Thom. 1992. "The African American Church: A Source of Empowerment, Mutual Help, and Social Change." In *Religion and Prevention in Mental Health*, ed. Robert Hess, Kenneth I. Maton, and Kenneth I. Pargament, 237–58. New York: Haworth.

Moran, Michael, Kevin J. Flannelly, Andrew J. Weaver, Jon A. Overvold, Winifred Hess, and Jo C. Wilson. 2005. "A Study of Pastoral Care, Referral, and Consultation Practices among Clergy in Four Settings in the New York City Area." *Pastoral Psychology* 53(3): 253–64.

Moulton, Benjamin E., Terrence D. Hill, and Amy Burdette. 2006. "Religion and Trends in Euthanasia Attitudes among U.S. Adults, 1977–2004." *Sociological Forum* 21(2): 249–72.

Murphy, Patricia E., Joseph W. Ciarrocchi, Ralph L. Piedmont, Sharon Cheston, Mark Peyrot, and George Fitchett. 2000. "The Relation of Religious Belief and Practices, Depression, and Hopelessness in Persons with Clinical Depression." *Journal of Consulting and Clinical Psychology* 68(6): 1102–6.

Musick, Marc. A. 1996. "Religion and Subjective Health among Black and White Elders." *Journal of Health and Social Behavior* 37(3): 221–37.

———. 2000. "Theodicy and Life Satisfaction among Black and White Americans." *Sociology of Religion* 61(3): 267–87.

Musick, Marc A., James House, and David R. Williams. 2004. "Attendance at Religious Services and Mortality in a National Sample." *Journal of Health and Social Behavior* 45(2): 198–213.

Neff, James Alan. 2006. "Exploring the Dimensionality of 'Religiosity' and 'Spirituality' in the Fetzer Multidimensional Measure." *Journal for the Scientific Study of Religion* 45(3): 449–59.

Neighbors, Harold W., Marc A. Musick, and David R. Williams. 1998. "The African American Minister as a Source of Help for Serious Personal Crises: Bridge or Barrier to Mental Health Care?" *Health Education and Behavior* 25(4): 759–77.

Nelson, Sioban. 2001. *Say Little, Do Much: Nurses, Nuns and Hospitals in the Nineteenth Century*. Philadelphia: University of Pennsylvania Press.

Nonnemaker, James, Clea A. McNeely, and Robert W. Blum. 2006. "Public and Private Domains of Religiosity and Adolescent Smoking Transitions: Evidence from the National Longitudinal Study of Adolescent Health." *Social Science and Medicine* 62(12): 3084–95.

Nooney, Jennifer, and Eric Woodrum. 2002. "Religious Coping and Church-Based Social Support as Predictors of Mental Health Outcomes: Testing a Conceptual Model." *Journal for the Scientific Study of Religion* 41(2): 359–68.

Numbers, Ronald L., and Darrel Amundsen. 1998. *Caring and Curing: Health and Medicine in the Western Religious Traditions*. Baltimore: Johns Hopkins University Press.

Numbers, Ronald L., and Ronald C. Sawyer. 1982. "Medicine and Christianity in the Modern World." In *Health/Medicine and the Faith Traditions*, ed. Martin E. Marty and Kenneth L. Vaux, 133–60. Philadelphia: Fortress Press.

Numrich, Paul David. 2005. "Complementary

and Alternative Medicine in America's 'Two Buddhisms.'" In *Religion and Healing in America*, ed. Linda Barnes and Susan S. Sered, 343–58. New York: Oxford University Press.

O'Donnell, Thomas J. 1970. "Medicine and Religion: An Overview." *Journal of the American Medical Association* 211(5): 815–17.

Orr, John, and Sherry May. 2000. *Religion and Health Services in Los Angeles: Reconfiguring the Terrain*. Los Angeles: University of Southern California Center for Religion and Civic Culture.

Pargament, Kenneth I. 1997. *The Psychology of Religion and Coping: Theory, Research, Practice*. New York: Guilford.

Pargament, Kenneth I., David S. Ensing, Kathryn Falgout, Hannah Olsen, Barbara Reilly, Kimberly van Haitsma, and Richard Warren. 1990. "God Help Me: Religious Coping Efforts as Predictors of the Outcomes to Significant Negative Life Events." *American Journal of Community Psychology* 18(6): 793–824.

Pargament, Kenneth I., Gina M. Magyar, Ethan Benore, and Annette Mahoney. 2005. "Sacrilege: A Study of Sacred Loss and Desecration and Their Implications for Health and Well-Being in a Community Sample." *Journal for the Scientific Study of Religion* 44(1): 59–78.

Pargament, Kenneth I., Bruce W. Smith, Harold G. Koenig, and Lisa Perez. 1998. "Patterns of Positive and Negative Religious Coping with Major Life Stressors." *Journal for the Scientific Study of Religion* 37(4): 710–24.

Parkum, Kurt H. 1985. "The Impact of Chaplaincy Services in Selected Hospitals in the Eastern United States." *Journal of Pastoral Care* 39(3): 262–69.

Payne, I. Reed, Allen E. Bergin, Kimberly A. Bielema, and Paul H. Jenkins. 1991. "Review of Religion and Mental Health: Prevention and Enhancement of Psychosocial Functioning." *Prevention in Human Services* 9(2): 11–40.

Pew Forum [Pew Forum for Religion and Public Life]. 2007. U.S. Religious Landscape Survey, May 8–August 13. religions.pewforum.org/. Accessed August 22, 2008.

Poindexter, Cynthia Cannon, Nathan L. Linsk, and R. Stephen Warner. 1999. "He Listens . . . and Never Gossips": Spiritual Coping without Church Support among Older, Predominantly African American Caregivers of Persons with HIV." *Review of Religious Research* 40(3): 230–43.

Pollner, Melvin. 1989. "Divine Relations, Social Relations, and Well-Being." *Journal of Health and Social Behavior* 30(1): 92–104.

Porter, Roy. 1993. "Religion and Medicine." In *Companion Encyclopedia of the History of Medicine*, ed. W. F. Bynum and Roy Porter, 1449–68. New York: Routledge.

Porterfield, Amanda. 2005. *Healing in the History of Christianity*. New York: Oxford University Press.

Powell, Lynda H., Leila Shahabi, and Carl E. Thoresen. 2003. "Religion and Spirituality: Linkages to Physical Health." *American Psychologist* 58(1): 36–52.

Prince, Thomas R. 1994. "Assessing Catholic Community Hospitals versus Nonprofit Community Hospitals, 1989–1992." *Health Care Management Review* 19(4): 25–37.

Rapp, Rayna. 1999. *Testing Women, Testing the Fetus: The Social Impact of Amniocentesis in America*. New York: Routledge.

Regnerus, Mark D., and Christian Smith. 2005. "Selection Effects in Studies of Religious Influence." *Review of Religious Research* 47(1): 23–50.

Reverby, Susan M. 1987. *Ordered to Care: The Dilemma of American Nursing, 1850–1945*. Cambridge: Cambridge University Press.

Reyes-Ortiz, Carlos A., Ivonne M. Berges, Mukaila A. Raji, Harold G. Koenig, Yong-Fang Kuo, and Kyriakos S. Markides. 2008. "Church Attendance Mediates the Association between Depressive Symptoms and Cognitive Functioning among Older Mexican Americans." *Journal of Gerontology Series A: Biological and Medical Sciences* 63(5): 480–86.

Rhoads, Paul. 1967. "Medicine and Religion: A New Journal Department." *Journal of the American Medical Association* 200(2): 162.

Risse, Guenter B. 1999. *Mending Bodies, Saving Souls: A History of Hospitals*. New York: Oxford University Press.

Rodrigues, Bartholomew, Deanna Rodrigues, and D. Lynn Casey. 2000. *Spiritual Needs and Chaplaincy Services: A National Empirical Study on Chaplaincy Encounters in Health Care Settings*. Medford, Ore.: Providence Health System.

Roof, Wade C. 2003. "Religion and Spirituality: Toward an Integrated Analysis." In *Handbook of the Sociology of Religion*, ed. Michele Dillon, 137–50. Cambridge: Cambridge University Press.

Rosenberg, Charles E. 1987. *The Care of Strangers: The Rise of America's Hospital System*. New York: Basic Books.

Rosner, Fred. 2001. "Religion and Medicine." *Archives of Internal Medicine* 161(15): 1811–12.

Ruggie, Mary. 2004. *Marginal to Mainstream: Alternative Medicine in America*. New York: Cambridge University Press.

Sakurai, Michele L. 2005. "Ministry of Presence: Naming What Chaplains Do at the Bedside." Ph.D. diss., San Francisco Theological Seminary, San Anselmo, Calif.

Salsman, John M., and Charles R. Carlson. 2005.

"Religious Orientation, Mature Faith, and Psychological Distress: Elements of Positive and Negative Associations." *Journal for the Scientific Study of Religion* 44(2): 201–9.

Sarna, Jonathan D. 1987. "The Impact of Nineteenth-Century Christian Missions on American Jews." In *Jewish Apostasy in the Modern World*, ed. Todd M. Endelman, 232–54. New York: Holmes and Meier.

Schieman, Scott, Karen van Gundy, and John Taylor. 2001. "Status, Role, and Resource Explanations for Age Patterns in Psychological Distress." *Journal of Health and Social Behavior* 42(1): 80–96.

Scott, Eric L., Albert A. Agresti, and George Fitchett. 1998. "Factor Analysis of the 'Spiritual Well-Being Scale' and Its Clinical Utility with Psychiatric Inpatients." *Journal for the Scientific Study of Religion* 37(2): 314–21.

Sherkat, Darren E., and Christopher G. Ellison. 1999. "Recent Developments and Current Controversies in the Sociology of Religion." *Annual Review of Sociology* 25:363–94.

Smith, Tom W. 2002. "Religious Diversity in America: The Emergence of Muslims, Buddhists, Hindus, and Others." *Journal for the Scientific Study of Religion* 41(3): 577–85.

Solari-Twadell, Phyllis A., and Mary A. McDermott. 1999. *Parish Nursing: Promoting Whole Person Health within Faith Communities*. Thousand Oaks, Calif.: Sage.

Starr, Paul L. 1982. *The Social Transformation of American Medicine*. New York: Basic Books.

Staten, Pat. 2003. "Spiritual Assessment Required in All Settings." *Hospital Peer Review* 28(4): 55–56.

Stevens, Rosemary. 1989. *In Sickness and in Wealth: American Hospitals in the Twentieth Century*. Baltimore: Johns Hopkins University Press.

Strawbridge, William J., Richard D. Cohen, Sarah J. Shema, and George A. Kaplan. 1997. "Frequent Attendance at Religious Services and Mortality over 28 Years." *American Journal of Public Health* 87(6): 957–61.

Svetkey, Laura P., Linda K. George, Bruce M. Burchett, Perri A. Morgan, and Dan G. Blazer. 1993. "Black/White Differences in Hypertension in the Elderly: An Epidemiologic Analysis in Central North Carolina." *American Journal of Epidemiology* 137(1): 64–73.

Taylor, Robert J., Christopher G. Ellison, Linda M. Chatters, Jeffrey S. Levin, and Karen D. Lincoln. 2000. "Mental Health Services in Faith Communities: The Role of Clergy in Black Churches." *Social Work* 45(1): 73–87.

Thiel, Mary M., and Mary R. Robinson. 1997. "Physicians' Collaborations with Chaplains: Difficulties and Benefits." *Journal of Clinical Ethics* 8(1): 94–103.

Thomas, Stephen, Sandra Quinn, Andrew Billingsley, and Cleopatra Caldwell. 1994. "The Characteristics of Northern Black Churches with Community Health Outreach Programs." *American Journal of Public Health* 84(4): 575–79.

Thune-Boyle, Ingela C., Jan A. Stygall, Mohammed R. Keshtgar, and Stanton P. Newman. 2006. "Do Religious/Spiritual Coping Strategies Affect Illness Adjustment in Patients with Cancer? A Systematic Review of the Literature." *Social Science and Medicine* 63(1): 151–64.

Troyer, Henry. 1988. "Review of Cancer among Four Religious Sects: Evidence That Lifestyles Are Distinctive Sets of Risk Factors." *Social Science and Medicine* 26(10): 1007–17.

Turner, Bryan S. 1987. *Medical Power and Social Knowledge*. London: Sage.

Uttley, Lois J. 2000. "How Merging Religious and Secular Hospitals Can Threaten Health Care Services." *Social Policy* 30(3): 4–13.

Vaillant, George, Janice Templeton, Monika Ardelt, and Stephanie E. Meyer. 2008. "The Natural History of Male Mental Health: Health and Religious Involvement." *Social Science and Medicine* 66(2): 221–31.

VandeCreek, Larry, and Loren Connell. 1991. "Evaluation of the Hospital Chaplain's Pastoral Care: Catholic and Protestant Differences." *Journal of Pastoral Care* 45(3): 289–95.

VandeCreek, Larry, and Marjorie A. Lyon. 1994–1995. "The General Hospital Chaplain's Ministry: Analysis of Productivity, Quality and Cost." *Caregiver Journal* 11(2): 3–10.

———. 1997. *Ministry of Hospital Chaplains: Patient Satisfaction*. New York: Haworth Pastoral Press.

Vandecreek, Larry, and Sue E. Mooney, eds. 2002. *Parish Nurses, Health Care Chaplains, and Community Clergy: Navigating the Maze of Professional Relationships*. New York: Haworth Press.

VandeCreek, Larry, Karolynn Siegel, Eileen Gorey, Sharon Brown, and Rhonda Toperzer. 2001. "How Many Chaplains Per 100 Inpatients? Benchmarks of Health Care Chaplaincy Departments." *Journal of Pastoral Care* 55(3): 289–301.

Vogel, Morris J. 1980. *The Invention of the Modern Hospital: Boston 1870–1930*. Chicago: University of Chicago Press.

Voorhees, Carolyn C., Frances A. Stillman, Robert T. Swank, Patrick J. Heagerty, David M. Levine, and Diane M. Baker. 1996. "Heart, Body, and Soul: Impact of Church-Based Smoking Cessation Interventions on Readiness to Quit." *Preventative Medicine* 25(3): 277–85.

Wachholtz, Amy B., Michelle J. Pearce, and Harold G. Koenig. 2007. "Exploring the Relationship between Spirituality, Coping, and Pain." *Journal of Behavioral Medicine* 30(4): 311–18.

Wallace, John M., Jr., and Tyrone A. Forman. 1998. "Religion's Role in Promoting Health and Reducing Risk among American Youth." *Health Education and Behavior* 25(6): 721–41.

Wallace, John M., Jr., and David R. Williams. 1997. "Religion and Adolescent Health-Compromising Behavior." In *Health Risks and Developmental Transitions during Adolescence*, ed. John Schulenberg, Jennifer L. Maggs, and Klaus Hurrelmann, 444–68. Cambridge: Cambridge University Press.

Weaver, Andrew J., and Christopher G. Ellison. 2004. "Featured CME Topic: Spirituality: 'Introduction.'" *Southern Medical Journal* 97(12): 1191–93.

Weaver, Andrew J., Amy E. Kline, Judith A. Samford, Lee Ann Lucas, David B. Larson, and Richard L. Gorsuch. 1998. "Is Religion Taboo in Psychology? A Systematic Analysis of Research on Religion in Seven Major American Psychological Association Journals: 1991–1994." *Journal of Psychology and Christianity* 17(3): 220–32.

Weaver, Andrew J., Harold G. Koenig, Kevin J. Flannelly, and Fred D. Smith. 2004. "A Review of Research on Chaplains and Community-Based Clergy in the *Journal of the American Medical Association*, *Lancet*, and the *New England Journal of Medicine*: 1998–2000." *Journal of Pastoral Care and Counseling* 58(4): 343–50.

Weaver, Andrew J., Judith A. Samford, David B. Larson, Lee Ann Lucas, Harold G. Koenig, and Patrick Vijayalakshmy. 1998. "A Systematic Review of Research on Religion in Four Major Psychiatric Journals, 1991–1995." *Journal of Nervous and Mental Disease* 186(3): 187–90.

White, Kenneth R. 2000. "Hospitals Sponsored by the Roman Catholic Church: Separate, Equal, and Distinct?" *Milbank Quarterly* 78(2): 213–39.

White, Kenneth R., and James W. Begun. 1998–1999. "How Does Catholic Sponsorship Affect Services Provided?" *Inquiry* 35(4): 398–407.

White, Kenneth R., James W. Begun, and Wenqiang Tian. 2006. "Hospital Service Offerings: Does Catholic Ownership Matter?" *Health Care Management Review* 31(2): 99–108.

White, Lerrill. 2003. "Federal Funding Preserved for CPE Programs." Association for Clinical Pastoral Education webpage. acpe.edu/AdminMedicare.html.

Wink, Paul, Michele Dillon, and Britta Larsen. 2005. "Religion as a Moderator of the Depression-Health Connection." *Research on Aging* 27(2): 197–220.

Wisnia, Saul. 2004. "Having Faith." *Paths of Progress* [Dana-Farber Cancer Institute], fall/winter, 15–19. dana-farber.org/abo/news/publications/pop/fall-winter-2004/faith.asp.

Woodberry, Robert. 1998. "When Surveys Lie and People Tell the Truth: How Surveys Oversample Church Attenders." *American Sociological Review* 63(1): 119–22.

Wuthnow, Robert, and Wendy Cadge. 2004. "Buddhists and Buddhism in the United States: The Scope of Influence." *Journal for the Scientific Study of Religion* 43(3): 361–78.

21

Health, Security, and New Biological Threats
Reconfigurations of Expertise

Stephen J. Collier, The New School

Andrew Lakoff, University of Southern California

In recent decades, a series of new biological threats has raised both technical and political questions about how to understand and manage disease risk. In this chapter we explore what role the social studies of medicine can play in analyzing these new disease risks. We focus in particular on recent critical scholarship that has examined how existing forms of biomedical and security expertise are being reconfigured in response to new threats such as emerging infectious disease and bioterrorism.[1] This work provides insight into how disease threats are being "problematized," and therefore it helps us diagnose some of the political, ethical, and technical conflicts that have arisen in response to new or newly perceived threats to health.

The chapter begins with an introduction to the issue of securing health as a problem for expert practitioners, and suggests how new disease threats cut across existing fields of expertise and authority. We then look at several domains in which new biological threats have been identified by public health experts, policy makers, and other public authorities: emerging infectious disease, bioterrorism, the life sciences, and food safety. In the third section we describe recent work in the social studies of medicine that has analyzed the new configurations of authority and expertise that have emerged in these domains. In the conclusion we reflect on the role of the critical, reflexive knowledge produced by the social studies of medicine in approaching this terrain.

Biosecurity Interventions

The World Health Organization's (WHO) annual world health report for 2007, *A Safer Future: Global Public Health Security in the 21st Century*, began by noting the success of public health measures during the twentieth century in dealing with great microbial scourges such as cholera and smallpox. But in recent decades, it continued, there had been an alarming shift in the "delicate balance between humans and microbes." A confluence of factors—demographic changes, economic development, global travel and commerce, and conflict—had "heightened the risk of disease outbreaks," ranging from new infectious diseases such as HIV/AIDS and drug-resistant tuberculosis to food-borne pathogens and bioterrorist attacks (WHO 2007, 1).

The WHO report proposed a framework, "public health security," for responding to this new landscape of threats that is striking in its attempt to bring together previously distinct technical problems and political domains. Some of the biological threats discussed in the report—particularly the use of bioweapons—have traditionally been taken up under the rubric of national security and approached by organizations concerned with national defense. Others, such as infectious disease, have generally been managed as problems of public health, whose history, though certainly not unrelated to conflict and military affairs, has been institutionally distinct (Fearnley 2008; King 2002).[2] The WHO proposal also sought to reconfigure existing approaches to ensuring health. The report emphasized a space of "global health" distinct from the predominantly national organization of both biodefense and public health. "In the globalized world of the 21st century," it argued, simply stopping disease at national borders is not adequate. Nor is it sufficient to respond to diseases after they have become established in a population. Rather, it is necessary to prepare for unknown outbreaks in advance, something that can be achieved only "if there is immediate alert and response to disease outbreaks and other incidents that could spark epidemics or spread globally and if there are national systems in place for detection and response should such events occur across international borders" (WHO 2007, 11). According to WHO, then, a functioning global health security apparatus would have to focus on preparing for catastrophic disease outbreaks anywhere in the world.

The WHO report is one among a range of recent proposals for securing collective health against new or newly recognized biological threats. Other prominent examples include the recent Pandemic and All-Hazards Preparedness Act in the United States, reports on "global biological threats" from prominent think tanks such as the RAND Corporation, new research facilities such as the National Biodefense Analysis and Countermeasures Center, and ambitious initiatives such as the Global Fund to Fight AIDS, Tuberculosis, and Malaria, and the President's Emergency Plan for AIDS Relief. These proposals build on a growing perception among diverse experts and officials—life scientists and public health officials, policy makers and security analysts—that new biological threats challenge existing ways of understanding and managing collective health and security. From the vantage point of such actors, the global scale of these threats crosses and confounds the boundaries of existing regulatory jurisdictions.

Moreover, their pathogenicity and mutability push the limits of current technical capacities to detect and treat disease. And the diverse sources of these perceived threats—biomedical laboratories, the industrial food system, global trade and travel—suggest a troubling growth of modernization risks that are produced by the very institutions meant to promote health, security, and prosperity. In response, proposals for new interventions seek to bring various actors and institutions into a common strategic framework.

An initial aim of this chapter is to map this emerging field of biosecurity interventions. As we use the term here, "biosecurity" does not refer exclusively—or even primarily—to practices and policies associated with national security, that is, to defense of the sovereign state against enemy attack. Rather, we refer to the various technical and political interventions—efforts to "secure health"—that have been formulated in response to new or newly perceived pathogenic threats. In examining these interventions, we do not focus on the character of disease threats per se, or on the social factors that exacerbate disease risk, but rather on the forms of expertise and the practices of intervention through which new disease threats are understood and managed. Thus, we describe interactions among the diverse experts and organizations that are being assembled in new initiatives to link health and security.[3] These include public health officials, policy experts, humanitarian activists, life scientists, multilateral agencies such as WHO, national health agencies such as the Centers for Disease Control (CDC), national security experts, physicians, veterinarians, and government officials. We have selected several recent case studies of settings in which biosecurity interventions are being articulated. This research indicates that expert approaches to new biological threats remain unsettled: "biosecurity" does not name a stable or clearly defined approach, but rather a number of overlapping and rapidly changing problem areas.

Domains of Biosecurity

The current concern with new biological threats has developed in at least four domains: emerging infectious disease, bioterrorism, the cutting-edge life sciences, and food safety. The first of these domains, emerging infectious disease, initially drew the attention of public health experts in the late 1980s in response to the AIDS crisis, the appearance of drug-resistant strains of tuberculosis and malaria, and outbreaks of new diseases such as Ebola virus (King 2002). Alarm about these disease threats emanated from various quarters, including scientific reports by prominent organizations such as the Institute of Medicine (1992), the reporting of science journalists such as Laurie Garrett (1994), and the scenarios of novelists such as Richard Preston (1997). For many observers, the emerging disease threat—particularly when combined with weakening public health systems—marked a troubling reversal in the history of public health. At just the moment when it seemed that infectious disease was about to be conquered, and that the critical health problems of the industrialized world now involved chronic disease and diseases of lifestyle, experts warned that we were witnessing a return of the microbe (Anderson 2004). This judgment seemed to be confirmed in ensuing years by the appearance of new diseases such as West Nile virus and SARS (severe acute respiratory syndrome), by the intensification of the global AIDS crisis, and by the unexpected resurgence of diseases such as tuberculosis and malaria. After considerable delay, we have recently seen the implementation of large-scale responses to these new infectious disease threats by governmental, multilateral, and philanthropic organizations.

A second domain in which biological threats have received renewed attention is in response to the prospect of bioterrorism. In the wake of the Cold War, U.S. national security officials began to focus on bioterrorism as one of a number of asymmetric threats. These officials hypothesized an association between rogue states, global terrorist organizations, and the proliferation of weapons of mass destruction (Alibek and Handelman 1999; Guillemin 2005; Miller, Engelberg, and Broad 2001). Revelations during the 1990s about Soviet and Iraqi bioweapons programs, along with the Aum Shinrikyo subway attack in 1995, lent a sense of credibility to calls for biodefense measures focused on bioterrorism. Early advocates of such efforts, including infectious disease experts

such as D. A. Henderson and national security officials such as Richard Clarke, argued that adequate preparation for a biological attack would require a massive infusion of resources into both biomedical research and public health response capacity.[4] More broadly, they claimed, it would be necessary to incorporate the agencies and institutions of the life sciences and public health into the national security establishment. The anthrax letters of 2001 intensified this demand for new biosecurity initiatives. The eventual success of the campaign is reflected in the exponential increase in total U.S. government spending on civilian biodefense research between 2001 and 2005, from $294.8 million to $7.6 billion.[5]

Third, developments in the cutting-edge life sciences have generated new concerns about the proliferation of technical capacities to create lethal organisms, for example, in fields like synthetic biology that promise dramatic advances in techniques of genetic manipulation (Garfinkel et al. 2007). Security experts along with some life scientists worry that existing biosafety protocols, which focus on material controls in laboratories, will not be sufficient to prevent intentional misuse as techniques of genetic manipulation become more powerful and routine, and as expertise in molecular biology becomes increasingly widespread. As a result, a number of new biosafety regulations have been imposed on research dealing with potentially dangerous pathogens. Meanwhile, intensive discussions about how to regulate the production of knowledge are underway among policy planners, life scientists, and security officials; and lawmakers have put in place new oversight mechanisms such as the National Science Advisory Board for Biosecurity.

Fourth, and with more pronounced effects in Europe than in the United States, a series of food safety crises has sparked anxieties about agricultural biosecurity and the contamination of the food supply. In Europe, outbreaks of BSE (bovine spongiform encephalopathy, known also as mad cow disease) and foot-and-mouth disease in the 1990s drew attention to the side effects of industrial meat production. In the wake of these outbreaks, controversies raged both about the failures of the regulatory system in detecting new pathogens and about the mass culling measures that were mobilized in response. Also in Europe, environmental activists put the problem of regulating genetically modified organisms at the top of the political agenda. In the United States, meanwhile, public outcry over food safety has been provoked by outbreaks of *E. coli* and by the presence of sick animals in the food supply, which led in early 2008 to the largest beef recall in the history of the meat industry.

In each of these domains, a series of events has turned the attention of policy makers, health experts, civic groups, and the media to new biological threats. At one level, these may usefully be seen as "focusing events" in Thomas Birkland's (1998) sense: they have raised public awareness of threats to health, and catalyzed action on the part of governments and other actors. However, it is important to underscore that the meaning of such focusing events is not self-evident; indeed, these events are characterized by substantial ambiguity. In all of them, we find that health experts, policy advocates, and politicians have competing visions about how to characterize the problem of biosecurity and about what constitute the most appropriate responses. Thus, we should ask of these events: what *kind* of biosecurity problem are they seen to pose, what techniques are used to assess the problem, and how are diverse responses justified?

In this light, it is worth examining more closely how these new or newly perceived threats to health have been "problematized" (Foucault 1994). This mode of analysis asks how a given event or situation has been constituted as an object of thought—whether through moral reflection, scientific knowledge, or political critique.[6] Such an approach, when turned to the field of biosecurity, makes neither broad prescriptions for the improvement of health and security, nor blanket denunciations of new biosecurity interventions. Rather, it examines how policy makers, scientists, and security planners have constituted potential future events as biosecurity threats, and have responded by criticizing, redeploying, or reworking existing elements.

Recent work in the critical studies of health and security indicates some of the ways in which the field of biosecurity is being problematized today. On the one hand, these studies examine the different *normative frameworks* through which the problem of biosecurity is approached: national defense, public health, or humanitarianism, for example. On the other hand, they examine the *styles of reasoning* through which uncertain threats to health are transformed into risks that can be known and acted upon: public health practices based on cost-benefit analysis, preparedness strategies that emphasize the mitigation of vulnerabilities, or precautionary approaches that seek to minimize catastrophic risk.[7] And these studies indicate how, in fields such as public health and biomedical research, expert frameworks are being reconfigured in relation to new problems of health and security. As we will see, tensions and conflicts over normative frameworks arise when existing apparatuses for managing threats to health no longer seem to work, and new ways of taking up problems are emerging.

New Intersections of Health and Security

Public Health Preparedness

We first turn to research on the encounter of traditional public health organizations with current demands for preparedness against catastrophic threats. At this conjuncture of different normative frameworks—"public health preparedness"—an existing set of practices, understandings, and institutions has been reconfigured as experts perceive and respond to new microbial threats.

The field of public health developed in the nineteenth century as a new way to understand and manage infectious disease (Coleman 1982; Rosen 1993).[8] In contrast to prior understandings of epidemics as unexpected and unpredictable misfortunes that beset human communities from without, early public health efforts traced disease to the immanent properties of the social field—sanitation practices, water supplies, forms of habitation and circulation—using statistical analysis of the incidence and severity of disease events across a population over time (Rabinow 1989; Rose 1999). Public health also provided an approach to evaluating responses to disease outbreaks in a population. For example, as historian George Rosen has noted, beginning in the early nineteenth century statistical techniques were used to evaluate inoculation strategies by weighing the probability of disease outbreaks against the probability of adverse effects from inoculation (Foucault 2007; Rosen 1993). Such cost-benefit analyses became the norm for assessing public health interventions. Historians of public health have documented a second key point of inflection: the bacteriological revolution of the late nineteenth century, at which point the "social" form of public health was confronted with a more technically oriented set of interventions focused on pathogen eradication (Fee and Porter 1992; Tomes 1998). The eradicationist orientation toward infectious disease reached its zenith with the global smallpox and polio campaigns of the 1960s and 1970s.

Public health institutions consolidated after World War II, but simultaneously, in parallel domains such as biodefense, experts began to recognize possible limits to the public health approach to microbial threats. Thus, Lyle Fearnley has shown that in the United States after World War II, as officials perceived existing infectious diseases to be successfully managed, biodefense experts, concerned about bioweapons attack, began to conceptualize outbreaks of infectious disease as anomalous events—that is, novel occurrences about which historical data do not exist, and about which little is known (Fearnley 2005b). And yet, well into the post–World War II period, techniques had not been established for assessing or managing such uncertain disease events. Thus, in responding to a possible swine flu epidemic in 1976, U.S. public health authorities did not have a paradigm for managing a future event whose likelihood and consequence were unknown, and therefore had a difficult time agreeing on appropriate response measures—for example, whether to undertake mass vaccination of the population (Lakoff 2008).

In recent decades, newly perceived threats to health—including bioterrorist threats such as a smallpox attack and emerging infectious diseases such as highly pathogenic avian influenza—have placed greater pressure on public health departments and national security officials to develop an approach to disease events not easily managed through the traditional tools of public health.

One prominent response to these new threats has been the articulation of preparedness practices among local public health jurisdictions in the United States—practices that have migrated from the national security and disaster management fields (Schoch-Spana 2004). In contrast to traditional public health practice, health preparedness does not draw on statistical knowledge of past events in order to design interventions. Rather, it employs imaginative techniques of enactment such as scenarios, exercises, and analytical models to simulate the occurrence of uncertain future threats.[9] The aim of such techniques is not to manage known disease but to address vulnerabilities in health infrastructure by, for example, strengthening hospital surge capacity, stockpiling drugs, exercising response plans, and vaccinating first responders. Such techniques of preparedness often do not provide a clear basis for cost-benefit analysis. Rather, they are aimed at developing the capability to respond to various types of potentially catastrophic biological events.

Calls for public health preparedness in the United States have escalated in recent years as public health institutions faced mounting concerns about, first, a possible bioterrorist attack and then, beginning in 2005, a devastating influenza pandemic. The U.S. Congress's 2006 Pandemic and All-Hazards Preparedness Act delegated a number of new health preparedness functions to local and national public health authorities. According to a group of biosecurity analysts, the legislation marked "a major milestone in improving public health and hospital preparedness for bioterrorist attacks, pandemics, and other catastrophes and for improving the development of new medical countermeasures, such as medicines and vaccines, against biosecurity threats" (Mair, Maldin, and Smith 2006). Preparedness has thus become a crucial interface between public health and national security.

But increased attention to and funding of health preparedness by no means implies consensus around a single approach. The existing institutions of public health are not easily reconciled with the new demands and norms of health preparedness, and there is considerable disagreement about the most appropriate way to achieve preparedness. One question is whether preparedness measures should focus on specific interventions against known agents such as anthrax and smallpox, or instead on generic measures that would be effective against currently unknown pathogens (Brent 2006; Fearnley 2005a). Another debate among experts surrounds the "dual use" potential of biodefense measures. Advocates of increased health preparedness argue that even in the absence of a bioterrorist attack, resources spent on strengthening public health infrastructure will be useful for managing other unexpected events, such as the outbreak of a "naturally" occurring infectious disease. However, the ideal of dual use faces many difficulties, in part because public health professionals often do not agree with security experts about which problems deserve attention, and how interventions should be implemented.[10] Such disagreements point to broader tensions provoked by the current intersection of public health and national security. Public health officials and national security experts promoting preparedness strategies often have very different ways of evaluating threats and responses. Critical studies of public health preparedness demonstrate some of the tensions that develop at this intersection.

We can take, as an example, the 2002–2003 Smallpox Vaccination Program, which has been studied by Dale Rose (2008). The Smallpox Vaccination Program, whose goal was to vaccinate up to ten million first responders, was initiated, in part, in response to the imaginative enactment of a catastrophic event. A June 2001 scenario-based exercise called "Dark Winter" convinced officials that the United States was highly vulnerable to a smallpox attack. This focus on smallpox intensified in the run-up to the second Iraq war, as Bush administration officials worried that Iraq might retaliate against a U.S. invasion with a smallpox attack in the United States. The vaccination campaign, Rose notes, was meant to "take smallpox off the table" as a threat to national security.

But here a problem arose around conflicting styles of reasoning—as well as conflicting political positions. Public health experts are trained to weigh the risks of disease against risks posed by vaccines. From this perspective, the expert committee charged with making vaccination recommendations to the CDC had trouble gauging the costs and benefits of smallpox vaccination. The likelihood of a smallpox attack was unknown, while the side effects of the vaccine could be fatal. As a consequence, the committee could not develop a recommendation for a vaccination program that was credible to the public health community. Moreover, the vaccination program faced resistance from public health workers—particularly hospital medical and nursing personnel—who were skeptical about the likelihood of a smallpox attack and who, in many cases, were reluctant to be enrolled in national security efforts. In the absence of convincing quantitative data about the program, they were unwilling to take the risks associated with vaccination. As a result of such technical and political conflicts, the vaccination program faltered.

A similar problem of normative conflict combined with political distrust has hindered federal efforts to build a nationwide health-monitoring system based on so-called syndromic surveillance, as Fearnley (2008a) has shown. Initially developed by local public health departments in response to an *E. coli* outbreak that went undetected by physicians, syndromic surveillance uses sources other than physicians' diagnostic reports—such as over-the-counter drug sales—to alert health authorities of possible disease outbreaks. In the late 1990s, national security experts began to explore the possibility of using this kind of system to detect a biological attack, given that physicians might not immediately recognize the symptoms caused by an unexpected or unknown pathogen. It soon became apparent, however, that national security officials and local public health experts had very different priorities in designing the system's algorithm—its mechanism for distinguishing normal from anomalous fluctuations in syndrome incidence. Rather than data quality and predictive value—emphasized by public health experts, who were accustomed to dealing with known, regularly occurring diseases—national security officials wanted a highly sensitive algorithm that would ensure the rapid detection of a wider range of potential disease outbreaks. Even though most of these signals of anomalous events would turn out to be insignificant, security officials believed that each must be treated as potentially catastrophic. In response, local public health experts argued that they did not have the epidemiological capacity to investigate the high number of signals that would inevitably result, and that resources needed for existing health problems would be wasted chasing after false positives. As one early developer of syndromic surveillance put it, in a trenchant critique of the contradictions inherent to the federal program: "We have 80 percent of the nation covered but we really have nothing covered" (Fearnley 2008b, 80)—since, in the absence of basic health infrastructure, even a highly sophisticated disease surveillance program would be useless.

Global Health and Emergency Response

Let us now turn to recent conjunctures of global health and emergency response. Here again, we can see the way in which new problems—such as emerging infectious disease—provoke multiple responses and tensions among experts. Contemporary articulations of global health security typically focus on globalization processes as a key source of new biological threats, claiming that the intensifying global circulation of humans, animals, and agricultural products—as well as knowledge and technologies—encourages the spread of novel and dangerous new diseases. In response to such threats, global health security advocates argue, it is necessary to rethink regulation and responsibility: given the global scale of the threat and its multiple sources, it is often unclear who has regulatory jurisdiction or responsibility for managing a given disease event. A good example of such an articulation of global health comes from an influential 2003 RAND Corporation report, *The Global Threat of New and Reemerging Infectious Disease*. The report defines emerging disease as one among a number of new threats to security that "do not stem from the actions of clearly defined individual states but from diffuse issues that transcend sovereign borders and bear directly on the effects of increasing globalization that challenge extant frameworks for thinking about national and international security" (Brower and Chalk 2003, 3).

Proposed responses to this new "global threat" have come from diverse organizations, with equally varied agendas. Multilateral agencies such as WHO are developing new preparedness-based approaches to potential outbreaks of infectious disease; humanitarian organizations such as Médecins Sans Frontières focus on the immediate problem of reducing human suffering in the context of emergencies; and philanthropic ventures such as the Gates Foundation seek to manage global health threats by developing and disseminating new biomedical interventions. Despite many differences in their approaches, these various efforts share what we might call an emergency modality of intervention (Calhoun 2004). The emergency modality does not involve long-term intervention into the social and economic determinants of disease. Rather, it emphasizes practices such as rapid medical response, standardized protocols for managing global health crises, surveillance and reporting systems, or simple technological fixes like mosquito nets or antimicrobial drugs. Such emergency-management techniques are characterized by their mobility: at least in principle, they can be deployed anywhere, regardless of the distinctive characteristics of a given setting.

There are several reasons why global health organizations are often drawn to an emergency modality. One is that when cast as acute emergencies, situations may galvanize public attention and resources in a way that long-term problems do not. Another is that—at least from the vantage of first-order actors—measures focused on mitigating potential emergencies are easier to implement than longer-term structural interventions. As Nicholas King writes, short-term, technically focused "emergency" measures have "the advantage of immensely reducing the scale of intervention, from global political economy to laboratory investigation and information management" (King 2004, 64). And as Michael Barnett notes, such measures seek to avoid the complex entanglements implied by longer-term interventions in development and public health that "are political because they aspire to restructure underlying social relations" and therefore provoke controversy that purely medical interventions do not (Barnett 2008, 137).

For these reasons, even experts who understand that developmental issues such as poverty and deteriorating health infrastructure are critical sources of global disease risk may propose narrower technical measures given the difficulty of implementing more ambitious schemes. In 1996, for example, molecular biologist Joshua Lederberg noted the connections between global inequality and threats to U.S. health security: "World health is indivisible, [and] we cannot satisfy our most parochial needs without attending to the health conditions of all the globe" (King 2004, 65). But the concrete interventions Lederberg advocated, such as networks of reference laboratories and global disease surveillance systems, were modest and, as he put it, "selfishly motivated"—that is, they were focused on protecting the United States from outbreaks rather than on addressing major problems of political and economic transformation in poorer parts of the world.

Medical anthropologist Daniel Halperin has pointed to the tendency of global health organizations to self-consciously avoid investment in basic public health infrastructures despite awareness that such investments would significantly reduce global infectious disease mortality. While billions of dollars have been earmarked to fight what are seen as disease emergencies, he notes, basic public health issues are often not of interest to major donors: "Shortages of food and basic health services like vaccinations, prenatal care and family planning contribute to large family size and high child and maternal mortality. Major donors like the President's Emergency Plan for AIDS Relief and the Global Fund to Fight AIDS, Tuberculosis and Malaria have not directly addressed such basic health issues. As the Global Fund's director acknowledged, '*We are not a global fund that funds local health*'" (Halperin 2008, emphasis added). In sum, given the temporal, political, and ethical structures of humanitarian biomedicine, issues of long-term care or endemic disease are difficult to assimilate into what Craig Calhoun (2008) calls the "emergency imaginary."

Critical studies of global health and security indicate that there are serious limitations to forms of intervention that focus only on emergency response—whether such response is based on a humanitarian imperative of sympathy for suffering strangers or on a security-based logic seeking to avert the spread of emergencies. As Calhoun has noted in an essay on the rise of "emergency" as a mode of justification for urgent global intervention, and on the limitations to such intervention: "There is a tension between responses rooted in simply providing care and responses linked to broader notions of human progress" (Calhoun 2008, 74). This tension relates to a difference in aims but also in forms of intervention: emergency response is acute, short-term, focused on alleviating what is conceived as a temporally circumscribed event; whereas "social" interventions—such as those associated with development policy—focus on transforming political-economic structures over the long term. Thus, in global health initiatives we find a contrast between possible modalities of intervention that parallels the one already described in U.S.-based biosecurity efforts: between acute emergency measures on the one hand and long-term approaches to health and welfare on the other. These approaches are based on distinct forms of technical reasoning that, in turn, suggest quite different ethical and political considerations—for instance, an attention to acute, short-term needs versus longer-term questions of development.

The emergency-management approach thus seeks to develop techniques for managing health emergencies that can work independently of political context and of socioeconomic conditions. This approach has become an increasingly central way of thinking about and intervening in global health threats. For example, Erin Koch has described the implementation of a TB-control program called DOTS (for Directly Observed Treatment, Short-Course) in post-Soviet Georgia. Part of the attraction of DOTS for nonstate funders is that it can seemingly be implemented without treating longer-term issues of social and economic development. Thus Koch quotes a doctor from a U.S.-based nongovernmental organization, who says: "[With DOTS] your TB program works under whatever conditions: in refugee camps, in prison, wherever. . . . If you do your program you can forget about the big social economic approach" (Koch 2008, 127). However, as Koch shows, the DOTS protocol for treatment of drug-resistant TB in "resource poor" settings like post-Soviet Georgia faces major hurdles. The economic situation has led to a massive deterioration of the public health infrastructure, making adherence to DOTS's strict diagnostic and treatment regimen nearly impossible. Compounding the problem in Georgia, the professional norms of Soviet-trained doctors are incommensurable with the technical practices required by DOTS: most doctors in Georgia have been trained in very different methods for managing TB and are therefore unwilling or unable to comply with the protocol's directives. The implication is not necessarily that DOTS is the wrong answer, but that it cannot be successfully implemented without attention to a broader range of questions concerning social development and health infrastructure. As a number of critics have argued, global biomedical interventions such as DOTS can work only if they are accompanied by serious efforts to create local and sustainable forms of public health assistance (Farmer 2001; Nguyen 2004).

A common problem in emergency-oriented response is that highly mobile protocols or devices are implemented without attention to what is necessary for these protocols to function in concrete settings. In his research on Médecins Sans Frontières (MSF) Peter Redfield has analyzed the impressive logistical capabilities of the organization, which enable it to rapidly respond to health emergencies around the globe. Redfield focuses on the container-sized "humanitarian kit," a ready-made device, transported in shipping containers, that has proven efficacious in acute health emergencies for immediate intervention irrespective of place. But Redfield's analysis indicates that the strengths of the humanitarian kit and of the emergency modality more generally—their independence from social and political context—become weaknesses as soon as the organization seeks to intervene in longer-term problems. He points to the challenges posed by a new MSF initiative to provide sustained treatment to patients with HIV/AIDS in Uganda: to what extent can the kit—and the ostensibly apolitical humanitarian project it is associated with—be assimilated to chronic disease? Given its traditional focus on acute intervention, MSF struggles to provide the long-term care necessary to adequately treat HIV/AIDS. Nor is the organization equipped to deal with social and economic problems that are outside the scope of biomedical intervention. As Redfield writes: "Finding jobs and forging new relationships were matters of keen interest for members of patient support groups. . . . Although sympathetic, MSF was poorly equipped

to respond to matters of poverty, unemployment and family expectations. The translation of treatment from rich to poor countries could not alter the structural imbalance between contexts in economic terms" (Redfield 2008, 164).

In their research on local responses to the threat of an avian influenza pandemic, Nick Bingham and Steve Hinchliffe describe a WHO-prescribed program of massive poultry culling in Cairo to mitigate the risk of H5N1 contagion. The program, based on an emergency-oriented protocol that was designed to be implemented automatically in the event of disease detection, is an example of the effort to develop a "standard, worldwide approach to dealing with 'out of place' biological entities" (Bingham and Hinchliffe 2008, 174). As in other standardized approaches, a lack of attention to the distinctive political and economic characteristics of the setting hinders the measures' potential effectiveness. Subsistence farmers' dependence on their poultry stocks for their livelihood, along with their lack of trust in the government, means that they are unlikely to comply with the mass culling directive: "Householders skeptical of the government's promises or level of compensation . . . successfully hid their birds, unwilling to let such valuable possessions be needlessly culled" (182). More broadly, the "contemporary project of worldwide integration and harmonization of biosecurity measures" exemplified by such mass culling programs "is fraught with risks however appealing it might sound" (191): it may fail to decrease the likelihood of a flu pandemic, while exacerbating problems of hunger and poverty. The uncertainties endemic to contemporary biosecurity threats such as avian flu point to the need to develop new ways of living with and managing the possibility of outbreaks that are more nuanced than current attempt efforts, which seek to achieve absolute security but do so at the expense of local well-being.

Health Security and Modernization Risks

The regulation of what Ulrich Beck (1992) calls "modernization risks" is another arena in which existing arrangements for managing health threats have been reconfigured. Beck argues that increasing dependence on complex systems and technical innovations for health and welfare has "systematically produced" new risks. In the domain of health, such risks are linked to modernization processes such as expanding trade, industrial food production, or advances in the life sciences. Of course, while such problems are not new, the recent intensification of these processes has created new uncertainties about the forms of expertise appropriate to understand and mitigate these risks.

The area of food safety provides an illustration. Again, to simplify a complex story: the modernization of food production over the last century through industrial agriculture and food processing has, in the richest countries, provided access to a relatively abundant and predictable supply of food. But this increase in "food security" through industrialization and rationalization has consistently generated new risks, and, in response, new efforts to manage these risks. Thus, the first wave of food industrialization in the late nineteenth century led to abuses and scandals that were addressed in the United States by Progressive Era reforms, including the founding of the Food and Drug Administration and an expansion of the responsibilities of the U.S. Department of Agriculture.

For a number of reasons, however, the food safety risks that have emerged in recent decades challenge existing regulatory apparatuses. First, the intensifying globalization of industrial food production has posed new difficulties, such as the problem of maintaining quality control over global food and drug production chains, as indicated by recent scandals over the regulation of ingredients for pet food, toothpaste, and blood thinner that are imported from China. Second, emerging pathogens such as BSE (mad cow disease) and virulent new strains of *E. coli* have cast doubt on the adequacy of existing protocols and organizations for regulating food safety.[11] Third, intervention into agricultural production at the molecular level (e.g., genetically modified soy and corn) has led to disputes about proper forms of regulation, particularly in areas where risks are unknown.

Modernization risks are often associated with disputes over the authority of expert knowledge.[12] In attempts to increase health security, such disputes are characterized by technical disagreements over how to evaluate potential threats: cost-benefit analyses versus "precautionary" approaches that emphasize worst-case scenarios, for example, or different models for assessing the risk of certain experiments in the life sciences. In the area of food safety, one well-known case concerns the regulation of genetically modified organisms (GMOs). In the 1990s the European Union sought to ban the import of GMOs, influenced by a movement toward "precautionary" regulation that argued that new technologies could be restricted even in the absence of conclusive evidence about the risks they posed. The United States, which beginning in the 1980s instituted the use of cost-benefit analysis for addressing environmental and health risks, challenged the EU's policy in the World Trade Organization, insisting that without quantitative risk assessment, the ban constituted an illegal restraint on trade.[13]

Similar questions about risk assessment have played out within national regimes of regulation. For example, Frédéric Keck (2008) has described how the outbreak of BSE in France cast doubt on existing approaches to regulating food safety. In the French regulatory system, he notes, food safety had previously been the responsibility of veterinarians, who sought to manage animal diseases according to a rationality of prevention. But the scandals around BSE triggered a reproblematization of food safety. Human mortality had to be avoided at all costs, pushing the government to favor a precautionary approach that emphasized uncertain but potentially catastrophic risks. In response to the BSE crisis, the existing authority of veterinarians was supplanted by a new French Food Safety Agency in which physicians played a leading role.

While these conflicts appear in technical disputes about methods of risk assessment, they often have much broader social and economic consequences: the politics of expertise relates to questions about the distribution of social goods—and, as Beck (1992) points out, of social "bads." Arguably, the WHO consensus that avian flu can be traced to the interaction of wild bird migration and domestic poultry has meant that measures to counteract avian flu—particularly culling techniques—have disproportionately harmed domestic growers and benefited large-scale poultry farms that international officials assume to be biosecure (Bingham and Hinchliffe 2008). An alternative hypothesis—that the spread of avian flu can be traced to the international circulation of poultry through legal or illegal trade, and to industrial poultry production and processing—has been largely ignored in international protocols to contain the disease, but would imply a very different set of measures.[14]

We also find conflicting frameworks for assessing and managing modernization risks in debates around regulation of the life sciences, particularly in light of concerns that new techniques of genetic manipulation could become instruments of bioterrorism. Debates about the regulation of the life sciences are not new. As scholars such as Susan Wright (1986) and Sheldon Krimsky (2005) have argued, current debates can be traced at least back to the 1970s, when civic and environmental groups in the United States raised questions about the social and ethical implications of scientific research at a number of levels. Biomedical scandals such as the Tuskegee Syphilis Experiment shaped an emergent field of bioethics, and the environmental movement drew attention to the risks of an accidental release of new pathogens created in laboratory environments (Jones 1989; Rothman 2003). As Wright (1986) has shown, molecular biologists managed to fend off these critiques, in part by shifting attention from the possibility of a pathogen release outside the lab to questions of laboratory safety. From this perspective, leading biologists argued, the most relevant measures were material controls in laboratories, and self-regulation by life scientists, who claimed that they were best able to judge the potential danger of experiments, thus excluding others from the assessment of risks.

More recently, however, this regime of material controls and self-regulation has been called into question. This is due in part to advances in techniques of genetic manipulation that have made it ever easier to engineer dangerous new pathogens. But it is also due to the increasing attention paid to bioterrorism, which has shifted the discussion about biosafety regulations. In the 1970s civic groups focused on whether well-meant scientific experiments could have unintended consequences. Today, by contrast, national security officials' focus is on the intentional malevolent use of scientific knowledge, a concern that has been voiced by some scientists, but that has predominantly come from the national security establishment, including think tanks such as the Center for Strategic and International Studies (CSIS).[15] From the national security perspective, advanced research in the life sciences may in the future make it possible to detect, characterize, and mitigate a bioterrorist attack. But such research may also introduce new threats. The question, for national security officials, is no longer one of material controls and self-regulation, but of regulating the production and circulation of dangerous knowledge on a global scale.

In this context, we find disputes over how to assess the threat posed by research in the life sciences. As Carlo Caduff (2008, 260) has noted, these conflicts often pit security officials, oriented to precautionary measures in the face of worst-case scenarios, against scientists, who defend norms of autonomy and free inquiry against what they perceive to be "provisional rules, vague obligations, and impossible demands [that] are systematically imposed on biomedical research in the name of national security." Underlying these explicit debates are often divergent assumptions about how scientific knowledge works, and what might make it "dangerous." Security officials tend to see scientific knowledge as easily abstracted from its context of production: once it is developed, they fear, it can be used anywhere to reproduce pathogenic organisms. But research in the social studies of science indicates that experiments considered "dangerous" may in fact depend on highly specific contexts that are difficult to reproduce (Vogel 2006, 2008).[16]

In her work on recent efforts to regulate potentially dangerous scientific knowledge, Vogel argues that most participants in discussions about such regulation assume that both the knowledge produced in advanced labs and the materials that they employ could easily be used elsewhere. As an example, she cites a report from CSIS that claims that if the results of research in the life sciences "are published openly, they become available to all—including those who may seek to use those results maliciously" (Epstein 2005). She also points to a 2004 National Academy of Sciences report, *Biotechnology Research in an Age of Terrorism* (National Research Council 2004), which argued that "it is unrealistic to think that biological technologies . . . can somehow be isolated within the borders of a few countries" (Vogel 2008, 234). But on the basis of three case studies—the Soviet anthrax program, the 2003 poliovirus synthesis, and the 2003 synthesis of phiX bacteriophage—Vogel shows that, in fact, the replication of such feats of biological engineering is extremely challenging, depending on tacit knowledge and complex research apparatuses. She proposes an alternative approach to assessing "dangerous knowledge" not in terms of isolated materials and knowledge but in terms of the sociotechnical assemblies required to make experiments actually work.

Caduff (2008) has made a similar point in his study of the recent laboratory synthesis of the 1918 flu virus at the Centers for Disease Control, which was conducted under stringent biosafety controls. Media coverage focused on the possibility that the publication of results from such experiments could arm potential bioterrorists. Caduff notes that such concerns rested on a questionable model of pathogenicity. Viral pathogenicity is a property not of a virus in isolation, but of an interaction between the virus and the host—that is, human beings. Since humans are not, with respect to the 1918 virus, a naïve population (influenza viruses of the H1N1 subtype are still circulating today), it is unlikely that a release of the virus would have the same effects as it did ninety years ago.

Toward Critical, Reflexive Knowledge

Although there is a great sense of urgency to address biosecurity problems—and while impressive resources have been mobilized to do so—there is no consensus about how to conceptualize these threats, or about what the most appropriate measures are to deal with them. This situation is recognized by some of the more reflective observers in the fields in question here. Thus, as Richard Danzig (2003) has argued in the case of bioterrorism, despite the striking increase in funding

for biodefense in the United States, there is still no "common conceptual framework" that might bring various efforts together and make it possible to assess their adequacy. Similarly, in a recent commentary on ambitious new initiatives to fight infectious disease on a global scale, Laurie Garrett (2007, 16) has noted that health leaders are just beginning to ask: "Who should lead the fight against disease? Who should pay for it? And what are the best strategies and tactics to adopt?"

There is no shortage of attempts to answer these questions. As we have seen, the intersection of public health and security is crowded with experts laying claim to authoritative knowledge about the most serious threats to health, and about the most appropriate responses to these threats. Political elites and policy experts make urgent calls to enact new biosecurity measures, whether for reasons of national security or global health, or in the name of a moral imperative to alleviate suffering. Meanwhile, technicians of various stripes, engaged in developing and implementing interventions, debate how to evaluate and improve existing measures. In analyzing the work of these first-order actors, recent work in the social studies of medicine has addressed the intersection of health and security in a different register. Such analyses do not advance claims about the urgency (or absence of urgency) of biological threats, nor do they offer direct solutions to biosecurity problems. Rather, they take these conflicting claims—and the disputatious claimants—as objects of inquiry.

A key insight of this line of research is that there are different kinds of biosecurity—that is, there are diverse ways that biosecurity can be problematized—and these different kinds of biosecurity entail not only different technical understandings of threats, but different underlying values.[17] From this vantage many of the disputes that emerge in the field are not simply matters of technical disagreement, of finding the right protocol, the right drug, or the right approach to risk assessment. Rather, these disputes revolve around questions that cannot be settled—or, indeed, even posed—by technical experts alone. One of the potential contributions of the approach we have outlined here, in this light, is to make these values—and tensions over conflicting values—

more explicit as objects of reflection (Collier and Lakoff 2008).[18]

Thus, culling programs imply a judgment about the value of human versus animal life: animals, it is assumed, can be sacrificed on a massive scale to avert deadly human disease, even if the risk of widespread outbreaks in humans is unknown (Keck 2008). Similarly, WHO protocols implicitly assume that the economic costs of culling domestic poultry in poor countries—a cost that falls disproportionately on the poor—is a "reasonable" price to pay for measures that may avert a global pandemic (Bingham and Hinchliffe 2008). But are such programs in fact reasonable, particularly when experts disagree about how effective culling will be in mitigating the risk of a pandemic? "Reasonable" will mean different things depending, in part, on the standard of rationality used in making assessments. But it will also depend on political and ethical judgments about how the costs and harms of biosecurity interventions can be justly distributed when the benefits are uncertain or highly diffused. Thus, disputes about vaccination programs are in part about technical risk assessment. But they are also disputes about the politics of risk that cannot be resolved in purely technical terms. How should known risks taken by first responders be weighed against the unknown benefits of the program for the national population in the event of a smallpox attack? How, as in the case of disease surveillance programs, should the resources of government be directed, and where does its responsibility lie? Is the primary imperative to respond through public health measures to known and regularly occurring disease? Or to take measures that may avert uncertain but catastrophic outbreaks? Such problems are most acute, perhaps, when the field of regulation is global. How to decide which measures to undertake in situations with tremendous needs, and limited resources?

These kinds of questions are crucial to address today, when responses to the problem of health and security are still taking shape. Doing so requires critical and reflexive knowledge that examines how technical efforts to increase biosecurity relate to the political and ethical challenges of what might be called "living with risk." Security—the freedom from fear or risk—always suggests an absolute demand; the demand for security has no inherent principle of limitation (Foucault 1997). There is no such thing as being too secure. Living with risk, by contrast, acknowledges a more complex calculus. It requires new forms of political and ethical reasoning that take into account questions that are often only implicit in discussions of biosecurity interventions. Making such questions explicit is one of the critical tasks ahead for researchers analyzing areas such as biosecurity, health preparedness, and the emergence of new biological threats.

Notes

We are grateful for suggestions made by Carlo Caduff, Lyle Fearnley, Paul Rabinow, Dale Rose, Anthony Stavrianakis, and Stefan Timmermans on earlier drafts of this chapter.

1. In this chapter we do not aim for a comprehensive survey of the social science research in these areas. Rather, we have selected a number of exemplary recent studies that engage with concrete settings in which debates about the intersection of health and security are taking place. This essay draws on, and extends, the analysis developed in the introduction to our edited volume *Biosecurity Interventions* (Lakoff and Collier 2008). Two important recent collections on public health and security in a global context are Bashford 2007 and Ali and Keil 2008.

2. For analyses of how early international health projects were linked to colonial administration, see Arnold 1993 and Anderson 2006.

3. For an analysis of assemblages as an object of critical social scientific inquiry, see Collier and Ong 2005 and Rabinow 2003.

4. For a detailed review of the developing concern with bioterrorism in the 1990s, see Wright 2006. As Wright argues, the very use of the term "weapons of mass destruction" to link nuclear weapons to biological weapons was a strategic act on the part of biodefense advocates. For a critical analysis of the logic of preemption in biodefense, see Cooper 2006.

5. It then declined slightly, to $5.37 billion, in 2006 (see Lam, Franco, and Schuler 2006). See Lentzos 2006 for a critical analysis of U.S. biosecurity measures.

6. For a new problematization to occur, Foucault writes, "something prior must have happened to introduce uncertainty, a loss of familiarity. That loss, that uncertainty is the result of difficulties in our previous way of understanding, acting, relating" (Foucault 1994).

7. For a discussion of "styles of reasoning" in scientific practice, see Hacking 2002.

8. For case histories of the rise of a "social" understanding of infectious disease, see Barnes 1995 and Delaporte 1986.

9. For discussions of preparedness and enactment, see Collier 2008; Collier and Lakoff 2008; Lakoff 2007.

10. See, for example, Cohen, Gould, and Sidel 1999.

11. For example, as Elizabeth Dunn writes, an outbreak of a deadly new strain of *E. coli* in the U.S. was "the product of a particular agro-industrial configuration which is highly concentrated and which produces an astronomical amount of food" (2007, 48).

12. Risk society, writes Beck (1992, 30), is characterized by "competing rationality claims, struggling for acceptance."

13. Sheila Jasanoff (2005) has argued that in these contests over the regulation of genetically modified organisms, one can see the characteristics of distinctive national "civic epistemologies." Other recent analyses have called into question the strict divide between European "precaution" and U.S. "risk assessment," and noted a significant shift in the European discussion away from precaution with the emergence of the "better regulation" agenda. See Weiner 2002 and Lofstedt 2004.

14. For a critical analysis of the migratory bird hypothesis of avian influenza transmission, see Gauthier-Clerc, Lebarbenchon, and Thomas 2007. See also Davis 2006.

15. See, for example, Garfinkel et al. 2007. For a critique, see Rabinow, Bennett, and Stavrianakis 2006.

16. For an empirical analysis of the working practices of regulators charged with overseeing biological research that poses new risks, see Lentzos 2006.

17. The line of research we have outlined here shares a concern with developing critical knowledge about contemporary biosecurity interventions. But it suggests that there is no single critical lens that would enable us to arrive at an overarching diagnosis of "biosecurity" today. In this sense, it diverges from critical studies that denounce what is claimed to be the increasing "securitization" or "militarization" of health. For basic texts on the "securitization," see Lipschutz 1995.

18. The proposition that critical analysis of technical expertise can yield insight into value orientations is a classic Weberian position (Weber 1949).

References

Ali, S. Harris, and Roger Keil, eds. 2008. *Networked Disease: Emerging Infections in the Global City.* New York: Wiley-Blackwell.

Alibek, Ken, and Stephen Handelman. 1999. *Biohazard: The Chilling True Story of the Largest Covert Biological Weapons Program in the World, Told from the Inside by the Man Who Ran It.* New York: Random House.

Anderson, Warwick. 2004. "Natural Histories of Infectious Disease: Ecological Vision in Twentieth-Century Bioscience." *Osiris* 19:39–61.

———. 2006. *Colonial Pathologies: American Tropical Medicine, Race, and Hygiene in the Philippines.* Durham, N.C.: Duke University Press.

Arnold, David. 1993. *Colonizing the Body: State Medicine and Epidemic Disease in Nineteenth-Century India.* Berkeley: University of California Press.

Barnes, David S. 1995. *The Making of a Social Disease: Tuberculosis in Nineteenth-Century France.* Berkeley: University of California Press.

Barnett, Michael. 2008. "Is Multilateralism Bad for Humanitarianism?" In *Multilateralism and Security Institutions in an Era of Globalization*, ed. Dimitris Bourantonis, Kostas Ifantis, and Panayotis Tsakonas. New York: Routledge.

Bashford, Alison, ed. 2007. *Medicine at the Border: Disease, Globalization and Security, 1850 to the Present.* Basingstoke, UK: Palgrave Macmillan.

Beck, Ulrich. 1992. *Risk Society: Towards a New Modernity.* London: Sage.

Bingham, Nick, and Steve Hinchliffe. 2008. "Mapping the Multiplicities of Biosecurity." In *Biosecurity Interventions: Global Health and Security in Question*, ed. Andrew Lakoff and Stephen J. Collier. New York: Columbia University Press.

Birkland, Thomas A. 1998. "Focusing Events, Mobilization, and Agenda Setting." *Journal of Public Policy* 18:53–74.

Brent, Roger. 2006. "In the Shadow of the Valley of Death." DSpace @ MIT. dspace.mit.edu/bitstream/handle/1721.1/34914/Valley2006.pdf?sequence=1. Accessed February 2008.

Brower, Jennifer, and Peter Chalk. 2003. *The Global Threat of New and Reemerging Infectious Diseases: Reconciling U.S. National Security and Public Health Policy.* Santa Monica, Calif.: RAND.

Caduff, Carlo. 2008. "Anticipations of Biosecurity." In *Biosecurity Interventions: Global Health and Security in Question*, ed. Andrew Lakoff and Stephen J. Collier. New York: Columbia University Press.

Calhoun, Craig. 2004. "A World of Emergencies: Fear, Intervention, and the Limits of Cosmopolitan Order." *Canadian Review of Sociology and Anthropology* 41(4): 373–95.

———. 2008. "The Imperative to Reduce Suffering: Charity, Progress, and Emergencies in the Field of Humanitarian Action." In *Humanitarianism in Question: Power, Politics, Ethics*, ed. Michael

Barnett and Thomas G. Weiss. Ithaca, N.Y.: Cornell University Press.

Cohen, H. W., R. M. Gould, and V. W. Sidel. 1999. "Bioterrorism Initiatives: Public Health in Reverse?" *American Journal of Public Health* 89:1629–31.

Coleman, William. 1982. *Death Is a Social Disease: Public Health and Political Economy in Early Industrial France.* Madison: University of Wisconsin Press.

Collier, Stephen J. 2008. "Enacting Catastrophe: Preparedness, Insurance, Budgetary Rationalization." *Economy and Society* 37:224–50.

Collier, Stephen J., and Andrew Lakoff. 2008. "Distributed Preparedness: Space, Security and Citizenship in the United States." *Environment and Planning D: Society and Space* 26:7–28.

Collier, Stephen J., and Aihwa Ong. 2005. "Global Assemblages, Anthropological Problems." In *Global Assemblages: Technology, Politics, and Ethics as Anthropological Problems*, ed. Aihwa Ong and Stephen J. Collier. Malden, Mass.: Blackwell.

Cooper, Melinda. 2006. "Pre-empting Emergence: The Biological Turn in the War on Terror." *Theory, Culture and Society* 23:113–35.

Danzig, Richard. 2003. *Catastrophic Bioterrorism: What Is to Be Done?* Washington, D.C.: Center for Technology and National Security Policy, National Defense University.

Davis, Mike. 2006. *The Monster at Our Door: The Global Threat of Avian Flu.* New York: Henry Holt.

Delaporte, François. 1986. *Disease and Civilization: The Cholera in Paris, 1832.* Cambridge, Mass.: MIT Press.

Dunn, Elizabeth. 2007. "*Escherichia coli*, Corporate Discipline and the Failure of the Sewer State." *Space and Polity* 11:35–53.

Epstein, Gerald L. 2005. "Security Controls on Scientific Information and the Conduct of Scientific Research." White paper of the Commission on Scientific Communication and National Security, Center for Strategic and International Studies. csis.org/publication/security-controls-scientific -information-and-conduct-scientific-research.

Farmer, Paul. 2001. *Infections and Inequalities: The Modern Plagues.* Berkeley: University of California Press.

Fearnley, L. 2008a. "Signals Come and Go: Syndromic Surveillance and Styles of Biosecurity." *Environment and Planning A* 40:1615–32.

———. 2008b. "Redesigning Syndromic Surveillance for Biosecurity." In *Biosecurity Interventions: Global Health and Security in Question*, ed. Andrew Lakoff and Stephen J. Collier. New York: Columbia University Press.

———. 2005a. "'From Chaos to Controlled Disorder': Syndromic Surveillance, Bioweapons, and the Pathological Future." Anthropology of the Contemporary Research Collaboratory. anthropos-lab.net/wp/publications/2007/08/workingpaperno5 .pdf.

———. 2005b. "Pathogens and the Strategy of Preparedness: Disease Surveillance in Civil Defense Planning." Anthropology of the Contemporary Research Collaboratory. anthropos-lab.net/wp/ publications/2007/01/fearn_pathogens.pdf.

Fee, Elizabeth, and Dorothy Porter. 1992. "Public Health, Preventative Medicine, and Professionalization." In *Medicine and Society: Historical Essays*, ed. Andrew Wear. Cambridge: Cambridge University Press.

Foucault, Michel. 1994. *Dits et Écrits, 1954–1988.* Paris: Gallimard.

———. 1997. "The Risks of Security." In *The Essential Works of Michel Foucault, 1954–1984*, vol. 3, ed. Paul Rabinow. New York: New Press.

———. 2007. *Security, Territory, Population: Lectures at the Collège de France, 1977–78.* New York: Palgrave Macmillan.

Garfinkel, Michele S., Drew Endy, Gerald L. Epstein, and Robert M. Friedman. 2007. "Synthetic Genomics: Options for Governance." *Industrial Biotechnology* 3:333–65.

Garrett, Laurie. 1994. *The Coming Plague: Newly Emerging Diseases in a World out of Balance.* New York: Farrar, Straus and Giroux.

———. 2007. "The Challenge of Global Health." *Foreign Affairs*, January/February, 14–38.

Gauthier-Clerc, M., C. Lebarbenchon, and F. Thomas. 2007. "Recent Expansion of Highly Pathogenic Avian Influenza H5N1: A Critical Review." *Ibis* 149:202–14.

Guillemin, Jeanne. 2005. *Biological Weapons from the Invention of State-Sponsored Programs to Contemporary Bioterrorism.* New York: Columbia University Press.

Hacking, Ian. 2002. *Historical Ontology.* Cambridge, Mass.: Harvard University Press.

Halperin, Daniel. 2008. "Putting a Plague in Perspective." *New York Times*, January 1.

Institute of Medicine. 1992. *Emerging Infections: Microbial Threats to Health in the United States.* Washington, D.C.: National Academy Press.

Jasanoff, Sheila. 2005. *Designs on Nature: Science and Democracy in Europe and the United States.* Princeton, N.J.: Princeton University Press.

Jones, James. 1989. "The Tuskegee Syphilis Experiment." In *Perspectives in Medical Sociology*, ed. Phil Brown. Belmont, Calif.: Wadsworth.

Keck, Frédéric. 2008. "From Mad Cow Disease to Bird Flu: Transformations of Food Safety in France." In

Biosecurity Interventions: Global Health and Security in Question, ed. Andrew Lakoff and Stephen J. Collier. New York: Columbia University Press.

King, Nicholas B. 2002. "Security, Disease, Commerce: Ideologies of Postcolonial Global Health." *Social Studies of Science* 32:763–89.

———. 2004. "The Scale Politics of Emerging Diseases." *Osiris* 19:62–76.

Koch, Erin. 2008. "Disease as Security Threat: Critical Reflection on the Global TB Emergency." In *Biosecurity Interventions: Global Health and Security in Question*, ed. Andrew Lakoff and Stephen J. Collier. New York: Columbia University Press.

Krimsky, Sheldon. 2005. "From Asilomar to Industrial Biotechnology: Risks, Reductionism and Regulation." *Science as Culture* 14:309–23.

Lakoff, Andrew. 2007. "Preparing for the Next Emergency." *Public Culture* 19 (2): 247–71.

———. 2008. "The Generic Biothreat, or How We Became Unprepared." *Cultural Anthropology* 23(3): 399–428.

Lakoff, Andrew, and Stephen J. Collier. 2008. *Biosecurity Interventions: Global Health and Security in Question.* New York: Columbia University Press.

Lam, Clarence, Crystal Franco, and Ari Schuler. 2006. "Billions for Biodefense: Federal Agency Biodefense Funding, FY2006-FY2007." *Biosecurity and Bioterrorism: Biodefense Strategy, Practice, and Science* 4:113–27.

Lederberg, J. 1996. "Infection Emergent." *Journal of the American Medical Association* 275:243–45.

Lentzos, Filippa. 2006. "Rationality, Risk and Response: A Research Agenda for Biosecurity." *BioSocieties* 1:453–64.

Lipschutz, Ronnie D. 1995. *On Security.* New York: Columbia University Press.

Lofstedt, Ragnar E. 2004. "The Swing of the Regulatory Pendulum in Europe: From Precautionary Principle to (Regulatory) Impact Analysis." Working Paper No. 04–07. AEI-Brookings Joint Center for Regulatory Studies. papers.ssrn.com/sol3/papers .cfm?abstract_id=519563.

Mair, Michael, Beth Maldin, and Brad Smith. 2006. "Passage of S. 3678: The Pandemic and All-Hazards Preparedness Act." Baltimore: University of Pittsburgh Medical Center, Center for Biosecurity.

Miller, Judith, Stephen Engelberg, and William J. Broad. 2001. *Germs: Biological Weapons and America's Secret War.* New York: Simon and Schuster.

National Research Council. 2004. *Biotechnology Research in an Age of Terrorism.* Washington, D.C.: National Academies Press.

Nguyen, Vinh-Kim. 2004. "Emerging Infectious Disease." In *Encyclopedia of Medical Anthropology: Health and Illness in the World's Cultures*, ed. Carol R. Ember and Melvin Ember. New York: Kluwer Academic.

Preston, Richard. 1997. *The Cobra Event: A Novel.* New York: Random House.

Rabinow, Paul. 1989. *French Modern: Norms and Forms of the Social Environment.* Cambridge, Mass.: MIT Press.

———. 2003. *Anthropos Today: Reflections on Modern Equipment.* Princeton, N.J.: Princeton University Press.

Rabinow, Paul, Gaymon Bennett, and Anthony Stavrianakis. 2006. "Response to 'Synthetic Genomics: Options for Governance.'" In *ARC Concept Note.* Berkeley, Calif.: Anthropology of the Contemporary Research Collaboratory.

Redfield, Peter. 2008. "Vital Mobility and the Humanitarian Kit." In *Biosecurity Interventions: Global Health and Security in Question*, ed. Andrew Lakoff and Stephen J. Collier. New York: Columbia University Press.

Rose, Dale. 2008. "How Did the Smallpox Vaccination Program Come About? Tracing the Emergence of Recent Smallpox Vaccination Thinking." In *Biosecurity Interventions: Global Health and Security in Question*, ed. Andrew Lakoff and Stephen J. Collier. New York: Columbia University Press.

Rose, Nikolas S. 1999. *Powers of Freedom: Reframing Political Thought.* Cambridge: Cambridge University Press.

Rosen, George. 1993. *A History of Public Health.* Baltimore: Johns Hopkins University Press.

Rothman, David J. 2003. *Strangers at the Bedside: A History of How Law and Bioethics Transformed Medical Decision Making.* New York: Aldine de Gruyter.

Schoch-Spana, Monica. 2004. "Bioterrorism: U.S. Public Health and Secular Apocalypse." *Anthropology Today* 20:1–6.

Tomes, Nancy. 1998. *The Gospel of Germs: Men, Women, and the Microbe in American Life.* Cambridge, Mass.: Harvard University Press.

Vogel, Kathleen. 2006. "Bioweapons Proliferation: Where Science Studies and Public Policy Collide." *Social Studies of Science* 36:659–90.

———. 2008. "Biodefense: Considering the Sociotechnical Dimension." In *Biosecurity Interventions: Global Health and Security in Question*, ed. Andrew Lakoff and Stephen J. Collier. New York: Columbia University Press.

Weber, Max. 1949. *The Methodology of the Social Sciences.* Glencoe, Ill.: Free Press.

Weiner, Jonathan B. 2002. "Precaution in a Multirisk World." In *Human and Ecological Risk Assessment: Theory and Practice*, ed. Dennis Paustenbach, 1509–31. New York: John Wiley and Sons.

WHO [World Health Organization]. 2007. *The World Health Report 2007: A Safer Future; Global Public Health Security in the 21st Century*. Geneva: WHO.

Wright, Susan. 1986. "Molecular Biology or Molecular Politics? The Production of Scientific Consensus on the Hazards of Recombinant DNA Technology." *Social Studies of Science* 16:593–620.

———. 2006. "Terrorists and Biological Weapons." *Politics and the Life Sciences* 25:57–115.

22

Health Social Movements
History, Current Work, and Future Directions

Phil Brown, Brown University

Crystal Adams, Brown University

Rachel Morello-Frosch, University of California–Berkeley

Laura Senier, University of Wisconsin–Madison

Ruth Simpson, Bryn Mawr College

The last several decades have seen a burgeoning movement in health activism in which patients, consumers, and other lay people, sometimes in conjunction with scientists and health-care professionals, have lobbied for a more active role in defining and finding solutions for health concerns. In the 1960s the women's health movement began challenging prevailing conceptions of medical authority, feminine sexuality, and reproductive rights, with consequent changes in medical research, practice, and standards. In the 1970s and 1980s mental health activists advocated for patients' rights, while AIDS activists fought to expand the funding and scope of research and treatment, as well as the role of patient-activists in research decisions. More recent health social movements have taken on issues such as medical service cutbacks, insurance restrictions, discrimination against the disabled, and, through the environmental justice movement, the unequal distribution of exposure to environmental hazards. This recent activism is noteworthy in part for the emergence of citizen-science alliances in which citizens and scientists collaborate on issues that

usually have been identified by laypeople. These movements have in turn spawned an increase in scholarly activity related to health activism. Over the past decade several thematic conferences and an increasing number of articles and special issues of scholarly journals have focused attention on health social movements: special streams at the 2001 and 2003 conferences of the Society for the Social Study of Science, a workshop at the American Sociological Association's Collective Behavior and Social Movements Section Conference in 2002, a Medical Social Movements symposium in Sweden in 2003 that led to a *Social Science and Medicine* special issue on patient-based social movements in 2006, a special issue of *Annals of the American Academy of Political and Social Science* on health and the environment in 2002 (edited by Phil Brown), the *Sociology of Health and Illness* 2004 annual monograph on health social movements (later a book edited by Phil Brown and Stephen Zavestoski), and a conference on social movements and health institutions at the University of Michigan in 2007 from which a volume will shortly be published.

In their campaigns, health activists routinely address the same issues that have long concerned medical sociologists. For example, in challenging traditional roles and systems of knowledge, members of health social movements are highly attuned to how the authority of experts and social institutions—such as medical professionals, health-care organizations, and government agencies—affects the health-care process. Like sociologists of health and illness, many activists seek to understand how health problems are socially constructed, so they can better grasp the trajectories of the illness experience and can improve conditions for patients. Campaigns for health and social justice focus attention on the social determinants of health and disease and criticize systematic injustices or patterns of inequality that negatively affect health and quality of life. Health social movements and the scholarly work that focuses on them thus cut across many of the core theoretical concerns of medical sociology, such as medicalization, stratification, authority, and empowerment.

But despite the concerns that health social movements share with medical sociologists, and despite the existence of a well-developed scholarly literature about the health social movements themselves, medical sociology has traditionally not incorporated the conceptual or methodological lessons of health activism and the health social movement literature. This is surprising, given that the public health literature has actively engaged in studies of health activism, especially in terms of community-based participatory research, where community groups and individuals are involved from the beginning of a research question through the entire process of research, dissemination, and policy application. There are a number of possible reasons for this apparent disconnect between health social movements and medical sociology. Conceivably, the traditional exclusion from medical sociology of the physiological and biological dimensions of disease (Timmermans and Haas 2008) has discouraged exploration of health social movements, where patients' accounts of symptoms and their contesting of medical definitions of disease play such central roles. Perhaps the current lack of attention to health social movements owes something to the early divide

described by Straus (1957) as the "the sociology *of* medicine" versus "sociology *in* medicine," a gulf that has narrowed but not disappeared (Bird, Conrad, and Fremont 2000). The degree to which health social movement researchers work closely with activists and their goals may seem to threaten the independent critical perspective valued by those who identify as sociologists *of* medicine. Similarly, sociologists *in* medicine, already on the defensive for their collaborative work with health-care professionals and institutions, may be reluctant to add health activists to that list. Of course, the reasons for the separate lives of health social movements and medical sociology may be more mundane: the realities of academic specialization and associated professional pressures impede mutual awareness across any number of scholarly disciplines and subfields. In that sense, the disconnect between medical sociology and the health social movement literature may simply result from want of routine contact—a situation we seek to change with this chapter.

Medical sociologists may often be unaware of the importance of health social movements for the sociological analysis of health and illness and associated actors and institutions. Yet studies of health social movements—particularly citizen-science alliances and other forms of community-based participatory research—have much to offer medical sociology conceptually and methodologically. First, health social movement research directs attention to a range of actors and institutions outside the traditional focus of medical sociology that nonetheless contribute to how diseases are perceived and addressed. Second, the literature on health social movements helps illuminate the development of patient identity—a process closely linked to health social movements that has profound consequences for the ways patients will interact with the medical system. Third, the existence of citizen-science alliances in health social movements and the use of community-based participatory research in the health social movement literature affords an opportunity to bridge (or avoid) some of the divides within medical sociology and sociology as a whole, such as the gap between theory and practice. Finally, because health social movements represent actors actively engaged in questioning, challenging, and exploring the existence and causes of disease, studying health social movements offers the opportunity to engage in vibrant, cutting-edge research.

In this chapter, after a brief introduction to health social movements, we explain in detail how attention to health social movements and the health social movement literature would enhance the ways medical sociologists approach their own theoretical, methodological, and practical- and policy-related challenges. Finally, we discuss the applications of health social movement research for medical sociology and illustrate its utility through a case study.

A Historical and Conceptual Outline of Health Social Movements

Drawing on Della Porta and Diani's definition of social movements (1998), we define health social movements as informal networks comprised of an array of formal and informal organizations, supporters, networks of cooperation, and media that mobilize specifically in response to issues of health-care policy and politics, medical research and practice, and medical and scientific belief systems. In doing so, health social movements challenge political power, professional authority, and personal and collective identity (Zavestoski et al. 2002; McCormick, Brown, and Zavestoski 2003).

Organized activism around health issues dates back to the Industrial Revolution, when activists within the settlement house movement crusaded against urban poverty and industrial hygienists sought to improve health and safety conditions for workers (Waitzkin 2000). Women led much of that early organizing and were leaders as well in the 1960s when women's health activists' challenge to medical authority significantly altered medical conceptions of feminine behavior and sexuality, broadened reproductive rights, expanded funding and services, influenced standards of care, and changed medical research and practice (Ruzek 1978; Ruzek, Olesen, and Clarke 1997; Morgen 2002). Beginning in the 1980s, AIDS activists fought for expanded funding for research and treatment, increased appreciation for and integration of alternative treatment approaches, and won major victories in the design

and execution of clinical trials (including the right of patient-activists to participate in decisions about allocation of research dollars and discussions about research design [see Epstein 1996]). Self-care and alternative care activists have broadened health professionals' awareness of people's ability to deal with health problems in ways not necessarily sanctioned by allopathic medicine (Goldstein 1999). Mental patients' rights activists obtained major reforms in mental health care, demanding recognition of basic human and civil rights of mental patients and their right to better treatment and to refuse treatment (Brown 1984). Occupational health and safety movements have brought medical and governmental attention to a wide range of ergonomic, radiation, chemical, and stress hazards in workplaces, leading to extensive regulation and the creation of the Occupational Safety and Health Administration and National Institute of Occupational Safety and Health (Rosner and Markowitz 1987).

More recently, health social movements have broadened their focus from patient rights and standards of medical care to health access and social justice inequalities, targeting health-care organizations and governmental agencies in the process. Citizens have fought against hospital closings, medical service cutbacks, and restrictions by insurers (Waitzkin 2001). Disability rights activists have won major advances in areas such as accessibility and job discrimination, and countered stigmas against people with disabilities (Shapiro 1993). Toxic waste activists have brought national attention to the health risks of chemicals, radiation, air pollution, and other hazards, helping obtain regulations and bans on toxics, and remediate many hazardous sites (Brown and Mikkelsen 1990; Brown 2007). Environmental justice activists have expanded on toxic waste activism by demonstrating the class and race inequalities of environmental burdens (Bullard 2000). Their early focus on the siting of hazardous waste facilities has expanded to show how low-income communities and communities of color also suffer from a lack of environmental amenities such as parks and open spaces (Agyeman 2005).

While many participants in health social movements have been lay people, health professionals have also formed advocacy groups around health issues. Physicians, for example, have organized to advance health care for the underserved, to seek a national health plan, and to oppose the nuclear arms race (McCally 2002).

Health Social Movements: A Typology

We can usefully categorize health social movements (HSMs) into three types according to their dominant goals (Brown et al. 2004).[1] Health access movements seek equitable access to health care and improved provision of health-care services. These include movements such as those seeking national health-care reform, increased ability to pick specialists, and coverage of the uninsured. Constituency-based health movements, such as the women's health movement, gay and lesbian health movement, and environmental justice movement, concentrate on health inequalities rooted in race, ethnicity, gender, class, sexuality, or a combination of these. They address unequal health outcomes, unequal oversight by the scientific community, and scientific findings that are weak or tainted by conflicts of interest. Embodied health movements address disease, disability, or the experience of illness by challenging accepted scientific and medical perspectives on etiology, diagnosis, treatment, and prevention. Embodied health movements often mobilize around "contested illnesses" (Brown 2007) that are either unexplained (or even unacknowledged) by current medical science or whose purported cause is disputed (such causes are often, but by no means always, environmental). Contested illnesses require activists to organize to achieve medical recognition, treatment, and research. Embodied health movements include the breast cancer movement, the AIDS movement, and the tobacco control movement. Some established embodied health movements, such as breast cancer activism, include constituents who are not ill, but who consider themselves at risk of disease. Regardless, embodied health movements make the biological body central to social movements, primarily in terms of the embodied experience of disease-affected people, as in the disability rights movement (Fleischer and Zames

2002), and women's health movements (Morgen 2002). While the examples we include in this chapter focus on controversies in environmental health, many HSMs address nonenvironmental issues. The broader breast cancer movement, for example, works to guarantee women access to treatment and patient involvement in treatment and research. In the realm of infectious disease, Lyme disease sufferers faced challenges in getting their illness recognized and addressed by the medical establishment (Weintraub 2008).

Our interest in embodied health movements developed during a period of conflict among schools of thought within the social movements field. Our focus on embodied health movements allowed us to draw from these schools of thought rather than become enmeshed in the conflict itself. Like resource mobilization theory (e.g., Jenkins 1983; McCarthy and Zald 1977), our conceptualization of embodied health movements emphasizes the importance of the development of social movement organizations, although we reject resource mobilization theory's emphasis on rational action, as it would downplay the importance of grievance in the formation of embodied health movements. We draw on the political opportunity approach (McAdam 1982; McAdam, McCarthy, and Zald 1996; Tilly 1978) to emphasize how changing political circumstances and alliances can affect the ability of an embodied health movement to gain attention and recognition, although we extend our focus to include arenas other than state and political bodies, such as science, medicine, and the individual illness experience. The frame alignment perspective (e.g., Benford and Snow 2000; Snow et al. 1986) has been useful for understanding how those involved in embodied health movements emphasize solutions and agendas that will resonate with the personal experiences, values, and expectations of potential supporters, although such frame alignment strategies are initially viable only among illness sufferers or those closely allied with them. Finally, we share with new social movement theory the goal of understanding social movements that are not well explained by traditional models, although we have found that its dismissal of the significance of social class in postindustrial societies (Fitzgerald and Rodgers 2000) does not ring true for many embodied health movements where unequal access to housing, transportation, and economic development are tightly connected to the understanding and experience of illness (Brown et al. 2003, Morello-Frosch et al. 2006).

Citizen-Science Alliances

Embodied health movements often involve citizen-science alliances in which activists collaborate with scientists and health professionals in pursuing treatment, prevention, research, and expanded funding. Citizen-science alliances represent the willingness of citizens and scientists to go beyond an us-versus-them paradigm in order to develop innovative organizational forms that can effectively address the social determinants of health. Citizens bring insights from their personal illness experience and scientists contribute their technical skills and knowledge. These alliances contribute to new knowledge, and they also challenge—and sometimes change—scientific norms by valuing the experience and knowledge of illness sufferers. Citizen-science alliances may be citizen initiated, professionally initiated, or created through a joint affinity model in which lay and researcher interests are aligned.

Examples of citizen-science alliances include AIDS activists who have sought a place at the scientific table so that their personal illness experiences can help shape research design (Epstein 1996). Breast cancer activists have been involved in federal and state review panels, as well as in democratizing foundations' funding processes (Brown et al. 2006). Asthma activists have cooperated with scientists in projects linking air pollution to respiratory illnesses in urban neighborhoods that house bus depots and transit hubs (Shepard et al. 2002). Citizen-science alliances have also been important in the environmental breast cancer, environmental justice, and environmental health movements, which are concerned with the role of chemical and industrial exposures in human health. Participants in these movements have become involved in a new form of activism that helps generate new evidence of the omnipresent chemical assault by petrochemicals, plastics, and other industrial sectors.

Community-based participatory research (CBPR) programs are the most far-reaching example of citizen-science alliances. In CBPR programs, members of an affected community engage in the research process alongside scientists, social scientists, medical professionals, and other researchers. Drawing on their own experiences as members of the affected community, they participate in the definition of research questions and design, assist in carrying out the study, help disseminate information back to the community and the broader public, and actively help shape resulting policies. CBPR is thus inclusive of all affected parties and all potential end-users of the research, including community-based organizations, public health practitioners, and local health and social services agencies (Shepard et al. 2002; Israel et al. 1998). More comprehensive citizen involvement in research often occurs as a social problem becomes more public and the accompanying social movement gains strength and momentum.

CBPR and citizen-science alliances can expose tensions associated with merging sociological scholarship with research connected to specific policy goals. This linking of sociological research and policy action understandably raises concerns about the researcher's ability to maintain objectivity and a critical perspective on the social phenomena under study. While such tensions exist, it is possible to manage them through more intensive dialogue with community participants about research methods and by an increased focus on research methods to improve the rigor and integrity of the overall study design. As a mode of knowledge production, CBPR broadens the research process by ensuring that stakeholders have access to the process and results of knowledge production. Researchers who work on CBPR projects and in citizen-science alliances must find ways to negotiate the tensions that arise in working with multiple stakeholders. Later in this chapter, we describe some specific challenges that have arisen in designing research that meets rigorous scientific standards while also addressing the needs and concerns of community stakeholders. Ultimately, CBPR advances the public good by producing scientifically rigorous research that also has significant policy applications.

Policy Ethnography

In our research, we have come to rely on policy ethnography (Brown et al., 2010), a form of extended, multisited ethnography that studies social movements by including organizational and policy analysis alongside ethnographic observations and interviews, and that operates with a policy goal in mind (in some cases, policy ethnographers themselves engage in policy advocacy). We developed this approach when traditional ethnography proved too limited for our particular research situations. What happens in one health social movement organization is related to larger social movement networks and also involves institutions such as science and government. Therefore, one cannot separately address science, activism, and policy. Policy ethnography offers a more holistic outlook that integrates micro-, meso-, and macrolevels of society, targets the centrality of social movement interaction with science, and situates movements within large, complex fields.

In our practice, policy ethnography combines ethnographic interview and observation material, background history on the organizations we study, current and historical policy analysis, evaluation of the scientific basis for policy making and regulation, and in some cases engaging in policy advocacy through ongoing collaborations with health social movements. While a good deal of ethnography may engage in the first four elements to some extent, policy ethnography suggests that integrating sociology scholarship with the practical policy applications of CBPR can reveal the broader impacts of health social movements in reshaping regulatory science and policy making to protect community health.

Health Social Movements and Medical Sociology

The challenges that health social movements pose to professional and disciplinary boundaries (through embodied health movements and citizen-science alliances) and the ways health social movements connect research directly to policy formation (through community-based participatory research) mean the health social movement literature is a rich resource for any medical sociologist. Here we discuss four ways that medical sociology can benefit from attention to the health social movement literature. First, the literature has helped to identify and explore the range of nonmedical actors and institutions that are involved in the process of defining, identifying, and responding to health issues, such as activists, government agencies, and researchers; particularly important here are scientists. Second, health social movements help us track and understand the development of patient identity, which is often directly connected to the actions of health social movements, even for patients who have not become activists themselves. Third, citizen-science alliances and CBPR demonstrate how to merge theory with practice, and how to merge critical perspectives with embedded research interests. Fourth, the dynamic nature of the health social movements allows medical sociologists to do innovative research on concepts of health and disease, the roles and relationships of patients and health-care professionals, and the development and implementation of health policy.

Health Social Movements: Extending the Range of Medical Sociology

A focus on health social movements makes clear that the meaning and existence of diseases and decisions about preventive and ameliorative courses of action derive in part from institutions and actors outside the traditional focus of medical sociology. Health-care policies derive not just from health-care professionals and institutions but also from the actions of social movement activists and the scientists with whom they engage. Government and medical action on AIDS, for example, was due in part to AIDS activists engaging with the scientific enterprise to push for faster action based on better information and faster review and approval of emerging treatment regimes. Similarly, the identification of tobacco as an unhealthy substance for users and bystanders owed much to a tobacco control movement, including work by groups such as Groups Against Smoker's Pollution (GASP), which criticized science for failing to adequately pursue the dangers of primary tobacco use and secondary smoke hazards, and pushed scientists to take up more research on second-hand smoke (Wolfson 2001).

The literature on health social movements thus reveals that scientists and social movement activists, through both conflict and cooperation, play a major role in health-care policy. Fully understanding the development and implementation of health policy often requires an appreciation of how social movements work and how scientific knowledge is created and disseminated, making the sociology of science and social movements literatures deeply relevant for sociologists of medicine. Interestingly, we find a considerable number of publications on health social movements in *Science, Technology, and Human Values*, the major science studies publication. CBPR, a strong influence on the health social movement approach, is broadly informed by new theoretical approaches to citizen involvement, local democracy, environmental justice, lay knowledge, sociology of risk, and the new intersection of medical sociology, environmental sociology, science studies, and social movements that we and others (e.g., Moore and Frickel 2006) are employing. Because activists increasingly participate directly in the scientific research on the illnesses that afflict them, social scientists studying these movements need to be prepared to extend ethnographic research into the labs and field research settings of the scientists who are central to the movements being studied.

Health social movements—and especially embodied health movements—encourage researchers to pay special attention to the role that science and the scientific perspective play in medicine. Embodied health movements demonstrate the degree to which medicine has adopted a scientific approach that privileges quantitatively measurable and generalizable evidence over that which is particular to individual patients and knowable only through their accounts. Modern patients may find themselves clinically sick in the absence of any experience of disease or, alternatively, experiencing symptoms while being told that medically they show no signs of illness—one example, Lyme disease (Weintraub 2008), is now accepted by scientists and clinicians as an emerging infectious disease. This sociologically driven perspective in medicine is relatively recent and represents

a break from a long medical tradition in which the patient's bodily experience of illness was the primary means of diagnosis.

Health social movements' unique interaction with science and medicine poses a radical challenge to the professional hegemony of scientific and medical authorities that adhere to the "dominant epidemiological paradigm"—a set of entrenched beliefs and practices about disease treatment and causation embedded within a network of institutions, including medicine, science, government, health charities and voluntaries, professional associations, journals, universities, and the media (Brown et al. 2006). Activists point out that scientists are often asked to weigh in on questions that are impossible to answer scientifically in the here and now—either because data do not exist, or because studies required to answer the question at hand are not feasible. When science is in flux, it is essential that scientists have a say in the discussion, but their scientific opinions cannot be the deciding factor for the resolution of health problems, precisely because the science is inconclusive. Further, activists claim that many scientists, especially those who embrace the dominant epidemiological paradigm, inappropriately frame political, moral, or ethical questions in scientific terms. Such framing may limit participation in scientific decision making to the traditional experts and thus remove the concerned public from the process. Finally, activists point out how the dominant epidemiological paradigm delegitimizes questions that cannot be framed in scientific terms. They seek to redefine scientific problems in a way that opens up democratic avenues for public participation in science, and to redirect scientific effort to address problems of public concern (Morello-Frosch et al. 2006). For example, community advocates seeking to address high asthma rates among urban communities of color argue that scientific research has focused too exclusively on etiologic factors and lost sight of a solutions-based approach that assesses the effectiveness of social interventions that expand access to better-quality housing. In some cases, health social movements respond by marshaling resources to conduct their own research and produce their own scientific knowledge, as Corburn (2005) describes in terms of linking air pollution and asthma, and lead poisoning from bridge sanding in Williamsburg, Brooklyn. In doing so, the movements democratize the production of scientific knowledge and then use that transformed science as the basis for demanding improved research, treatment, and prevention, as well as calling for stricter and more protective policies and regulations. Movements also use that transformed science to demand structural changes in the political economy that reduce risk of the disease and facilitate research. Indeed, one of the common features of embodied health movements is that they often initiate new scientific directions in advance of medical science.

Health Social Movements and Patient Identity

The health social movement literature can also help medical sociologists better understand the development of patient identity, which in turn affects how patients come to perceive their own conditions and participate in their own care. Embodied health movements depend on the emergence of a collective identity, what we term a "politicized illness experience," as a mobilizing force. When institutions of science and medicine, correctly or incorrectly, fail to offer disease accounts that are consistent with individuals' experiences of illness, or when science and medicine offer accounts of disease that individuals are unwilling to accept, people may adopt an identity as aggrieved illness sufferers and progress to collective action.

For example, although lay perceptions of etiology may not be borne out by scientific investigation, in certain instances, hypothesized links between environmental exposures and human disease have been found to have some support, although these associations are often not immediately recognized (Gee and Stirling 2003). But even if evidence does not ultimately confirm a connection, the politicized illness experience may still be an understandable reaction to researcher or government resistance to a comprehensive research program or to public involvement in that research.

For environmental justice groups, urban asthma sufferers epitomize such a politicized illness experience (Shepard et al. 2002). Similarly, the environmental breast cancer movement has been an exceptional locale for such a politicized transformation (McCormick, Brown, and Zavestoski 2003). In both these cases, sufferers' etiologic perceptions challenged the dominant epidemiological paradigm, which focused on individual factors and downplayed or ignored environmental causation.

Patients that move from being isolated, individual sufferers to active members in a health social movement often find that their self-concept changes as well. For those diagnosed with illnesses for which there are well-established activist movements, those movements may very well shape the way patients perceive their illness and their relationship to medical institutions and health-care professionals, even without direct involvement in the health social movement. By attending to the health social movement literature, medical sociology can gain valuable insight into the roles that science and social movements play in the concepts, actors, and institutions that are central to their field, and the ways that scholars of social movements and science and technology studies are contributing to the medical sociology discourse.

Bridging Gaps via Health Social Movements

Community-based participatory research of health social movements avoids many of the divisions that exist within medical sociology (and sociology generally), variously described as the gap between theory and practice, the *of* medicine/*in* medicine divide (Straus 1957), and the different though not inevitably divergent paths of public, professional, critical, and policy sociology (Burawoy 2004). In CBPR, theory and practice are tightly linked, each informing the other. For researchers involved in the very movement they are analyzing, the disciplinary advancement of professional sociology and the service element of public sociology work together organically (and thus, strictly speaking, do not need to be bridged). Indeed, in his 2004 presidential address to the American Sociological Association, Burawoy identified CBPR studies of health social movements as having "married all four sociologies through collaboration with citizen groups around [various] illnesses" (Burawoy 2004, 16).

CBPR thus provides many examples of how to avoid the divide between theory and practice, and between our lives as professional sociologists and the action we may take in the public sphere. For example, scholars studying policy-relevant issues are likely at some point to be asked to take a stand or to provide information and expertise to community collaborators. In our experience with a toxic-contaminated community in Rhode Island, the academic partnership led to successful legislation that provided home equity loans to homeowners who could not qualify on the open market due to their homes' contamination. Our efforts were appreciated not only by the community partners, but also by federal government officials in the Environmental Protection Agency and the National Institute of Environmental Health Sciences (Senier et al. 2008). In the teaching component of our academic life, we have integrated CBPR approaches in educating students in an ongoing research group, as well as conducting service learning in undergraduate classes (Senier et al. 2006). Blending professional and public sociologies through CBPR is a beneficial community service, but also has benefits for researchers. In our own work as scholars in a larger collaboration on breast cancer and environmental justice, which has a strong component of biomonitoring and household exposure, we have learned much about sociological research, including its intersection with the promotion of environmental public health. Our CBPR work is not only a service for community groups but has also produced high-quality research that has been received well in medical sociology, as well as in environmental public health. Specifically, community groups have pointed to important contaminants for sampling and have been critical in preparing the community for research participation and in recruiting participants, aiding in research design, guiding the process of dissemination and education, and directing policy applications.

Integrating community involvement and scholarly research can challenge and benefit research design. A good example of community involvement in research design occurred in our work on the Northern California Household Exposure Study, a project that involved university researchers, Communities for a Better Environment (an environmental justice organization in Richmond, California), and Silent Spring Institute (a community-oriented nonprofit organization focusing on women's health and the environment that was founded by a breast cancer movement organization). The project entails air and dust sampling for a wide range of endocrine-disrupting chemicals and other pollutants, with an expressed purpose of providing scientific data to support Communities for a Better Environment in their efforts to stop the expansion of production activities of a nearby oil refinery. Our initial sampling protocol entailed a random sample of forty homes in Richmond. However, Communities for a Better Environment encouraged the research collaborative to accept some households as volunteers for the study, since the organization had worked hard to mobilize a base that wanted to integrate sampling data into their organizing efforts to address refinery emissions. Despite initial methodological concerns about accepting volunteers, the research collaborative revised its recruitment protocol by setting aside twenty of the forty slots for volunteers, realizing that some of the volunteers might also be among those randomly selected. Thus the research collaborative learned how democratizing the process of designing study protocols may improve the rigor, relevance, and reach of the broader research enterprise.

The CBPR literature on health social movements (e.g., Shepard et al. 2002; Corburn 2005; Agyeman 2005; Sze 2007) is similarly helpful in surmounting the diverging perspectives of "sociology of medicine" and "sociology in medicine." Because it focuses on issues and problems that the medical establishment itself has identified as important, sociology in medicine has been assessed as insufficiently critical of the actors and institutions it serves. At first glance, CBPR would seem vulnerable to the same critique, given its close affiliation with the participants inside and outside health social movements. However, health social movements (and embodied health movements in particular) are themselves engaged in challenging tradition, giving the entire enterprise an inherently critical perspective. Also, researchers are using CBPR work in multiple settings and with multiple groups, collaborating with laypeople and community groups on one side, and mainstream institutions and professionals on the other (Senier et al. 2008). This involvement with multiple interests and perspectives helps the researcher maintain a critical eye on all facets of the process, and provides a useful example of how medical sociology can pursue the research interests of specific groups while maintaining a critical perspective on the entire enterprise.

Cutting-Edge Medical Sociology

This community involvement in our own professional sociological research process demonstrates a fourth way that work on health social movements can benefit medical sociology: medical sociologists who participate in health social movements have the opportunity to be engaged not only with activism, but also with forms of science that are new and innovative to which they might not otherwise have access. Direct involvement with the actors and activities of health social movements can lead to a sociology of medicine that is especially current and dynamic in its theory, concepts, methods, and findings.

The use of policy ethnography for health social movements, for example, has led researchers into interesting and new hybrid spaces where the work of science, policy making, and social change take place. Science is increasingly being conducted outside laboratories, and policy is being devised beyond policy chambers. Social movement groups also cross multiple sector boundaries, as conveyed in concepts like boundary movements (Brown et al. 2004) and interpenetration (Wolfson 2001). Boundary movements are a combination of social movements and their constituent organizations, including some or all of the following: individual activists, outside supporters, scientists, academics, legislators, government officials, government agencies (usually parts of them), and foundations. With so many components, they blur traditional distinctions, such as those between movement and nonmovement actors and between laypeople and professionals.

Five characteristics define boundary movements. First, they attempt to reconstruct the line that separates science from nonscience. They push science in new directions and participate in scientific processes as a means of bringing previously unaddressed issues to clinical and bench scientists. Second, they blur the boundary between experts and laypeople. Some activists informally become experts by arming themselves with medical and scientific knowledge that can be employed in conflicts with health-care providers or environmental health regulators. Others gain a more legitimate form of expertise by collaborating with scientists and medical experts in research. Third, boundary movements often have state allies. For example, the tobacco control office of a public health department might be part of an anti-tobacco movement in tandem with a nonprofit organization or a political group (Wolfson 2001). Fourth, boundary movements transcend the traditional conceptions (i.e., boundaries) of what is or is not a social movement by moving fluidly between lay and expert identities and across organizational forms. Fifth, boundary movements use "boundary objects," which overlap social worlds and are malleable enough to be used for different purposes by different parties (Star and Griesemer 1989). For instance, a mammography machine is a diagnostic tool for science, a symbol of unequal health-care access to black activists, and for environmental breast cancer activists, a symbol of overemphasis on mammography and of the false claim that mammography is a form of disease prevention.

When studying human burdens of chemicals, Altman (2008) found herself crossing many boundaries and entering many spaces between boundaries. She observed a social movement organization's press conference at the Maine state house, watched community organizers pack glass specimen collection jars in the offices of an Alaskan environmental health and justice organization, and attended science-intensive discussions in a rural Appalachian high school auditorium. The use of policy ethnography in the health social movement literature, with its at once broad and intricate perspective, can help medical sociologists identify and explore similar hybrid spaces that shape health concepts and policies, and that may otherwise go unnoticed.

This attention to ongoing health social movements that involve multiple perspectives and actors engaged in contesting traditional sources of authority allows researchers to examine the twists and turns of policy as it happens. For example, in studying the environmental breast cancer movement, researchers sat benchside with breast cancer scientists, entered surgical suites as patients underwent mastectomies, marched alongside survivors and women living with breast cancer at public rallies, and examined how policy makers allocated money for etiological research. Such research could explain how local groups on Long Island were more likely to link up with status quo allies, including Republican lawmakers, while more radical groups like Breast Cancer Action took direct action, engaging in demonstrations and challenging mainstream breast cancer organizations (Brown et al. 2006).

Case Study: Biomonitoring/ Household Exposure Activism

We illustrate how health social movement literature can contribute to the objectives of medical sociology with a brief description of a CBPR project on the use of biomonitoring in health social movements concerned with the possibilities of household exposure to chemicals. The project exemplifies the way HSMs connect to public health, in that in the absence of specific disease, personal exposure monitoring serves as the surveillance so central to public health.

Recently, environmental exposure science has evolved from measuring contaminants in outdoor environments to measuring chemicals in human bodies and the household environments in which they live (Altman et al. 2008). Biomonitoring, the study of the presence and concentration of chemicals in humans, usually by the measurement of breast milk, blood, urine or breath, has the potential to identify the links between chemical exposure and health (NAS 2006). Household exposure studies, too, are undertaken to identify chemical exposure patterns in the hopes of providing insight on the health impacts of chemical exposure. While scientists hope this empirical data will lead to scientifically valid conclusions, the immediate

impacts of these techniques reach beyond the scientific realm and into the lay sphere where these studies are being conducted. Health social movements have recently begun to initiate and draw on these studies to buttress their claims that, in spite of a lack of evidence of the effects of most environmental pollutants, chemicals pose a threat to the livelihood of people and the environments in which they live, work, and play.

Organizations that integrate exposure studies into their movement activities exhibit the defining characteristics of embodied health movements: the centrality of the biological body, challenges to existing medical/scientific knowledge and practice, and citizen-science alliances. These organizations encourage the development of a proactive stance that questions and challenges parties adhere to the dominant epidemiological paradigm. Particularly among communities in the most contaminated environments, awareness of widespread chemical exposure can often lead to political engagement to confront the institutions responsible for contamination, remediation, or prevention. The "Is It in Us?" network of environmental health groups around the country that conducted human biomonitoring of 250 people in seven states is one such example (Coming Clean Network 2008). Communities for a Better Environment in California, with whom we partner, also uses household exposure work to advance their opposition to high emissions levels from a major oil refinery. These examples are part of a phenomenon we call advocacy exposure assessment.

Health social movements that are empowered to marshal scientific knowledge are born from the personal and collective realization that biological ills arise in part from social ills, and that the resolution of both lies in cooperation. When health social movements, in collaboration with their science and community partners, play a dominant role in conducting exposure studies, they infuse them with a sense of relevance for study participants, and exposure studies become avenues by which the lay public becomes empowered to adopt an activist stance. When a study participant receives results from a health social movement organization that values the right of an individual to receive their results, a previously remote problem becomes real and deeply salient to the person. Even among environmental activists educated about environmental issues, chemical contamination is transformed from an abstract issue into a personal concern when chemical body burden or toxic trespass in the home is revealed to study participants and the broader public.

Changes in perception and action orientation toward one's household and community often accompany this altered awareness, as indicated by a quote from an environmentally conscious participant to whom we reported personal household chemical exposures in the Northern California Household Exposure Study:

Researcher: So what were your thoughts or feelings the first time you read the information packet that was mailed to you?

Participant: I was in shock. I was stunned. I mean, I was really kind of traumatized by the information because having lived in this unit for—I guess it had been three and a half years when I got that information—and proceeding the way I do trying to use non-toxic things, the number of problem chemicals from my home was just an utter shock . . . so, then I kind of stepped back and thought, "Ok, well, there is no real difference, probably, it's just that I had this information."

This participant's initial reaction is at the heart of the most common criticism of exposure studies: the release of results in the context of scientific uncertainty can initially surprise study participants, who become aware of the ubiquity of chemical exposures in their everyday lives. Public health practitioners who abide by a clinical ethics approach contend that a researcher has an ethical obligation to inform subjects about their personal exposure results only when action can be taken (Brody et al. 2007). Communication of exposure results that are more consistent with the CBPR paradigm assumes that research results belong to study participants themselves. These tensions over participants' right to know are especially salient when there is scientific uncertainty and the health implications of exposure results are not clear. In situations where the clinical relevance

of exposures is well understood (as in the case of lead, for example) right-to-know conflicts are less likely to arise. However, in cases where the implications of exposures results are contested, scientists are more likely to withhold exposure results from participants.

Citizen-science alliances utilizing household exposure studies are emerging at a time when many are critical of the authoritative claims made by scientists. But far from challenging scientific validity, citizen-science alliances reach dual empowerment: scientists learn about personal and community impact of illness experience from affected people, and citizens learn about the state of the science. The use of biomonitoring and household exposure studies among health social movements touches on many significant topics in medical sociology, from lay-professional conflict, illness experience, and the political economy of health to privacy, confidentiality and right-to-know issues. Because of the myriad issues involved and the increasingly blurred boundaries between sectors, our policy ethnography approach has allowed us to make sense of and manage the messy dynamics of health social movement's use of exposure studies.

Conclusion

In sum, the multifaceted area of health social movements allows medical sociology to incorporate many of its core components. Through health social movements, medical sociologists can get a more intricate picture of the process through which diseases are defined (or dismissed). By examining health social movements, medical sociologists understand how patients perceive themselves as sufferers of specific illnesses and how they define their own relationship to the medical enterprise and medical authority. Further, health social movements turn a necessary spotlight on the role that science plays in the development of disease concepts and health policy. More fundamentally, health social movements (and particularly embodied health movements) help highlight the degree to which the epistemological assumptions of science have come to be part of the dominant epidemiological paradigm in ways that frequently go unnoticed and unexamined, until patients in embodied health movements begin to challenge them.[2]

While our biomonitoring case study focused on environmentally caused disease, contested illnesses and embodied health movements are conceptually broader categories that are also relevant to disease movements not associated explicitly with the environment. Those wrestling with any contested illness share problems of classification as they struggle to define the boundaries of an illness and show how it is distinct from established diseases. Contested illnesses of all sorts also share problems of etiology, as patients, health-care professionals, and other interested parties attempt to identify possible causes of the condition (environmental, genetic, or otherwise). By the same token, embodied health movements of all types—not merely those associated with environmental causes—involve conflicts between the individual's experience of illness and the existing scientific measures that may or may not endorse that experience (Barker 2005; Brown et al. 2001).

The health social movement literature is also unique for its strong emphasis on CBPR and use of policy ethnography. Together these research approaches can help to provide a more comprehensive account of the development of disease concepts and links to health policy. In addition, by bringing researchers from a variety of fields into direct contact with the challenges posed by health social movement activists, CBPR is a dynamic source of new perspectives and ideas for any field, medical sociology included. Finally, by blending research activities with service to health social movements, CBPR allows the researcher to blend seamlessly and rewardingly the often-separate worlds of theory and practice in ways that are beneficial to all involved. In the case of health social movements, the practical approach of community-based participatory research contributes new theoretical richness. This produces a valuable guide to how medical sociology can simultaneously serve itself and the public good, in ways that transcends the gap between "in" and "of." As an outcome, we arrive at research that pursues questions of interest to the medical establishment, but also to patients and others who interact with that establishment, and that retains always its own sociological agenda and perspective.

Notes

1. These categories are ideal types and do not cover the universe of health social movements (Epstein 2007). Some movements fall into more than one category, such as the women's health movement, a constituency-based movement that contains elements of both access health social movements (e.g., in seeking more health services for women) and embodied health social movements (e.g., in challenging assumptions about psychiatric diagnoses for premenstrual symptoms). Similarly, environmental justice organizing motivated by the disproportionate emergence of environmentally linked illnesses among marginalized communities shares features of both embodied health social movements and constituency-based health social movements.

2. "Patients" here includes "prepatients." Health social movements often involve not only those who have been diagnosed with the illness but also those who worry, for various reasons, that they might one day be diagnosed.

References

Agyeman, Julian. 2005. *Sustainable Communities and the Challenge of Environmental Justice.* New York: NYU Press.

Altman, Rebecca Gasior. 2008. "Chemical Body Burden and Place-Based Struggles for Environmental Health and Justice: A Multi-Sited Ethnography." Ph.D. diss., Brown University.

Altman, Rebecca Gasior, Julia Brody, Ruthann Rudel, Rachel Morello-Frosch, Phil Brown, and Mara Averick. 2008. "Pollution Comes Home and Pollution Gets Personal: Women's Experience of Household Toxic Exposure." *Journal of Health and Social Behavior* 49:417–35.

Barker, Kristen. 2005. *The Fibromyalgia Story: Medical Authority and Women's Worlds of Pain.* Philadelphia: Temple University Press.

Benford, Robert D., and David Snow. 2000. "Framing Process and Social Movements: An Overview and Assessment." *Annual Review of Sociology* 26:611–39.

Bird, Chloe, Peter Conrad, and Allen Fremont. 2000. "Medical Sociology at the Millennium." In *Handbook of Medical Sociology*, ed. Chloe Bird, Peter Conrad, and Allen Fremont, 1–10. Upper Saddle River, N.J.: Prentice Hall.

Brody, Julia Green, Rachel Morello-Frosch, Phil Brown, Ruthann A. Rudel, Rebecca Gasior Altman,

Margaret Frye, Cheryl C. Osimo, Carla Perez, and Liesel M. Seryak. 2007. "Is It Safe? New Ethics for Reporting Personal Exposures to Environmental Chemicals." *American Journal of Public Health* 97:1547–54.

Brown, Phil. 1984. "The Right to Refuse Treatment and the Movement for Mental Health Reform." *Journal of Health Policy, Politics, and Law* 9:291–313.

———. 2007. *Toxic Exposures: Contested Illnesses and the Environmental Health Movement.* New York: Columbia University Press.

Brown, Phil, Sabrina McCormick, Brian Mayer, Stephen Zavestoski, Rachel Morello-Frosch, Rebecca Gasior Altman, and Laura Senier. 2006. "'A Lab of Our Own': Environmental Causation of Breast Cancer and Challenges to the Dominant Epidemiological Paradigm." *Science, Technology, and Human Values* 31:499–536.

Brown, Phil, and Edwin J. Mikkelsen. 1990. *No Safe Place: Toxic Waste, Leukemia, and Community Action.* Berkeley: University of California Press.

Brown, Phil, Rachel Morello-Frosch, Stephen Zavestoski, Laura Senier, Rebecca Altman, Elizabeth Hoover, Sabrina McCormick, Brian Mayer, and Crystal Adams. 2010. "Field Analysis and Policy Ethnography: New Directions for Studying Health Social Movements." In *Social Movements and the Development of Health Institutions,* ed. M. Zald, J. Banaszak-Holl, and S. Levitsky. New York: Oxford University Press.

Brown, Phil, Stephen Zavestoski, Theo Luebke, Joshua Mandelbaum, Sabrina McCormick, and Brian Mayer. 2003. "The Health Politics of Asthma: Environmental Justice and Collective Illness Experience in the United States." *Social Science and Medicine* 57:453–64.

Brown, Phil, Stephen Zavestoski, Sabrina McCormick, Joshua Mandelbaum, Theo Luebke, and Meadow Linder. 2001. "A Gulf of Difference: Disputes over Gulf War–Related Illnesses." *Journal of Health and Social Behavior* 42:235–57.

Brown, Phil, Stephen Zavestoski, Sabrina McCormick, Brian Mayer, Rachel Morello-Frosch, and Rebecca Gasior Altman. 2004. "Embodied Health Movements: New Approaches to Social Movements in Health." *Sociology of Health and Illness* 26:50–80.

Bullard, Robert D. 2000. *Dumping in Dixie: Race, Class, and Environmental Quality.* 3rd ed. Boulder, Colo.: Westview Press.

Burawoy, Michael. 2004. "Public Sociologies: Contradictions, Dilemmas, and Possibilities." *Social Forces* 82:1603–18.

Coming Clean Network. 2008. "Is It in Us?" isitinus. org/home.php.

Corburn, Jason. 2005. *Street Science: Community Knowledge and Environmental Health Justice.* Cambridge, Mass.: MIT Press.

Della Porta, Donatella, and Mario Diani. 1998. *Social Movements: An Introduction.* Malden, Mass.: Blackwell.

Epstein, Steven. 1996. *Impure Science: AIDS, Activism, and the Politics of Knowledge.* Berkeley: University of California Press.

———. 2007. "Patient Groups and Health Movements." In *The Handbook of Science and Technology Studies,* ed. Edward J. Hackett, Olga Amsterdamska, Michael Lynch, and Judy Wajcman, 499–539. Cambridge, Mass.: MIT Press.

Fitzgerald, Kathleen J., and Diane M. Rodgers. 2000. "Radical Social Movement Organizations: A Theoretical Model." *Sociological Quarterly* 41:573–92.

Fleischer, Doris, and Frieda Zames. 2002. *The Disability Rights Movement: From Charity to Confrontation.* Philadelphia: Temple University Press.

Gee, David, and Andrew Stirling. 2003. "Late Lessons from Early Warnings: Improving Science and Governance under Uncertainty and Ignorance." In *Precaution: Environmental Science and Preventive Public Policy,* ed. Joel Tickner, 195–214. Washington, D.C.: Island Press.

Goldstein, Michael. 1999. *Alternative Health Care: Medicine, Miracle, or Mirage?* Philadelphia: Temple University Press.

Israel, Barbara, Amy J. Schulz, Edith A. Parker, and Adam B. Becker. 1998. "Review of Community-Based Research: Assessing Partnership Approaches to Improving Public Health." *Annual Review of Public Health* 19:173–202.

Jenkins, J. Craig. 1983. "Resource Mobilization Theory." *Annual Review of Sociology* 9:527–53.

Krimsky, Sheldon. 2000. *Hormonal Chaos: The Scientific and Social Origins of the Environmental Endocrine Hypothesis.* Baltimore: Johns Hopkins University Press.

McCarthy, John D., and Mayer N. Zald. 1977. "Resource Mobilization and Social Movements." *American Journal of Sociology* 92:64–90.

McAdam, Doug. 1982. *Political Process and the Development of Black Insurgency, 1930–1970.* Chicago: University of Chicago Press.

McAdam, Doug, John D. McCarthy, and Mayer N. Zald, eds. 1996. *Comparative Perspectives on Social Movements: Political Opportunities, Mobilizing Structures, and Cultural Framings.* Cambridge: Cambridge University Press.

McCally, Michael. 2002. "Medical Activism and Environmental Health." *Annals of the American Academy of Political and Social Science* 584:145–58.

McCormick, Sabrina, Julia Brody, Phil Brown, and Ruth

Polk. 2004. "Lay Involvement in Breast Cancer Research." *International Journal of Health Services* 34:625–46.

McCormick, Sabrina, Phil Brown, and Stephen Zavestoski. 2003. "The Personal Is Scientific, the Scientific Is Political: The Public Paradigm of the Environmental Breast Cancer Movement." *Sociological Forum* 18:545–76.

Moore, Kelly, and Scott Frickel, eds. 2006. *The New Political Sociology of Science: Institutions, Networks, and Power.* Madison: University of Wisconsin Press.

Morello-Frosch, Rachel, Manuel Pastor Jr., James L. Sadd, Carlos Porras, and Michele Prichard. 2005. "Citizens, Science, and Data Judo: Leveraging Secondary Data Analysis to Build a Community-Academic Collaborative for Environmental Justice in Southern California." In *Methods in Community-Based Participatory Research for Health*, ed. Barbara A. Israel, Eugenia Eng, Amy J. Schulz, and Edith A. Parker, 371–92. San Francisco: Jossey-Bass.

Morello-Frosch, Rachel, Stephen Zavestoski, Phil Brown, Rebecca Gasior Altman, Sabrina McCormick, and Brian Mayer. 2006. "Embodied Health Movements: Responses to a 'Scientized' World." In *The New Political Sociology of Science: Institutions, Networks, and Power*, ed. Kelly Moore and Scott Frickel. Madison: University of Wisconsin Press.

Morgen, Sandra. 2002. *Into Our Own Hands: The Women's Health Movement in the United States, 1969–1990.* New Brunswick, N.J.: Rutgers University Press.

NAS [National Academy of Sciences]. 2006. *Human Biomonitoring for Environmental Chemicals.* Washington, D.C.: NAS.

Rosner, David, and Gerald Markowitz. 1987. *Dying for Work: Workers' Safety and Health in Twentieth-Century America.* Indianapolis: Indiana University Press.

Ruzek, Sheryl Burt. 1978. *The Women's Health Movement: Feminist Alternatives to Medical Control.* New York: Praeger.

Ruzek, Sheryl Burt, Virginia L. Olesen, and Adele E. Clarke, eds. 1997. *Women's Health: Complexities and Differences.* Columbus: Ohio State University Press.

Senier, Laura, Rebecca Gasior Altman, Rachel Morello-Frosch, and Phil Brown. 2006. "Research and Action for Environmental Health and Environmental Justice: A Report on the Brown University Contested Illnesses Research Group." *Collective Behavior and Social Movements Newsletter* (American Sociological Association).

Senier, Laura, Benjamin Hudson, Sarah Fort, Elizabeth

Hoover, Rebecca Tillson, and Phil Brown. 2008. "Brown Superfund Basic Research Program: A Multistakeholder Partnership Addresses Real-World Problems in Contaminated Communities." *Environmental Science and Technology* 42(13): 4655–62.

Shapiro, Joseph. 1993. *No Pity: People with Disabilities Forging a New Civil Rights Movement.* New York: Random House.

Shepard, Peggy M., Mary E. Northridge, Swati Prakash, and Gabriel Stover. 2002. "Preface: Advancing Environmental Justice through Community-Based Participatory Research." *Environmental Health Perspectives* 110, suppl. 2:139–40.

Snow, David, E. Burke Rochford, Steven K. Worden, and Robert D. Benford. 1986. "Frame Alignment Processes, Micromobilization, and Movement Participation." *American Sociological Review* 51:464–81.

Star, Susan Leigh, and James R. Griesemer. 1989. "Institutional Ecology, 'Translations' and Boundary Objects: Amateurs and Professionals in Berkeley's Museum of Vertebrate Zoology, 1907–39." *Social Studies of Science* 19(3): 387–420.

Straus, Robert. 1957. "The Nature and Status of Medical Sociology." *American Sociological Review* 22(2): 200–204.

Sze, Julie. 2007. *Noxious New York: The Racial Politics of Urban Health and Environmental Justice.* Cambridge, Mass.: MIT Press.

Tilly, Charles. 1978. *From Mobilization to Revolution.* Reading, Mass.: Addison-Wesley.

Timmermans, Stefan, and Steven Haas. 2008. "Towards a Sociology of Disease." *Sociology of Health and Illness* 30(5): 659–76.

Waitzkin, Howard. 2000. *The Second Sickness: Contradictions of Capitalist Healthcare.* Updated ed. Lanham, Md.: Rowman and Littlefield.

———. 2001. *At the Front Lines of Medicine: How the Health Care System Alienates Doctors and Mistreats Patients.* Lanham, Md.: Rowman and Littlefield.

Weintraub, Pamela. 2008. *Cure Unknown: Inside the Lyme Epidemic.* New York: St. Martin's Press.

Wolfson, Mark. 2001. *The Fight against Big Tobacco: The Movement, the State, and the Public's Health.* New York: Aldine de Gruyter.

Zavestoski, Stephen, Phil Brown, Meadow Linder, Brian Mayer, and Sabrina McCormick. 2002. "Science, Policy, Activism, and War: Defining the Health of Gulf War Veterans." *Science, Technology, and Human Values* 27:171–205.

23

The Application of Biomarker Data to the Study of Social Determinants of Health

Regina A. Shih, RAND Corporation

Meenakshi M. Fernandes, Abt Associates

Chloe E. Bird, RAND Corporation

Medical sociologists have a shared goal of examining relationships of race, class, and gender inequity and health to ultimately reduce the burden associated with morbidity and mortality. For decades, much of the medical sociological research on health disparities focused on psychological outcomes, self-rated health, or mortality (Bird, Conrad, and Fremont 2000). Sociological studies of health have typically lacked the biological measures necessary to identify physiologic mechanisms by which life experiences—specifically, psychosocial stressors—get under the skin and affect physical and mental health. Such work can only infer the physiologic pathways involved in health outcomes.

Biological measures of physiologic function do exist and are increasingly used in the medical, clinical, and immunology fields as screening tools for diagnosis and as markers for disease severity (Ahmed and Thornalley 2003; Committee on Developing Biomarker-Based Tools for Cancer Screening Diagnosis and Treatment 2007; Forum on Neuroscience and Nervous System Disorders 2008; Munoz and Gange 1998; Pepe et al. 2001). Known more simply as biomarkers, these biological measures assess the byproducts of the body's responses to physiological processes that lead to identifiable health outcomes. As biomarker data

are increasingly available, our overall aim is to raise awareness of the role of biomarkers in the advancement of medical sociology research. Research linking social factors, biomarkers of physiological processes, and health outcomes offers medical sociologists an unprecedented opportunity to test and refine models of health and illness, and to present findings using outcomes that are of interest to a larger audience of health researchers and practitioners.

In this chapter, we introduce and discuss the use of biomarkers in the study of health and health disparities. We begin by defining biomarkers and briefly describing the benefits they provide to medical sociology. Next, we introduce the physiological effects of psychosocial stressors encountered in the social environment. From this foundation, we review the multisystem evidence for the physiological responses to stressors, focusing on the relationship between biomarkers of stress and disease trajectories in the immune, cardiovascular, and central nervous systems. We then proceed with an overview of large-scale medical sociology studies that incorporate biomarkers, and a discussion of key issues surrounding the use of biomarker data in medical sociology research. We conclude with some thoughts on the future directions for biomarkers in medical sociology research, and on how such research can inform policy.

Introduction to Biomarkers

Biomarker data in the context of medical sociology can provide insight into the inner workings of the body's responses to psychosocial stressors—from depression to racial discrimination. As we discuss later in this chapter, such stressors have documented effects on physiologic function and may contribute to morbidity and mortality. While biomarkers have wide versatility across many broad disciplines such as genetic epidemiology and environmental health, we focus on biomarkers of stress as it relates to health. By using biomarkers, medical sociologist researchers can test the hypothesized mechanism relating health and social risk factors. An observed change in a biomarker due to change in stressor exposure lends credence to the physiological effects of these more distal social risk factors of interest to medical sociologists.

In the past decade, medical sociology studies using biomarker data have strengthened or refuted various theories on how sociological stressors may influence physiological functioning or disease. The measurement of biomarkers themselves has improved as well, resulting in better insight into the physiological processes of how external social factors get under our skin. Studies that longitudinally track biomarkers have progressed to the point that some measures considered markers of functioning are now recognized as also early markers for disease diagnosis. Perhaps the most exciting advances have occurred in the field of genetic epidemiology, where certain genetic mutations are now identifiable biomarkers that indicate genetic susceptibility to psychosocial stressors, disease, and resistance to effective disease treatment.

By demonstrating how social processes impact disease trajectories through intermediate outcomes such as high blood pressure, inflammation, or high cholesterol, which are commonly of interest to clinicians and medical researchers, new research incorporating biomarkers can speak to a larger audience. Moreover, such studies could provide more intervention options to circum-

vent the adverse impacts of stressors on health. For example, a study relating the impact of living in a disadvantaged neighborhood to health outcomes may be more widely accepted and more actionable if it also demonstrates some of the physiologic pathways through which the effect occurs. Similarly, a study demonstrating the clinical pathways through which pollution and neighborhood disadvantage act together to influence health could draw attention to both problems and contribute to a larger transdisciplinary dialogue on the confluence of environmental and social determinants of health.

Biomarker Definition

Although some researchers use the term biomarkers (or biological markers) to refer to all physiological or functional measurements of health, including weight, height, and mobility, in this chapter we employ the National Library of Medicine medical subject headings definition, which is more restrictive:

> Measurable and quantifiable biological parameters (e.g., specific enzyme concentration, specific hormone concentration, specific gene phenotype distribution in a population, presence of biological substances) which serve as indices for health—and physiology-related assessments such as disease risk, psychiatric disorders, environmental exposure and its effects, disease diagnosis, metabolic processes, substance abuse, pregnancy, cell line development, epidemiologic studies, etc. (National Library of Medicine 2009)

Common biospecimen sources of biomarkers include blood, saliva, and urine. Commonly studied biomarkers from these biospecimens include hormones, enzymes, and genes, the primary actors in human physiology. While we do not discuss the many biomarker measures for genetic mutations, it is important to note that the field of epigenetics is of relevance to medical sociology. For example, exposure to a psychosocial stressor, environmental agent, or behavioral change may result in the modification of the activation of certain genes, or epigenetic change in expression of a protein, that code for a specific hormone or enzyme (National Human Genome Research

Institute 2009). Altered protein expression can have a variety of consequences. For example, it could have immediate effects on a physiological system(s); arise as an individual ages; or increase susceptibility to infection or disease. Table 23.1 provides examples of commonly studied biomarkers, the physiological system with which they are most commonly affiliated, and the biospecimen source from which they can be measured.

Benefits to the Study of Social Determinants of Health

Biomarker data provide alternative measures of health status to the traditional sources, such as self-reported measures, self-reported symptoms or functioning, and vital records and clinical records. Generally, biomarker data may provide insight for sociological investigations in four ways.

First, biomarkers are unlikely to possess some of the reporting biases by sociodemographic characteristics that occur with self-report data. Biomarkers avoid the problem of individuals using different comparison groups to assess their health and are less biased than self-reports of medical history. Self-reported health is often assessed by asking questions such as, "Has a doctor ever diagnosed you with diabetes?" and the answer is often influenced by differential access to care and quality of care. Such problems in data quality could affect investigations exploring differences by gender, race/ethnicity, SES, or age. Thus, integrating

objective measures such as biomarkers may make population research more compelling to a broader audience of researchers and policy makers (Mc-Dade, Williams, and Snodgrass 2007).

Second, biomarkers can be used in conjunction with other health status measures such as self-reported disease or clinical records. For example, a young adult may report "excellent" health, but a blood sample may reveal a high cholesterol or insulin level (McDade, Williams, and Snodgrass 2007), both of which can track quite stably into adulthood and are well-established risk factors for heart disease (Bao, Srinivasan, and Berenson 1996; Li, Srinivasan, and Berenson 2004). Thus, biomarkers can provide information beyond the awareness of the respondent and potentially identify those who are at increased risk for the development of a particular disease (Willis and Weinstein 2001).

Third, biomarkers may be a preferred data source if the study aim is to understand causal links and pathways. Biomarkers are well suited to addressing questions such as, How does social environment factor X affect the biological pathway to disease Y? To the extent that biomarkers have been used in clinical diagnoses, there is less misclassification of disease presence and severity compared to self-reported health. For example, a CD4 count from a blood draw is a more valid and reliable indicator of HIV/AIDS presence and severity than self-reported survey responses. Similarly, biomarkers (such as cotinine) may allow researchers to conduct a more accurate assessment

Table 23.1. Common biomarkers and biospecimen sources

	Example biomarkers	Biospecimen source
Physiological system		
Immune system	Secretory IgA	Saliva
Metabolic system	Hemoglobin A1C	Blood
Sympathetic nervous system	Norepinephrine, epinephrine	Urine
Endocrine system	Cortisol, serum dehydroepiandrosterone sulfate	Blood, urine, or saliva
Cardiovascular system	Serum high-density lipoprotein, total cholesterol	Blood
Inflammation system	Interleukin-6, C-reactive protein, albumin, fibrinogen	Blood
Other factors		
Environmental exposures	Lead, arsenic	Blood, bone, or hair
Genetic susceptibility	Genetic polymorphisms	DNA in serum, hair root, fingernail clipping, or cheek cell sample

of how related health behaviors (such as smoking during pregnancy) are linked to external social factors and certain health outcomes.

Fourth, biomarkers may be most useful when the effects of a disease process or risk factors do not occur immediately but over longer periods of time, as is the case for many chronic diseases such as diabetes. Without prospective biomarker data, it is difficult to define the beginning, duration, and intensity of exposure to risk factors. Biomarkers can also indicate cumulative exposure or cumulative risk for disease, for instance, hemoglobin A1c (HbA1c) is a commonly used biomarker for assessing chronic elevated blood glucose levels that is a better measure of diabetes risk than simple one-time blood glucose measures.

Physiological Effects of Stressors in the Social Environment

Differential exposure to the recurring stressors of daily life can contribute to health disparities. Stressors can be defined as psychological or social stimulators of a stress response. Selye's seminal work on the General Adaptation Syndrome first linked stressors to physiologic processes and disease, identifying both a protective and damaging physiological effect of stress (Selye 1951). The field of stress research has progressed substantially, especially within the last decade, with pioneering work on new biomarkers of stress responses, and on the interaction of genes and environment.

Definition of Stressors and Stress Response

As events and exposures that provoke a physiological and psychological stress response, stressors may range from racial discrimination or caring for an ill family member to exposure to an act of violence. However, the perceived psychological impact of stressors varies by individual, resulting in different vulnerabilities and associated health outcomes. Factors that may protect against stressors and elicit a muted response could include high SES; presence of positive social support from one's partner, family, and social network; or variations in perception of the social stressor (e.g.,

positive affect). Thus, researchers distinguish *stressors* from *perceived stressors*.

Both stressors and the stress response can be acute or chronic. The stress response is a natural reaction to stressors that confers a beneficial evolutionary advantage for survival. In fact, some stress is to a certain extent an unavoidable and necessary component of life, for example, exercise is a form of stressing the body to create and maintain physical conditioning. Similarly, exposure to stressful events or experiences can maintain controlled stress responses and protect against future exposures, as is the intention of training exercises such as boot camp. However, a persistent stress response can influence the development of health problems when the stress response overreacts or does not turn off and reset itself (McEwen 1998).

Physiological Responses to Stressors

The human body responds to stressors in a complex hierarchy of physiologic control and feedback systems. Although organ systems such as the cardiovascular system can function autonomously, their activities are also regulated and coordinated by higher-level control systems—the sympathetic nervous system and the hypothalamic pituitary adrenal (HPA) axis—which are governed by the central nervous system.

During exposure to stressors, the HPA axis and sympathetic nervous system respond in a cascade of biological processes that begin in a brain structure, the hypothalamus. The hypothalamus then signals the adrenal glands to release a catecholamine called adrenaline (also called epinephrine) and cortisol. Adrenaline works to prepare the body for action through the triggered release of several chemicals such as fibrinogen, endorphins, glucose, and fatty acids (McEwen and Stellar 1993). Cortisol promotes the conversion of muscle to fat and blocks insulin from taking up valuable glucose. This ability to activate an acute flight-or-fight response, which promotes survival in the face of stressors in the environment, is referred to as allostasis (Karlamangla et al. 2002; Sterling and Eyer 1988). Cortisol and adrenaline return to baseline levels after the stressor withdraws.

Figure 23.1 presents an overarching theoretical framework by which stressors, individual characteristics such as race/ethnicity, and social factors such as social support influence perceived stress, stress responses, and resulting health outcomes. The curved double-headed arrows indicate that individual characteristics are correlated with social factors and exposure to chronic stressors. Single-headed arrows suggest causal relationships: individual characteristics (e.g., sex and age) and social factors influence the development of perceived stress, physiological stress responses, and subsequent outcomes that can be assessed with biomarkers measures. For simplicity in the figure, points at which individual characteristics and social factors may modify relationships are marked with bold block arrows. For instance, an individual's SES level may influence the extent to which the individual perceives a stressor to be dangerous. Dashed arrows indicate reciprocal relationships: morbidity can influence perceived stress and the physiological stress response, which can create exacerbation loops. In addition, chronic stressors may directly affect physiological stress responses without requiring a mental perception that circumstances are stressful.

Stressors and Allostatic Load

Allostasis, as we have seen, refers to the ability of the body to activate neuronal, endocrine, and immune processes in response to external stress. While allostatic responses are an evolutionary survival mechanism, they can become less efficient with repeated exposures to a stressor. The cumulative biological burden or wear and tear resulting from inefficient allostatic responses is referred to as *allostatic load* (McEwen and Stellar 1993) and can have consequential impacts on physiology and health. For instance, elevated adrenaline levels stimulate fat deposition and insulin resistance and increase the risk for osteoporosis via osteoblast inhibition and calcium absorption (Canalis 1996). Elevated cortisol levels influence neuronal death in the hippocampus, a key brain structure involved in many neurological disorders (Sapolsky, Krey, and McEwen 1986).

Allostatic load encompasses three possible stress responses: (1) lack of adaptation to chronic stress or repeated stressors of the same type; (2) inability to shut off allostatic responses after the exposure to the stressor is eliminated; and (3) inadequate response in some allostatic systems that

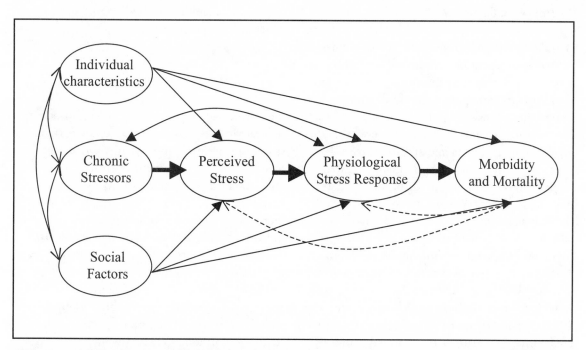

Figure 23.1. Theoretical framework for chronic exposure to stressors, perceived stress, and physiological stress responses (adapted from Glei et al. 2007)

triggers compensation by other systems (McEwen 1998; McEwen and Stellar 1993). Collectively referred to as dysregulation, these responses are characterized by elevated or reduced levels of biomarkers that reflect the functioning of the HPA axis, sympathetic nervous system, cardiovascular system, immune system, and metabolic and endocrine processes, leading to increased risk for chronic disease. Numerous epidemiological studies have linked allostatic dysregulation to hypertension, obesity, atherosclerosis, and mortality risk (Goldman et al. 2005; McEwen 1998; McEwen and Stellar 1993; Seeman et al. 2008). High allostatic load has also been found to influence mental health conditions such as depression, anxiety, self-regulatory behavior, and cognitive function (McEwen 2000; Seeman, Singer, et al. 1997). The extent to which allostatic dysregulation is linked with disease development is influenced by many factors such as genes, early development, and health behaviors such as diet, exercise, and cigarette and alcohol consumption (McEwen and Seeman 1999). Each of these factors may influence the reactivity and efficiency of physiologic systems in response to stress.

Allostatic Load Biomarkers

Biomarkers related to allostatic load include serum dehydroepiandrosterone sulfate (DHEA-S, a functional antagonist of cortisol), urinary cortisol, urinary norepinephrine and epinephrine, serum high-density lipoprotein (HDL), total cholesterol concentrations, and plasma glycosylated hemoglobin (a measure of glucose levels over time) (McEwen 1998; Seeman, McEwen, et al. 1997). While they can all be obtained from blood, they reflect different physiological systems that are activated by the HPA axis. Traditionally, allostatic load is defined by dichotomizing each biomarker and counting the number of biomarkers exceeding a certain threshold to give an overall allostatic load score. Allostatic load has expanded to include other biomarkers such as interleukin-6 (IL-6) and interferon gamma that may be associated with inflammation in response to stressors.

Since the concept of allostatic load was first introduced, a number of concerns about its validity have risen of which two are particularly important. First, there is a dearth of studies that have directly measured stress- and stressor-exposure-related multisystem physiological dysregulation in response to chronic stress. While the MacArthur Study of Successful Aging has made great contributions to the assessment of allostatic load, studies to date have had only one wave of biomarker data and thus have not investigated dynamic changes that are purported to occur in the build up of allostatic load. Longitudinal biomarker data, which would allow researchers to assess allostatic load trajectories as a process rather than simply as an intermediary state during the disease process, is only now becoming available in several population-based samples. Second, the thresholds used to dichotomize biomarker measures in the construction of allostatic load in the first studies did not have a clinical basis. However, more recent studies employing established clinical cut points for each biomarker address this concern (Merkin et al. 2009; Seeman et al. 2008).

As allostatic load has increased our scientific understanding of how psychological and physical stressors influence health from a multisystem perspective, there is promise for the development of related indices for specific conditions that will improve our ability to predict and prevent declines in functional health.

Stress over the Lifespan

The effects of stress can be observed throughout the human lifespan, although they are particularly salient during early and late life. Organ development and the development of the stress response are programmed from very early in life and can be affected by external factors such as stress in utero and during early postnatal development. As individuals age, vulnerability may again increase due to organ deterioration and the accumulation of stress over the lifespan.

Recent perinatal epidemiology research suggests that maternal stress during pregnancy stimulates placental secretion of corticotrophin-releasing hormone (CRH), which then stimulates the release of cortisol in utero (Seckl 2004). Dysregulation of cortisol in utero has been linked with various infant and child outcomes, including preterm birth, low birth weight, and reduced cognitive ability (Field, Diego, and Hernandez-Reif 2006; Talge, Neal, and Glover 2007). Moreover, the dysregulation that occurs in utero may extend to hormonal and immunological responses to stressors after birth that are determined by early life changes, or "perinatal programming" of the HPA axis (Welberg and Seckl 2001).

The life-course model posits that exposures early in life, including stress, are formative and predictive of later health outcomes (Barker 1995; Ben-Shlomo and Kuh 2002; Hayward and Gorman 2004). One potential mechanism of promoting resiliency and reducing the negative effects associated with psychosocial stress is by buffering against stress in early life through controlled exposures. This "stress inoculation" may occur through maternal-child interactions or through stimulating and supportive family environments during early childhood (Bremner and Narayan 1998; Liu et al. 1997).

Stress that occurs during childhood is a strong predictor of health conditions in adulthood, such as coronary heart disease (Kaplan and Manuck 1999; Pollitt et al. 2007; Poulton et al. 2002), mental health (Heim et al. 2000; Teicher, Tomoda, and Andersen 2006), and poor cognitive function (Richards and Wadsworth 2004). Most studies focus on more acute stressors such as acts of sexual abuse or domestic violence, but others consider chronic stress due to conditions of family life adversity. A study of the Atherosclerosis Risk in Communities cohort found that low childhood social class and education were associated with higher levels of inflammatory markers such as c-reactive protein (CRP), fibrinogen, white blood cell count, and von Willebrand factor, although only among whites. However, in this study, adult SES was still more strongly related to inflammation than childhood SES (Pollitt et al. 2007). Animal studies have been a valuable source of information on the development of stress responses. In young rats, more handling (positive support) resulted in more glucocorticoid receptors throughout the lifespan than for non-handled rats (Meaney et al. 1988). The presence of more receptors heightens the sensitivity to the inhibitory effects of glucocorticoids, which in turn increases the responsivity of the HPA axis to subsequent stressors (Meaney et al. 1996). A review of forty-nine studies published between 1966 and 2003 suggested that low childhood SES and accumulative stress insults were risk factors for adult coronary heart disease (Pollitt, Rose, and Kaufman 2005).

Because immune function declines with age, older adults experience dysregulation of immune reactions to stressful events to which they might have responded more effectively at younger ages (Kiecolt-Glaser and Glaser 1999). Chronic stress over the life cycle may lead to prolonged release of cortisol and amino acids (Lupien et al. 2007; Lupien et al. 1998; McCarty 1985; McEwen and Stellar 1993; Sapolsky 1999; Sapolsky, Krey, and McEwen 1986; Wilkinson, Peskind, and Raskind 1997). In addition, proinflammatory cytokines such as IL-6 may play a role, since production increases with age and may be a marker of chronic inflammation. Thus, inflammation may be a key biological mechanism through which lifelong stress acts synergistically with age to increase risk for cardiovascular disease, arthritis, diabetes, and disability (Butcher and Lord 2004; Ferrucci et al. 1999).

Psychosocial Factors and the Central Nervous System

As the central system of the stress response, the central nervous system (CNS) initiates a behavioral and physiological response to a perceived stressor. Stress responses can result in structural-level (brain structure volumes) and chemical-level (neurotransmitters) alterations in the brain, the main organ of the CNS. These changes are mediated by glucocorticoid and catecholamine stress hormones, in addition to pro-inflammatory cytokines that respond during the fight-or-flight stress.

Due to difficulties in collecting biomarker measures related to CNS function and in diagnosing psychopathologies, research using biomarker measures to elucidate the role of psychosocial stressors on the CNS has primarily used animal models. Increased stress levels in animals have been found to influence the structure of neurons and ultimately of brain structure (McEwen 2008). Observed changes that occur in response to both acute and chronic stress are concentrated in the hippocampus, a structure of the brain involved in cognitive function, including memory; the amygdala, which in involved in emotion; and the orbitofrontal cortex, which is involved in executive functioning or decision making (Cook and Wellman 2004; Vyas, Rao, and Chattarji 2002).

Biomarkers of CNS function can be obtained from cerebral spinal fluid through a lumbar puncture or spinal tap. However, this procedure is invasive and involves some risk. While no biomarkers in urine or blood are considered to be reliable measures of central nervous system functioning, neuroimaging such as positron emission topography (PET) or magnetic resonance imaging (MRI) have been used to measure brain changes in response to stress on a structural or functional level. In addition, cognitive, psychiatric, and neurological scales have been validated as measures of brain or psychiatric functioning.

Several recent studies have linked allostatic load from cumulative exposure to stress with the development of psychopathology. The hypothesis driving these studies suggests that stress-induced changes in the hippocampus and amygdala may lead to dysfunctional processing of information, with implications for the development of delusions, for example, in bipolar disorder or schizophrenia (Kapczinski et al. 2008; Koob 2008). A complicating factor is whether stressors' effects on the development of psychopathology simultaneously illicit hormonal changes that affect brain structure changes. Brain changes can occur concurrently with psychopathology such that amygdala volume increases after the first episode of depression, and hippocampal volume decreases (Frodl et al. 2003; MacQueen et al. 2003). This reflects a disciplinary difference: some sociology researchers focus on psychopathology as a stressor itself, and psychiatric epidemiologists mostly focus on psychopathology as a health endpoint potentially caused by stressors.

Psychosocial Factors and the Immune System

The validity of biomarkers such as IL-6 and serum immunoglobulin A (s-IgA) has supported investigations of the impact of acute and chronic stress on the immune system. Early studies on immune function and psychosocial stress typically involved experimental designs with relatively small samples. Several reviews broadly summarize key studies conducted in the last three decades (Cohen 2000; Kiecolt-Glaser and Glaser 2002; Segerstrom and Miller 2004). Substantial research on humans that has ensued supports evidence of a relationship between psychological stress and decreases in immune system function. A consistent and important finding from this literature has been that exposure to short-term acute stressors generates transient immune responses, while more chronic long-term exposure to stressors provokes immune function declines and prolonged dysregulation (Cohen, Miller, and Rabin 2001; Kiecolt-Glaser and Glaser 2002).

The complex mechanisms through which psychosocial stress shapes immune system function are moderated by the endocrine system. Acute social stress is positively associated with stress hormone secretion of catecholamines, which bind to receptors on white blood cells and regulate immune function (Glaser et al. 1994). Secretion of cortisol (a glucocorticoid) due to stress may overstimulate the immune system, leading to a propensity for the immune system to attack its own host body in the form of asthma, diabetes, and multiple sclerosis (McEwen and Lasley 2003). Another pathway is through the stress-induced production of proinflammatory cytokines, specifically IL-6.

Two well-known studies have examined the association between short-term acute stress or transient stressors (lasting from days to weeks) and immune function. The first focused on medical students between major exam periods. Students reporting higher levels of distress leading up to major exams showed changes in several immune markers (e.g., decreased lymphocyte, or white blood cell proliferation) that were consistent with immunosuppression (Glaser et al. 1987). Students with preexam stress were also at greater risk for viral infections, herpes recurrence, and allergic reactions (Marshall et al. 1998). The second study found that individuals with a greater number of stressful life events or higher levels of acute psychological distress suffered a greater incidence and severity of colds (Cohen et al. 1998). In contradiction to the widely held assumption that reporting greater cold symptoms simply reflected reporting bias due to psychological distress, objective measures of severity of infection such as viral shedding and mucus production confirmed self-reported data. The apparent physiological pathway in this instance was greater production of IL-6 messenger, which may have been triggered by higher cortisol levels (Cohen et al. 1999).

Chronic stress lasting months or years has also been shown to affect immune function. Chronic stressors associated with immune dysfunction include social isolation, job strain, unemployment, and chronic stressful life events (Kawakami et al. 1997; Muller, Lugg, and Quinn 1995). As an example of the relationship between chronic stress and immune responses, acting as the primary caregiver to a spouse with Alzheimer's disease was associated with increased psychological distress and prolonged endocrine and immune dysregulation, including delayed wound healing and muted immune responses to vaccinations (Glaser et al. 1999; Kiecolt-Glaser et al. 1991; Kiecolt-Glaser et al. 1995; Rojas et al. 2002). These factors could help explain the greater incidence of all-cause mortality among the aged caregiver population (Kiecolt-Glaser and Glaser 2002). Individuals reporting more stressful life events had lower s-IgA concentrations, which could potentially increase one's susceptibility to an upper respiratory tract infection (Phillips et al. 2006).

Numerous studies have also shown that psychosocial stress in the form of depression can reduce immune function (Herbert and Cohen 1993). Depression activates the HPA system and inflammatory responses (Black, Markides, and Ray 2003; Ford et al. 2004; Kiecolt-Glaser and Glaser 2002). This results in increased cortisol, catecholamine, and cytokine production, as well as increased insulin resistance. Thus, elevated depressive symptoms have been implicated in the pathway to Type 2 diabetes, an immune-inflammatory disease. It is important to note that this may be explained in part by metabolic and behavioral risk factors that are associated with depression, including physical inactivity, a high-calorie diet, and smoking. However, a recent study found negligible contributions of health behaviors and inflammatory markers (IL-6 and CRP) to attenuate the association between depression and subsequent diabetes (Golden et al. 2008). It should be noted that diabetes may also increase the risk for subsequent depression (De Jonge and Rodger 2006; Maraldi et al. 2007; Polsky et al. 2005). However, the effects of diabetes on development of depression may operate through psychological stress associated with managing diabetes, or with complications and comorbidities (Golden et al. 2008; Maraldi et al. 2007).

Psychosocial Factors and the Cardiovascular System

The cardiovascular literature draws extensively from the work of social and clinical epidemiologists who examine the associations of psychosocial stressors with cardiovascular biomarkers, cardiovascular reactivity, and cardiovascular disease in numerous large prospective studies. Replication of studies presented here using biomarker measures to capture cardiovascular risk can improve our understanding of the mechanisms whereby psychosocial stress ultimately leads to cardiovascular outcomes. Established effects of acute stress on cardiovascular functioning include: (1) increased heart rate and blood pressure, also referred to as cardiovascular reactivity, resulting in increased work for the heart, need for oxygen, and cardiovascular morbidity; (2) constriction of coronary arteries, reducing blood supply to the heart muscle at a time when more oxygen is needed; (3) increased electrical excitability and lowered threshold for arrhythmias, a common cause of sudden death; (4) damage to the endothelial lining of coronary arteries that increases the likelihood of plaque formation and rupture, which can cause a heart attack; and (5) increased "stickiness" of platelets and other clotting factors, resulting in increased likelihood of a clot that could occlude a coronary artery (Rozanski, Blumenthal, and Kaplan 1999).

These effects are thought to be mediated primarily by increased activity of the sympathetic nervous system. For example, chronic stress leading to episodes of depression can result in increased cortisol levels, which could increase cholesterol and glucose levels and accelerate atherosclerosis (Steptoe 2007). Some recent studies suggest that chronic psychosocial stress may be associated with inflammatory biomarkers such as IL-6 and CRP levels, although findings are not consistent (Ford and Erlinger 2004; Penninx et al. 2003; Steptoe, Kunz-Ebrecht, and Owen 2003; Tiemeier 2003). However, these inflammatory markers play a crucial role in the pathway to cardiovascular disease (Ferrucci et al. 1999; Redwine et al. 2000; Taaffe et al. 2000; Vgontzas et al. 2005, 1999), including atherosclerotic heart disease and greater mortality risk in patients with existing cardiovascular disease (Libby, Ridker, and Maseri 2002; Ridker, Hennekens, et al. 2000; Ridker, Rifai, et al. 2000; Ross 1999).

Low SES is associated with both perceived low social status and psychosocial stress, which contribute to increased risk of poor cardiovascular outcomes. Multiple studies have found that low SES is associated with subclinical changes in vasculature, even adjusting for poor health behaviors such as smoking (Chen and Miller 2007; Yan et al. 2006), and also with changes in systemic inflammation as measured by fibrogen and CRP (Jousilahti et al. 2003). Experimental manipulation of subordinate status in studies of female primates and of humans resulted in higher levels of cortisol, more fearful vigilance, increased risk for atherosclerosis, and higher cardiovascular reactivity (Mendelson, Thurston, and Kubzansky 2008; Mendes 2001; Shively, Laber-Laird, and Anton 1997).

Recent research has also examined neighborhood-level indicators of SES and stress with inflammatory markers relevant to cardiovascular disease (Peterson et al. 2008). After adjusting for individual-level SES and behavioral risk factors, lower community-level SES was associated with higher proinflammatory biomarker IL-6, although not with CRP. In another study, higher exposure to urban neighborhood psychosocial hazards was associated with higher odds of negative cardiovascular events, even after adjusting for individual-level risk factors for cardiovascular disease (Augustin et al. 2008). These hazards included high violent crime rates, off-site liquor licenses, and calls to city agencies about street problems.

Work-related stress is another active area of research in relation to cardiovascular disease. For example, numerous studies have indicated that high psychological demand in combination with low control over decisions (i.e., job strain) increases cardiac risk (e.g., in terms of smoking, blood pressure, and cholesterol) and cardiac-related mortality (Theorell and Karasek 1996). Similarly, work characterized as high-demand but low-reward is associated with increasing atherosclerosis risk (Lynch et al. 1997). In another study, self-reported persistent stress and low occupational class were independently predictive of pulmonary embolism (Rosengren et al. 2008).

Chronic stress associated with anxiety or depression has also been linked with the development of heart disease in healthy populations and increased mortality in patients with existing coronary artery disease, particularly after a heart attack (Kawachi et al. 1994; Rozanski, Blumenthal, and Kaplan 1999). Social conflict and instability on a societal scale have also been shown to increase cardiovascular morbidity and mortality. For instance, life expectancy in Russia fell sharply during the four-year period immediately following the collapse of communism. Cardiovascular disease accounted for more than 75 percent of the decline in life expectancy (Notzon et al. 1998).

Mediating, Confounding, and Effect Modification Factors in Psychosocial Stress Responses

Variables that influence the relationship between social stressors and health can act as mediators, confounders, or effect modifiers. For example, individuals with low social support or those living in areas with harmful environmental exposures may be more vulnerable to psychosocial stressors.

Individual Characteristics

There is considerable variation in the magnitude of a physiological response to a stressor depending on an individual's perception of the stressor. Personality characteristics may buffer or magnify the health effects of perceived stressors. For instance, personality characteristics such as a sense of humor can influence the relationship between psychosocial stress and s-IgA (an immunoglobulin antibody found in mucosal areas) (Valdimarsdottir and Stone 1997). High negative affect and diminished T-cell proliferation independently predicted stress-induced suppression of immune function in response to the hepatitis B vaccination (Marsland et al. 2002). Self-efficacy has been found to be related to the adoption of risk behaviors, and also has an independent role in the physiological stress response (O'Leary 1992). Another coping mechanism is the adoption of health behaviors to alleviate stress. Stressed individuals report less quality sleep, more alcohol and tobacco use, poor nutritional intake, and less physical activity, each of which is key to immune, cardiovascular, and central nervous system functioning. To the extent that they are malleable, one's disposition or negative affect and poor health behaviors are all targets for potential interventions thatpromote resilience to social stressors (Gallo and Matthews 1999; Richman et al. 2007; see also Ross and Mirowsky, this volume).

Social Factors

Social isolation and social support are both particularly powerful predictors of development and progression to poor health outcomes, including cardiovascular disease (Andre-Petersson et al. 2007; Cohen et al. 1998; House, Landis, and Umberson 1988; Uchino, Cacioppo, Kiecolt-Glaser 1996). The magnitude of these associations is substantial and often equals or exceeds that of well-established risk factors (Rozanski, Blumenthal, and Kaplan 1999). For example, in a prospective study of male health professionals, socially isolated men had twice the risk of mortality from cardiovascular disease of those with the largest and most varied social networks (Kawachi et al. 1996). In a prospective study of heart attack patients, lack of emotional support was related to both in-hospital mortality and cardiac-related mortality during the six months following the attack.

In addition, social factors related to coping resources (e.g., social support) may mediate or offset the effects of stress on physiological dysregulation. One of the first studies in this area found that medical students who reported more loneliness or less social support had larger declines in immune function both during and between stressful testing periods (Kiecolt-Glaser et al. 1984). Similarly, the caregiver spouses of people with Alzheimer's disease with the least social support in caring for their spouse had higher resting epinephrine levels and significant decreases in cellular adhesion molecules on lymphocytes compared to caregiver spouses with more support (Mills et al. 1999). Cellular adhesion is crucial to lymphocytes' ability to migrate to a site of active infection. In cardiovascular processes, positive social support may mediate the negative physiological effects of social stressors by influencing cardiovascular reactivity or high blood pressure (Holt-Lunstad, Smith, and Uchino 2008).

Environmental Factors

Individuals who experience contextual stressors such as low SES, poor neighborhood quality, and high residential segregation also tend to live in areas where they are exposed to higher levels of environmental toxins (Evans and Kantrowitz 2002). These environmental exposures may mask or exacerbate the negative effects of these contextual-level stressors (Gouveia and Fletcher 2000; Jerrett et al. 2004). For instance, environmental lead exposure, even at low levels, has been consistently associated with poor cardiovascular functioning (peripheral or vascular resistance) and higher risk for cardiovascular disease (hypertension) (Gump et al. 2007; Navas-Acien et al. 2007). Ambient air pollution has also been consistently linked with subclinical atherosclerosis, cardiovascular mortality, and asthma (Diez Roux et al. 2008). Yet, individuals with higher exposures to lead and ambient air pollution also tend to live in areas where they encounter more stressors that affect cardiovascular and immune system functioning. Thus, the independent effects of social stressors and environmental toxins are often difficult to disentangle.

Genetic Factors

Psychiatric, cardiovascular, and immune disorders that manifest in response to stressors may be partially mediated by genetic susceptibility. A hypothesized mechanism is the diathesis-stress hypothesis (Zubin and Spring 1977), which states that innate susceptibility to psychiatric disorders is driven by a combination of biological or genetic vulnerabilities, but that the disorder must be elicited by an environmental stressor. Environmental stressors in this context most frequently refer to stressful life events, although the definition has been extended to other realms, such as obstetrical complications or perinatal infection, that increase risk for disorders like autism or schizophrenia in the presence of innate (e.g., genetic) vulnerability (Mittal, Ellman, and Cannon 2008). In particular, a landmark study by Caspi and colleagues (2003) demonstrated an association between the short allele of the serotonin transporter gene (5-HTT LPR) and major depression. Children who possessed this short allele were more vulnerable to stressful experiences and developed major depression in adulthood at higher rates than those who did not possess the short allele. Interactions between genetic markers and environmental exposures are of great interest in current research. This is due in part to the considerable importance and attention to genetic biomarkers within the last decade with the development of new study methods, such as linkage disequilibrium and candidate loci identification in genome-wide association studies.

Incorporating Biomarker Data in Medical Sociology Research

Longitudinal Epidemiological Studies with Biomarkers

Most data sets designed by social scientists with appropriate measures of socioeconomic status do not contain physiological data. In Table 23.2, we provide a sample of longitudinal studies that facilitate the analysis of biomarkers and health trajectories. Some studies have included biomarkers from the beginning of the study, and others have incorporated them in later waves of data collection after initial recruitment. The majority of studies focus on adults, although biomarker data have become more common for child and ado-

lescent study populations. A variety of sampling designs among surveys is evident, perhaps a factor of the population of interest or of cost. Data that provide geographic identifiers for respondent home addresses at the census tract or street address allow for the incorporation of additional contextual measures.

The National Health and Examination Survey (NHANES) has provided many rich insights into health and health disparities. Physiological, medical, and laboratory test measures are available for respondents who participated in the Medical Examination Component. For example, in our study that assessed the relationship between neighborhood SES and stress, neighborhood SES was independently associated with a higher cumulative biological risk profile among blacks, with weaker results for whites and Mexican Americans (Bird, Seeman, et al. 2009). The risk profile measure incorporated nine biomarkers, including CRP, glycated hemoglobin, and albumin, while the neighborhood SES measure was a composite of neighborhood measures of income, employment, and education. Other recent studies that have incorporated biomarker measures from the NHANES include studies of cognitive function and obesity (Delpierre et al. 2009; Nguyen et al. 2009).

While most research to date using the Women's Health Initiative (WHI) study data has been primarily medical, this is another strong data set for medical sociology research. The sample consists of women ages fifty to seventy-nine across the United States and can support ancillary studies that span more than a decade. The WHI consists of the observational study (OS) arm and the clinical trial (CT) arm. Participants in the OS provide some biomarker measures at select years, with more detailed measures collected for 6 percent of the CT sample. One of our ongoing projects with the WHI examines the role of neighborhood factors in cardiovascular function and the development of coronary heart disease, and looks at whether this association is mediated by poor health behaviors that may be facilitated by living in a low SES neighborhood environment. Other factors that are being assessed include economic segregation, street connectivity, and social support. Our recent work finds that

Table 23.2. Examples of longitudinal U.S. epidemiological studies with biospecimens/biomarker data

Study name	Coverage	Approximate sample size[a] and target age group[b]	Year of first enrollment	Unit[c]	Survey Design[d]	Biospecimens/biomarkers	Geocoding	Unique survey features
Framingham Heart Study	Framingham, Mass.	5,000 adults ages 30–62	1948	P	G; LT	Blood, MRI of heart and brain, CT scans of heart and bone	N/A	Multigenerational
Health and Retirement Study	National	22,000 adults ages 50 and older	1992	P	LT	Saliva, blood; spirometry starting in 2006	Home street address	Spouse respondents, cognitive function, labor market participation
Los Angeles Family and Neighborhood Study	Los Angeles County	3,000 households	2000–2001	P	LT	Blood, saliva; spirometry starting in 2008	Home and work street addresses	Neighborhood measures
Multiethnic Study of Atherosclerosis	6 field centers	6,800 adults ages 45–84	2000–2002	P	LT	Blood, urine, ultrasounds	Home street address	Cardiovascular risk measures
National Children's Study	National	100,000 children	Pilot in 2009	C/P	LT	Blood, urine, hair, nails, saliva, buccal cells	Home street address	Environmental exposures
National Health and Nutrition Examination Survey	National	7,800 adults[e]	1959–1962	P	CS	Blood, urine	Home census tract	Medical examination component
National Longitudinal Study of Adolescent Health	National	90,000 7th–12th graders	1994–1995 school year	S	LT	Saliva, urine, blood	Home and school street addresses	Psychosocial environment, social networks, health, and risk behaviors
Nurses' Health Study	11 states	122,000 married nurses ages 30–35	1976	C	LT	Toenail, blood, urine	Home street address	Work stress, social networks, and social support measures
Women's Health Initiative	National	162,000 women ages 50–74	1993–1998	C	LT	Blood, urine	Home street address	Vitamin D/calcium, diet modification, and hormone therapy trials

a. Sample size at baseline, if the survey is longitudinal
b. For enrollment
c. S = school, P = population, C = clinic
d. LT = longitudinal, CS = cross-sectional, G = multigenerational
e. Children and youth interviews in later waves
N/A = Not Applicable

Reference websites: Framingham Heart Study (*framinghamheartstudy.org/about/history.html*); Health and Retirement Study (*hrsonline.isr.umich.edu/*); Los Angeles Family and Neighborhoods Study (*lasurvey.rand.org/*); Multi-Ethnic Study of Atherosclerosis (*mesa-nhlbi.org/*); National Children's Study (*nationalchildrensstudy.gov/*); National Health and Nutrition Examination Survey (*cdc.gov/nchs/nhanes/cyclei_iii.htm*); National Longitudinal Study of Adolescent Health (*nichd.nih.gov/health/topics/add_health_study.cfm*); Nurses' Health Study (*channing.harvard.edu/nhs/index.php/history/*); Women's Health Initiative (*whiscience.org/*)

living in a neighborhood with low socioeconomic status was independently associated with greater cardiovascular heart disease risk (Bird, Shih, et al. 2009). Many of these environmental measures used in conjunction with the WHI data have been computed from the RAND Center for Population Health and Health Disparities Data Core.

Biomarker Collection

Several key interrelated considerations determine what types of biomarkers to use in a study, and how often to collect them: burden and invasiveness to the study participant, logistical feasibility, costs, and ethical considerations. (Finch, Vaupel, and Kinsella 2001). Djuric and colleagues (2008) have published a technical review of the logistics of collecting stress biomarker data in the context of health disparities research.

BURDEN AND INVASIVENESS

The choice of a valid biomarker requires understanding the biological process for the body's absorption and metabolism of an exposure, and physiological response to an exposure. There are different sources from which to collect a sample (blood, urine, etc.) that have different implications for both participant burden and a study's budget and feasibility. In the rapidly evolving field of biomarker measurement, multiple approaches are continuously being validated to improve validity, increase feasibility, reduce costs associated with data collection and analysis, and prevent degradation of the sample during storage.

After a potential biomarker has been deemed a valid measure for a health outcome of interest, researchers must consider burden and invasiveness to the study participant. Some biomarker collection is so invasive it turns participants away from providing biomarker data and participating in a study. Population- or school-based studies are less supportive of invasive biomarker collection than are studies where collection occurs at a clinic. Study administrators should adopt the least invasive way of collecting a biomarker. When possible, genetic data can be obtained with a buccal cell sample from a cheek swab rather than by a blood draw, often ensuring better consent and

participation rates. However, if other biomarker data are desired (e.g., CRP, glycosolated Hb A1C, glucose, and Epstein-Barr virus), a cheek swab may not be sufficient, and blood specimens will be required.

The collection of some biomarkers may not be feasible because they incur significant participant burden. For instance, hormone biomarker levels may fluctuate over the course of the day and therefore require multiple collections. Since it may be onerous for a participant to provide saliva multiple times a day, researchers may have to sacrifice validity and goldstandard procedures for less frequently collected saliva samples. Burden and logistic feasibility are often directly tied to compliance, which has ramifications for how validly a biomarker measures physiological functioning. For example, if diurnal cortisol levels are not measured within key time intervals in the morning and evening according to the protocol, they may not be a valid measure of an individual's reactivity to stress. To obtain the highest quality sample with high fidelity to established collection protocols, clear instructions at appropriate reading levels should be provided to the respondent. Surveys also often use incentive payments to improve participation rates and adherence to the guidelines for proper biospecimen collection.

LOGISTICAL FEASIBILITY

Logistics surrounding biomarker data collection also include issues related to sampling, processing, shipping, storage, and analysis. Some blood assays can be obtained through finger sticks or from dried blood samples. Others require larger blood draws and more rapid transition to the processing step, potentially limiting collection efforts in rural areas. Logistics such as adding stabilizers to preserve cell structure at the processing stage, the time window for processing, and the ideal temperature for shipping and storage all depend on both the biomarker of interest and the biospecimen (Holland et al. 2003; Tworoger and Hankinson 2006; Vaught 2006). Logistical feasibility also depends on the sampling scheme. Surveys that can support medical sociology inquiries tend to be either population based or a combination of population-based and clinic-based designs. Biomarkers obtained from clinical samples may not be externally valid to the greater population at large, in which case a population-based study is more appropriate for external validity. Thus, the key study hypotheses and extent of desired generalizability of biomarker findings should drive the choice of sampling design.

COSTS

The survey administrator must determine if adding a biomarker measure to a survey is worth the cost. Newer biomarkers that have been studied less extensively tend to be more expensive but may provide novel evidence in a less-studied field. The desire for large, prospectively collected data that are representative bears great economic costs. Logistics, burden, invasiveness, and costs of analyzing biomarkers must be balanced against the potential to provide novel research findings. To control costs, a pilot study can be conducted before launching a full-scale biomarker collection effort, or a substudy can be conducted of a small proportion of study participants who are willing to provide biomarker data.

ETHICAL CONSIDERATIONS

Medical sociologists are often interested in health disparities among disadvantaged subpopulations. Sampling from ethnic enclaves or disadvantaged populations will benefit from strong relationships and communication between the respondent and the study's data collectors from the very inception of the study. Collecting biomarkers requires special considerations for participant consent and privacy, and the respondents must fully understand the procedure and issues associated with storing and analyzing their samples. Separate consent can be provided for biological specimens, with options provided to the participant for how those specimens can be used and stored. Disadvantaged populations should not feel pressured to provide biospecimens because of monetary compensation or other incentives (Schulte and Sweeney 1995). Careful attention should be paid to institution review board (IRB) requirements for biomarker collection, especially for those that are genetic in nature. Human subjects review includes specific guidelines for the collection and analysis of human tissue. As specific guidelines vary across federal agencies, researchers collecting or working with biomarker data should consult their institution's IRB before proceeding.[1]

Future Directions for Biomarkers in Medical Sociology

Recent advances in computational capacity and software algorithms and the decreasing cost and complexity of collecting and analyzing biological data have opened new avenues for transdisciplinary collaboration. By collaborating with biomedical researchers to study biological and sociological pathways, medical sociologists can shed light on the shared goal to understand how risk of disease and death is differentially acquired over the life course.

Several methodological considerations could be incorporated into future research in order to clarify causal pathways. While most research to date on physiological functioning has been conducted on healthy populations, it is likely that the relatively small immune effects of psychosocial factors have greater consequences for more biologically vulnerable persons such as the elderly, the very young, or individuals with inherited or acquired biological vulnerabilities. Sociological models that ignore interactions with vulnerability factors will yield inconsistent results that may underestimate the impact of social factors. More attention is also needed to mediating factors such as negative affect, coping resources such as perceived self-efficacy or adoption of coping health behaviors, and positive social support. With some exceptions, conceptual models used in many studies have lacked the sophistication of including these intermediate variables, which may provide alternative explanations for the association between psychosocial factors and biomarkers. Advanced biostatistical modeling such as structural equation models that hypothesize causal pathways may help to distinguish direct effects for each psychosocial stressor, from indirect pathways through other correlated social and biological risk factors. Longitudinal studies can also provide critical information on the timing of exposure to stressors and periods of vulnerability to stressors, especially in the case of acute stressors.

Research involving biomarkers offers an array

of exciting possibilities for advancing the study of health in general, and for medical sociology in particular. If medical sociologists incorporate biomarkers into research models, sociological studies will be able to use biomarkers as: (1) predictors of baseline health to examine how social circumstances and social processes play into trajectories of health and longevity; (2) outcomes to study the impact of social contexts on health without having to collect data on illness trajectories or mortality patterns over decades; and (3) a means of understanding how social factors affect multiple physiological systems, to ultimately identify key intervention points to bolster protection against the effects of psychosocial stress. By incorporating biomarkers into our theories and research on the social patterning of health, illness, and mortality, sociologists can shed new light on the underlying processes and engage in a transdisciplinary discussion on the social determinants of health, increasingly called for by the National Institutes of Health Office of Behavioral and Social Sciences Research.

How Can Biomarker Studies Inform Policy?

Medical sociology research involving biomarkers may have a greater potential to inform policy in part because it can demonstrate the impact of social disparities and actionable social factors on illness trajectories with known social and economic costs and consequences. Using biomarkers can allow sociological work to speak to a larger audience of researchers, policy makers, and clinicians. The ability to connect findings to previously established health consequences of altered biomarker levels allows researchers to make a more credible case to policy makers on a range of implied health effects (such as projected increases in rates of cardiovascular disease and diabetes) that would traditionally have required much longer follow-up periods.

While some research findings directly change the course of policy, more often data are used to make smaller course corrections or to support narrower decisions. Some examples include changes at the neighborhood level or with an employer. Communities, cities, and even states can

apply information on how strongly contextual-level risk factors relate to health as demonstrated through biomarkers to ultimately inform building development and housing policies. Examples of policies that could influence community health include those that regulate housing density, mass transit, and green space. Demonstrating whether and how mutable neighborhood characteristics relate to individual and population health should be of interest for policy makers.

Similarly, intervention studies could be used to support workplace health and the adoption of policies that facilitate positive health behaviors. For example, if medical sociologists could demonstrate that particular workplace policies regarding the types of food available and facilitation of exercise (e.g., providing accessible stairways as well as hallways suitable for brisk walking, and encouraging walking or even stretching breaks) are associated with improved cardiovascular profiles, that evidence could provide employers with the business case to invest in workplace health in order to reduce health insurance costs and productivity losses due to illness and absenteeism.

Using biomarkers to clarify biological pathways by which disease processes occur in response to psychosocial stressors may help determine points for intervention and treatment. In addition, biomarker research may help to identify vulnerable populations for which specific interventions and treatments may be most effective. Clinicians and public health researchers can determine whether there are subpopulations that are genetically susceptible to disease, or subgroups for whom a treatment may be most effective (e.g., cancer treatment, hypertension management).

Using biomarkers to understand the biological pathway from sociological risk factor to health endpoint supports evidence toward causality, or at least makes it plausible, and reduces the possibility that what is observed is purely selection or an ecological finding with no real individual-level basis. Incorporating biomarker research into medical sociology can also speak to whether, and to what extent, different approaches to redress a social problem are likely to be effective. Thus, understanding the biological process can help clarify the costs of primary versus secondary prevention and the likely health outcomes of each. Secondary prevention cannot eliminate health disparities, as its benefits are often too little and too late. Individuals may have acquired increased biologic risk for poor health and have an altered health trajectory with a worse prognosis than those who have not reached the same level of biologic dysregulation.

Healthcare policy alone cannot eliminate racial/ethnic or socioeconomic disparities in health. Bridging biomarker research and medical sociology is a translational effort to bring the biological mechanism discussion to a more contextual level with the ultimate goal of informing policy decisions on an ecological level.

Note

1. For a list from the National Institutes of Health of online bioethics resources, see bioethics.od.nih.gov/humantissue.html.

References

Ahmed, N., and P. J. Thornalley. 2003. "Quantitative Screening of Protein Biomarkers of Early Glycation, Advanced Glycation, Oxidation and Nitrosation in Cellular and Extracellular Proteins by Tandem Mass Spectrometry Multiple Reaction Monitoring." *Biochemical Society Transactions* 31(pt 6): 1417–22.

Andre-Petersson, Lena, Gunnar Engstrom, Bo Hedblad, Lars Janzon, and Malmo Rosvall. 2007. "Social Support at Work and the Risk of Myocardial Infarction and Stroke in Women and Men." *Social Science and Medicine* 64(4): 830–41.

Augustin, Toms, Thomas A. Glass, Bryan D. James, and Brian S. Schwartz. 2008. "Neighborhood Psychosocial Hazards and Cardiovascular Disease: The Baltimore Memory Study." *American Journal of Public Health* 98(9): 1664–70.

Bao, Weihang, Sathanur R. Srinivasan, and Gerald S. Berenson. 1996. "Persistent Elevation of Plasma Insulin Levels Is Associated with Increased Cardiovascular Risk in Children and Young Adults: The Bogalusa Heart Study." *Circulation* 93(1): 54–59.

Barker, D. J. 1995. "Intrauterine Programming of Adult Disease." *Molecular Medicine Today* 1(9): 418–23.

Ben-Shlomo, Yoav, and Diana Kuh. 2002. "A Life Course Approach to Chronic Disease Epidemiology: Conceptual Models, Empirical Challenges and Interdisciplinary Perspectives." *International Journal of Epidemiology* 31(2): 285–93.

Bird, Chloe E., Peter Conrad, and Allen M. Fremont. 2000. *Handbook of Medical Sociology.* Upper Saddle River, N.J.: Prentice Hall.

Bird, Chloe E., Teresa Seeman, Jose J. Escarce, Ricardo Basurto-Davila, Brian Finch, Tamara Dubowitz, Melonie Heron, Lauren Hale, Sharon S. Merkin, Margaret Weden, and Nicole Lurie. 2009. "Neighbourhood Socioeconomic Status and Biological 'Wear and Tear' in a Nationally Representative Sample of U.S. Adults." *Journal of Epidemiology and Community Health* [epub ahead of print]. jech.bmj.com/content/early/2009/09/16/jech.2008.084814.full.pdf.

Bird, Chloe E., Regina Shih, Christine Eibner, Beth Ann Griffin, Mary Slaughter, Eric A. Whitsel, Karen L. Margolis, Jose J. Escarce, Adria Jewell, Charles Mouton, and Nicole Lurie. 2009. "Neighborhood SES and Incident CHD among Women." *Journal of General Internal Medicine Abstracts* 24, suppl. 1: S127.

Black, Sandra A., Kyriakos S. Markides, and Laura A. Ray. 2003. "Depression Predicts Increased Incidence of Adverse Health Outcomes in Older Mexican Americans with Type 2 Diabetes." *Diabetes Care* 26(10): 2822–28.

Bremner, J. Douglas, and Meena Narayan. 1998. "The Effects of Stress on Memory and the Hippocampus throughout the Life Cycle: Implications for Childhood Development and Aging." *Development and Psychopathology* 10(4): 871–85.

Butcher, Stephen K., and Janet M. Lord. 2004. "Stress Responses and Innate Immunity: Aging as a Contributory Factor." *Aging Cell* 3(4): 151–60.

Canalis, E. 1996. "Clinical Review 83: Mechanisms of Glucocorticoid Action in Bone: Implications to Glucocorticoid-Induced Osteoporosis." *Journal of Clinical Endocrinology and Metabolism* 81(10): 3441–47.

Caspi, Avshalom, Karen Sugden, Terrie E. Moffitt, Alan Taylor, Ian W. Craig, HonaLee Harrington, Joseph McClay, Jonathan Mill, Judy Martin, Anthony Braithwaite, and Richie Poulton. 2003. "Influence of Life Stress on Depression: Moderation by a Polymorphism in the 5-Htt Gene." *Science* 301(5631): 386–89.

Chen, Edith, and Gregory E. Miller. 2007. "Stress and Inflammation in Exacerbations of Asthma." *Brain Behavior and Immunity* 21(8): 993–99.

Cohen, Joan I. 2000. "Stress and Mental Health: A Biobehavioral Perspective." *Issues in Mental Health Nursing* 21(2): 185–202.

Cohen, Sheldon, William J. Doyle, and David P. Skoner. 1999. "Psychological Stress, Cytokine Production, and Severity of Upper Respiratory Illness." *Psychosomatic Medicine* 61(2): 175–80.

Cohen, Sheldon, Ellen Frank, William J. Doyle, David P. Skoner, Bruce S. Rabin, and Jack M. Gwaltney Jr. 1998. "Types of Stressors That Increase Susceptibility to the Common Cold in Healthy Adults." *Health Psychology* 17(3): 214–23.

Cohen, Sheldon, Gregory E. Miller, and Bruce S. Rabin. 2001. "Psychological Stress and Antibody Response to Immunization: A Critical Review of the Human Literature." *Psychosomatic Medicine* 63(1): 7–18.

Committee on Developing Biomarker-Based Tools for Cancer Screening Diagnosis and Treatment. 2007. *Cancer Biomarkers: The Promises and Challenges of Improving Detection and Treatment*, ed. S. J. Nass and H. L. Moses. Washington, D.C.: National Academies Press.

Cook, Susan C., and Cara L. Wellman. 2004. "Chronic Stress Alters Dendritic Morphology in Rat Medial Prefrontal Cortex." *Journal of Neurobiology* 60(2): 236–48.

De Jonge, Desleigh M., and Sylvia A. Rodger. 2006. "Consumer-Identified Barriers and Strategies for Optimizing Technology Use in the Workplace." *Disability and Rehabilitation Assistive Technology* 1(1/2): 79–88.

Delpierre, Cyrille, Valerie Lauwers-Cances, Geetanjali D. Datta, Lisa Berkman, and Thierry Lang. 2009. "Impact of Social Position on the Effect of Cardiovascular Risk Factors on Self-Rated Health." *American Journal of Public Health* 99(7): 1278–84.

Diez Roux, Ana V., Amy H. Auchincloss, Tracy G. Franklin, Trivellore Raghunathan, R. Graham Barr, Joel Kaufman, Brad Astor, and Jerry Keeler. 2008. "Long-Term Exposure to Ambient Particulate Matter and Prevalence of Subclinical Atherosclerosis in the Multi-Ethnic Study of Atherosclerosis." *American Journal of Epidemiology* 167(6): 667–75.

Djuric, Zora, Chloe E. Bird, Alice Furumoto-Dawson, Garth Rauscher, Mack Ruffin, Raymond Stowe, Katherine Tucker, and Christopher Masi. 2008. "Biological Markers of Psychological Stress in Health Disparities Research." *Open Biomarkers Journal* 1:17–19.

Evans, Gary W., and Elyse Kantrowitz. 2002. "Socioeconomic Status and Health: The Potential Role of Environmental Risk Exposure." *Annual Review of Public Health* 23:303–31.

Ferrucci, L., T. B. Harris, J. M. Guralnik, R. P. Tracy, M. C. Corti, H. J. Cohen, B. Penninx, M. Pahor, R. Wallace, and R. J. Havlik. 1999. "Serum Il-6 Level and the Development of Disability in Older Persons." *Journal of the American Geriatrics Society* 47(6): 639–46.

Field, Tiffany, Miguel Diego, and Maria Hernandez-Reif. 2006. "Prenatal Depression Effects on the Fetus and Newborn: A Review." *Infant Behavior and Development* 29(3): 445–55.

Finch, Caleb E., James W. Vaupel, and Kevin G. Kinsella. 2001. *Cells and Surveys: Should Biological Measures Be Included in Social Science Research?* Washington, D.C.: National Academy Press.

Ford, Daniel E., and Thomas P. Erlinger. 2004. "Depression and C-Reactive Protein in U.S. Adults: Data from the Third National Health and Nutrition Examination Survey." *Archives of Internal Medicine* 164(9): 1010–14.

Ford, Julian D., Robert L. Trestman, Karen Steinberg, Howard Tennen, and Scott Allen. 2004. "Prospective Association of Anxiety, Depressive, and Addictive Disorders with High Utilization of Primary, Specialty and Emergency Medical Care." *Social Science and Medicine* 58(11): 2145–48.

Forum on Neuroscience and Nervous System Disorders. 2008. *Neuroscience Biomarkers and Biosignatures: Converging Technologies, Emerging Partnerships: Workshop Summary*. Washington, D.C.: National Academies Press.

Frodl, Thomas, Eva M. Meisenzahl, Thomas Zetzsche, Christine Born, Markus Jager, Constanze Groll, Ronald Bottlender, Gerga Leinsinger, and Hans-Junger Moller. 2003. "Larger Amygdala Volumes in First Depressive Episode as Compared to Recurrent Major Depression and Healthy Control Subjects." *Biological Psychiatry* 53(4): 338–44.

Gallo, Linda C., and Karen A. Matthews. 1999. "Do Negative Emotions Mediate the Association between Socioeconomic Status and Health?" *Annals of the New York Academy of Sciences* 896:226–45.

Glaser, Ronald, D. K. Pearl, J. K. Kiecolt-Glaser, and W. B. Malarkey. 1994. "Plasma Cortisol Levels and Reactivation of Latent Epstein-Barr Virus in Response to Examination Stress." *Psychoneuroendocrinology* 19(8): 765–72.

Glaser, Ronald, Bruce Rabin, Margaret Chesney, Sheldon Cohen, and Benjamin Natelson. 1999. "Stress-Induced Immunomodulation: Implications for Infectious Diseases?" *Journal of the American Medical Association* 281(24): 2268–70.

Glaser, Ronald, J. Rice, J. Sheridan, R. Fertel, J. Stout, C. Speicher, D. Pinsky, M. Kotur, A. Post, M. Beck, et al. 1987. "Stress-Related Immune Suppression: Health Implications." *Brain Behavior and Immunity* 1(1): 7–20.

Glei, Dana, Noreen Goldman, Yi-Li Chuang, and Maxine Weinstein. 2007. "Do Chronic Stressors Lead to Physiological Dysregulation? Testing the Theory of Allostatist Load." *Psychosomatic Medicine* 69:769–76.

Golden, Sherita H., Mariana Lazo, Mercedes Carnethon, Alain G. Bertoni, Pamela J. Schreiner, Ana V. Diez Roux, Hochang B. Lee, and Constantine Lyketsos. 2008. "Examining a Bidirectional Association between Depressive Symptoms and Diabetes."

Journal of the American Medical Association 299(23): 2751–59.

Goldman, Noreen, Dana A. Glei, Christopher Seplaki, I-Wen Liu, and Maxine Weinstein. 2005. "Perceived Stress and Physiological Dysregulation in Older Adults." *Stress* 8(2): 95–105.

Gouveia, Nelson, and Tony Fletcher. 2000. "Time Series Analysis of Air Pollution and Mortality: Effects by Cause, Age and Socioeconomic Status." *Journal of Epidemiology and Community Health* 54:750–55.

Gump, Brooks B., Jacki Reihman, Paul Stewart, Ed Lonky, Tom Darvill, and Karen A. Matthews. 2007. "Blood Lead (Pb) Levels: A Potential Environmental Mechanism Explaining the Relation between Socioeconomic Status and Cardiovascular Reactivity in Children." *Health Psychology* 26(3): 296–304.

Hayward, Mark D., and Bridget K. Gorman. 2004. "The Long Arm of Childhood: The Influence of Early-Life Social Conditions on Men's Mortality." *Demography* 41(1): 87–107.

Heim, Christine, D. Jeffrey Newport, Stacey Heit, Yolanda P. Graham, Molly Wilcox, Robert Bonsall, Andrew H. Miller, and Charles B. Nemeroff. 2000. "Pituitary-Adrenal and Autonomic Responses to Stress in Women after Sexual and Physical Abuse in Childhood." *Journal of the American Medical Association* 284(5): 592–97.

Herbert, Tracy B., and Sheldon Cohen. 1993. "Depression and Immunity: A Meta-Analytic Review." *Psychological Bulletin* 113(3): 472–86.

Holland, Nina T., Martyn T. Smith, Brenda Eskenazi, and Maria Bastaki. 2003. "Biological Sample Collection and Processing for Molecular Epidemiological Studies." *Mutation Research* 543(3): 217–34.

Holt-Lunstad, Julianne, Timothy W. Smith, and Bert N. Uchino. 2008. "Can Hostility Interfere with the Health Benefits of Giving and Receiving Social Support? The Impact of Cynical Hostility on Cardiovascular Reactivity during Social Support Interactions among Friends." *Annals of Behavioral Medicine* 35(3): 319–30.

House, James S., Karl R. Landis, and Debra Umberson. 1988. "Social Relationships and Health." *Science* 241(4865): 540–45.

Jerrett, M., R. T. Burnett, J. Brook, P. Kanaroglou, C. Giovis, N. Finkelstein, and B. Hutchison. 2004. "Do Socioeconomic Characteristics Modify the Short Term Association between Air Pollution and Mortality? Evidence from a Zonal Time Series in Hamilton, Canada." *Journal of Epidemiology and Community Health* 58(1): 31–40.

Jousilahti, P., V. Salomaa, V. Rasi, E. Vahtera, and T. Palosuo. 2003. "Association of Markers of Systemic Inflammation, C Reactive Protein, Serum Amyloid a, and Fibrinogen, with Socioeconomic Status." *Journal of Epidemiology and Community Health* 57(9): 730–33.

Kapczinski, Flavio, Eduard Vieta, Ana C. Andreazza, Benicio N. Frey, Fabiano A. Gomes, Juliana Tramontina, Marcia Kauer-Sant'anna, Rodrigo Grassi-Oliveira, and Robert M. Post. 2008. "Allostatic Load in Bipolar Disorder: Implications for Pathophysiology and Treatment." *Neuroscience and Biobehavioral Reviews* 32(4): 675–92.

Kaplan, Jay R., and Stephen B. Manuck. 1999. "Status, Stress, and Atherosclerosis: The Role of Environment and Individual Behavior." *Annals of the New York Academy of Sciences* 896:145–61.

Karlamangla, Arun S., Burton H. Singer, Bruce S. McEwen, John W. Rowe, and Teresa E. Seeman. 2002. "Allostatic Load as a Predictor of Functional Decline. Macarthur Studies of Successful Aging." *Journal of Clinical Epidemiology* 55(7): 696–710.

Kawachi, Ichiro, Graham A. Colditz, Alberto Ascherio, Eric B. Rimm, Edward Giovannucci, Meir J. Stampfer, and Walter C. Willett. 1996. "A Prospective Study of Social Networks in Relation to Total Mortality and Cardiovascular Disease in Men in the USA." *Journal of Epidemiology and Community Health* 50(3): 245–51.

Kawachi, Ichiro, David Sparrow, Pantel S. Vokonas, and Scott T. Weiss. 1994. "Symptoms of Anxiety and Risk of Coronary Heart Disease. The Normative Aging Study." *Circulation* 90(5): 2225–29.

Kawakami, N., T. Tanigawa, S. Araki, A. Nakata, S. Sakurai, K. Yokoyama, and Y. Morita. 1997. "Effects of Job Strain on Helper-Inducer (Cd4+Cd29+) and Suppressor-Inducer (Cd4+Cd45ra+) T Cells in Japanese Blue-Collar Workers." *Psychotherapy and Psychosomatics* 66:192–98.

Kiecolt-Glaser, Janice K., Jason R. Dura, Carl E. Speicher, O. Joseph Trask, and Ronald Glaser. 1991. "Spousal Caregivers of Dementia Victims: Longitudinal Changes in Immunity and Health." *Psychosomatic Medicine* 53(4): 345–62.

Kiecolt-Glaser, Janice K., Warren Garner, Carl Speicher, Gerald M. Penn, Jane Holliday, and Ronald Glaser. 1984. "Psychosocial Modifiers of Immunocompetence in Medical Students." *Psychosomatic Medicine* 46(1): 7–14.

Kiecolt-Glaser, Janice K., and Ronald Glaser. 1999. "Chronic Stress and Mortality among Older Adults." *Journal of the American Medical Association* 282(23): 2259–60.

———. 2002. "Depression and Immune Function: Central Pathways to Morbidity and Mortality." *Journal of Psychosomatic Research* 53(4): 873–76.

Kiecolt-Glaser, Janice K., P. T. Marucha, W. B. Malarkey, A. M. Mercado, and Ronald Glaser. 1995. "Slowing of Wound Healing by Psychological Stress." *Lancet* 346(8984): 1194–96.

Koob, George F. 2008. "Alcoholism, Corticotropin-Releasing Factor, and Molecular Genetic Allostasis." *Biological Psychiatry* 63(2): 137–38.

Li, Shenghu, Wei Chen, Sathanur R. Srinivasan, and Gerald S. Berenson. 2004. "Childhood Blood Pressure as a Predictor of Arterial Stiffness in Young Adults: The Bogalusa Heart Study." *Hypertension* 43(3): 541–46.

Libby, Peter, Paul M. Ridker, and Attilio Maseri. 2002. "Inflammation and Atherosclerosis." *Circulation* 105(9): 1135–43.

Liu, Dong, Josie Diorio, Beth Tannenbaum, Christian Caldji, Darlene Francis, Alison Freedman, Shakti Sharma, Deborah Pearson, Paul M. Plotsky, and Michael J. Meaney. 1997. "Maternal Care, Hippocampal Glucocorticoid Receptors, and Hypothalamic-Pituitary-Adrenal Responses to Stress." *Science* 277(5332): 1659–62.

Lupien, S. J., F. Maheu, M. Tu, A. Fiocco, and T. E. Schramek. 2007. "The Effects of Stress and Stress Hormones on Human Cognition: Implications for the Field of Brain and Cognition." *Brain and Cognition* 65(3): 209–37.

Lupien, Sonia J., Mony de Leon, Susan de Santi, Antonio Convit, Chaim Tarshish, N. P. V. Nair, Mira Thakur, Bruce S. McEwen, Richard L. Hauger, and Michael J. Meaney. 1998. "Cortisol Levels during Human Aging Predict Hippocampal Atrophy and Memory Deficits." *Nature Neuroscience* 1(1): 69–73.

Lynch, John, Niklas Krause, George A. Kaplan, Jaakko Tuomilehto, and Jukka T. Salonen. 1997. "Workplace Conditions, Socioeconomic Status, and the Risk of Mortality and Acute Myocardial Infarction: The Kuopio Ischemic Heart Disease Risk Factor Study." *American Journal of Public Health* 87(4): 617–22.

MacQueen, Glenda M., Stephanie Campbell, Bruce S. McEwen, Kathryn Macdonald, Shigeko Amano, Russell T. Joffe, Claude Nahmias, and L. Trevor Young. 2003. "Course of Illness, Hippocampal Function, and Hippocampal Volume in Major Depression." *Proceedings of the National Academy of Sciences Online (US)* 100(3): 1387–92.

Maraldi, Cinzia, Stefano Volpato, Brenda W. Penninx, Kristine Yaffe, Eleanor M. Simonsick, Elsa S. Strotmeyer, Matteo Cesari, Stephen B. Kritchevsky, Sara Perry, Hilsa N. Ayonayon, and Marco Pahor. 2007. "Diabetes Mellitus, Glycemic Control, and Incident Depressive Symptoms among 70- to 79-Year-Old Persons: The Health, Aging, and Body Composition Study." *Archives of Internal Medicine* 167(11): 1137–44.

Marshall, Gailen D., Jr., Sandeep K. Agarwal, Camille

Lloyd, Lorenzo Cohen, Evelyn M. Henninger, and Gloria J. Morris. 1998. "Cytokine Dysregulation Associated with Exam Stress in Healthy Medical Students." *Brain Behavior and Immunity* 12(4): 297–307.

Marsland, A. L., E. A. Bachen, S. Cohen, B. Rabin, and S. B. Manuck. 2002. "Stress, Immune Reactivity and Susceptibility to Infectious Disease." *Physiology and Behavior* 77(4/5): 711–16.

McCarty, R. 1985. "Sympathetic-Adrenal Medullary and Cardiovascular Responses to Acute Cold Stress in Adult and Aged Rats." *Journal of the Autonomic Nervous System* 12(1): 15–22.

McDade, Thomas W., Sharon Williams, and J. Josh Snodgrass. 2007. "What a Drop Can Do: Dried Blood Spots as a Minimally Invasive Method for Integrating Biomarkers into Population-Based Research." *Demography* 44(4): 899–925.

McEwen, Bruce S. 1998. "Protective and Damaging Effects of Stress Mediators." *New England Journal of Medicine* 338(3): 171–79.

———. 2000. "Protective and Damaging Effects of Stress Mediators: Central Role of the Brain." *Progress in Brain Research* 12:225–34.

———. 2008. "Central Effects of Stress Hormones in Health and Disease: Understanding the Protective and Damaging Effects of Stress and Stress Mediators." *European Journal of Pharmacology* 583(2/3): 174–85.

McEwen, Bruce S., and Elizabeth N. Lasley. 2003. "Allostatic Load: When Protection Gives Way to Damage." *Advances in Mind-Body Medicine* 19(1): 28–33.

McEwen, Bruce S., and Teresa E. Seeman. 1999. "Protective and Damaging Effects of Mediators of Stress: Elaborating and Testing the Concepts of Allostasis and Allostatic Load." *Annals of the New York Academy of Sciences* 896:30–47.

McEwen, Bruce S., and Eliot Stellar. 1993. "Stress and the Individual: Mechanisms Leading to Disease." *Archives of Internal Medicine* 153(18): 2093–2101.

Meaney, Michael J., David H. Aitken, Chayann van Berkel, Seema Bhatnagar, and Robert M. Sapolsky. 1988. "Effect of Neonatal Handling on Age-Related Impairments Associated with the Hippocampus." *Science* 239(4841, pt. 1): 766–68.

Meaney, Michael J., Josie Diorio, Darlene Francis, Judith Widdowson, Patricia LaPlante, Christian Caldji, Shakti Sharma, Jonathan R. Seckl, and Paul M. Plotsky. 1996. "Early Environmental Regulation of Forebrain Glucocorticoid Receptor Gene Expression: Implications for Adrenocortical Responses to Stress." *Developmental Neuroscience* 18(1/2): 49–72.

Mendelson, Tamar, Rebecca C. Thurston, and Laura D. Kubzansky. 2008. "Affective and Cardiovascular

Effects of Experimentally-Induced Social Status." *Health Psychology* 27(4): 482–89.

Mendes, I. A. 2001. "Experiencing and Coping with Situations of Professional Stress." *Revista de Latino-Americana Enfermagem* 9(2): 1.

Merkin, S. S., R. Basurto-Davila, A. Karlamangla, C. E. Bird, N. Lurie, J. Escarce, and T. Seeman. 2009. "Neighborhoods and Cumulative Biological Risk Profiles by Race/Ethnicity in a National Sample of U.S. Adults: NHANES III." *Annals of Epidemiology* 19(3): 194–201.

Mills, Paul J., Henry Yu, Michael G. Ziegler, Thomas Patterson, and Igor Grant. 1999. "Vulnerable Caregivers of Patients with Alzheimer's Disease Have a Deficit in Circulating Cd62l- T Lymphocytes." *Psychosomatic Medicine* 61(2): 168–74.

Mittal, Vijay A., Lauren M. Ellman, and Tyrone D. Cannon. 2008. "Gene-Environment Interaction and Covariation in Schizophrenia: The Role of Obstetric Complications." *Schizophrenia Bulletin* 34:1083–94.

Muller, H. K., D. J. Lugg, and D. Quinn. 1995. "Cell Mediated Immunity in Antarctic Wintering Personnel; 1984–1992." *Immunology and Cell Biology* 73(4): 316–20.

Munoz, Alvaro, and Stephen J. Gange. 1998. "Methodological Issues for Biomarkers and Intermediate Outcomes in Cohort Studies." *Epidemiologic Reviews* 20(1): 29–42.

National Human Genome Research Institute. 2009. "Epigenomics." genome.gov/27532724.

National Library of Medicine. 2009. "National Library of Medicine—Medical Subject Headings: Biological Markers." nlm.nih.gov/cgi/mesh/2009/MB_cgi?mode=andindex=14776andfield=allandHM=andII=andPA=andform=andinput=.

Navas-Acien, Ana, Eliseo Guallar, Ellen K. Silbergeld, and Stephen J. Rothenberg. 2007. "Lead Exposure and Cardiovascular Disease: A Systematic Review." *Environmental Health Perspectives* 115(3): 472–82.

Nguyen, Xuan-Mai T., John Lane, Brian R. Smith, and Ninh T. Nguyen. 2009. "Changes in Inflammatory Biomarkers across Weight Classes in a Representative U.S. Population: A Link between Obesity and Inflammation." *Journal of Gastrointestinal Surgery* 13(7): 1205–12.

Notzon, Francis C., Yuri M. Komarov, Sergei P. Ermakov, Christopher T. Sempos, James S. Marks, and Elena V. Sempos. 1998. "Causes of Declining Life Expectancy in Russia." *Journal of the American Medical Association* 279(10): 793–800.

O'Leary, Ann. 1992. "Self-Efficacy and Health: Behavioral and Stress-Physiological Mediation." *Cognitive Therapy and Research* 16(2): 229–45.

Penninx, Brenda W., Stephen B. Kritchevsky, Kristine Yaffe, Anne B. Newman, Eleanor M. Simonsick, Susan Rubin, Luigi Ferrucci, Tamara Harris, and Marco Pahor. 2003. "Inflammatory Markers and Depressed Mood in Older Persons: Results from the Health, Aging and Body Composition Study." *Biological Psychiatry* 54(5): 566–72.

Pepe, Margaret S., Ruth Etzioni, Ziding Feng, John D. Potter, Mary L. Thompson, Mark Thornquist, Marcy Winget, and Yutaka Yasui. 2001. "Phases of Biomarker Development for Early Detection of Cancer." *Journal of the National Cancer Institute* 93(14): 1054–61.

Peterson, Ulla, Gunnar Bergstrom, Mats Samuelsson, Marie Asberg, and Ake Nygren. 2008. "Reflecting Peer-Support Groups in the Prevention of Stress and Burnout: Randomized Controlled Trial." *Journal of Advanced Nursing* 63(5): 506–16.

Phillips, Anna C., Douglas Carroll, Phil Evans, Jos A. Bosch, Angela Clow, Frank Hucklebridge, and Geoff Der. 2006. "Stressful Life Events Are Associated with Low Secretion Rates of Immunoglobulin A in Saliva in the Middle Aged and Elderly." *Brain Behavior and Immunity* 20(2): 191–97.

Pollitt, Ricardo A., Jay S. Kaufman, Kathryn M. Rose, Ana V. Diez-Roux, Donglin Zeng, and Gerardo Heiss. 2007. "Early-Life and Adult Socioeconomic Status and Inflammatory Risk Markers in Adulthood." *European Journal of Epidemiology* 22(1): 55–66.

Pollitt, Ricardo A., Kathryn M. Rose, and Jay S. Kaufman. 2005. "Evaluating the Evidence for Models of Life Course Socioeconomic Factors and Cardiovascular Outcomes: A Systemic Review." *BMC Public Health* 5(7). biomedcentral.com/content/pdf/1471-2458-5-7.pdf.

Polsky, Daniel, Jalpa A. Doshi, Steven Marcus, David Oslin, Aileen Rothbard, Niku Thomas, and Christy L. Thompson. 2005. "Long-Term Risk for Depressive Symptoms after a Medical Diagnosis." *Archives of Internal Medicine* 165(11): 1260–66.

Poulton, Richie, Avshlom Caspi, Barry J. Milne, W. Murry Thomson, Alan Taylor, Malcolm R. Sears, and Terrie E. Moffitt. 2002. "Association between Children's Experience of Socioeconomic Disadvantage and Adult Health: A Life-Course Study." *Lancet* 360(9346): 1640–45.

Redwine, Laura, Richard L. Hauger, J. Christian Gillin, and Michael Irwin. 2000. "Effects of Sleep and Sleep Deprivation on Interleukin-6, Growth Hormone, Cortisol, and Melatonin Levels in Humans." *Journal of Clinical Endocrinology and Metabolism* 85(10): 3597–3603.

Richards, M., and M. E. J. Wadsworth. 2004. "Long Term Effects of Early Adversity on Cognitive Function." *Archives of Disease in Childhood* 89(10): 922–27.

Richman, Laura S., Gary G. Bennett, Jolynn Pek, Ilene Siegler, and Redford B. Williams Jr. 2007. "Discrimination, Dispositions, and Cardiovascular Responses to Stress." *Health Psychology* 26(6): 675–83.

Ridker, Paul M., Charles H. Hennekens, Julie E. Buring, and Nader Rifai. 2000. "C-Reactive Protein and Other Markers of Inflammation in the Prediction of Cardiovascular Disease in Women." *New England Journal of Medicine* 342(12): 836–43.

Ridker, Paul M., Nader Rifai, Meir J. Stampfer, and Charles H. Hennekens. 2000. "Plasma Concentration of Interleukin-6 and the Risk of Future Myocardial Infarction among Apparently Healthy Men." *Circulation* 101(15): 1767–72.

Rojas, Isolde-Gina, David A. Padgett, John F. Sheridan, and Phillip T. Marucha. 2002. "Stress-Induced Susceptibility to Bacterial Infection during Cutaneous Wound Healing." *Brain Behavior and Immunity* 16(1): 74–84.

Rosengren, A., M. Freden, P. O. Hansson, L. Wilhelmsen, H. Wedel, and H. Eriksson. 2008. "Psychosocial Factors and Venous Thromboembolism: A Long-Term Follow-Up Study of Swedish Men." *Journal of Thrombosis and Haemostasis* 6(4): 558–64.

Ross, Russell. 1999. "Atherosclerosis Is an Inflammatory Disease." *America Heart Journal* 138(5, pt. 2): S419–20.

Rozanski, Alan, James A. Blumenthal, and Jay Kaplan. 1999. "Impact of Psychological Factors on the Pathogenesis of Cardiovascular Disease and Implications for Therapy." *Circulation* 99(16): 2192–2217.

Sapolsky, Robert M. 1999. "Glucocorticoids, Stress, and Their Adverse Neurological Effects: Relevance to Aging." *Experimental Gerontology* 34(6): 721–32.

Sapolsky, Robert M., Lewis C. Krey, and Bruce S. McEwen. 1986. "The Neuroendocrinology of Stress and Aging: The Glucocorticoid Cascade Hypothesis." *Endocrine Reviews* 7(3): 284–301.

Schulte, P. A., and M. H. Sweeney. 1995. "Ethical Considerations, Confidentiality Issues, Rights of Human Subjects, and Uses of Monitoring Data in Research and Regulation." *Environmental Health Perspectives* 103, suppl: 369–74.

Seckl, Jonathan R. 2004. "Prenatal Glucocorticoids and Long-Term Programming." *European Journal of Endocrinology* 151(3): U49–62.

Seeman, Teresa E., Bruce S. McEwen, Burton H. Singer, Marilyn S. Albert, and John W. Rowe. 1997. "Increase in Urinary Cortisol Excretion and Memory Declines: Macarthur Studies of Successful Aging." *Journal of Clinical Endocrinology and Metabolism* 82(8): 2458–65.

Seeman, Teresa E., Sharon S. Merkin, Eileen Crimmins, Brandon Koretz, Sue Charette, and Arun S. Karlamangla. 2008. "Education, Income and Ethnic Differences in Cumulative Biological Risk Profiles in a National Sample of U.S. Adults: NHANES III (1988–1994)." *Social Science and Medicine* 66(1): 72–87.

Seeman, Teresa E., Burton H. Singer, John W. Rowe, Ralph I. Horwitz, and Bruce S. McEwen. 1997. "Price of Adaptation: Allostatic Load and Its Health Consequences; Macarthur Studies of Successful Aging." *Archives of Internal Medicine* 157(19): 2259–68.

Segerstrom, Suzanne C., and Gregory E. Miller. 2004. "Psychological Stress and the Human Immune System: A Meta-Analytic Study of 30 Years of Inquiry." *Psychological Bulletin* 130(4): 601–30.

Selye, Hans. 1951. "The General Adaptation Syndrome and the Diseases of Adaptation." *American Journal of Medicine* 10(5): 549–55.

Shively, Carol A., Kathy Laber-Laird, and Raymond F. Anton. 1997. "Behavior and Physiology of Social Stress and Depression in Female Cynomolgus Monkeys." *Biological Psychiatry* 41(8): 871–82.

Steptoe, Andrew. 2007. *Depression and Physical Illness.* New York: Cambridge University Press.

Steptoe, Andrew, S. R. Kunz-Ebrecht, and N. Owen. 2003. "Lack of Association between Depressive Symptoms and Markers of Immune and Vascular Inflammation in Middle-Aged Men and Women." *Psychological Medicine* 33(4): 667–74.

Sterling, P., and J. Eyer. 1988. "Allostasis: A New Paradigm to Explain Arousal Pathology." In *Handbook of Life Stress, Cognition and Health*, ed. S. Fisher and J. Reason, 631–51. New York: Wiley and Sons.

Taaffe, Dennis R., Tamara B. Harris, Luigi Ferrucci, John Rowe, and Teresa E. Seeman. 2000. "Cross-Sectional and Prospective Relationships of Interleukin-6 and C-Reactive Protein with Physical Performance in Elderly Persons: Macarthur Studies of Successful Aging." *Journals of Gerontology Series A: Biological and Medical Sciences* 55(12): M709–15.

Talge, Nicole M., Charles Neal, and Vivette Glover. 2007. "Antenatal Maternal Stress and Long-Term Effects on Child Neurodevelopment: How and Why?" *Journal of Child Psychology and Psychiatry* 48(3/4): 245–61.

Teicher, Martin H., Akemi Tomoda, and Susan L. Andersen. 2006. "Neurobiological Consequences of Early Stress and Childhood Maltreatment: Are Results from Human and Animal Studies Comparable?" *Annals of the New York Academy of Sciences* 1071:313–23.

Theorell, Tores, and Robert A. Karasek. 1996. "Current

Issues Relating to Psychosocial Job Strain and Cardiovascular Disease Research." *Journal of Occupational Health Psychology* 1(1): 9–26.

Tiemeier, Henning. 2003. "Biological Risk Factors for Late Life Depression." *European Journal of Epidemiology* 18(8): 745–50.

Tworoger, Shelley S., and Susan E. Hankinson. 2006. "Collection, Processing, and Storage of Biological Samples in Epidemiologic Studies: Sex Hormones, Carotenoids, Inflammatory Markers, and Proteomics as Examples." *Cancer Epidemiology, Biomarkers and Prevention* 15(9): 1578–81.

Uchino, Bert N., John T. Cacioppo, and Janice K. Kiecolt-Glaser. 1996. "The Relationship between Social Support and Physiological Processes: A Review with Emphasis on Underlying Mechanisms and Implications for Health." *Psychological Bulletin* 119(3): 488–531.

Valdimarsdottir, Heiddis B., and Arthur A. Stone. 1997. "Psychosocial Factors and Secretory Immunoglobulin A." *Critical Reviews in Oral Biology and Medicine* 8(4): 461–74.

Vaught, Jimmie B. 2006. "Blood Collection, Shipment, Processing, and Storage." *Cancer Epidemiology, Biomarkers and Prevention* 15(9): 1582–84.

Vgontzas, Alexandros N., Edward O. Bixler, H. M. Lin, Paolo Prolo, G. Trakada, and George P. Chrousos. 2005. "Il-6 and Its Circadian Secretion in Humans." *Neuroimmunomodulation* 12(3): 131–40.

Vgontzas, Alexandros N., Dimitris A. Papanicolaou, Edward O. Bixler, Angela Lotsikas, Keith Zachman, Anthony Kales, Paolo Prolo, Ma-Li Wong, Julio Licinio, Philip W. Gold, Ramon C. Hermida, George Mastorakos, and George P. Chrousos. 1999. "Circadian Interleukin-6 Secretion and Quantity and Depth of Sleep." *Journal of Clinical Endocrinology and Metabolism* 84(8): 2603–7.

Vyas, Ajai, Rupshi Mitra, B. S. Shankaranarayana Rao, and Sumantra Chattarji. 2002. "Chronic Stress Induces Contrasting Patterns of Dendritic Remodeling in Hippocampal and Amygdaloid Neurons." *Journal of Neuroscience* 22(15): 6810–18.

Welberg, L. A., and Jonathan R. Seckl. 2001. "Prenatal Stress, Glucocorticoids and the Programming of the Brain." *Journal of Neuroendocrinology* 13(2): 113–28.

Wilkinson, Charles W., Elaine R. Peskind, and Murray A. Raskind. 1997. "Decreased Hypothalamic-Pituitary-Adrenal Axis Sensitivity to Cortisol Feedback Inhibition in Human Aging." *Neuroendocrinology* 65(1): 79–90.

Williams, Redford B., Douglas A. Marchuk, Ilene C. Siegler, John C. Barefoot, Michael J. Helms, Beverly H. Brummett, Richard S. Surwit, James D. Lane, Cynthia M. Kuhn, Kishore M. Gadde, Allison Ashley-Koch, Ingrid K. Svenson, and Saul M. Schanberg. 2008. "Childhood Socioeconomic Status and Serotonin Transporter Gene Polymorphism Enhance Cardiovascular Reactivity to Mental Stress." *Psychosomatic Medicine* 70(1): 32–39.

Willis, Robert, and Maxine Weinstein. 2001. "Stretching Social Surveys to Include Bioindicators: Possibilities for the Health and Retirement Study, Experience from the Taiwan Study of the Elderly." In *Cells and Surveys: Should Biological Measures Be Included in Social Research?* ed. C. E. Finch, J. W. Vaupel, and K. Kinsella. Washington, D.C.: National Academies Press.

Yan, Lijing L., Kiang Liu, Martha L. Daviglus, Laura A. Colangelo, Catarina I. Kiefe, Stephen Sidney, Karen A. Matthews, and Philip Greenland. 2006. "Education, 15-Year Risk Factor Progression, and Coronary Artery Calcium in Young Adulthood and Early Middle Age: The Coronary Artery Risk Development in Young Adults Study." *Journal of the American Medical Association* 295(15): 1793–1800.

Zubin, Joseph, and Bonnie Spring. 1977. "Vulnerability: A New View of Schizophrenia." *Journal of Abnormal Psychology* 86(2): 103–26.

24

Gene-Environment Interaction and Medical Sociology

Sara Shostak, Brandeis University

Jeremy Freese, Northwestern University

The boundaries between sociology and biology have long been sites of tension and contestation (Anderson 1967; Pescosolido 2006).[1] In part, these contestations emerge from a concern that biological accounts of the production of human difference pose a threat to sociology's defining focus on social and environmental causes of human health and social outcomes (Duster 2006). Medical sociologists have been at the vanguard of efforts to find productive modes of engagement between the social sciences and contemporary human genetics. Increasingly, these efforts center on gene-environment interaction. We consider here two domains of social scientific inquiry that address gene-environment interaction vis-à-vis health and illness. First, we discuss analyses of the social implications of research on gene-environment interaction, including studies of public understandings and beliefs about genetic and environmental causes of health and social outcomes. Second, we consider research that uses information about genetics and gene-environment interaction as a lever to reveal mechanisms of social and social psychological causation of health and illness. Taken together, this work points to the importance of moving past the assumption of an essential tension between genetic and social (or other environmental) explanations for health and illness toward more integrative analyses that can encompass multiple and simultaneous forms of causation, including the "looping effects" (Hacking 1995) of genetic categories and the enduring influence of fundamental causes of health and illness, especially as capacities for intervention change (Link and Phelan 1995; Freese and Lutfey, forthcoming).

Genes, Environments, and Health

At the turn of the century, gene-environment interaction emerged at the center of research funded by the National Institutes of Health (NIH) (Schwartz and Collins 2007), as well as in the human sciences more broadly (Rutter, Moffitt, and Caspi 2006).[2] As just one measure of its currency at the NIH, in 2006, health and human services secretary Mike Leavitt announced that the president's budget proposal for fiscal year 2007 would include $68 million for the Genes and Environment Initiative, an NIH research effort to combine genetic analysis and environmental technology development to understand how gene-environment interactions contribute to the etiology of common diseases.[3] The prominent role of the concept of gene-environment interaction in this initiative was highlighted in the press release that announced it: "Differences in our genetic makeup certainly influence our risks of developing various illnesses.... We only have to look at family medical histories to know that is true. But whether a genetic predisposition actually makes a person sick depends on the *interaction between genes and the environment*" (NIEHS 2006 [emphasis added]).

In the United Kingdom, the UK Biobank represents a massive investment on the part of the Medical Research Council, the Wellcome Trust, and the Department of Health, with the goal of elucidating "the complex interplay of genetic and environmental factors involved in the aetiology of common diseases" (Tutton, Kaye, and Hoeyer 2004, 284). Gene-environment interaction is also of great interest in the private sector. In the United States, the GEI is to be "accelerated" by the efforts of a public-private partnership, the Genetic Association Information Network (GAIN), a joint venture between the NIH, Pfizer Pharmaceuticals, and the biotech company Affymetrix.

Social scientists also increasingly are taking up questions about gene-environment interaction. Indeed, one of the ironies of the success of the Human Genome Project is that it highlights the imperative for sophisticated conceptualizations and measures of the social environment, long the jurisdiction of sociology (Pescosolido 2006; Perrin and Lee 2007). While not explicitly focused on gene-environment interaction, the recent call for a "sociology of disease," which would incorporate biomarkers into studies of the experience of trajectories of illness, likewise points to the need for knowledge about the intersections of social and biological pathways (Timmermans and Haas 2008). With the inclusion of DNA and biomarker data in large-scale social science data sets (Weinstein, Vaupel, and Wachter 2008; Finch, Vaupel, and Kinsella 2000), the opportunities for sociologists to study gene-environment interaction will proliferate rapidly in the coming years. Likewise, sociologists already have given consideration to social implications of gene-environment interaction, pointing to many concerns and opportunities for the years ahead.

Social Implications of Research on Gene-Environment Interaction

Human genetics has been centrally concerned with understanding how genes work as causes of development and of disease and has turned only recently to studies of gene-environment interaction. As knowledge claims diffuse beyond the laboratory, they may serve as warrants for individual and collective action and transform social policies and institutions. Medical sociology offers at least three important vantage points on the social implications of genetic research—geneticization, biosociality, and public understanding of genetics.

Geneticization

As introduced by Lippman (1991, 19), geneticization refers to "an ongoing process by which differences between individuals are reduced to their DNA codes, with most disorders, behaviours, and physiological variations defined, at least in part, as genetic in origin." Geneticization is both "a way of thinking" about human differences, especially in the context of health and illness, and also "a way of doing," as genetic technologies are "applied to diagnose, treat, and categorize conditions previously identified in other ways" (Lippman 1998). Like many words that end in *-tion*, geneticization refers simultaneously to a social process and to its results (Hacking 1999, 36).

Much as with "medicalization" (Conrad 1992), there has been disagreement over whether the concept of geneticization is primarily "a heuristic tool" in a moral debate (ten Have 2001) or maintains sufficient neutrality to serve empirical research (Hedgecoe 1998).[4] Writing on geneticization often centers on a number of interlocking concerns about genetics as a "dominant discourse" (Lippman 1991, 18) with myriad potential negative social implications. These concerns include *genetic reductionism*, in which a complex understanding of the causes of human development is displaced by one in which genes are perceived as the "true cause" of difference (Sloan 2000, 17); *genetic determinism*, in which genes are taken as inevitably implying traits and behaviors (Lippman 1992; Nelkin and Lindee 2004; Rothman 2001); *genetic essentialism*, in which genetics becomes a dominant way to talk about fundamental life issues such as "guilt and responsibility, power and privilege, intellectual or emotional status"

(Nelkin and Lindee 2004, 16); and *genetic fatalism*, the belief that if a trait or behavior has a genetic etiology, then it is fixed and unchangeable (Alper and Beckwith 1993).[5]

In the context of health and illness, sociologists have been especially concerned about the possibility that such dynamics will contribute to the individualization of health and illness, with social, political, and economic etiological explanations relegated to secondary status or discredited altogether (Conrad 1999; Duster 2003, 2006; Hedgecoe 2001; Lippman 1991; Rothman 2001). Duster (2003) argues that extensive public sector investment in genetic research will disproportionately and negatively impact blacks by diverting attention and resources away from social environmental factors that contribute to increasing rates of lung cancer and cardiovascular disease in the African American population (see also Chaufan 2007). Related, social scientists have been leading critics of the potential of genetic information to reify social categories such as race, especially in the context of biomedical research (Duster 2005; Lee, Mountain, and Koenig 2001; Ossorio and Duster 2005). Recent work has considered also whether geneticization will result in increased stigmatization of people affected by mental illness or their relatives (Phelan 2005).

The consequences of scientists' emerging focus on gene-environment interaction for geneticization remains contingent upon how gene-environment interaction is conceptualized (Shostak 2003) and materialized in the lab (Hall 2005; Landecker, n.d.), articulated in biomedical texts (Hedgecoe 2001) and practices (Cunningham-Burley and Kerr 1999), and reported to the public (Horwitz 2005). At each of these sites, research highlights the multiplicity (Mol 2002) of the concept of gene-environment interaction and, concomitantly, the challenges of predicting its implications. For example, Shostak (2003) demonstrates that in the environmental health sciences, gene-environment interaction historically has been the focus of two very different lines of inquiry, one focused on how individual genetic susceptibilities predispose individuals to illness under specific environmental conditions, and the other focused on how environmental conditions affect genes and gene expression. Adding

further complexity, how scientists in either line of research define "the environment" varies widely and may include the interior of a cell (as the environment of DNA) and the interior of a human body (as the environment of cells, organs, and organ systems), as well as the ambient environment (air, water, and soil) and the social environment (Shostak 2003). The complexities involved in defining, operationalizing, and measuring environmental influences on health may enhance "the allure of specificity" of genetic explanations (Conrad 1999).[6] Further, Hedgecoe (2001) describes a "narrative of enlightened geneticization" which accepts a role for environmental factors in disease etiology, while consistently prioritizing genetic causes, Such narratives of "enlightened geneticization" appear to be replicated in popular media coverage of research on gene-environment interaction, which selectively emphasizes genetic influences, while largely ignoring environmental causes (Horwitz 2005). This is concordant with the tendency toward "genetic optimism" which characterizes the reporting of genetics research, especially in the United States (Conrad 2001).[7]

At the same time, there is evidence that the social environment shapes understandings and uses of genetic information. Ethnographic and cross-national investigations have found that local knowledge (Rapp 1999), national contexts (Parthasarathy 2007; Prainsack and Siegal 2006; Remennick 2006), and everyday understandings of risk, kinship, and inheritance (Gibbon 2007; Richards and Ponder 1996) shape how people understand and make use of genetic information in daily life. Indeed, even in the context of prenatal genetics, arguably the clinical setting where genetic testing is most standardized and routinized, social factors shape both the use of genetic technologies and the interpretation of test results (Franklin and Roberts 2006; Lock et al. 2006; Markens, Browner, and Press 1999; Rapp 1999; Whitmarsh et al. 2007). Social scientists have highlighted also how the daily practices of diagnosis and disease management may mitigate geneticization, even for conditions with simple genetic etiologies such as hereditary polycystic kidney disease, a life-threatening, autosomal dominant trait for which genetic testing is available (Cox and Starzomski 2004). More broadly, existing discourse, public opinion, and organizational arrangements may strongly condition the potential consequences of findings of genetic influence (Shostak, Conrad, and Horwitz 2008).

The expanding focus of the life sciences on complex biological systems (Fujimura 2005; Kitano 2002) and epigenetics (Feinberg 2008) can be expected to continue to challenge how social scientists think about gene-environment interaction and its social implications. Broadly speaking, epigenetics highlights processes by which cellular environments can modify genetic expression. The key insight of epigenetics is that gene expression can be altered by environmental exposures, even without changes in the actual sequence of DNA, and that these patterns of gene expression and regulation are heritable (Francis et al., 1999; Meaney 2001). Thus, scientists are increasingly focused on how social and historical factors can be seen as interacting directly with DNA, although how to operationalize such factors in laboratory settings (Landecker, n.d.) and how to connect social science data to such biologically fine-grained processes are major challenges. Meanwhile, the concept of biosociality raises questions about how genetic information may further blur boundaries between categories such as nature and culture, genes and environments.

Biosociality

In articulating the concept of "biosociality," anthropologist Paul Rabinow argued that advances in biological knowledge would yield new forms of collective identity and an increasingly efficacious orientation of individuals toward themselves as material entities. Consequently, "nature will be known and remade through technique and will finally become artificial, just as culture becomes natural" (1996, 99). In addition, Rabinow predicted, a variety of microlevel political practices and discourses embedding genetic information in social life would make the new genetics a potent force in reshaping society (98–99). In part, this is because the identification of genetic risks simultaneously will destabilize extant subjectivities and contribute to the emergence of new biosocial individual and group identities, which are defined

not by traditional subject positions, but rather as sites defined by their relation to means, norms, and other measures of probabilistic risks (100).[8]

These new identities are expected to serve as the basis for innovative forms of social organization and interaction, as biosocial groups "will have medical specialists, laboratories, narratives, traditions, and a heavy panoply of pastoral keepers to help them experience, share, intervene in and 'understand' their fate" (Rabinow 1996, 102). Groups of persons at risk for illness or their family members and allies are reshaping and reorienting social movement organization and advocacy (Callon and Rabeharisoa 2003; Gibbon 2007), relationships between citizens and the state (Epstein 2007; Heath, Rapp, and Taussig 2004; Petryna 2002), and modes of capital production and economies, which increasingly rely on innovative relationships between disease advocacy groups and scientists (Heath, Rapp, and Taussig 2004; Novas 2007, 2008; Silverman 2008; Sunder Rajan 2006). Research on biosociality focuses also on how genetics fosters the reworking of extant identities, especially race and ethnicity (Abu El-Haj 2007; Atkinson, Glasner, and Greenslade 2007; Gibbon and Novas 2008; Hacking 2006; Nelson 2008; Reardon 2004).

In highlighting how genetic information enables new forms of human organization and agency, the concept of biosociality stands in stark contrast to the assumption of genetic fatalism and calls attention to how individuals make use of genetic information in specific environments. For example, Rose and colleagues (Novas and Rose 2000; Rose 2007) argue that genetic information creates new obligations to act on knowledge to protect health, maximize quality of life, and optimize life chances. In support of this argument, and reminiscent of Parsons's conceptualization of the sick role (1951), Condit and colleagues (2006) find that while laypeople do not hold individuals responsible for their genetic endowments, they still expect individuals to work to override negative genetic predispositions to whatever extent they are able. Thus, at least with respect to health, the rise of genetic science need not be coterminous with feelings of hopelessness or inefficacy. Rather, genetic research has secured enormous public funding precisely due to hopes that understanding genetic causation will lead to the development of improved capacity for intervention, as seen especially today in the hope that genetics will yield a new era of personalized medicine (Novas 2007; Sunder Rajan 2006).

Thus, biosociality highlights the role of social relations in shaping social and material consequences of genetic variation. Indeed, for medical sociologists, a key insight of the literature on biosociality is that genetic causation of health and illness depends not just on the causality of genes or gene-environment interactions, but on the causality associated with social action based on scientific knowledge claims about genes. For example, increasingly, one response to diagnosis is to contribute to collective efforts to increase and improve the scientific study of one's illness; healthy individuals with genetic predispositions now lobby the state to fund scientists to discover knowledge that can be translated into new technologies that will intervene to prevent their genes from causing pathological consequences (Epstein 1996; Novas 2007; Petryna 2002; Silverman 2008). This trend points to the importance of research on how people understand genes and environments as causes of health and illness.

Public Understandings and Beliefs about Genetics, Environments, Health, and Illness

Assessing public perceptions and opinions provides an important means of understanding how people interpret social problems such as health inequalities, and how they respond to policy initiatives regarding health and illness (Schnittker, Freese, and Powell 2000). Traditionally, public opinion research has investigated attributions for health and social outcomes by considering genetics, environmental factors, and individual behavior as independent causes. Innovation in this area is clearly warranted to explore public understandings of gene-environment interaction and its implications for health and social policy.

Of course, there are many groups within "the public" with varying interests and perspectives regarding the causes of health and illness. Much of the early research on beliefs about genes as causes of health and illness focused on attitudes toward genetic testing for specific conditions. Such studies were largely clinically oriented and tended to draw on highly selected nonprobability samples of individuals from families affected by illnesses with genetic etiology (e.g., Lafayette et al. 1999; Lerman et al. 1994). While these studies provide important insights about how people in families affected by specific illnesses conceptualize genetic risk for those illnesses, they do not assess uses of genetic attributions more broadly.

Research on attitudes toward genetic testing also has been undertaken to assess racial/ethnic differences in use of genetic testing. This research indicates that African Americans and Latinos are more eager than are whites to avail themselves of both prenatal and adult genetic testing (Singer, Antonucci, and Hoewyk 2004, 41). One might infer that endorsement of genetic testing reflects underlying beliefs about genes as causes for these traits. Importantly, however, the study questions asserted the importance of genes for the disease outcome *as a premise to the question*, and therefore this work does not speak directly to beliefs about the importance of genes for individual health or social outcomes (33).

On the whole, surveys of representative samples of the U.S. population make plain that a strong majority of Americans regard genes as important determinants of health, illness, and other life outcomes. Over 90 percent of U.S. respondents report genetic makeup as at least somewhat important for physical illness, and almost two-thirds report the same for success in life (Shostak et al. 2009). Additionally, belief in the importance of genetics for particular outcomes may be increasing. For example, in 1979, 36 percent of respondents reported that heredity was more important than the environment in determining whether or not a person was overweight, while in 1995, 63 percent of respondents attributed "being substantially overweight" to genetics (Singer, Corning, and Lamias 1998, 637–38).[9] That said, it is unclear whether there has been any overall shift toward belief in genetics, as widespread notions of the importance of "breeding," "constitution," or "inborn character" predate the discovery of DNA (Kevles 1985).

Additionally, people appear to believe that the causal importance of genetics varies for different outcomes, in that the attribution of genetic influence does not rule out perception of the importance of other factors (Parrott, Silk, and Condit 2003), including both the environment and, especially, individual behavior (Condit et al. 2004, 260–61). For example, when asked to partition pie charts to represent the relative contribution of genes, the physical environment, the social environment, and personal action, participants assigned to "genes" 71 percent of etiologic responsibility for height, 41 percent for weight, 54 percent for breast and prostate cancer, 26 percent for talent, and 40 percent for mental abilities (Parrott, Silk, and Condit 2003). Additionally, when asked to compare the role of genes and individual behaviors in determining health outcomes, generally people assigned a greater role to personal behavior (Condit et al. 2004). Poll data similarly indicate that endorsement of genetics as an explanation for health and social outcomes varies by the outcome of interest and, possibly, perceptions of individual responsibility for specific outcomes. For example, in a 1995 Harris poll (n = 1005), 90 percent of respondents attributed success in life to learning and experience (vs. 8 percent to "genes you inherit"), while 63 percent of respondents attributed being substantially overweight to genetics (vs. 32 percent who chose learning and experience) (Singer, Corning, and Lamias 1998).

What outcomes are regarded as "more genetic" may be influenced by a cultural schema, at least in the United States, in which individual characteristics perceived as closer to the body are seen as more strongly caused by genetics. A recent study of genetic attributions for individual outcomes found that physical health is perceived as more strongly genetically influenced than is mental health; mental health is perceived as more strongly genetically influenced than is personality; and personality is seen as more strongly genetically influenced than is success in life (Shostak et al. 2009). Such a cultural schema may reflect the legacy of Cartesian dualism, which insists that the causes of bodily states, such as physical illness, are to be located in the body (Scheper-Hughes and Lock 1987). In addition, many people have a strong notion of individual will as a causal force independent from either genetics or environ-

ment, which could be seen as more important for social outcomes (Condit et al. 2004).

While research has considered the possibility of various sorts of social cleavages in beliefs about genes as causes of health and social outcomes, race/ethnic differences have received the most attention. This focus emerges in part from concerns about eugenics (Kevles 1985; Duster 2003) and the possibility that genetic information again could be used to reify racial classifications (Omi and Winant 1994; Duster 2005), undermine progressive policies, and promote discriminatory programs (for reviews, see Condit and Bates 2005; Condit et al. 2004). Reflecting on such abuses, social scientists have hypothesized that the historical use of biological claims to justify racial inequality will prompt minorities to be more skeptical of genetics. Using vignette data from the General Social Survey, Schnittker, Freese, and Powell (2000, 1109, 1112) found that blacks are less likely than whites to endorse genetic explanations of mental illness. In contrast, however, Shostak and colleagues find that blacks and Latinos rated genetic makeup on average as more important for a set of individual attributes than did whites. Black respondents were relatively more averse than whites to endorsing genetic makeup as important to individual differences in intelligence—the outcome for which historical abuse arguably has been most pervasive and invidious—but that was the only instance in their analysis in which a socially disadvantaged group evinced greater aversion to genetic explanation (Shostak et al. 2009). In an analysis of General Social Surveys since 1990, Hunt (2007) found that blacks were not less likely than whites to regard "innate ability" as important to explaining black-white differences in socioeconomic attainment (12.0 percent of whites and 12.2 percent of blacks).[10]

Despite the conventional wisdom that perceptions of the relative significance of genes and environments as causes of health and illness will be consequential for health and social policy, only a very few studies consider the relationship between beliefs about genetic causes and specific policy attitudes. Shostak and colleagues (2009) find that belief in the importance of genetics for individual differences in outcomes are associated with support for health policies predicated on genetic causes being important, such as supporting human genetics research and genetic screening before marriage. Regarding beliefs in the genetic basis of group differences, Jayaratne and colleagues find that belief in the genetic basis of racial differences is associated with more negative attitudes toward blacks and less support for social policies to help blacks (Jayaratne et al. 2006; see also Keller 2005).[11] In contrast, genetic attributions for differences in sexual orientation are associated with greater tolerance toward gay men and lesbians, as measured by attitudes toward whether gays should marry, whether gay couples should adopt, and whether gay people should be allowed to teach elementary school (Jayaratne et al. 2006; see also Tygart 2000).

We have much to learn about how people make sense of theories and data about gene-environment interaction. As the social sciences increasingly are considering the relevance of gene-environment interaction to outcomes of longstanding sociological interest (Freese 2008), it is imperative that future research on public beliefs and opinions about genetics include questions on this broadening range of outcomes and their associations with orientations to specific health and social policies. Such policies will have a critical role in determining the consequences of knowledge about gene-environment interactions, as they shape the opportunities that people have both to make use of medical interventions and treatments developed using this knowledge and to avoid identified health risks (Link and Phelan 1995; Lutfey and Freese 2005).

Gene-Environment Interaction and Social Causation of Health and Illness

As noted previously, social environmental conditions have historically often been interpreted as competing with genetics in the explanation of disease. The notion that lung cancers were invariably genetically determined—and so any relationship between smoking and lung cancer had to reflect a common genetic cause—was the main alternative used to justify doubt that smoking causes cancer (Brandt 2007). Today, funding for research into the possibility that genetic dif-

ferences may explain part of the observed racial disparities in health has been decried by some who believe this delays attention to the obviously fundamental role of socioeconomic differences, unequal treatment in the health-care system, and discrimination-related stressors (Sankar et al. 2004; Chaufan 2007). Sociological writing on the contingency and capriciousness of diagnostic processes may likewise be seen as contradictory to research attempting to document associations between genetic differences and diagnoses (Brown 1995; Zavestoski et al. 2004).

More recently, there has been stronger emphasis on constructive and integrative engagement between genetics and social science (Pescosolido 2006). This has been exemplified by the push for including "biomarkers" in social science data resources (Singer and Ryff 2001; Finch, Vaupel, and Kinsella 2000; Timmermans and Haas 2008; Weinstein, Vaupel, and Wachter 2008). For those who study disease, of course, biological measurement is already fundamental; if anything, it is remarkable how much epidemiology and social science have accomplished with self-report surveys. In thinking about how biomarkers may be incorporated into social research, a key distinction needs to be drawn between measures of genotype and measures of cortisol, immune response, allostatic load, or other of what Freese, Li, and Wade (2003) call "proximate" biomarkers. The latter are interesting to social scientists primarily for their role as mediating variables, that is, in elucidating the actual physiological process by which life circumstances get under the skin. Genotypic measures, by contrast, are quintessential *moderators*. While epigenetics provides ways in which external processes can influence the cellular expression of genes, the genotype itself is not influenced by life circumstances, even though the two interact in the production of health and other phenotypic outcomes.

Although discourse about genetic causes in much of social science is heavily freighted by a false moral equation of genetics with inevitability, this is much less the case in health research, which has always been premised on the possibility of salutary manipulation of the body. A favorite example for illustrating the pervasive interpenetration of genes and environments in disease etiology is phenylketonuria (PKU). Classic PKU is caused by an autosomal recessive genetic variant on chromosome 12, and those with PKU lack an enzyme needed to break down the amino acid phenylalanine. Consequently, phenylalanine accumulates in tissue and causes progressive, irreversible cognitive impairments, among other problems. PKU is thus a genetically determined disease for which severe negative health outcomes were once inevitable. For decades, it has been known that if someone with PKU adheres to a diet low in phenylalanine, the accumulation can be avoided and the negative consequences of the condition can be minimized. In other words, PKU is a genetically determined condition whose consequences medical science has transformed to being largely environmentally determined.

At the same time, MacDonald et al. (2008) find that, for children with PKU, lower maternal education is associated with higher child blood phenylalanine, apparently as a result of poorer adherence to a low phenylalanine diet (see also Russell, Mills, and Zucconi 1988). Consequently, while no one regrets our being able to treat PKU, this knowledge may have created an education-related disparity where none existed before. As science increases the possible leverage that humans have over their genes, socioeconomic factors may become relevant for understanding variation in the utilization of knowledge, technology, and ultimately outcomes.

With PKU, a drug to reduce blood phenylalanine levels was approved by the FDA in 2007 (sapropterin dihydrochloride; brand name Kuvan). Nothing is yet known about the consequences of this treatment for socioeconomic differences in children's blood phenylalanine levels. Thinking abstractly, however, one can imagine that such an innovation might reduce inequalities if it reduces the importance of dietary adherence and is widely utilized. On the other hand, it could increase inequalities if it is utilized primarily by advantaged individuals who are already most likely to have good adherence. Medical innovations that increase population health may increase or decrease disparities as they do so; what consequence innovations do have depends on the technology they supercede and on the barriers to utilizing the innovation. What will prove

to be the key barriers for utilizing innovations from genetics research remains largely unknown, although a strong lesson from the existing literature on health disparities would be not to exaggerate the importance of financial resources per se (Mirowsky and Ross 2003; Cutler, Deaton, and Lleras-Muney 2006).

Another example of the fundamental interaction between genetics and social environment in disease is provided by diabetes. Diabetes is commonly divided into Types 1 and 2, with the former characterized by inability to produce insulin and the latter by relative deficiency or insulin resistance. Onset for Type 1 is typically in childhood, while onset of Type 2 is typically in adulthood and appears strongly linked to obesity. Rates of obesity have increased dramatically in recent decades, and of course this change cannot be attributed to underlying genetic changes in the population; it is rightly characterized as a social epidemic (Christakis and Fowler 2007; Martin 2008). At the same time, obesity is strongly heritable, with genetic differences implicated in level of caloric intake, physical activity, and the weight change of those with similar caloric intake and activity (Faith and Kral 2006). Consequently, concordance of identical twins for diabetes in U.S. society is higher for Type 2 diabetes than for Type 1 (Dean and McEntyre 2004). In societies where obesity is rare, Type 2 diabetes is rare. The environmental changes that have resulted in contemporary Western lifestyles have thereby created associations between genotypes and diabetes risk that did not exist before.

Over many years, the elevated blood sugar levels in diabetes lead to increased risk for a wide variety of vascular-related complications, and so the basic goal of diabetes treatment is typically to emulate normal blood sugar levels as closely as possible. Using ethnographic data, Lutfey and Freese (2005) compare two diabetes clinics serving very different SES populations and are able to articulate an array of possible reasons why lower SES diabetes patients may have more difficulty maintaining normal glucose levels. Others have suggested that psychological traits like cognitive ability and conscientiousness also may be important for managing chronic conditions with sustained and complex treatment regimens

(Goldman and Smith 2002). While few would dispute the importance of environments for understanding variation in either cognitive ability or conscientiousness, behavioral genetics has produced strong evidence that genetic differences are influential as well (Plomin and Caspi 1999; Plomin and Spinath 2002). If so, then as disease consequences become amenable to treatment by personal management, one may see a shift whereby the importance of genes related to the disease itself becomes less important for ultimate consequences, but genes related to the psychology of managing disease become more important (Freese 2006). In other words, the relevance of genetics for medical outcomes is not restricted to genetic effects on physiological processes, and, when disease risk and treatment depends strongly on individual behavior, understanding genetic differences in behavioral tendencies may be a vital part of developing interventions.

The conventional way of determining the overall contribution of genetic variation to population variation in a phenotypic characteristic has been to compare pairs of individuals with known genetic relatedness, especially monozygotic twins (MZ; identical) and dizygotic twins (DZ; fraternal). Given certain assumptions, the higher correlation of MZ twins is taken as evidence of genetic influence, with the estimated magnitude of genetic influence increasing as the difference in correlations increases (see Schaffner 2006 a, b for an especially lucid overview). When genes and environments interact, saying that some percentage of the outcome "is genetic" loses coherence, and heritability estimates seem instead best interpreted as an imperfect but informative indicator of genetic influence. In this respect, substantial heritability estimates have been observed not only for a wide range of health and psychological measures, but also for items of such longstanding sociological interest as educational attainment, earnings, divorce, and voting (Behrman et al. 1980; McGue and Lykken 1992; Fowler, Baker, and Dawes 2008). To be sure, criticism of twin studies exists, including debate among sociologists (Horwitz et al. 2003; Freese and Powell 2003). However, many have concluded that there is no evidence of problems severe enough that twin studies would pervasively produce evidence of substantial ge-

netic influence when none existed (see detailed arguments in Kendler and Prescott 2006; Rutter 2006).

Studies of variation in estimated heritability across different populations—or in the same population at different times—can be used to provide broad information about gene-environment interactions. Boardman (2009) finds that more aggressive policies against cigarette use (e.g., higher taxes, stronger restrictions on advertising) are associated with lower heritability of daily smoking but not lower heritability of smoking onset. Given evidence of the success of aggressive policies in reducing onset overall, Boardman interprets this result as suggesting that existing antismoking policies may be most effective for those whose smoking initiation is least associated with underlying genetic causes. As a different example, Guo and Stearns (2002) find that the heritability of adolescent vocabulary score is higher in families with higher income (see also Turkheimer et al. 2003). Because genetic differences apparently matter more in wealthier families, Guo and Stearns speculate that richer environments better allow children to develop their differing genetic potential (cf. Perrin and Lee 2007).

While such findings are intriguing, comparing heritability estimates across groups is a rough tool for studying how genes moderate the effects of environments. Even when model assumptions are met, heritability estimates still measure only the proportion of overall variation resolved by genetic variability. Groups may differ in the heritability of an outcome because of differences in the effects of genes, but also because of differences in the overall level of genetic variation, environmental variation, or variation in measurement error. In the Guo and Stearns (2007) study, for example, the difference in heritability between the highest and lowest income groups was less than 0.1, and the heritability differences between the highest and lowest education groups were nearly this large in the opposite direction. In the end, the conclusions to be drawn from such indirect methods about the interaction of genes and social environments are likely quite limited.

For this reason, more enthusiasm currently surrounds the direct utilization of molecular genetic measures for studying gene-environment interactions. The remarkably rapid drop in the cost of these measures has accelerated the effort to integrate them into existing social science data resources. To give one concrete example, in 2006 the Wisconsin Longitudinal Study planned an initiative to assay 4,500 cases for variants of a single gene (APOE) associated with Alzheimer's disease (Bertram and Tanzi 2008). Two years later, after all data were collected and the salivary samples were prepared to be submitted for assaying, the initiative had grown to include 6,800 participants and variants of more than ninety different single nucleotide polymorphisms (SNPs), and yet the estimated overall cost of assaying had declined slightly.[12] Sociologists interested in health will have vastly greater opportunities to incorporate molecular genetic data into their work.

As an example of a study of gene-environment interaction led by a medical sociologist, Pescosolido and colleagues (2008) found support for their hypothesis that the association between a variant of the gene GABRA2 and being diagnosed with alcoholism may be highest for individuals from disadvantaged backgrounds or low social support. Their results highlight the possibility that molecular genetic data may contribute to understanding the wide variation in the physical and mental health consequences of social adversity. Shanahan and colleagues (2008) have argued also that sociologists should be leaders in exploring how gene-environment interaction may require methods for assessing complex configurations of environmental characteristics (and, for that matter, configurations of genes). In other words, the consequences of genetic differences may be suppressed or accentuated less by particular environmental conditions than by the presence of multiple conditions that together provide special contexts of vulnerability or resilience.

Molecular genetic data may also be used to provide some leverage into famously difficult causal questions in social science research on health. In particular, as more becomes known about genetic determinants of health conditions, possibilities increase for being able to infer that the only reason some genetic variant would be associated with a social outcome like education and earnings is indirectly, via the effect of the genetic variant on health. In such a case, one could then use genotypic information as an instrumental variable to disentangle the causal effect of the genetically influenced health condition on socioeconomic outcomes from the effect of socioeconomic outcomes on health (Ding et al. 2009; see also Ebrahim and Davey Smith 2008). To cite an analogous example, a genetic variant that influences levels of c-reactive protein in blood was used to examine direction of causality issues in the association between c-reactive protein and insulin resistance (Lawlor et al. 2008). Roughly, because any influence of insulin resistance on c-reactive protein does not change the gene, any association between the gene and insulin resistance can instead be attributed to the influence of c-reactive protein on insulin resistance. Using full siblings who differ on the genes in question makes this an even stronger possible research design by eliminating the possibility of confounding the correlations among parent genes, child genes, and family environment (Fletcher and Lehrer 2008).

While molecular genetic data thus provides immense and exciting scientific opportunity for medical sociologists, the importance of caution in interpreting findings prior to replication must be emphasized. The extent of replication failure in medical genetics has been a source of regular lament (Ahsan and Rundle 2003; Taioli and Garte 2002). The particular reasons for such failures are many, but important among them is that having a large number of genetic measures and a large number of environmental measures yields a very large number of potential interactions that can be analyzed, especially when those analyses can be carried out for different subgroups and different outcomes. While methods of correcting for multiple significance tests exist, the number of tests underlying a presented result can be difficult for researchers to determine (and impossible for reviewers).

Given that statistical interactions are already notorious for replication problems when genes are not involved, reported gene-environment interactions should perhaps be approached even more gingerly than should reported main effects of genetic differences (Rutter 2006). Worse, many social science data resources are effectively unique with respect to some questions they can be used to address, making direct replication across samples far more difficult than in many medical studies. Moffitt, Caspi, and Rutter (2005) provide an especially lucid guide to the proper theoretical justification motivating a search for a gene-environment interaction, and they caution strongly against "overreacting" to one study in advance of replication. When evidence for gene-environment interaction is appropriately adducted, researchers must also caution against unwarranted privileging of the "genetic" side of the interaction, and indeed often diseases described in the scientific literature as "complex genetic disorders" might just as easily be characterized as "complex environmental disorders."[13]

Conclusions

A longstanding strength of medical sociology is its theoretical and methodological diversity. Thus, it is no surprise to see medical sociologists at the forefront of widely varied approaches to the study of gene-environment interaction. Such efforts include historical excavations of the concept of gene-environment interaction, ethnographic studies of the operationalization of gene-environment interaction in specific laboratories, analyses of biomedical texts and newspaper reporting, surveys of public beliefs and attitudes about genes and environments as causes of health and social outcomes, and new forms of sociological research which directly incorporate genotypic data. Taken together, these inquiries underscore the importance of understanding health and illness as shaped by genes in interaction with multiple environments—social, economic, physical, biological. Genes and environments become embodied as health and illness in and through social processes that are conditioned by dimensions of social structure (Bearman, Martin, and Shostak 2008). Research about gene-environment interactions provides medical sociologists with another warrant—and another set of tools—for elucidating the complex causes of health and illness.

Notes

We thank Miranda Waggoner for providing research assistance.

1. This chapter draws on work that appeared originally in Freese and Shostak (2009).

2. A key word search using "gene-environment interaction" in PubMed generates 28 articles on the topic published from 1974 to 1989, 18 from 1990 to 1995, 85 from 1995 to 2000, and 243 from 2001 to 2005.

3. This represents a $40 million increase above the $28 million already planned for these efforts in the NIH budget, a significant allocation in relative scarcity at the NIH.

4. An alternative analytic frame is provided in writing on "molecularization," which refers to the reorientation of the life sciences to the submicroscopic level (de Chadarevian and Kamminga 1998; Kay 1993). Some authors prefer "molecularization" because it lacks the negative valence often associated with "geneticization" (Hedgecoe 1998), while others use it to describe how genes and environments both are increasingly known and governed at the molecular level (Shostak 2005).

5. For example, in an experimental investigation of the consequences of genetic information in a clinical context, participants presented with results for what was called a "genetic" test for heart disease perceived the disease to be less preventable than those assigned to the unspecified test condition (Senior, Marteau, and Weinman 2000).

6. This may occur even as scientists recognize that "there is no one single fact of the matter about what a gene is" (Keller 2001, 139)

7. The frame of genetic optimism consists of three components: (1) a gene for the disorder exists; (2) it will be found; and (3) this will be good (Conrad 2001).

8. Related, Clarke and colleagues use the concept of "technoscientific identities" to refer broadly to identities based in biomedical science and technology, including genomics (Clarke et al. 2003, 182–83).

9. Changes in the wording of the question and the structure of response options also may have contributed to this change (Singer, Corning, and Lamias 1998, 638).

10. Academic discussions of heritability regularly point out that evidence of the importance of genetics for explaining individual differences is not evidence of the importance of genetics for explaining group differences (e.g., Schaffner 2006a, b). To our knowledge, no published study has considered how the same people respond to questions about individual and group differences in the same trait.

11. The direction of causality here is unclear, and belief in genetic differences between oneself and an outgroup does not inevitably imply negative attitudes.

12. This information about the Wisconsin Longitudinal

Study was provided by personal communication with Robert M. Hauser and Taissa S. Hauser, January 2009.

13. We thank Peter Conrad for this point.

References

Abu El-Haj, Nadia. 2007. "The Genetic Reinscription of Race." *Annual Review of Anthropology* 36:283–300.

Ahsan, Hasan, and Andrew Rundle. 2003. "Measures of Genotype vs. Gene Products: Promise and Pitfalls in Cancer Prevention." *Carcinogenesis* 24:1229–34.

Alford, John, Carolyn Funk, and John R. Hibbing. 2005. "Are Political Orientations Genetically Transmitted?" *American Political Science Review* 99:153–67.

Alper, Joseph S., and Jon Beckwith. 1993. "Genetic Fatalism and Social Policy: The Implications of Behavioral Genetics Research." *Yale Journal of Biology and Medicine* 66:511–24.

Anderson, Robert G., III. 1967. "On Genetics and Sociology (II)." *American Sociological Review* 32:997–99.

Atkinson, Paul, Peter Glasner, and Helen Greenslade, eds. 2007. *New Genetics, New Identities*. London: Routledge.

Bearman, Peter, Molly Martin, and Sara Shostak, eds. 2008. Special issue on genetics and social structure. *American Journal of Sociology* 114, suppl. 1:v–S316.

Behrman, Jere R., Zdenek Hrubec, Paul Taubman, and Terence J. Wales. 1980. *Socioeconomic Success: A Study of the Effects of Genetic Endowments, Family Environment, and Schooling*. New York: North-Holland.

Bertram, Lars, and Rudolph E. Tanzi. 2008. "Thirty Years of Alzheimer's Disease Genetics: The Implications of Systematic Meta-analyses." *Nature Reviews Neuroscience* 9:768–78.

Boardman, Jason. 2009. "State-Level Moderation of Genetic Tendencies to Smoke." *American Journal of Public Health* 99:480–86.

Brandt, Allan. 2007. *The Cigarette Century: The Rise and Fall of the Drug That Defined America*. New York: Basic Books.

Brown, Phil. 1995. "Naming and Framing: The Social Construction of Diagnosis and Illness." *Journal of Health and Social Behavior*, suppl. 1:34–52.

Callon, Michel, and Vololona Rabeharisoa. 2003. "Research 'in the Wild' and the Shaping of New Social Identities." *Technology in Society* 25:193–204.

Chaufan, Claudia. 2007. "How Much Can a Large Population Study on Genes, Environments, Their Interactions and Common Diseases Contribute to the Health of the American People?" *Social Science and Medicine* 65:1730–41.

Christakis, Nicholas A., and James H. Fowler. 2007. "The Spread of Obesity in a Large Social Network over 32 Years." *New England Journal of Medicine* 357:370–79.

Clarke, Adele E., Janet K. Shim, Laura Mamo, Jennifer R. Fosket, and Jennifer Fishman. 2003. "Biomedicalization: Technoscientific Transformations of Health, Illness, and U.S. Biomedicine." *American Sociological Review* 68:161–94.

Condit, Celeste M. 1999. "How the Public Understands Genetics: Non-deterministic and Non-discriminatory Interpretations of the 'Blueprint' Metaphor." *Public Understanding of Science* 8:169–80.

Condit, Celeste M., and Benjamin R. Bates. 2005. "How Lay People Respond to Messages about Genetics, Health, and Race." *Clinical Genetics* 68:97–105.

Condit, Celeste M., Nneka Ofulue, and Kristine M. Sheedy. 1998. "Determinism and Mass-Media Portrayals of Genetics." *American Journal of Human Genetics* 62:979–84.

Condit, Celeste M., Roxanne L Parrott, Tina M. Harris, John Lynch, and Tasha Dubriwy. 2004. "The Role of 'Genetics' in Popular Understandings of Race in the United States." *Public Understanding of Science* 13:249–72.

Condit, Celeste M., Roxanne Parrott, and Tina M. Harris. 2006. "Laypeople and Behavioral Genetics." In *Wrestling with Behavioral Genetics: Science, Ethics, and Public Conversation*, ed. Erik Parens, Audrey R. Chapman, and Nancy Press, 286–308. Baltimore: Johns Hopkins University Press.

Conrad, Peter. 1992. "Medicalization and Social Control." *Annual Review of Sociology* 18:209–32.

———. 1999. "A Mirage of Genes." *Sociology of Health and Illness* 21:228–41.

———. 2001. "Genetic Optimism: Framing Genes and Mental Illness in the News." *Culture, Medicine and Psychiatry* 25:225–47.

Cox, Susan M., and Rosalie C. Starzomski. 2004. "Genes and Geneticization? The Social Construction of Autosomal Dominant Polycystic Kidney Disease." *New Genetics and Society* 23:137–66.

Cunningham-Burley, Sarah, and Anne Kerr. 1999. "Defining the 'Social': Toward an Understanding of Scientific and Medical Discourses on the Social Aspects of the New Human Genetics." *Sociology of Health and Illness* 21:647–68.

Cutler, David M., Angus Deaton, and Adriana Lleras-Muney. 2006. "The Determinants of Mortality." *Journal of Economic Perspectives* 20:97–120.

Dean, Laura, and Johanna McEntyre. 2004. *The Genetic Landscape of Diabetes*. Bethesda, Md.: National Center for Biotechnology Information.

de Chadarevian, Soraya, and Harmke Kamminga, eds.

1998. *Molecularizing Biology and Medicine: New Practices and Alliances, 1910s–1970s*. Amsterdam: Harwood Academic.

Ding, Weili, Steven F. Lehrer, J. Niels Rosenquist, and Janet Audrain-McGovern. 2009. "The Impact of Poor Health on Academic Performance: New Evidence Using Genetic Markers." *Journal of Health Economics* 28:578–97.

Duster, Troy. 2003. *Backdoor to Eugenics*. 2nd ed. New York: Routledge.

———. 2005. "Race and Reification in Science." *Science* 307:1050–51.

———. 2006. "Comparative Perspectives and Competing Explanations: Taking on the Newly Configured Reductionist Challenge to Sociology." *American Sociological Review* 71:1–15.

Ebrahim, Shah, and George Davey Smith. 2008. "Mendelian Randomization: Can Genetic Epidemiology Help Redress the Failures of Observational Epidemiology?" *Human Genetics* 123:15–33.

Epstein, Steven. 1996. *Impure Science: AIDS, Activism and the Politics of Knowledge*. Berkeley: University of California Press.

———. 2007. *Inclusion: The Politics of Difference in Medical Research*. Chicago: University of Chicago Press.

Faith, Myles S., and Tanja V. E. Kral. 2006. "Social Environmental and Genetic Influences on Obesity and Obesity-Promoting Behaviors: Fostering Research Integration." In *Genes, Behavior, and the Social Environment*, ed. Lyla M. Hernandez and Dan G. Blazer, 236–80. Washington, D.C.: National Academies Press.

Farrer, Lindsay A., Adrienne Cupples, Jonathan L. Haines, Bradley Hyman, Walter A. Kukull, Richard Mayeux, Richard H. Myers, Margaret A. Pericak-Vance, Neil Risch, and Cornelia M. van Duijn. 1997. "Effect of Age, Sex and Ethnicity on the Association between Apolipoprotein E Genotype and Alzheimer's Disease: A Meta-analysis." ApoE and Alzheimer's Disease Meta-Analysis Consortium. *Journal of the American Medical Association* 278:1349–56.

Feero, W. Gregory, Alan E. Guttmacher, and Francis S. Collins. 2008. "The Genome Gets Personal—Almost." *Journal of the American Medical Association* 299:1351–52.

Feinberg, Andrew P. 2008. "Epigenetics at the Epicenter of Modern Medicine." *Journal of the American Medical Association* 299:1345–50.

Finch, Caleb E., James W. Vaupel, and Kevin Kinsella. 2000. *Cells and Surveys: Should Biological Measures Be Included in Social Science Research?* Washington, D.C.: National Academies Press.

Fletcher, Jason M., and Steven F. Lehrer. 2009. "Using Genetic Lotteries within Families to Examine the Causal Impact of Poor Health on Academic Achievement." National Bureau of Economic Research Working Paper. ssrn.com/abstract=1434663.

Fowler, James H., Laura A. Baker, and Christopher T. Dawes. 2008. "Genetic Variation in Political Participation." *American Political Science Review* 102:233–48.

Francis, Darlene, Josie Diorio, Dong Liu, Michael J. Meaney. 1999. "Nongenomic Transmission across Generations of Maternal Behavior and Stress Responses in the Rat." *Science* 286:1155–58.

Franklin, Sarah, and Celia Roberts. 2006. *Born and Made: An Ethnography of Preimplantation Genetic Diagnosis*. Princeton, N.J.: Princeton University Press.

Freese, Jeremy. 2006. "The Analysis of Variance and the Social Complexities of Genetic Causation." *International Journal of Epidemiology* 35:534–36.

———. 2008. "Genetics and the Social Science Explanation of Individual Outcomes." *American Journal of Sociology* 114, suppl. 1: S1–35.

Freese, Jeremy, Jui-Chung Allen Li, and Lisa D. Wade. 2003. "The Potential Relevances of Biology to Social Inquiry." *Annual Review of Sociology* 29:233–56.

Freese, Jeremy, and Karen Lutfey. Forthcoming. "Fundamental Causality: Challenges of an Animating Concept in Medical Sociology." *Handbook of the Sociology of Health, Illness, and Healing*, ed. Bernice Pescosolido, Jack K. Martin, Jane McLeod, and Anne Rogers. New York: Springer.

Freese, Jeremy, and Brian Powell. 2003. "Tilting at Twindmills: Rethinking Sociological Responses to Behavioral Genetics." *Journal of Health and Social Behavior* 44:130–35.

Freese, Jeremy, and Sara Shostak. 2009. "Genetics and Social Inquiry." *Annual Review of Sociology* 35:107–28.

Fujimura, Joan H. 2005. "Postgenomic Futures: Translations across the Machine-Nature Border in Systems Biology." *New Genetics and Society* 24:195–226.

Gibbon, Sahra. 2007. *Breast Cancer Genes and the Gendering of Knowledge: Science and Citizenship in the Cultural Context of the "New" Genetics*. Basingstoke, Eng.: Palgrave Macmillan.

Gibbon, Sahra, and Carlos Novas. 2008. *Biosocialities, Genetics and the Social Sciences: Making Biologies and Identities*. London: Routledge.

Gieryn, Thomas F. 1999. *Cultural Boundaries of Science: Credibility on the Line*. Chicago: University of Chicago Press.

Goldman, Dana, and James Smith. 2002. "Can Patient

Self-Management Help Explain the SES Health Gradient?" *Proceedings of the National Academy of Sciences* 99:10929–34.

Guo, Guang, Michael Roettger, and Tianji Cai. 2008. "The Integration of Genetic Propensities into Social Control Models of Delinquency and Violence among Male Youths." *American Sociological Review* 73:543–68.

Guo, Guang, and Elizabeth Stearns. 2002. "The Social Influences on the Realization of Genetic Potential for Intellectual Development." *Social Forces* 80:881–910.

Guo, Guang, Yuying Tong, and Tianji Cai. 2008. "Gene by Social-Context Interactions for Number of Sexual Partners among White Male Youths: Genetics-Informed Sociology." *American Journal of Sociology* 114:S36–66.

Hacking, Ian. 1995. "The Looping Effects of Human Kinds." In *Causal Cognition: A Multidisciplinary Debate*, ed. Dan Sperber, David Premack, 351–83. Oxford: Oxford University Press.

———. 1999. *The Social Construction of What?* Cambridge, Mass.: Harvard University Press.

———. 2006. "Genetics, Biosocial Groups, and the Future of Identity." *Daedalus* 135(4): 81–95.

Hall, Edward. 2005. "The 'Geneticization' of Heart Disease: A Network Analysis of the Production of New Genetic Knowledge." *Social Science and Medicine*, 60:2673–83.

Heath, Deborah, Rayna Rapp, and Karen Sue Taussig. 2004. "Genetic Citizenship." In *A Companion to the Anthropology of Politics*, ed. D. Nugent and J. Vincent, 152–67. London: Blackwell.

Hedgecoe, A. 1998. "Geneticization, Medicalisation and Polemics." *Medicine, Healthcare and Philosophy* 1:235–43.

———. 2001. "Schizophrenia and the Narrative of Enlightened Geneticization." *Social Studies of Science* 31:875–911.

———. 2002. "Reinventing Diabetes: Classification, Division and the Geneticization of Disease." *New Genetics and Society* 21:7–27.

Hernandez, Lyla M., and Dan G. Blazer. 2006. *Genes, Behavior, and the Social Environment: Moving beyond the Nature/Nurture Debate*. Washington, D.C.: National Academies Press.

Horwitz, Allan V. 2005. "Media Portrayals and Health Inequalities: A Case Study of Characterizations of Gene x Environment Interactions." *Journal of Gerontology Series B: Psychological and Social Sciences* 60B: 48–52.

Horwitz, Allan V., Tami Videon, Mark Schmitz, and Diane Davis. 2003. "Rethinking Twins and Environments: Possible Social Sources for Presumed Genetic Influences in Twin Research." *Journal of Health and Social Behavior* 44:111–29.

Hunt, Matthew O. 2007. "African American, Hispanic, and White Beliefs about Black/White Inequality, 1977–2004." *American Sociological Review* 72:390–415.

Jayaratne, Toby Epstein, Oscar Ybarra, Jane P. Sheldon, Tony N. Brown, Merle Feldbaum, Carla A. Pfeffer, and Elizabeth M. Petty. 2006. "White Americans' Genetic Lay Theories of Race Differences and Sexual Orientation: Their Relationship with Prejudice toward Blacks, and Gay Men and Lesbians." *Group Processes and Intergroup Relations* 9:77–94.

Kay, Lily E. 1993. *The Molecular Vision of Life: Caltech, the Rockefeller Foundation and the New Biology*. Oxford: Oxford University Press.

Keller, Evelyn Fox. 2001. *The Century of the Gene.* Cambridge, Mass.: Harvard University Press.

Keller, Johannes. 2005. "In Genes We Trust: The Biological Component of Psychological Essentialism and Its Relationship to Mechanisms of Motivated Social Cognition." *Journal of Personality and Social Psychology* 88:686–702.

Kendler, Kenneth S., and Carol A. Prescott. 2006. *Genes, Environment and Psychopathology: Understanding the Causes of Psychiatric and Substance Use Disorders.* Boston: Guilford Press.

Kevles, Daniel. 1985. *In the Name of Eugenics: Genetics and the Uses of Human Heredity.* Cambridge, Mass.: Harvard University Press.

Kitano, Hiroaki. 2002. "Systems Biology: A Brief Overview." *Science* 295:1662–64.

Lafayette, DeeDee, Diane Abuelo, Mary Ann Passero, and Umadevi Tantravahi. 1999. "Attitudes toward Cystic Fibrosis Carrier and Prenatal Testing and Utilization of Carrier Testing among Relatives of Individuals with Cystic Fibrosis." *Journal of Genetic Counseling* 8:17–36.

Landecker, Hannah. "Epigenetics and the Experimental Formalization of the Environment." Typescript. Author files.

Lawlor, Debbie A., Roger M. Harbord, Jonathan A. C. Sterne, Nic J. Timpson, and George Davey Smith. 2008. "Mendelian Randomization: Using Genes as Instruments for Making Causal Inferences in Epidemiology." *Statistics in Medicine* 27:1133–63.

Lerman, Caryn, Mary Daly, Agnes Masny, and Andrew Balshem. 1994. "Attitudes about Genetic Testing for Breast-Ovarian Cancer Susceptibility." *Journal of Clinical Oncology* 12:843–50.

Lee, Sandra S., Johanna Mountain, and Barbara J. Koenig. 2001. "The Meanings of 'Race' in the New Genomics: Implications for Health Disparities Research." *Yale Journal of Health Policy, Law and Ethics* 33:53–59.

Link, Bruce G., and Jo Phelan. 1995. "Social Conditions

as Fundamental Causes of Disease." *Journal of Health and Social Behavior*, suppl.: 80–94.

Lippman, Abby J. 1991. "Prenatal Genetic Testing and Screening: Constructing Needs and Reinforcing Inequities." *American Journal of Law and Medicine* 17:15–50.

———. 1992. "Led (Astray) by Genetic Maps: The Cartography of the Human Genome and Health Care." *Social Science and Medicine* 35:1469–76.

———. 1998. "The Politics of Health: Geneticization Versus Health Promotion." In *The Politics of Women's Health: Exploring Agency and Autonomy*, ed. Susan Sherwin, 64–82. Philadelphia: Temple University Press.

Lock, Margaret. 2005. "Eclipse of the Gene and the Return of Divination." *Current Anthropology* 46: S47–70.

Lock, Margaret, Julia Freeman, Rosemary Sharples, and Stephanie Lloyd. 2006. "When It Runs in the Family: Putting Susceptibility Genes in Perspective." *Public Understanding of Science* 15:277–300.

Lutfey, Karen, and Jeremy Freese. 2005. "Toward Some Fundamentals of Fundamental Causality: Socioeconomic Status and Health in the Routine Clinic Visit for Diabetes." *American Journal of Sociology* 110:1326–72.

MacDonald, A., P. Davies, A. Daly, V. Hopkins, S. K. Hall, D. Asplin, C. Hendriksz, and A. Chakrapani. 2008. "Does Maternal Knowledge and Parent Education Affect Blood Phenylalanine Control in Phenylketonuria?" *Journal of Human Nutrition and Dietetics* 21:351–58.

Markens, Susan, Carole. H. Browner, and Nancy Press. 1999. "'Because of the Risks': How U.S. Pregnant Women Account for Refusing Prenatal Screening." *Social Science and Medicine* 49:359–69.

Martin, Molly A. 2008. "The Intergenerational Correlation in Weight: How Genetic Resemblance Reveals the Social Role of Families." *American Journal of Sociology* 114, suppl. 1: S67–105.

McGue, Matt, and David T. Lykken. 1992. "Genetic Influence on Risk of Divorce." *Psychological Science* 3:368–73.

Meaney, Michael J. 2001. "Maternal Care, Gene Expression, and the Transmission of Individual Differences in Stress Reactivity across Generations." *Annual Review of Neuroscience* 24:1161–92.

Mirowsky, John, and Catherine E. Ross. 2003. *Education, Social Status, and Health*. New York: Aldine de Gruyter.

Moffitt, Terrie E., Avshalom Caspi, and Michael Rutter. 2005. "Strategy for Investigating Interactions between Measured Genes and Measured Environments." *Archives of General Psychiatry* 62:473–81.

Mol, Annemarie. 2002. *The Body Multiple: Ontology in Medical Practice*. Durham, N.C.: Duke University Press.

NIEHS [National Institute of Environmental Health Sciences]. 2006. "Two NIH Initiatives Launch Intensive Efforts to Determine Genetic and Environmental Roots of Common Diseases." Press release. niehs.nih.gov/news/releases/2006/gei.cfm.

Nelkin, Dorothy, and M. Susan Lindee. 2004. *The DNA Mystique: The Gene as a Cultural Icon*. New ed. Ann Arbor: University of Michigan Press.

Nelson, Alondra. 2008. "Bio Science: Genetic Genealogy Testing and the Pursuit of African Ancestry." *Social Studies of Science* 38:759–78.

Novas Carlos. 2007. "Genetic Advocacy Groups, Science and Biovalue: Creating Political Economies of Hope." In *New Genetics, New Identities*, ed. Paul Atkinson, Peter Glasner, and Helen Greenslade, 11–27. London: Routledge.

———. 2008. "Patients, Profits and Values: Myozyme as an Exemplar of Biosociality." In *Biosocialities, Genetics and the Social Sciences*, ed. Sahra Gibbon and Carlos Novas, 136–56. London: Routledge.

Novas, Carlos, and Nikolas Rose. 2000. "Genetic Risk and the Birth of the Somatic Individual." *Economy and Society* 29:485–513.

Omi, Michael, and Howard Winant. 1994. *Racial Formation in the United States: From the 1960s to the 1990s*. 2nd ed. New York and London: Routledge.

Ossorio, Pilar, and Troy Duster. 2005. "Race and Genetics: Controversies in Biomedical, Behavioral, and Forensic Sciences." *American Psychologist* 60:115–28.

Parrott, Roxanne L., Kami J. Silk, and Celeste Condit. 2003. "Diversity in Lay Perceptions of the Sources of Human Traits: Genes, Environments, and Personal Behaviors." *Social Science and Medicine* 56:1099–1109.

Parrott, Roxanne L., Kami J. Silk, Megan R. Dillow, Janice Raup Krieger, Tina Harris, and Celeste M. Condit. 2005. "The Development and Validation of Tools to Assess Genetic Discrimination and Genetically Based Racism." *Journal of the National Medical Association* 97:980–90.

Parsons, Talcott. 1951. *The Social System*. Glencoe, Ill.: Free Press.

Parthasarathy, Shobita. 2007. *Building Genetic Medicine: Breast Cancer, Technology, and the Comparative Politics of Health Care*. Cambridge, Mass.: MIT Press.

Perrin, Andrew J., and Hedwig Lee. 2007. "The Undertheorized Environment: Sociological Theory and the Ontology of Behavioral Genetics." *Sociological Perspectives* 50:303–22.

Pescosolido, Bernice. 2006. "Of Pride and Prejudice: The Role of Sociology and Social Networks in Integrating the Health Sciences." *Journal of Health and Social Behavior* 47:189–208.

Pescosolido, Bernice, Brea L. Perry, J. Scott Long, Jack K. Martin, John I. Nurnberger Jr., John Kramer, and Victor Hesselbrock. 2008. "Under the Influence of Genetics: How Transdisciplinarity Leads Us to Rethink Social Pathways to Illness." *American Journal of Sociology* 114, suppl. 1: S171–201.

Petryna, Adryana. 2002. *Life Exposed: Biological Citizens after Chernobyl*. Princeton, N.J.: Princeton University Press.

Phelan, Jo C. 2005. "Geneticization of Deviant Behavior and Consequences for Stigma: The Case of Mental Illness." *Journal of Health and Social Behavior* 46:307–22.

Plomin, Robert, and Avshalom Caspi. 1999. "Behavioral Genetics and Personality." In *Handbook of Personality: Theory and Research*, 2nd ed., ed. Lawrence. A. Pervin and Oliver P. John, 251–76. New York: Guilford.

Plomin, Robert, and Frank M. Spinath. 2002. "Genetics and General Cognitive Ability." *Trends in Cognitive Sciences* 6:169–76.

Prainsack, Barbara, and Gil Siegal. 2006. "The Rise of Genetic Couplehood? A Comparative View of Premarital Genetic Testing." *BioSocieties* 1:17–36.

Rabinow, Paul. 1996. "Artificiality and Enlightenment: From Sociobiology to Biosociality." In *Essays on the Anthropology of Reason*, ed. Paul Rabinow, 91–111. Princeton, N.J.: Princeton University Press.

Rapp, Rayna. 1999. *Testing Women, Testing the Fetus: The Social Impact of Amniocentesis in America*. New York: Routledge.

Reardon, Jennifer. 2004. *Race to the Finish: Identity and Governance in an Age of Genomics*. Princeton, N.J.: Princeton University Press.

Remennick, Larissa. 2006. "The Quest for the Perfect Baby: Why Do Israeli Women Seek Prenatal Genetic Testing?" *Sociology of Health and Illness* 28:21–53.

Richard, Martin, and Maggie Ponder. 1996. "Lay Understanding of Genetics: A Test of a Hypothesis." *Journal of Medical Genetics* 33:1032–36.

Rose, Nikolas. 2007. *The Politics of Life Itself: Biomedicine, Power, and Subjectivity in the Twenty-First Century*. Princeton, N.J.: Princeton University Press.

Rothman, Barbara Katz. 2001. *The Book of Life: A Personal and Ethical Guide to Race, Normality, and the Implications of the Human Genome Project*. Boston, Mass.: Beacon Press.

Russell, F. F., B. C. Mills, and T. Zucconi. 1988. "Relationship of Parental Attitudes and Knowledge to Treatment Adherence in Children with PKU." *Pediatric Nursing* 14:514–16.

Rutter, Michael. 2006. *Genes and Behavior: Nature-Nurture Interplay Explained*. Malden, Mass.: Blackwell.

———. 2007. "Gene-Environment Interdependence." *Developmental Science* 10:12–18.

Rutter, Michael, Terrie E. Moffit, and Avshalom Caspi. 2006. "Gene-Environment Interplay and Psychopathology: Multiple Varieties but Real Effects." *Journal of Child Psychology and Psychiatry* 47(3/4): 226–61.

Sankar, Pamela, Mildred K. Cho, Celeste M. Condit, Linda M. Hunt, Barbara Koenig, Patrick Marshall, Sandra Soo-Jin Lee, and Paul Spicer. 2004. "Genetic Research and Health Disparities." *Journal of the American Medical Association* 291:2985–89.

Schaffner, Kenneth F. 2006a. "Behavior: Its Nature and Nurture, Part 1." In *Wrestling with Behavioral Genetics: Science, Ethics, and Public Conversation*, ed. Erik Parens, Audrey R. Chapman, and Nancy Press, 3–39. Baltimore: Johns Hopkins University Press.

———. 2006b. "Behavior: Its Nature and Nurture, Part 2." In *Wrestling with Behavioral Genetics: Science, Ethics, and Public Conversation*, ed. Erik Parens, Audrey R. Chapman, and Nancy Press, 40–73. Baltimore: Johns Hopkins University Press.

Scheper-Hughes, Nancy, and Margaret M. Lock. 1987. "The Mindful Body: A Prolegomenon to Future Work in Medical Anthropology." *Medical Anthropology Quarterly* 1:6–41.

Schnittker, Jason, Jeremy Freese, and Brian Powell. 2000. "Nature, Nurture, Neither, Nor: Black-White Differences in Beliefs about the Causes and Appropriate Treatment of Mental Illness." *Social Forces* 72:1101–32.

Schwartz, David, and Francis S. Collins. 2007. "Environmental Biology and Human Disease." *Science* 316:695–96.

Senior, Victoria, Theresa M. Marteau, and John Weinman. 2000. "Impact of Genetic Testing on Causal Models of Heart Disease and Arthritis: An Analogue Study." *Psychology and Health* 14:1077–88.

Shanahan, Michael J., and Scott M. Hofer. 2005. "Social Context in Gene-Environment Interactions: Retrospect and Prospect." *Journals of Gerontology Series B: Psychological and Social Sciences* 60B: 65–76.

Shanahan, Michael J., Lance D. Erickson, Stephen Vaisey, and Andrew Smolen. 2007. "Helping Relationships and Genetic Propensities: A Combinatoric Study of DRD2, Mentoring, and Educational Continuation." *Twin Research and Human Genetics* 10:285–98.

Shanahan, Michael J., Stephen Vaisey, Lance D. Erickson, and Andrew Smolen. 2008. "Environmental Contingencies and Genetic Propensities: Social Capital, Educational Continuation, and a Dopamine Receptor

Polymorphism." *American Journal of Sociology*, suppl. 1: S260–86.

Shostak, Sara. 2003. "Locating Gene-Environment Interaction: At the Intersections of Genetics and Public Health." *Social Science and Medicine* 56(11): 2327–42.

———. 2005. "The Emergence of Toxicogenomics: A Case Study of Molecularization." *Social Studies of Science* 35(3): 367–403.

Shostak, Sara, Peter Conrad, and Allan V. Horwitz. 2008. "Sequencing and Its Consequences: Path Dependence and the Relationships between Genetics and Medicalization." *American Journal of Sociology* 114, suppl. 1: S287–316.

Shostak, Sara, Jeremy Freese, Bruce G. Link, and Jo C. Phelan. 2009. "The Politics of the Gene: Social Status and Beliefs about Genetics for Individual Outcomes." *Social Psychology Quarterly* 72:77–93.

Silverman, Chloe. 2008. "Brains, Pedigrees, and Promises: Lessons from the Politics of Autism Genetics." In *Biosocialities, Genetics and the Social Sciences*, ed. Sahra Gibbon and Carlos Novas, 38–55. London: Routledge.

Singer, Burton H., and Carol D. Ryff. 2001. *New Horizons in Health: An Integrative Approach*. Washington, D.C.: National Academies Press.

Singer, Eleanor, Toni Antonucci, and John Van Hoewyk. 2004. "Racial and Ethnic Variations in Knowledge and Attitudes about Genetic Testing." *Genetic Testing* 8:31–43.

Singer, Eleanor, Amy D. Corning, and Mark Lamias. 1998. "Trends: Genetic Testing, Engineering, and Therapy: Awareness and Attitudes." *Public Opinion Quarterly* 62:633–64.

Sloan, Philip R. 2000. "Completing the Tree of Descartes." In *Controlling Our Destinies: Historical, Philosophical, Ethical, and Theological Perspectives on the Human Genome Project*, ed. Philip R. Sloan, 1–25. Notre Dame, Ind.: University of Notre Dame Press.

Stockdale, Alan. 1999. "Waiting for the Cure: Mapping the Social Relations of Human Gene Therapy Research." *Sociology of Health and Illness* 21:579–96.

Sunder Rajan, K. 2006. *Biocapital: The Constitution of Postgenomic Life*. Durham, N.C.: Duke University Press.

Taioli, Emanuela, and Seymour Garte. 2002. "Covariates and Confounding in Epidemiologic Studies Using Metabolic Gene Polymorphisms." *International Journal of Cancer* 100:97–100.

ten Have, Henk. 2001. "Genetics and Culture: The Geneticization Thesis." *Medicine, Health Care and Philosophy* 4:295–304.

Thompson, Charis. 2005. *Making Parents: The Ontological Choreography of Reproductive Technologies*. Cambridge, Mass.: MIT Press.

Timmermans, Stefan, and Steven Haas. 2008. "Toward a Sociology of Disease." *Sociology of Health and Illness* 30:659–76.

Turkheimer, Eric, Andreana Haley, Mary Waldron, Brian D'Onofrio, and Irving I. Gottesman. 2003. "Socioeconomic Status Modifies Heritability of IQ in Young Children." *Psychological Science* 14:623–28.

Tutton, Richard, Jane Kaye, and Klaus Hoeyer. 2004. "Governing UK Biobank: The Importance of Ensuring Public Trust." *Trends in Biotechnology* 22:284–85.

Tygart, C. E. 2000. "Genetic Causation Attribution and Public Support of Gay Rights." *International Journal of Public Opinion Research* 12:259–75.

Wailoo, Keith. 2003. "Inventing the Heterozygote: Molecular Biology, Racial Identity, and the Narratives of Sickle Cell Disease, Tay-Sachs, and Cystic Fibrosis." In *Race, Nature, and the Politics of Difference*, ed. Donald S. Moore, Anand Pandian, and Jake Kosek, 325–53. Durham, N.C.: Duke University Press.

Weinstein, Maxine A., James W. Vaupel, and Kenneth W. Wachter. 2008. *Biosocial Surveys*. Washington, D.C.: National Research Council.

Whitmarsh, Ian, Arlene M. Davis, Debra Skinner, and Donald B. Bailey Jr. 2007. "A Place for Genetic Uncertainty: Parents Valuing an Unknown in the Meaning of Disease." *Social Science and Medicine* 65:1082–93.

Zavestoski, Stephen, Phil Brown, Sabrina McCormick, Brian Mayer, Maryhelen D'Ottavi, and Jaime Lucove. 2004. "Patient Activism and the Struggle for Diagnosis: Gulf War Illnesses and Other Medically Unexplained Physical Symptoms in the U.S." *Social Science and Medicine* 58:161–75.

25

Biotechnology and the Prolongation of Life
A Sociological Critique

Bryan S. Turner, The Graduate Center, City University of New York

Puzzles surrounding health, longevity, and death have preoccupied the human mind throughout history, but the question "Can we live forever?" has a decidedly contemporary resonance, since modern medicine holds out the actual possibility rather than the merely fantastic promise of longevity. Furthermore, contemporary medicine offers us longevity without disability and infirmity. In one sense, the issues surrounding aging are quite simple: can we be happy, healthy, and chronologically old, or is physical deterioration and death necessarily a depressing and destructive experience? Is death ultimately inescapable? A number of popular science books—*How to Live Forever or Die Trying* (Appleyard 2007), *The Living End* (Brown 2008), and *The Immortalists* (Friedman 2008)—have recently explored the issues of life prolongation through the application of modern biotechnological inventions. The optimistic answer to the question about indefinite survival looks toward medical science and technology to secure survival without aging. Optimists are in search of a medical utopia that can not only prolong life indefinitely but also eliminate its attendant discomforts and disabilities. The optimism is of course not new. Nikolai Fedorov (1828–1903) argued in *What Was Man Created For* (1990) that with the application of science, human transcendence was possible. Death was not an inevitable outcome of human life but an avoidable evil. Thus the struggle against nature should have primacy over the social struggle, and

he realized that to overcome the scarcity imposed by nature, human beings would have to colonize space. By contrast, there is a well-established tradition of critical responses to the promises of medical science, challenging the view that humans can achieve almost complete control over their environment and rejecting the assumption that they could control their own biological evolution and destiny (Dubos 1959). The pessimistic response to utopian thought argues that technology cannot ultimately solve the problems of old age and that in some circumstances technology actually compounds our difficulties. In the contemporary debate about aging, the optimists are represented by scientists such as the Cambridge biogerontologist Aubrey de Grey, who in *Ending Aging* (2008) treats aging as an engineering problem, advocating a plan to eradicate death from aging through SENS—"Strategies for Engineered Negligible Senescence." The pessimistic view, which he has dubbed the "pro-aging stance," induces the populace to accept aging and its negative outcomes as both natural and unavoidable. The optimists argue that any commitment to the inevitability of death rests on implicit and often hidden religious assumptions about "nature."

Rejuvenation sciences claim to provide a range of solutions to resolve the problems of old age itself (as opposed to solving issues arising from age-related diseases). De Grey believes that recent developments—for example, in microbiology and its related technologies—offer the possibility that death could be eliminated. To deny this possibility is simply irrational. Those who hold a negative perception on the life-extension project are accused of possessing a conservative outlook, being unnecessarily reluctant to embrace social change, and being constrained by rigid religious conceptions of the human life span, all of which restrict the potential offered by antiaging technology.

Of course the controversial but simple question "Can we live forever?" has a variety of answers. We can in fact distinguish various possible forms of survival (Callahan 2009). The first is basically the existing situation, involving a relatively long life in historical terms but with all the disability and immobility that characteristically goes with aging. This situation may be tolerable for the individual but costly for society with rising health-care costs. The second possibility might be an extension of life with relatively little disability and a quick death. In this case, medical science would have successfully overcome many geriatric diseases without finally providing us immortality. From an individual point of view, this outcome is clearly desirable. We could also imagine simply decelerated aging, which would mean slowing down the aging process, and finally there might be arrested aging, in which the aging process could be delayed or deferred for an indefinite period. The immediate medical goal of the immortalists is a version of arrested aging in which the inconvenience of morbidity could be more or less eliminated and immortality could be delivered through extensive geriatric engineering. This final outcome is clearly problematic because it is costly from an economic perspective, and it may also be disturbing for the individual, given a range of psychological problems that might follow life extension, such as boredom, depression, and despair. As a matter of fact, significant improvements in life expectancy have already been taking place in the developed world throughout the twentieth century, and decelerated and compressed aging both look feasible in the twenty-first century. In the light of these medical options, the developed societies have urgently to develop radical social policies toward aging, because the consequences of the demographic transition or "secular shift," in whatever form, are far-reaching and fundamental (Laslett 1995).

The immortalist objective to give us both youthfulness and longevity is a utopian ambition. However, we need to take the ambition and the dream seriously. From a sociological perspective, immortalism as a program tells us a lot about the society in which we live, especially its subjective individualism, its obsession with technological solutions, and its overwhelming confidence in scientific advance. The medical dream of a long and trouble-free life tells us a lot about the baby-boomer generation, its continuing influence, and its reluctance to leave the historical stage. The immortalist program also brings to our attention a range of exciting and imaginative aspects of medical technology and research that *may* in the long term have a radical impact on the human life cycle. For example, any discussion about the life-extension project brings into view the possibility of a posthuman society (Fukuyama 2002). However, there is a more challenging literature associated with the Transhumanist Association which claims that we are close to manufacturing posthuman beings who will be so radically transformed by medical science that they will be no longer unambiguously human according to our contemporary standards. Cybernetics and informatics will, alongside biomedicine, produce enhanced beings that will be immortalized by such technological advances (Hayles 1999). Although this debate may look like science fiction from the perspective of conventional medical sociology, these developments should, in my view, become an aspect of sociological research, because these technologies already impinge on our lives and they are reshaping existing concepts of mind and body. As we will see in this chapter, the transhumanist agenda has in fact an elegant and persuasive philosophical defense (Bostrom 2005) that deserves sociological scrutiny.

The Body and Aging as Engineering Problems

In 1967 Christiaan Barnard performed the first heart transplant operation at the Grote Schuur Hospital. Similar experiments had been conducted on chimpanzees, and in the majority of these early heart transplant operations, the patients died shortly afterward. Despite Barnard's technical brilliance, his patient died eighteen days after the operation from pneumonia. At the time, heart transplants were often regarded as medical gimmickry, and they were condemned as expensive technology solutions for a limited number of patients in a world where the mass of humanity, especially in Africa, lived relatively short lives with depressingly high levels of poverty and morbidity. Almost half a century later, we regard organ transplants as routine low-risk procedures, and medical science is now experimenting with hearts and other organs that can be cultivated in the laboratory with modern genetic technologies. In the context of the prolongevity debate, a heart transplant can be regarded as a technique for extending life, and such procedures can be seen as relevant to the goal of living indefinitely.

Heart transplant operations can be perceived as tangible proof of the project to treat the aging body as simply a defective machine, which was anticipated by an unusual partnership between the famous flyer Charles Lindbergh and Alexis Carrel, the founder of tissue culture, who in developing experimental medicine had grown human tissue outside the body. Having successfully flown across the Atlantic in 1927, Lindbergh wanted to enlist experimental medicine to cure his sister-in-law, who suffered from a damaged mitral valve in her heart. Lindbergh's response to her condition was to think of the defective heart valve as one might respond to a defective oil pump in an airplane engine. When Lindbergh established a working relationship with Carrel, the engineer and the experimental scientist dreamt of the possibility of removing the heart from a sick patient, repairing it, and implanting the restored organ in the patient (Friedman 2008). One outcome of Lindbergh's professional involvement with Carrel at the Experimental Surgery Division of the Rockefeller Institute was his conclusion that death was simply the avoidable consequence of failed bodily machines.

The notion that we can regard the ailing body as a defective machine has a long history, but it is only in recent times with the development, for example, of nanotechnology that the prospects of an engineering solution to aging begin to gain greater recognition and prominence. An engi-

neering solution to the contingency of life can be regarded as compatible with Cartesianism, in which the body as a physical object is merely an extension of the person (Turner 2008). Much of this experimental work rests on the research of K. Eric Drexler. Born in Oakland, California, in 1955, Drexler completed his early research at the Massachusetts Institute of Technology (MIT) and participated in National Aeronautics and Space Administration summer studies in 1975 and 1976 on space colonies. During the 1970s, he began to develop ideas about the applications of molecular nanotechnology. In *Engines of Creation* (1986) he proposed to construct a nanoscale "assembler" which would be able to build a copy of itself with the use of an arm and a computer. This development could lead eventually to the efficient mass production of nanomachines. Because assemblers can copy themselves, such nanoproducts would have low marginal costs. With Christine Petersen, Drexler founded the Foresight Institute in 1986 to prepare for nanotechnology, and in 2005 he joined Nanorex to participate in their projects to develop molecular software. Drexler's work has been criticized because currently there is no way to build his proposed assembler, and while Drexler and his colleagues have produced some designs for simpler machines, the design tasks remain formidable. Finally, there are no reliable procedures to distinguish between the failures and successes of possible applications of these designs.

Despite these damaging criticisms, the potential applications of nanotechnology are significant. In medical procedures, Drexler proposes that nanocomputers would give surgery much greater precision and speed. Such machines could also be employed to help the immune system more accurately identify and combat cancer cells. These nanohealth machines could in principle be implanted to correct the failures of the aging body, thereby finally fulfilling what we might call the iatro-engineering dreams of Lindbergh. Drexler's machines could assist in the development of cryonics—freezing bodies for a future medical restoration of life—in which the resuscitation of frozen patients would require considerable corporeal reconstruction and repair. Finally, Drexler demonstrated in *Nanosystems* (1992) that these assemblers are consistent with the known laws of chemistry, and the possible medical applications of these developments were considered in some detail by Robert A. Freitas in *Nanomedicine* (1999). It is assumed that the first assembler will be built within the next decade.

One might reasonably predict that some aspects of today's prolongation gimmickry—cryonics and nanoprotein machines—will become routine procedures in the next fifty years. Some version of Aubrey de Grey's engineering solutions to the causes of aging—cell depletion, cell excess, mutations of the chromosome, mitochondrial mutations, cellular debris, and cross-linking—may also become commonplace procedures for prolonging human life. Many of the other recommendations for delaying aging—cosmetic surgery, vitamin supplements, dietary regimes, exercise, a modest consumption of red wine, and so forth—are already accepted without much public controversy. The more questionable solutions, such as the massive calorie restriction recommended by some pathologists—possibly as a solution for diabetes—may also become standard practice but in some modified form (Mason 2006). Even a more advanced and reliable version of cryonics might become part of mainstream medical technology. Some medical conditions such as single-gene disorders, Huntington's disease, cystic fibrosis, and sickle cell anaemia will be in the front row of targets for genetic interventions, and other conditions will be rapidly added to the list of treatable problems.

We might also reasonably assume that, regardless of any ethical or economic objections, these technological inventions and their applications are probably unstoppable and inevitable for four reasons. The first is the obvious quest for economic profit. Prolonging life—whether in the conventional form of geriatric tourism, cosmetics, diets, vitamins, and exercise routines, or in more experimental medical regimes—is already a feature of global business, and with aging populations business opportunities will only increase around an emerging global retirement industry. Stem-cell research offers significant opportunities for regenerative medicine. Second, the desire of human beings to live longer is a more or less permanent feature of human society, from ancient China to modern-day America. Third, even if legislation in the United States sought to curb certain forms of medical research—such as stem-cell research—other countries such as Singapore would provide a safe haven for such scientific experimentation. Finally, there is a specific driving force that will be characteristic of the next three decades—the aging of the baby-boom generation, which has enjoyed a lifetime of consumerism and relative affluence. Despite their aging and imminent retirement, boomers are now reluctant to relinquish their significant acquisitions of property and power (Kinsley 2008). In the short term, we may expect life expectancy in the developed world to approach one hundred years, but in the long term, life expectancy may simply keep increasing with improvements in the standard of living and in conjunction with new medical technologies. In the twenty-first century, life expectancy may extend well beyond 120 years for elite social groups.

Is the indefinite prolongation of life socially desirable, as opposed to being merely in the interests of the individual? To answer this question, let us start by making a basic economic assumption that scarcity is unavoidable and hence conflicts over resources are inescapable. Scarcity is the basic assumption of economics as a science, and without that assumption one could not understand such phenomena as competition, rational choice, or inequality. Some natural resources such as water and fossil fuels may be scarce simply because they are inadequate for human need. Therefore, extending life in a context of scarcity must result in increased social competition, if not social conflict. The prolongation of life by an immortalist social movement will increase social conflict between generations and between the long-living elite and the short-living majority. The elite will be constituted of the rich, primarily from the northern hemisphere, and the majority of the poor will be located in the southern hemisphere and their life span will actually decrease as a consequence of poverty, social deprivation, and infectious diseases. Over time these medical technologies—such as stem-cell therapies, organ transplants, nanomedicine, and cryonics—will become cheaper and more effective, and therefore available to a wider range of social groups. But we cannot expect these treatments to become universally available at affordable prices. In the modern world, it is now possible to treat conditions such as AIDS/HIV with modern drugs, thereby controlling many of the opportunistic conditions such as pneumonia that eventually kill the victims of this disease, but these drugs have not been available in much of Africa and Asia at an affordable price. If in some future world there is an effective antiaging drug, it is unlikely that this drug will be available in the impoverished, deprived, and war-torn areas of such an unequal world.

Transhumance

There is the possibility of a more radical and challenging future, which will be the unintended consequences of modern medical technology. Elsewhere I have argued that our humanity is defined by our vulnerability, which is simply a consequence of being a perishable organism that ages and is subject to inescapable morbidity and mortality (Turner 2006). Vulnerability—from the Latin word for "wound"—defines a shared human world of risk with which we can cope through a shared culture. Collective institutions—law, government, religion, and family—are social mechanisms that offer some respite from our ontological vulnerability. Life-extension medicine promises to solve the problem of our vulnerability by paradoxically creating a posthuman world. The contemporary life-extension movement is driven by a profoundly individualist ideology that offers individual solutions but largely ignores many of the social consequences—generational conflict, the exhaustion of basic resources, and massive regional inequalities. One might argue of course that our contemporary situation is in any case characterized by violence, inequality, and scarcity and that medical technology is at least one solution to our vulnerability. However, a significant increase in the immortals in a world of declining fertility rates and existing scarcities would result in a posthuman world in which the only long-term solution to scarcity would be either a radical reduction in the human population or the colonization of outer space. In other words, the prolongevity movement has to offer some alternative to a Malthusian future. Given these economic assumptions about scarcity, pessimistic conclusions about the impact of

life extension on resources, social capital, and social harmony appear inevitable. However, in the literature on transhumance, a range of proposals begins to address some of these issues. For example, transhumanist philosophy has produced a number of responses to the argument that longevity would create psychological malfunctioning. Because the immortalist worldview is what we might call a fix-it ideology, their proposal is that we can live in a posthuman world provided we have the correct brain-enhancing antidepressant drugs. A prolonged existence could be tolerable with the appropriate pills. Such an argument assumes that human mental functions and psychology would not change significantly. However, a posthuman society will have individuals of greatly enhanced intelligence, and it would be technologically possible to upload the brain into an electronic medium such as an electronic chip. These posthuman uploads would not suffer from biological senescence and they would not be a significant drain on scarce resources. Uploading would also solve the problem of cryonic patients, whose brains could be copied into a computerized system. These proposals are related to developments in artificial intelligence. Rodney Brooks (2002), a founding fellow of the American Association for Artificial Intelligence and director of the Artificial Intelligence Laboratory at MIT, argues that humans are simply "wetware" organic machines that could be duplicated with metal and silicon, and hence prolongevity could be achieved through processes related to or resembling uploading and duplicating. The possibility of creating transhuman existence raises the possibility of a future society composed of humans who are subject to decay and extinction and posthuman beings that are equipped with superior intelligence and blessed with technological immortality (Kurzweil 1999). Would such a world resemble the futuristic nightmare of Stanley Kubrick's *2001: A Space Odyssey*?

Theories of Aging

While transhuman theory may appear implausible, it has the merit of bringing into focus the nature of aging and forces us to reconceptualize often-sterile debates about the greying of populations. It brings into critical focus the question, What is aging? Contemporary genetic thinking about aging has been significantly influenced by Thomas Kirkwood in such publications as *Time of Our Lives* (1999) and "The End of Age" (2001). The Kirkwood view of aging argues that it is the consequence of limited investments in somatic maintenance and repair, owing to competing priorities in reproductive investments. Longevity is programmed by the settings of genes relating to repair and maintenance. Aging is the outcome of damaged cells and tissues that have accumulated through the life course, and thus a great variety of mechanisms contributes to the aging process. The principal genes determining longevity are related to these maintenance functions, such as antioxidant enzymes. It follows from these assumptions that the maximum human life span is not fixed and determined but malleable, for example, through the limitation of exposure to cellular damage.

Kirkwood's reinterpretation of existing biological theories has important implications for the social and commercial exploitation of biogerontology. Following Kirkwood's approach, the aim of biomedicine is to enhance the ability of an individual "to imitate the immortal germinal line" (Moreira and Palladino 2008, 37). These scientific developments quite specifically support antiageist social policies, holding out the promise of achieving a better fit between individual mortality and social functioning. These developments suggest that we should regard our biological constitution as merely a somatic vehicle for reproducing the genetic line. Furthermore, the notion that we are simply constituted by the disposable soma is the ultimate definition of human vulnerability. The thrust of the medical program of the prolongevity movement is that we can in fact delay the disposability of the soma by invasive and determined medical engineering, that is, through rejuvenative medicine (de Grey 2008).

The Baby Boomers and the Demographic Transition

What is problematic about the current prolongevity debate is that it rarely addresses the political economy of aging—who will pay for it, what will the unintended consequences on the environment be, how will it influence family life, and how would it change the balance of power between generations or indeed between nations? One reason for the absence of any serious attempt to understand the social consequences of living forever is that the ideological underpinnings of the immortalist movement are largely individualistic and are thereby consistent with the values of the baby-boom generation that has celebrated youth, youthfulness, and success. In the drab postwar years of rationing and restrictions, the baby-boom generation brought a new zest for life and enjoyment, but it became a movement that was shaped by the consumer boom of the 1970s. Although the immortalist case is often wrapped up in a moral claim about the unacceptable fact of death—how can we let thousands of people die each year globally of old age?—the immortalist ethos is essentially private and personal. It is not overly concerned with issues of justice, dependency, or economic growth. The prospect of significantly extending the expectation of life in the affluent societies of the northern hemisphere by the application of medical research on stem cells has clear Malthusian implications for the world as a whole. There is a close relationship between poverty and injustice, and therefore we should take this Malthusian question seriously if we are to understand the relationship between human rights and poverty. The transhumance argument that, as the costs of rejuvenative medicine declined, these therapeutic interventions would become widely available to the public and gross inequalities between the rich and the poor would diminish is not convincing. Inequalities in morbidity and mortality have not diminished with technological improvements in medicine. Although it is at this stage merely sociological speculation, one can nevertheless assume that, if successful on a large scale, the life-extension project would produce a range of major socioeconomic and environmental problems. Increasing world inequality between the rejuvenated, immortalized North and the naturally aging senescent South would further inflame the resentment of deprived social groups against wealthy aged populations. As the AIDS/HIV epidemic takes a significant toll on life expectancy in many impoverished African societies, the differences in the demographic profile between the North and South are becoming extreme. Life extension in the North implies increasing environmental degradation, global warming, and consequently further depletion of natural resources. In addition to social class conflicts over limited resources, there may be intergenerational conflicts, including conflicts over jobs, retirement benefits, and pensions. Much sociological research on generational relations has rejected the idea that increasing life expectancy will lead to intergenerational conflict, but the life-extension project raises issues about such generational equity not covered by the current discussion. Whereas eighteenth-century political economists like Thomas Malthus and the Marquis de Condorcet realized that there was an important connection between the organic perfection of Man (to use their language) and the improvement of society, the modern immortalist movement pays scant attention to the social conditions that would be necessary to sustain large cohorts of human beings enjoying a prolongation of life (Turner 2009).

There is a paradox in scientific discourses of rejuvenation. On the one hand, there is a wish to prolong life; on the other, there is an indifference to the means to prevent premature death. Assuming a link between wealth and health, it is unjust to value some lives more than others, that is, to value the addition of extra years to already long lives rather than adding extra years to those whose lives are relatively short as a result of poverty. While life expectancy in many African societies is declining as a consequence of poverty, authoritarian governments, new wars based on warlordism and drug barons, and the AIDS epidemic, lives in many northern-hemisphere societies are being extended. The prospect of further life extension will simply increase this global gap between the rich and the poor. Considerations about existing inequality should moderate arguments about the health rights of the elderly to live longer, regardless of the unintended consequences for other communities.

However, moral standards regarding human life are constantly challenged by new technologies (Latour 2002) that affect the foundation of human rights. If death by old age is perceived as pathological, it is likely that older adults will compete with other age cohorts for access to scarce medical resources. If instead death in old age is considered normal, then premature deaths in underdeveloped countries would in turn be interpreted as a priority since they are incongruent with the current norms defining the "natural" life span. Queuing for resources is thus central to the tensions emerging from the life-extension project, because it establishes a hierarchy among humans that determines medical care. The question is, Upon what shared values, if any, is queuing organized within the project of immortalist longevity?

Intergenerational Exchange

We should consider the issues of prolongation and social rights against the more general issues of social solidarity and security. These questions point to the likelihood that we should look at pensions from the perspective of intergenerational exchanges and the question of generational equity. It is well recognized that the welfare states of northern Europe have rested on an explicit social contract between generations. This modern contractual welfare state is based on intergenerational transfers of resources through taxation and social expenditure. In addition to this public or formal contract, there is an informal and domestic contract between generations within households. Generally speaking, the state works to reinforce and sustain the informal contractual arrangements operating within households. With the aging of Western populations, declining fertility, and compulsory retirement, there has been increasing political pressure to modify the generational contract. Critics of the existing arrangements have argued that the baby boomers or the "welfare generation" has captured the welfare state and its resources, ensuring that social funding is directed away from the young to the elderly (Thomson 1996). The social construction of a demographic imperative is based on the economic assumption that welfare has become an unacceptable public burden. Lobby groups in the United States have campaigned against public expenditure on the elderly, promoting instead the idea of personal responsibility and obligation within the family. Fears about a social burden have also been associated with the idea that there is growing conflict between generations over the unequal distribution of resources.

The debate about intergenerational reciprocity can be usefully divided into two competing positions (Williamson, McNamara, and Howling 2003). There is the generational equity argument that each generation should take care of itself rather than relying on other generations or the state. Privatization of resources is one logical outcome of this position. The alternative is generational interdependence, which emphasizes the diversity of emotional, cultural, and economic exchanges between generations and, in criticizing the emphasis on economic exchange, integrationist arguments draw attention to the social importance of reciprocity norms. By contrast, the equity framework arose in the 1980s as a response to the perception of a growing economic crisis attendant upon radical demographic changes. This framework was associated with a number of conservative institutions such as the Cato Institute and the Olin Foundation. It also had an advocacy wing organized by AGE (Americans for Generational Equity). Their argument was based on the findings of empirical research that suggested that, while the economic status of the elderly had been improving, that of their children had been declining. This framework argued that existing provisions were unfair and more importantly unaffordable (Marmor, Cook, and Scher 1999). Dependency ratios between workers and pensioners, it was claimed, showed that current welfare arrangements could not be sustained indefinitely into the twenty-first century and immediate action was required to provide for these demographic changes. It was in this context that some economists predicted that age wars would replace class wars as the elderly use their political influence through interest groups such as the American Association of Retired Persons to steer resources toward pensions and health care and away from educational investments for younger generations (Thurow 1996). As age conflict increases, the possibilities for age integration declines.

The interdependency or integration framework arose essentially as a critique of these pessimistic predictions about generational conflict. The interdependency position recognized that the elderly do not function politically as an integrated and coherent category but are divided, like the rest of the population, by class, gender, and ethnicity. The interests of rich and poor elderly do not necessarily coincide. Furthermore, there is little evidence that the elderly vote as a block, and often the interests of different age groups coincide. For example, in the early 1980s young and old opposed cuts to education and health programs (Minkler 1991). A recent analysis of data from the British Retirement Plans Survey undertaken by the Office for National Statistics on behalf of the Department of Social Security found that parents who help their children are more likely to receive support, children respond to parents in need, and divorced fathers are the least likely to be involved in exchanges with children (Grundy 2005). Finally, it is unrealistic to expect each generation to be responsible for itself, because this ignores changing fortunes brought about by historical contingency. The generation of the Depression faced unusually hard circumstances that shaped its entire future (Elder 1974). Similarly, we may speculate that the current credit crisis and the turmoil in the U.S. financial and housing markets in 2008–2009 will have a significant impact on young families who are currently struggling with a global financial meltdown not of their making (Edmunds and Turner 2005). Research on generations clearly demonstrates that historical contingency means that we cannot assume a level playing field between one generation and another, and hence the idea of fairness is not easily applied in these circumstances (Edmunds and Turner 2002). The problem with the equity perspective is that it makes little or no allowance for those vulnerable social groups who do not have the resources to cope with exceptional circumstances such as natural disasters, economic crises, or social turmoil. In all of these circumstances, it is very difficult to see how social justice between generations could be achieved. Any significant prolongation of life within the immortalist framework will certainly intensify conflicts in the public arena over scarce resources, even where these public conflicts may be absent within the family itself.

Despite the cogency of the interdependency standpoint, the equity lobby has been successful, because the simple logic of its appeal to individualism resonates with the neoconservative climate that was sustained long after the departure of political leaders such as President Reagan and Prime Minister Thatcher. The political appeal to responsibility and personal choice against compulsory measures remains a potent aspect of the view that generational interests are on a collision course. While sociologists have generally supported the notion that intergenerational reciprocity, even with the decline of traditional family structures, is a significant aspect of modern societies, tensions over resources will inevitably persist, mainly because there is the suspicion that older, retired generations are parasitic on younger, employed generations. With the credit crunch, there has been much talk about the need for a reassertion of values and moral guidelines to stem the greed that has become associated with the consumer boom of the 1990s. The emerging focus on morality may also provide ammunition for the integration argument.

Conclusion: The Right to Longevity?

Scientific research seeking to prolong human life has generated a number of criticisms. Two questions—one empirical and the other normative—dominate current debates about life extension: Can we live forever? and Should we live forever? The first question emerges mainly from the field of biomedical sciences, concentrating on the feasibility of biological engineering as a method capable of prolonging life, on the protection of consumers from quackery, and on maintaining the credibility of biomedical science (Binstock 2003, 2004). The second or normative question is primarily embedded in the fields of humanities and social sciences, being concerned with social and ethical issues (Vincent 2003). The works of Francis Fukuyama (2002) and Leon Kass (2002) have been particularly influential in recent years, both contesting the virtues of prolonging life beyond the "normal" human life span.

Rejuvenation sciences will not be easy to regulate because of the mixed and often contradictory outcomes they have for individuals and for societies. Legislative regulation to limit or to control the scope of antiaging technology would not be easily enforced for political reasons. In addition, it is perfectly rational for an aging individual to embrace the opportunities to extend life, even where the technology may have negative consequences for society as a whole. Stem-cell research is a good example of this problem. It is reasonable for an individual to wish to add extra years to his or her "natural" life span, even if this means spending much time distracted by geriatric disease and discomfort, while waiting for anticipated future cures for existing morbidity. Contrary to the immortalist promise of good health in old age, it is more plausible to imagine a common situation where elderly individuals are enjoying significantly longer lives but with mounting problems from their (as yet) incurable and threatening conditions such as Parkinsonism and Alzheimer's disease. In that case, societies will be exposed to the phenomenon of decompressed morbidity—when disabilities are compressed into the final stages of life—and hence the social costs of longevity will be significant.

In addition to these economic consequences, the moral arguments against the life-extension project are considerable, even though such an enhancement of the life span is at present remote. If antiaging technology can in principle make it possible to live forever, technology will corrode existing ethical systems, because the conventional relationships between the ethical life, the good society, and the management of the body are being dissolved by advances in medical sciences. Medical regulation of the body does not, for example, presuppose any personal responsibility for conduct, apart from compliance with a medical regime. The new biotechnology breaks the traditional connection between morals and longevity, because we can in principle solve most of life's troublesome issues by medical interventions. While medical science encourages me to manage my body carefully, it also promises to solve my problems when things go wrong. The uneasiness that many have with this project can be understood through the moral legacy of religions on current value systems. For religious institutions, which constantly participate in debates over values, the life-extension project presents a serious challenge, because the traditional theology of the Christian churches presumed the achievement of personal salvation and the enjoyment of eternal life on the basis of being virtuous and without sin. Rejuvenation sciences promise not an eternal sacred life but an eternal, or at least extended, secular life. The life expectancy of an individual is not based on moral worth, but on the outcome of a political debate about the allocation of sufficient resources to meet the research goals of the life-extension project.

An aging process of this magnitude will also have a significant impact on the viability of the state, since the tax base will be seriously eroded because there will be an imbalance between the working population and retirees. Even if retirement is postponed or made more flexible, there is a serious issue about how the productive population will be replenished as dependency ratios increase in the developed world. Longevity for the privileged generation will curtail the employment opportunities of the young and increase the possibility of tensions between the generations. The citizenship claims of the elderly will no longer match their contributions to the system. One solution to this problem for developed societies is to continue to import labor from the less developed world. There is currently a large army of Filipino domestic workers in Singapore and the Gulf States, providing services to families with elderly relatives, while Mexican migrants both legal and illegal supply the labor market of the U.S. Southwest. North African and more recently east European migration has been important in the labor markets of the European Union. Japan, which has historically resisted inward migration, has become increasingly dependent on Korean and Chinese labor. There are other solutions that involve delaying entry into the labor market, for example, by providing universal access to higher education and abolishing the retirement age. Another solution is to shorten the working week in order to guarantee more opportunities for employment for all. Another prospect is the development of some form of social storage by sending the elderly to gated communities outside their homeland. This strategy is already employed by Japan, for example, where many Japanese retirees

are now in retirement compounds in Thailand and Malaysia enjoying leisure activities and medical services at competitive prices. The major solution in many of the Anglo-Saxon economies—the United States, United Kingdom, Australia, Canada, and New Zealand—has been an attempt to dismantle the postwar welfare capitalist system of social security primarily through the privatization of pension schemes (Blackburn 2002).

Because economists have generally regarded the aging of the developed world as an important threat to continuing global economic growth, there is considerable interest in the commercial possibilities of stem-cell research as a feature of regenerative medicine (World Bank 1994). Companies operating in the Caribbean and Southeast Asia are already offering regenerative medicine as part of holiday packages, designed to alleviate the negative consequences of degenerative diseases such as multiple sclerosis or diabetes. These social and medical transformations imply an interesting change from early to late modernity. In the early stages of capitalism, the social role of medical science was to improve health care, thereby making the working class healthy and efficient. The application of medical science was to produce an efficient labor force, but late capitalism does not necessarily need a large labor force at full employment, because technology has made labor more efficient. In the new biotechnological environment, disease is no longer a negative force in the economy but on the contrary an aspect of the factors of production. The economy can capitalize on disease by keeping people alive longer. It is thus very likely that the economic interests of the corporate world will have an important role in funding antiaging technology. The new approach to the science of aging has resulted in a merger between the biomedicine business and governmentality, encouraging citizens to exercise responsibility for their own aging and the dependency of their relatives. One implication of Kirkwood's science of aging is that the diseases of the elderly are avoidable, being amenable to social and political interventions. Kirkwood had pointed out that aging is primarily a disease peculiar to human societies, since animals in the wild rarely live long enough to experience aging. Because "death is a preventable and unnecessary event" (Moreira and

Palladino 2008, 40), the new gerontology opens up huge commercial possibilities to improve lifestyle and diet to enhance the repair of the body and to delay its ultimate disposability.

In conclusion, any extension of life must be considered alongside the reform of society. This issue of individual improvement and social reform was the important message of the Enlightenment reformers such as Thomas Paine, William Godwin, Mary Wollstonecraft, and Marquis de Condorcet around the time of the French Revolution. The organic perfection of Man, they argued, could only occur alongside a radical reform of society, including the abolition of the aristocracy and the monarchy, the extension of the franchise to women, the improvement of agriculture, and the reform of education. Although the pessimistic criticism of the reformers often appeared to be triumphant in the writings of Edmund Burke and Jeremy Bentham, democratic improvement in Europe and North America did in fact take place—wages improved, famine became a rarity, women got the vote, and adult literacy became universal. In the twenty-first century, the extension of life must also take place alongside a revival of civil society and citizenship, the refashioning of public institutions, the enhancement in pensions, and a more equitable system of general taxation. Furthermore, these reforms to manage the consequences of extended longevity more adequately cannot be confined to nation-states. A global strategy is required to deal with aging populations, declining natural resources, and global warming. The principal sociological criticism of the immortalist agenda is that it does not engage with the issue of social reform that is the legacy of the political economy emerging from the original debate around Malthus. If from an economic point of view scarcity is an inevitable aspect of human society, where will we find the resources to sustain the deeply aged without damaging the life chances of people in developing societies and without an erosion of the opportunities of youth in the developed world?

Note

Aspects of this chapter first appeared in Alex Dumas and Bryan S. Turner, 2007, "The Life-Extension Project:

A Sociological Critique," *Health Sociological Review* 16:5–17.

References

Appleyard, Bryan. 2007. *How to Live Forever or Die Trying: On the New Immortality.* New York: Simon and Schuster.

Binstock, R. H. 2003. "The War on Anti-Aging Medicine." *Gerontologist* 43 (1): 4–14.

———. 2004. "Anti-Aging Medicine and Research: A Realm of Conflict and Profound Societal Implications." *Journal of Gerontology Series A: Biological and Medical Sciences* 59(6): 523–33.

Blackburn, Robin. 2002. *Banking on Death or Investing in Life: The History and Future of Pensions.* London: Verso.

Bostrom, Nick. 2005. "In Defence of Posthuman Dignity." *Bioethics* 19(3): 202–14.

Brooks, Rodney A. 2002. *Flesh and Machines: How Robots Will Change Us.* New York: Vintage Books.

Brown, Guy. 2008. *The Living End: The Future of Death, Aging and Immortality.* London: Macmillan.

Callahan, David. 1987. *Setting Limits: Medical Goals in an Aging Society.* New York: Simon and Shuster.

———. 2009. "Life Extension: Rolling the Technological Dice." *Society* 46(3): 214–20.

Cooper, M. 2006. "Resuscitations: Stem Cells and the Crisis of Old Age." *Body and Society* 12(1): 1–23.

de Grey, Aubrey, with Michael Rae. 2008. *Ending Aging: The Rejuvenation Breakthroughs That Could Reverse Human Aging in Our Lifetime.* London: St. Martin's Press.

Drexler, Eric. 1986. *Engines of Creation: The Coming Era of Nanotechnology.* New York: Doubleday.

———. 1992. *Nanosystems: Molecular Machinery, Manufacturing and Computation.* New York: John Wiley and Sons.

Dubos, René. 1959. *Mirage of Health: Utopias, Progress and Biological Change.* London: George Allen and Unwin.

Dumas, Alex, and Bryan S. Turner. 2006. "Age and Ageing: The Social Worlds of Foucault and Bourdieu." In *Foucault and Ageing*, ed. Jason L. Powell and A. Wahidin, 145–55. New York: Nova Science.

Edmunds, June, and Bryan S. Turner. 2002. *Generations, Culture and Society.* Buckingham, Eng.: Open University Press.

———. 2005. "Global Generations: Social Change in the Twentieth Century." *British Journal of Sociology* 56(4): 559–77.

Elder, Gary H., Jr. 1974. *Children of the Great Depression: Social Change in Life Experience.* Chicago: University of Chicago Press.

Fedorov, Nikolai. 1990. *What Was Man Created For?* New York: Hyperion.

Freitas, Robert A. 1999. *Basic Capabilities*. Vol. 1 of *Nanomedicine*. Georgetown, Tex.: Landes Bioscience.

Friedman, David M. 2008. *The Immortalists: Charles Lindbergh, Dr. Alex de Carrel, and Their Daring Quest to Live Forever*. New York: Harper Perennial.

Fukuyama, Francis. 2002. *Our Posthuman Future: Consequences of the Biotechnology Revolution*. New York: Farrar, Straus and Giroux.

Grundy, E. 2005. "Reciprocity in Relationships: Socio-Economic and Health Influences on Intergenerational Exchanges between Third Age Parents and Their Adult Children in Great Britain." *British Journal of Sociology* 56(2): 233–55.

Hayles, N. Katherine. 1999. *How to Become Posthuman: Virtual Bodies in Cybernetics, Literature and Informatics*. Chicago: University of Chicago Press.

Kass, Leon. 2002. *Human Cloning and Dignity: The Report of the President's Council on Bioethics*. New York: PublicAffairs.

Kinsley, Michael. 2008. "Mine Is Longer Than Yours." *New Yorker*, April 7, 38–43.

Kirkwood, Thomas. 1999. *Time of Our Lives: The Science of Human Aging*. Oxford: Oxford University Press.

———. 2001. "The End of Age." BBC Reith Lecture. bbc.co.uk/radio4/reith2001/.

Kurzweil, Ray. 1999. *The Age of Spiritual Machines: When Computers Exceed Human Intelligence*. New York: Penguin Books.

Laslett, Peter. 1995. "Necessary Knowledge: Age and Aging in the Societies of the Past." In *Aging in the Past: Demography, Society and Old Age*, ed. David L. Kertzer and Peter Laslett, 3–77. Berkeley: University of California Press.

Latour, Bruno. 2002. "Morality and Technology: The End of the Means." *Theory, Culture and Society* 19 (5/6): 247–60.

Marmor, T. R., F. L. Cook, and S. Scher. 1999. "Social Security and the Politics of Generational Conflict." In *The Generational Equity Debate*, ed.

J. B. Williamson, E. R. Kingson, and D. M. Watts-Roy, 185–203. New York: Columbia University Press.

Mason, Michael. 2006. "One for the Ages: A Prescription That May Extend Life." *New York Times*, October 31, supercentarian.com/archive/cr.htm.

Minkler, M. 1991. "Generational Equity and the New Victim Blaming." In *Cultural Perspectives on Aging*, ed. M. Minkler and C. Estes, 67–79. Amityville, N.Y.: Baywood Press.

Moody, R. H. 2006. "Who's Afraid of Life Extension?" hrmoody.com/art5.html.

Moreira, Tiago, and Paolo Palladino. 2008. "Squaring the Curve: The Anatomo-Politics of Ageing, Life and Death." *Body and Society* 14(3): 21–47.

Thomson, D. 1996. *Selfish Generations? How Welfare States Grow Old*. Cambridge: White Horse Press.

Thurow, Lester C. 1996. "The Birth of a Revolutionary Class." *New York Times Magazine*, May 19, 46–47.

Turner, Bryan S. 2006. *Vulnerability and Human Rights*. University Park: Pennsylvania State University Press.

———. 2008. *The Body and Society: Explorations in Social Theory*. London: Sage.

———. 2009. *Can We Live Forever? A Sociological and Moral Inquiry*. London: Anthem Press.

Vincent, John. 2003. "What Is at Stake in the 'War on Anti-Ageing Medicine.'" *Ageing and Society* 23:675–84.

———. 2006. "Ageing Contested: Anti-Ageing Science and the Cultural Construction of Old Age." *Sociology* 40(4): 681–98.

Williamson, John B., Tay K. McNamara, and Stephanie A. Howling. 2003. "Generational Equity, Generational Interdependence and the Framing of the Debate over Social Security Reform." *Journal of Sociology and Social Welfare* 30(3): 3–14.

World Bank. 1994. *Averting the Old Age Crisis: Policies to Protect the Old and Promote Growth*. Oxford: Oxford University Press.

Contributors

John Abraham, PhD, is professor of sociology at University of Sussex.

Dolores Acevedo-Garcia, PhD, is associate professor, Bouve College of Health Sciences, and associate director, Institute on Urban Health Research, at Northeastern University and adjunct associate professor of society, human development, and health, Harvard School of Public Health.

Crystal Adams, MA, is a graduate student in sociology at Brown University.

jimi adams, PhD, is assistant professor of sociology in the School of Social and Family Dynamics at Arizona State University.

Gary L. Albrecht, PhD, is a fellow of the Royal Belgian Academy of Science and Arts; extraordinary guest professor of social sciences, University of Leuven, Belgium; and professor emeritus of public health and of disability and human development at the University of Illinois at Chicago.

Renee R. Anspach, PhD, is associate professor of sociology, University of Michigan.

Kristin K. Barker, PhD, is associate professor of sociology, Oregon State University.

Lisa M. Bates, SM, ScD, is assistant professor in the Departments of Epidemiology and Population and Family Health at the Columbia University Mailman School of Public Health.

Peter S. Bearman, PhD, is the Cole Professor of Social Science at Columbia University.

Marc Berg, MA, MD, PhD, is a partner at Plexus Medical Group and professor at the Institute of Health Policy and Management, Erasmus University Rotterdam, the Netherlands.

Chloe E. Bird, PhD, is senior sociologist at the RAND Corporation and professor of sociology and policy analysis at Pardee RAND Graduate School.

Phil Brown, PhD, is professor of sociology and environmental studies at Brown University.

Wendy Cadge, PhD, is associate professor of sociology at Brandeis University.

Kathleen A. Cagney, PhD, is director of the National Opinion Research Center's Population Research Center and associate director of NORC's Center on Aging, University of Chicago.

Stephen J. Collier, PhD, is assistant professor of international affairs at the New School.

Peter Conrad, PhD, is Harry Coplan Professor of Social Sciences at Brandeis University.

Tamara Dubowitz, MSc, SM, ScD, is an associate policy researcher at the RAND Corporation.

Brian Fair is a PhD candidate in the Department of Sociology at Brandeis University.

Meenakshi M. Fernandes, PhD, is senior analyst in the Social and Economic Policy Group at Abt Associates.

Allen M. Fremont, MD, PhD, is a natural scientist and sociologist at the RAND Corporation and a practicing physician with clinical academic appointments at University of California–Los Angeles and the West Los Angeles Veterans Affairs Medical Center.

Jeremy Freese, PhD, is professor of sociology at Northwestern University.

Ichiro Kawachi, MD, PhD, is professor of social epidemiology and chair of the Department of

Society, Human Development, and Health at Harvard School of Public Health.

Andrew Lakoff, PhD, is associate professor of sociology at University of Southern California.

Martha E. Lang, PhD, is the coordinator of Lesbian, Gay, Bisexual, Transgender, Queer, and Allied Resources and visiting assistant professor of sociology/anthropology at Guilford College.

ManChui Leung is a graduate student at the Department of Sociology, University of Washington, and the former HIV/AIDS director at the Asian and Pacific Islander American Health Forum.

Donald W. Light, PhD, is professor of social and behavioral medicine at the University of Medicine and Dentistry of New Jersey.

Bruce Link, PhD, is professor of epidemiology and sociomedical sciences at the Columbia University Mailman School of Public Health and a research scientist at the New York State Psychiatric Institute.

Gina S. Lovasi, PhD, is assistant professor in epidemiology at the Columbia University Mailman School of Public Health.

Peter Mendel, PhD, is a social scientist at the RAND Corporation.

John Mirowsky, PhD, is professor of sociology at the University of Texas at Austin.

Rachel Morello-Frosch, PhD, MPH, is associate professor with the Department of Environmental Science, Policy, and Management and the School of Public Health at the University of California–Berkeley.

Jo Phelan, PhD, is associate professor of epidemiology and sociomedical sciences at the Columbia University Mailman School of Public Health.

Patricia P. Rieker, PhD, is adjunct professor of sociology at Boston University and associate professor of psychiatry at Harvard Medical School.

David A. Rier, PhD, is senior lecturer, Department of Sociology and Anthropology, Bar-Ilan University, Ramat-Gan, Israel.

Stephanie A. Robert, PhD, is professor of social work at the University of Wisconsin-Madison.

Catherine E. Ross, PhD, is professor of sociology at the University of Texas at Austin.

W. Richard Scott, PhD, is professor of sociology emeritus at Stanford University.

Clive Seale, PhD, is professor of medical sociology at Barts and the London School of Medicine and Dentistry, Queen Mary, University of London.

Laura Senier, MPH, PhD, is assistant professor in the Department of Community and Environmental Sociology and the Department of Family Medicine at the University of Wisconsin-Madison.

Regina A. Shih, PhD, is an associate behavioral/social scientist at the RAND Corporation and adjunct instructor at the George Washington University School of Public Health and Human Services.

Sara Shostak, PhD, is assistant professor of sociology at Brandeis University.

Ruth Simpson, PhD, is visiting professor of sociology and environmental studies at Bryn Mawr College.

Cheryl Stults, PhD, is lecturer in sociology at Santa Clara University.

David T. Takeuchi, PhD, is associate dean of research and professor of sociology and social work at University of Washington School of Social Work.

Stefan Timmermans, PhD, is professor of sociology at the University of California–Los Angeles.

Bryan S. Turner, LittD, is the Presidential Professor of Sociology at the City University of New York Graduate Center.

Emily Walton, PhD, is a Robert Wood Johnson Health and Society Scholars postdoctoral fellow at the University of Wisconsin.

Margaret M. Weden, PhD, is a social scientist at the RAND Corporation and director of the RAND Population Research Center Data and Information Core.

Teun Zuiderent-Jerak, MA, MA, PhD, is assistant professor of science and technology studies at the institute of Health Policy and Management, Erasmus University Rotterdam, the Netherlands.

Index

Tritter, Jonathan Q., 171
tuberculosis (TB)
    discovery of, 150
    outbreak risk, 363–65, 370
    pharmaceuticalization and, 299
    residential segregation and, 98
    SES and, 4, 7
    See also DOTS; Roth, Julius
Tufts Centre, 302
Turner, Bryan S., 200, 435–45
Turner, R. Jay, 204
Turra, Cassio M., 109
Tutton, Richard, 419
twins, 26–27, 425, 426

Ubeda, Luis, 135
Udry, J. Richard, 203
UK Biobank, 419
Ulrich, Esther, 221–22
UN Convention on the Rights of
    Persons with Disabilities, 192,
    201
UPIAS (Union of the Physically
    Impaired against Segregation),
    194, 197
Upjohn, 293, 294
urinary incontinence, 183

vaccination, 7, 82, 364, 367, 368,
    375, 405
van der Gaag, M., 21
van der Heide, Agnes, 221
van der Kroef, C., 293
Vanderpool, Harold Y., 346
van Gennep, Arnold, 168
Varshney, Ashutosh, 29
Vega, William A., 111
Verbrugge, Lois M., 56

veterans, 59, 165, 192, 198, 203. *See
    also* Gulf War syndrome
Veterans Health Administration, 260,
    274, 277, 280
Viagra (sildenafil), 290, 291
Villanueva-Russell, Yvonne, 314
Ville, Isabelle, 168
Vincent, John, 443
Vioxx, 294
Vlahov, David, 133
Vogel, Kathleen, 373–74

Wachs, Faye L., 64
Wade, Lisa D., 203, 424
Wagner, Todd H., 183
Walston, Stephen, L., 260
Walter, Tony, 213
Walton, Emily, 92–102
Ward, Katie J., 167, 185
Waring, Justin, 326, 327
Weber, Max, 147, 194, 214, 275,
    342, 376n18
Weden, Margaret M., 124–37
weight
    education and, 33, 35, 36, 45
    genetics and, 422, 423
    medicalization and, 241
    race and, 98, 110–11
    social networks and, 82–85, 167
    See also anorexia; obesity
Welberg, L. A., 401
Wellman, Barry, 128
Wen, Ming, 128
Wennberg, John E., 324
West, Candace, 61, 233, 235
Westberg, Granger, 351
West Nile virus, 365
Wheaton, Blair, 125

Whitley, Rob, 23
WHO. *See* World Health
    Organization
Wilkinson, Richard G., 11
Windish, Donna M., 316
Wingard, Deborah L., 56
Winkleby, Marilyn, 65
Wisconsin Longitudinal Study, 13,
    427
Wolf, Leslie E., 218
Women's Health Initiative (WHI),
    406
Wong, Rebecca, 112
Wood, Phillip, 193
Woolcock, M., 18, 27
World Bank, 192, 195, 201
World Health Organization (WHO)
    avian flu response, 371, 372–73,
        375
    disease classifications, 193–94,
        202
    global health and, 363–64, 369
    rankings and studies, 58, 192,
        195, 304
    See also International Obesity
        Task Force
Wright, Susan, 373, 375n4

Yoshida, Karen K., 167

Zelizer, Viviana A., 211
Zero Population Growth, 242
Zhang, Wenquan, 135
Zimmerman, Don H., 61
Zola, Irving, 194–95, 198, 200, 204,
    277
Zuckerman, Adam, 80, 85
Zuiderent-Jerak, Teun, 324–35